P9-BYB-746

The Female Body

A Head-to-Toe

Guide to Good Health

and Body Care—

At Any Age

The Female Body

an owner's manual

By Peggy Morgan, Caroline Saucer, Elisabeth Torg
and the Editors of **PREVENTION** Magazine Health Books

Rodale Press, Inc., Emmaus, Pennsylvania

Notice

This book is intended as a reference volume only, not as a medical manual. The information given here is designed to help you make informed decisions about your health. It is not intended as a substitute for any treatment that may have been prescribed by your doctor. If you suspect that you have a medical problem, we urge you to seek competent medical help.

Copyright © 1996 by Rodale Press, Inc.

Cover photograph copyright © 1996 by Robert Whitman
Illustrations copyright © 1996 by Narda Lebo

All rights reserved. No part of this publication may be reproduced or transmitted in any form or by any means, electronic or mechanical, including photocopying, recording or any other information storage and retrieval system, without the written permission of the publisher.

Prevention is a registered trademark of Rodale Press, Inc.

Printed in the United States of America on acid-free ∞, recycled paper ♻

Portions of "Emotions" on page 93 are adapted from "Tame Your Temper" by Paula M. Siegel, in *Healthy Woman* magazine. Copyright © 1995 by Paula M. Siegel. Reprinted by permission.

Library of Congress Cataloging-in-Publication Data

The Female body : an owner's manual : a head-to-toe guide to
    good health and body care—at any age / the editors of
Prevention Magazine Health Books
        p.   cm.
        Includes index
        ISBN 0–87596–290–4 hardcover
        ISBN 0–87596–400–1 paperback
        1. Women—Health and hygiene. 2. Medicine, Popular.
I. Prevention Magazine Health Books.
RA778.F435 1996
613'.04244—dc20   96–13237

Distributed in the book trade by St. Martin's Press

2   4   6   8   10   9   7   5   3   1   hardcover
2   4   6   8   10   9   7   5   3   1   paperback

—— OUR MISSION ——
We publish books that empower people's lives.
 RODALE BOOKS ——

The Female Body: An Owner's Manual
Editorial Staff

Senior Managing Editor: Edward Claflin

Writers: Peggy Morgan, Caroline Saucer, Elisabeth Torg

Nutrition Writer: Holly McCord, R.D.

Assistant Research Manager: Carol Svec

Head Researcher: Anita Small

Researchers and Fact-checkers: Susan E. Burdick, Derria Byrd,
    Christine Dreisbach, Valerie Edwards-Paulik, Carol J. Gilmore,
    Lois Hazel, Kristina Orchard-Hays, Kathryn Piff, Sandra
    Salera-Lloyd, Bernadette Sukley, Michelle M. Szulborski

Book and Cover Designer: Debra Sfetsios

Cover Photographer: Robert Whitman

Illustrator: Narda Lebo

Associate Art Director: Elizabeth Otwell

Technical Artists: Thomas P. Aczel, J. Andrew Brubaker

Studio Manager: Joe Golden

Photo Editor: Susan Pollack

Senior Copy Editor: Susan G. Berg

Copy Editor: Kathy Diehl

Production Manager: Helen Clogston

Manufacturing Coordinator: Patrick T. Smith

Office Staff: Roberta Mulliner, Julie Kehs, Bernadette Sauerwine,
    Mary Lou Stephen

PREVENTION Magazine Health Books

Vice-President and Editorial Director: Debora T. Yost

Art Director: Jane Colby Knutila

Research Manager: Ann Gossy Yermish

Copy Manager: Lisa D. Andruscavage

Board of Advisers for Rodale Women's
Health Books

Marie Leslie Borum, M.D.
Assistant professor of medicine in the Division of Gastroenterology
and Nutrition at the George Washington University Medical Center in Washington, D.C.

Trudy L. Bush, Ph.D.
Professor of epidemiology and preventive medicine at the University of Maryland School of Medicine at Baltimore and principal
investigator for the Heart and Estrogen/Progestin Replacement
Study and for the Postmenopausal Estrogen/Progestin Intervention (PEPI) Safety Follow-Up Study at the Johns Hopkins
Women's Research Core in Lutherville, Maryland

Diana L. Dell, M.D.
Assistant professor of obstetrics and gynecology at the Duke University Medical Center in Durham, North Carolina, past-president
of the American Medical Women's Association (AMWA) and co-director of its Breast and Cervical Cancer Physician Training
Project

Leah J. Dickstein, M.D.
Professor and associate chair for academic affairs in the Department of Psychiatry and Behavioral Sciences, associate dean for
faculty and student advocacy at the University of Louisville
School of Medicine in Kentucky and past-president of the American Medical Women's Association (AMWA)

Jean L. Fourcroy, M.D., Ph.D.
President of the American Medical Women's Association (AMWA)
in Alexandria, Virginia, and past-president of the National Council of Women's Health in New York City

Jean A. Hamilton, M.D.
Betty Cohen chair on Women's Health and director of the Institute
for Women's Health at the Medical College of Pennsylvania and
Hahnemann University

Debra Ruth Judelson, M.D.
Senior partner with the Cardiovascular Medical Group of Southern California in Beverly Hills and fellow of the American College
of Cardiology

JoAnn E. Manson, M.D.

Associate professor of medicine at Harvard Medical School and
co-director of women's health at Brigham and Women's Hospital
in Boston

Irma Mebane-Sims, Ph.D.

Epidemiologist at the National Heart, Blood and Lung Institute
of the National Institutes of Health in Bethesda, Maryland, and
clinical trials researcher of heart disease and hormones in
menopausal-aged women; board member of the Society for the
Advancement of Women's Health Research

Mary Lake Polan, M.D., Ph.D.

Professor and chairman of the Department of Gynecology and
Obstetrics at Stanford University School of Medicine in California

Yvonne S. Thornton, M.D.

Visiting associate physician at the Rockefeller University Hospital
in New York City and director of the perinatal diagnostic testing
center at Morristown Memorial Hospital in New Jersey

Lila A. Wallis, M.D.

Clinical professor of medicine at Cornell University Medical College in New York City and director of "Update Your Medicine," a
series of continuing medical educational programs for physicians
at Cornell University Medical College in New York City

Judith N. Wasserheit, M.D.

Director of the Division of Sexually Transmitted Diseases and
Prevention of the National Center for HIV/STD and TB Prevention at the Centers for Disease Control and Prevention in Atlanta

Anne Colston Wentz, M.D.

Adjunct professor of obstetrics and gynecology at Johns Hopkins
University School of Medicine in Baltimore and former special
assistant in the contraceptive development branch of the Center
for Population Research at the National Institute of Child Health
and Human Development at the National Institutes of Health in
Bethesda, Maryland

Contents

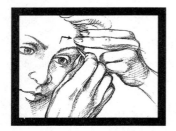

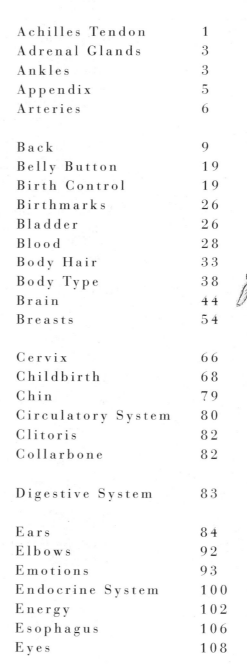

Introduction   xii

Your Body

Achilles Tendon   1
Adrenal Glands   3
Ankles   3
Appendix   5
Arteries   6

Back   9
Belly Button   19
Birth Control   19
Birthmarks   26
Bladder   26
Blood   28
Body Hair   33
Body Type   38
Brain   44
Breasts   54

Cervix   66
Childbirth   68
Chin   79
Circulatory System   80
Clitoris   82
Collarbone   82

Digestive System   83

Ears   84
Elbows   92
Emotions   93
Endocrine System   100
Energy   102
Esophagus   106
Eyes   108

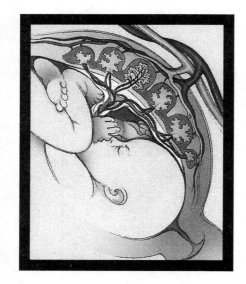

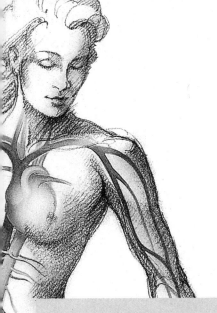

Fallopian Tubes   118
Fat   120
Feet   131
Fertility   141
Fingernails   146

Gallbladder   151
Gums   154
Gynecological Exam   159

Hair   162
Hands   165
Heart   168
Hips   177
Hormones   182

Intestines   183

Jaw   185
Joints   187

Kidneys   190
Knees   192

Larynx and
    Vocal Cords   197
Lips   201
Liver   204
Lungs   206
Lymphatic System   216

Medical Tests   218
Menopause   227
Menstrual Cycle   237
Moles   246
Mouth   248
Muscular System   250

Where to find
illustrated guides to
your body systems:

System	Page
Circulatory System	80
Digestive System	83
Endocrine System	100
Lymphatic System	216
Muscular System	250
Nervous System	258
Reproductive System	322
Respiratory System	324
Skeletal System	358
Urinary System	418

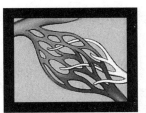

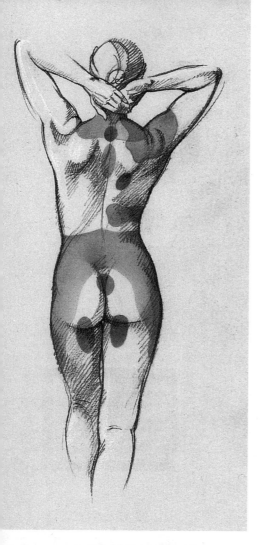

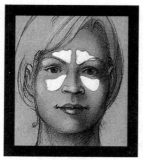

Neck	252
Nervous System	258
Nose	260
Nutrition	266
Ovaries	285
Pain Relief	290
Pancreas	304
Pelvis	309
Pregnancy	309
Rectum	320
Reproductive System	322
Respiratory System	324
Ribs	326
Salivary Glands	327
Scalp	328
Sex	330
Sexually Transmitted Diseases	341
Shins	346
Shoulders	348
Sinuses	352
Skeletal System	358
Skin	360
Skull	377
Spine	379
Spleen	388
Stomach	389
Stress	392
Sweat Glands	395
Tailbone	397
Tear Ducts	398
Teeth	399

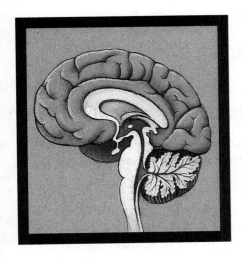

Throat   406
Thyroid   408
Toenails   410
Tongue   411
Tonsils   415

Underarms   417
Urinary System   418
Urine   420
Uterus   421

Vagina   427
Veins   431
Vulva   435

Wrists   436

Toning Your Body

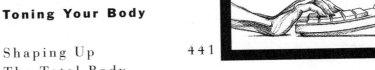

Shaping Up   441
The Total Body-
   Shaping Workout   443
Abdominals   450
Biceps   452
Buttocks   454
Calves   455
Chest   456
Forearms   458
Neck   459
Shoulders   460
Thighs   461
Triceps   464

Aerobic
   Conditioning   466
Five Super Videos   468
Index   470

The Female Body

Introduction

JUST ASK.

There are lots of books about women's health. But none like this one.

You can tell some of the things that make this book different just by looking ahead a few pages. There you'll find practical, useful, down-to-earth advice from leading doctors and women's health experts. You'll discover that their tips are easy to follow. Their explanations are straightforward—free from medical jargon. Their advice is as specific as it can be (though, of course, how you take it is up to you).

Whether they're suggesting how to prevent a yeast infection, how to treat muscle aches, how to fend off cramps or burn fat quickly, theirs are words to the wise. And that's good, because women are wise. We already know a lot about our bodies and how they work. We've mastered the basics of being women.

But we also know that there have been some very significant breakthroughs in doctors' understanding of women's health in the past few years. We have many more personal health care choices from puberty right through and after menopause—choices such as whether we should take the Pill, how to best meet our calcium needs, the pluses and minuses of hormone replacement therapy, the surest form of breast exam—even which questions to ask our doctors.

Where do you find the answers? You can ask your doctor, of course—but does that doctor (male or female) really have time to answer all the questions you have? You can look things up in a medical encyclopedia—but those explanations of chemistry and anatomy don't add up to the everyday advice you're probably seeking. And you can always ask your friends or female relatives—but are their solutions appropriate for you?

Be assured, you're not the only woman with these questions. Others share your concerns—and yes, even some of your doubts and confusion about what's best for you and what you should be doing to protect your health at this time in your life. With so many concerns in common, it only made sense for us to ask experts the thousands of questions you have—and then bring their answers together in one common place that we all can share.

This book is that place. So if there's something you've been wondering about your health, just ask. Chances are very good that you'll find the answers here.

How did we go about getting those answers?

A team of dedicated researchers and writers spent thousands of hours interviewing women's health care experts and combing through the most recent research. We talked to hundreds of doctors, teachers, researchers, midwives, therapists, nutritionists and nurses. We asked each of them what *you* want to know about. Not you, personally, of course—but women like you, of many ages, married and single, older and younger, with children and without.

From all that research and all those interviews came the book you hold in your hands. It's an A-to-Z guide to the entire universe of a woman's body—with clearly explained, authoritative, up-to-date information on what you can do to prevent disease and what steps you can take to heal yourself.

Turn to the Contents or the Index, and you'll quickly see that this is far more than an anatomy book. Yes, *The Female Body: An Owner's Manual* discusses every part of your body, but it also tells you what can go wrong and what you can do to prevent it from happening. You'll also find chapters with authoritative information, tips and advice about fertility, pregnancy, menopause, nutrition, weight loss, body toning and other topics that are critical to women's health care.

In addition, you'll find some illustrated two-page sections that are devoted to the ten "systems" in your body. So, for instance, you can turn to "Muscular System" if you have aching muscles; "Endocrine System" if you're wondering about hormonal changes; "Circulatory System" if you're troubled with varicose veins. From there you'll be guided to the chapter or the special box that helps answer your questions.

The Female Body: An Owner's Manual is more than a body book. It's a book that puts *you* in charge of your health.

Debora T. Yost
Vice-President and Editorial Director
Prevention Magazine Health Books

Your Body

Achilles Tendon

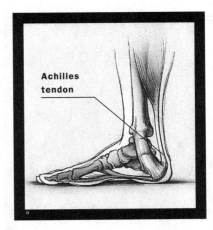

Normal foot position, with the sole flat and the Achilles tendon extended.

WHEN YOUR ACHILLES TENDON IS in good shape, it's as reliable as the spring on a trampoline. You can use it to kick up your heels or to dig them in. If you leap in the air for joy, spring for a jump shot, twirl in a pirouette or execute a double flip, count on that mighty tendon to soften the jolt when you come down.

This fat, six-inch-long bundle of fibers is the strongest and thickest tendon in your whole body. In a way, it merely does what all tendons do: It connects muscle to bone. But its location gives it added importance. This is the crucial tissue that connects your calf muscles to the heel bone of your foot. A little bit of mistreatment can make it hurt like the dickens.

"If that tendon is tight, it's easily injured," says James McGuire, D.P.M., director of physical therapy and instructor in the Department of Orthopedics at the Foot and Ankle Institute of Pennsylvania College of Podiatric Medicine in Philadelphia.

Regular stretching and wearing the right kinds of shoes will help your Achilles tendon stay flexible. But if you overuse it or overstretch it, you're risking trouble.

Here are some tactics to keep your Achilles tendon limber and pain-free.

Avoid high heels. High-heeled shoes take the greatest toll on the tendon. "Women who spend a great deal of time in them—and then perform exercises in flat sneakers or walk around the house barefooted for extended periods of time—are prone to tendinitis," says Dr. McGuire. When Achilles tendinitis sets in, the heel cord becomes swollen and inflamed, causing aching, soreness or pain.

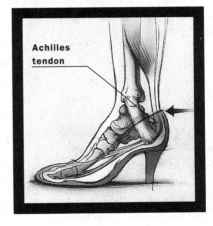

When your heel is raised, the Achilles tendon is compressed.

The problem is, when you wear pumps or high heels, you tilt your heel up in your shoe and compress your Achilles tendon as shown in the illustration above. Then, when you try to lower your heel, the tendon protests.

"High heels can shorten the heel cord dramatically," observes William Case, P.T., president of Case Physical Therapy in Houston. "I remember one young woman who walked on her tiptoes when she took off her heels—she couldn't let her feet go flat."

Kick the same-height habit. Even if you can't get away with wearing flat shoes all the time, you can come up with a number of creative ways to finesse dress shoes.

"Do some cross-training," says Case.

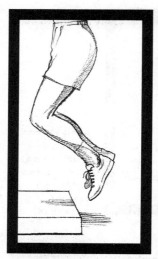

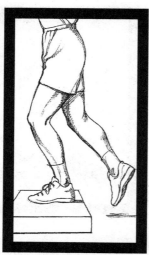

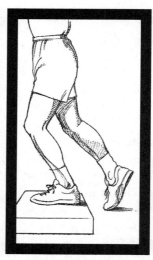

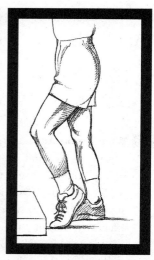

To avoid injury in step aerobics, jump up to the riser with both feet.

Descend with one foot, keeping it close to the riser.

Place the toe near the riser, then lower the heel.

Descend with the second foot, repeating the toe-heel motion.

"Don't always wear the same height heel day after day." Alternate high heels with flats and low heels during the work week—then wear sneakers on weekends. "Remember, the lower the heel, the less stress on the Achilles."

Lift your sole. If you're making the move to flatter dress shoes, you can ease the shock of the new by putting a heel lift in your flatter shoes. "Using a heel lift can also help you make the change from high heels at work into sneakers at the gym," says Dr. McGuire.

Warm up for action. Before any exercise that puts strain on your Achilles tendon,

warm up first. That means giving yourself time for some low-speed activity that doesn't make your heart race. "Do at least five low-intensity minutes on a stationary bike or take a slow five-minute walk outside or on a treadmill," suggests Reba Schecter, director of exercise physiology at Canyon Ranch health spa in Lenox, Massachusetts. She advises that you stretch your Achilles twice during your workout—a few times after you warm up, then again after you finish.

Tend it with ice. "If your Achilles tendon is sore, ice it," suggests Dr. McGuire. Ice will numb the pain and help alleviate any inflammation.

Use a cold gel pack or an ice bag. Or put a bag of dried beans or dried split peas in the freezer and use that as an ice pack. You'll need a towel to protect your skin from getting overchilled. Wrap the Achilles area in the towel, then apply the cold pack directly over the tendon. Apply ice three times a day for no more than 15 minutes, until the soreness is gone. If pain persists for several days, he suggests that you see your doctor.

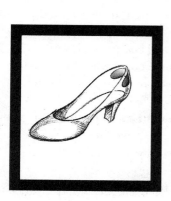

Some women have worn heels so often for so long that they've developed a "pump bump"—a hard, bony enlargement where the shoe hits the Achilles tendon. One way to relieve a pump bump is with a U-shaped heel pad, available at any drugstore.

Adrenal Glands

THE ADRENALINE RUSH IS FAMOUS. Stress or danger sends signals to the adrenal glands, adrenaline pours out and we spring into the fight or suddenly take flight.

Churning out adrenaline isn't the only job your adrenal glands do, though. These two small glands located at the top of each kidney also churn out hormones that regulate your blood sugar level, keep your blood volume where it should be and contribute to normal sexual development.

When these glands malfunction, several health problems can arise. If the glands are overactive and you produce too much of the steroid hormone cortisol, you may have Cushing's syndrome, according to Kay McFarland, M.D., professor of medicine at the University of South Carolina School of Medicine in Charleston.

Cushing's usually causes unexplained weight gain—particularly behind the neck or around the collarbone and at the abdomen. Also, the syndrome may cause a ruddy complexion, facial hair and dark purplish stripes on the abdomen, buttocks and armpits. The disease can be treated with surgery or medication, says Dr. McFarland.

Another problem, Addison's disease, develops when the adrenals stop producing steroid-based hormones, particularly cortisol. Low blood pressure, darkening of the skin, weakness, lethargy and abdominal pain can all signal Addison's disease. The disease can be treated by taking replacement hormones two times a day, says Dr. McFarland.

See also Endocrine System

Ankles

IT'S A POWERFUL BUT DELICATE FEAT of foot engineering.

Your ankle is the hinge that joins your leg to your foot as well as the joint that moves them. In fact, the big bumps you feel on each side of your ankle are the junctures where two leg bones meet the heel bone. Inside that structure is a complex web of ligaments, tendons and muscles that protects the ankle.

If you wrench your foot to one side, stretching or tearing one of the ligaments that connects the leg bone to the ankle bone, you'll get a sprain—the most common type of ankle injury. There are infinite ways to do that—catching a high heel, stepping off a curb the wrong way or wrenching your ankle as you dash to catch a train.

Here are some things you can do to keep your ankles strong and make sure the sprain and pain stay mainly under rein.

Stand like a stork. "One of the reasons we trip and fall is because our sense of balance isn't good," says Steven I. Subotnick, D.P.M., former professor of biomechanics and surgery at California College of Podiatric Medicine and a sports podiatrist in private practice in Hayward, California. You can improve your sense of balance with an exercise that will also help strengthen your ankles. "Take off your shoes and stand like a stork on one leg." While you're perched on one leg, bend the other one up behind you.

"Close your eyes while you do the exercise," he suggests. "Hold the pose for up to a minute." Then switch legs and do the same thing on the other foot. He suggests doing the stork exercise a couple of times a day to im-

New Angles on Ankle Looks

Your ankles feel fine. But when you look in a full-length mirror, you wish the sturdy things were a little less stout. Is there anything you can do about thick ankles?

"If you tend to store fat in the lower leg area, you can reduce by reducing your overall body fat levels," says Rebecca Gorrell, fitness instructor and wellness education director at Canyon Ranch in Tucson, Arizona. She recommends "eating a low-fat, high-carbohydrate diet with adequate protein and doing a combination of aerobics and strength training."

In the meantime, while the fat melts, follow these tips for slimming the look of your ankles from nationally syndicated fashion columnist Patricia McLaughlin.

- **Cover your ankles with boots.**
- **Choose black stockings to narrow ankle appearance.**
- **Wear fashionably "clunky" shoes. "They make your ankles look relatively small by comparison," says McLaughlin.**
- **Or wear fashionably heavy socks. "Thick, heavy wool socks that you push down around your ankles make a virtue out of mass," she says.**

prove your balance and lessen your chances of stumbling.

Build your calves. The calf muscles make up an important muscle group that controls and gives support to the ankle. Both strength and flexibility here are important, explains Reba Schecter, director of exercise physiology at Canyon Ranch health spa in Lenox, Massachusetts. One way to make calf muscles stronger is with a heel-raise exercise.

Stand on the stairs, facing up, with the balls of your feet on one step. Your feet should be parallel and a few inches apart. Hold the railing for balance. Slowly rise up on your toes, then lower your heels gently as far as you can with control. Repeat the strengthener 8 to 10 times. Do it three times a week, with a day or two between sessions, Schecter advises. Your calf muscles should feel pleasantly fatigued after each set. As the fatigue lessens, increase the repetitions until you get to a maximum of 12.

Flex your calves. The same position can be used for flexibility. As you gently lower your heels, go to the point where you feel a moderate stretch in your calves. Hold the stretch 10 to 30 seconds. According to Schecter, the count depends on how well you can control the stretch—you shouldn't stretch to the point of feeling unbalanced.

Repeat the stretch three to four times. Do it after the calf-strengthening exercise—or after any other exercise that works the calves, such as walking or cycling.

Coddling a Sprain

The ligaments that unite our bones and protect our joints are like taffy. If you stretch them, they stay stretched. So even if you only have a mild sprain, it can take two to three weeks for the ligament to lose its pulled-taffy shape and become a normally acting fiber again.

You can help the healing process by doing these things.

RICE it. RICE stands for *rest*, *ice*, compression and *elevation*. Rest means staying off your feet and using crutches if necessary. Ice means applying ice to the injured part of your ankle—for 15 to 20 minutes every 2 to 4 hours during the first 48 to 72 hours, says William Case, P.T., president of Case Physical

Therapy in Houston and certified in sports physical therapy. (Use a towel under the ice to avoid frostbite.)

Compression means wrapping your ankle to control swelling. To wrap your foot properly, you'll need a long elastic compression bandage 1½ inches wide (such as an Ace bandage). Here's the procedure: Starting at the base of your toes—but leaving your toes exposed—wrap the elastic bandage once around the end of your foot. Then walk the bandage up your leg; overlap half the width of the bandage with the next wrap. Continue wrapping around your foot, overlapping half the bandage width each time. Lessen the tension of the bandage as you wrap up your foot and over your ankle going up your leg to the base of your calf. Make sure that no one area gets too much tension or too much overlap. Get around your ankle as best you can; you can leave your heel exposed.

Elevation means propping up your ankle (above the level of your heart) to prevent swelling.

RICE your ankle for one to two days, until the swelling goes down and you're not in pain. If the ankle doesn't improve or you're still in pain, call your doctor.

Pedal to strength. Even if you've injured your ankle, you can still strengthen it as it heals. After any pain and swelling have subsided, usually a week or two after a sprain, start using a stationary bike, suggests Case.

When you're using the bike to build up your ankle, set the tension on minimum to medium, he suggests. Then, start pedaling for 5 minutes at a time twice a day. Gradually work up to 10 minutes of biking three times a day. Eventually, you can work up to 15 to 20 minutes on the bike.

See also Muscular System, Skeletal System

Appendix

YOU MIGHT SAY THAT THE APPENDIX is like holding a Republican party sign-up drive at an Aerosmith concert or slapping on Right Guard before you jump in a sauna—that is, pretty useless.

Even after all those years of medical research, doctors are still baffled by this narrow, finger-shaped tube that branches off the large intestine. It's unique, as far as body parts go, in that it has absolutely no known function.

But that doesn't mean you can disregard it. If the ambulance siren is blaring, there's a good chance someone's on her way to the hospital with appendicitis: it's the most common abdominal surgical emergency in developed countries.

Diagnosis of this gut-kicker isn't easy, partly because the position of the appendix can vary. Most people have an appendix that projects out of the colon at the lower right-hand side of the abdomen. Other people have an appendix behind or below the first part of the colon or in front of or behind the ileum, which is part of the small intestine.

A Hurt Attack

A classic symptom of appendicitis is pain in the stomach area around the belly button and in the lower right area of the abdomen. If your appendix is acting up, the pain will be constant and aggravated by movement. Other symptoms are nausea, vomiting and low-grade fever. If you do have persistent discomfort, especially around the lower right side of your belly, you should notice whether you also have loss of appetite or nausea soon after. A combination of these symptoms within a 12- to 24-hour period means that you should give your doctor a call.

If a doctor suspects appendicitis, you can be certain she'll recommend an appendectomy as soon as possible. Your appendix can rupture within hours of becoming inflamed and infected. A ruptured appendix could lead to peritonitis, an inflammation of the abdominal organs that is sometimes fatal if not treated with antibiotics.

Just who gets this great big pain in their side? In a Swedish study of over 7,000 patients who had operations for suspected appendicitis, researchers found that the age of peak risk was 10 to 14 years. The incidence of appendicitis was about 1 in 1,000—and more common among males than females. The study also showed that doctors diagnosed men's appendicitis more accurately than women's—because there are some gynecological diseases that can mimic appendicitis.

One way to help avoid unnecessary surgery is for your doctor to do an ultrasound of the area. In a study of 110 patients admitted to the U.S. Naval Hospital in San Diego with suspected appendicitis, ultrasound-derived diagnoses had an 85 percent accuracy rate. But there's also evidence that ultrasound diagnosis sometimes misses appendicitis—so even with the technology, you need a doctor who has knowledge about symptoms.

Arteries

A MIGHTY RED RIVER FLOWS FROM your heart to all your limbs, branching into creeks, rivulets and estuaries that carry fresh blood to every part of your body.

Each of the arteries that snakes through your system is sheathed and swathed like a muscle-bound snake. From the hefty aorta that leaves your heart to the tiny vessels called arterioles that thread the tips of your hands and toes, the entire network of blood-carrying vessels is well-protected. Two outer layers shield the exterior of each artery and arteriole. Inside those layers is a jacket of muscle and a leotard of elastic tissue. As the vessel surges and subsides with blood, each pulse is regulated by the smooth muscles that help do the grunt work of pushing blood on its way. Speeding its course through the body is the silky-smooth lining of the artery called the endothelium.

It's a great system. But like every mighty river, from the Mississippi to the Monongahela, there's just one problem—silt. In arteries, that silt is composed of free-floating globules of fat (or lipids) and the potential saboteur of the whole system, nasty cholesterol.

Tunnel Damage

No matter how well we treat our arteries—eating low-fat food, getting plenty of exercise, watching blood pressure—nearly all of us eventually get some blemishes on the inner lining of our arteries. These minor aberrations are hardly enough to interfere with the blood flow. But even the smallest of blemishes may eventually throw your blood off course.

What causes these blemishes? "We just don't know precisely what it is," says Malcolm Perry, M.D., professor and chief of vascular surgery at Texas Tech University in Lubbock. "But something happens to the artery lining that results in the conversion of smooth muscle cells to fatty lipid-bearing cells."

There are a number of likely suspects, notes Dr. Perry. Cell-damaging agents in cigarette smoke—called mutagens—may inflict the first damage. Or the cholesterol molecules in high-fat diets could launch a secret assault. High blood pressure could be partially to blame—or the family genes might make it easier for some people to have damaged vessels than others.

"Once that break in the lining happens, whatever the cause, a whole cascade of events occurs," says Edward S. Cooper, M.D., professor of medicine at the University of Pennsylvania School of Medicine in Philadelphia and past president of the American Heart Association. Disklike blood components called platelets rush in to seal the lining shut. As they're repairing the artery, the platelets further roughen the inner surface, causing turbulent blood flow.

Meanwhile, the surface turns knobby, easily snagging fat molecules that hang on and stay within the roughed-up sides like rust in a pipe. That congregation of fat—collectively called an atheroma—eventually makes up a dense, artery-clogging substance called plaque. As plaque narrows the arteries at these points, the result is a condition called atherosclerosis.

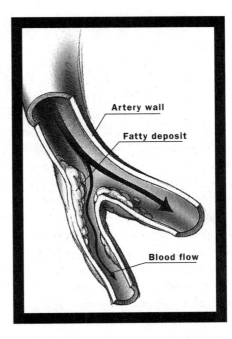

The buildup of fatty deposits along artery walls creates plaque— which interferes with blood flow.

Artery wall

Fatty deposit

Blood flow

The Clot Thickens

In the narrowed artery it doesn't take much of an obstruction to jam up the tunnel and stop the flow. A small blood clot can dam up the works. Though the clot can occur in any part of the body—because arteries are everywhere—certain sites are more vulnerable than others.

"They most commonly involve the coronary arteries that serve the heart, the carotid artery to the brain and the femoral artery to the lower legs," says Dr. Perry. If the clot occurs in one of the arteries that feeds the heart muscle, you're at risk for coronary artery disease.

"It's critical when a clot suddenly closes one of those narrowed arteries to the heart or brain," says Dr. Perry. "Heart attack and stroke are the most common causes of sudden death, next to trauma." Because it sets the stage for these life-threatening occurrences, arterial disease indirectly claims half of all the citizens of the Western world.

Going with the Flow

For many people, risks rise with age because the arteries begin to get stiff and less flexible. The result is the condition called arteriosclerosis, better known as hardening of the arteries. When atherosclerosis teams up with arteriosclerosis, you have a life-threatening conspiracy—because the clogged up artery doesn't have the flexibility to expand when it needs to.

Often arterial disease pads stealthily into place before you have an inkling of trouble. "It begins in childhood—even adolescents have fatty streaks forming on their arteries," says JoAnn E. Manson, M.D., associate professor of medicine at Harvard Medical School and co-director of women's health at Brigham and Women's Hospital in Boston.

With a few precautions arterial disease doesn't have to catch you by surprise. Here are some things you can do to prevent it.

Favor fresh veggies. "There have been decades of studies that showed without fail the protective effects eating vegetables has on the arteries," says Dr. Perry.

Among the substances that seem to lend protective power are vegetables that contain the so-called antioxidants—most prominently, vitamin C, vitamin E and beta-carotene. The antioxidants have a protective effect on cells, helping capture "free radicals," chemically unstable oxygen molecules that can do a lot of cell damage. It has been shown that the antioxidant vitamins also help prevent arterial damage.

Many fresh fruits and vegetables are good sources of one key antioxidant, vitamin C. If you choose fruits and vegetables that are orange, yellow or dark green, you're also getting the benefit of beta-carotene, which turns to vitamin A in your body. True, you could take supplements, but researchers have found that you don't get the same beneficial effects. Fruits and vegetables contain other micronutrients that are healthful.

"It doesn't seem to be as simple as taking one beta-carotene capsule or a vitamin C tablet," says Dexter L. Morris, M.D., Ph.D., vice chairman and assistant professor of emergency medicine at the University of North Carolina at Chapel Hill School of Medicine. "It's more complicated than that."

"Nothing's really proven for sure, but the message is to eat five to nine servings of fruits and vegetables every day," says Dr. Manson.

Leaf through your menu. You'll get another benefit beyond vitamin C and beta-carotene from dark green, leafy vegetables, researchers say. These valuable leafy greens also give you a B vitamin called folate. (The supplement form is called folic acid.)

Folate isn't an antioxidant, but it lowers levels of an amino acid called homocysteine that has shown up in the blood of people with arterial disease. When the Centers for Disease Control and Prevention in Atlanta sponsored a review of 38 studies on the subject, researchers found that people who had arterial health problems often had high homocysteine levels and low folate levels. They also discovered—in 11 of the studies—that folic acid lowered homocysteine levels.

Some of the investigators who did the study found it so convincing that they now take the recommended 400 micrograms of folate in supplement form, says investigator Carol J. Boushey, R.D., Ph.D., assistant professor of food and nutrition at Southern Illinois University at Carbondale. "I drink orange juice and fix legumes for dinner to get mine." Just a cup of orange juice and a cup of raw spinach will get you halfway to your folate goal. Add a bean-and-broccoli salad, and you've met your daily requirement for folate.

Stub out cigs. "Smoking is turning out to be even more important than we thought 20 or 30 years ago," says Dr. Cooper. "It's very likely that even passive smoke might be harmful."

It's never too late to stop, however, according to Dr. Manson. When you do, your blood pressure and carbon monoxide levels immediately drop. After three to five years you reduce your risk of coronary heart disease to the level of a person who never smoked.

Tone up for your arteries. You firm up your arms and tighten your abs when you weight train, and you help your body burn fat when you do aerobics. For your arteries, either kind of exercise can help keep the red pipelines toned, flexible and fat-free.

Exercise is famous for elevating HDLs, or high-density lipoproteins, the "good" cholesterol that protects against artery-clogging plaques. Exercise also helps lower blood pressure. "But the good effects of exercise go even beyond what we can measure—like blood pressure and HDLs," says Dr. Cooper. "It can probably unclog at least some of the fat from our arteries."

Counter claudication. Exercise is also turning out to be better therapy than surgery for the arterial bad news known as claudication. The word comes from the Greek word for limp. People who have claudication must often stop to rest their aching calves. The pain comes from narrowed, clogged-up arteries in the legs, and surgery is sometimes needed to clear up the condition.

But exercise may be a good alternative. "There have been several good studies showing that people with this condition get better on exercise therapy than they do with surgery to clean out the artery," says Dr. Perry.

See also Circulatory System

Back

FIVE YEARS AGO, MARGARET'S BACK kicked up painfully and she panicked. She's an active woman, and a bad back seemed to threaten all her favorite pursuits—long hikes, daily aerobics classes, bike rides down sleepy morning streets. She cut down on her exercise just a smidgen. Then she trekked from doctor to doctor, searching for a diagnosis and a cure.

But the diagnosis she finally got seemed vague: The doctor said she was suffering from muscle strain. The cure—ibuprofen and modifying her exercise program—seemed, well, wishy-washy. And the pain got worse, no matter what she did. Even bed rest didn't help. Then, when she resumed her workouts, the meanest pain of all—sciatica—started traveling from her back, along one side, from her buttock to her foot.

Margaret decided to give up all exercise until the sciatica subsided. Some days later, she took a ten-minute tentative nonpower-walk. In the days that followed, she gradually increased her pace and walked longer distances. Eventually, she resumed biking, hiking and even aerobics classes. True, she didn't take double aerobics classes, and she carefully alternated activities instead of stressing the same muscles. But the woman who thought her exercising days were over was cured. Her back pain never flared up again.

Why didn't it? What exactly had happened? What cured her? And what had caused the pain in the first place?

She was never really sure. Both the cause of the problem and the reason for her recovery were a double mystery to Margaret.

A History of Mysteries

Far from being an isolated case, Margaret's experience with back pain is typical. As often as 80 percent of the time, the cause of back pain is a mystery, says John D. Loeser, M.D., professor of neurologic surgery and director of the Pain Center at the University of Washington School of Medicine in Seattle. "We can't make a definite diagnosis except for a small fraction of the people who come to the office."

With 31 million people in the United States bearing the burden of bad backs, plenty of doctors are looking for answers. Only the common cold prompts more office visits than the common backache. In fact, 70 percent of American women will have back pain sometime in their lives—usually before they're 50.

Of course, it's understandable that a part of the anatomy with so many complex moving parts would prove to be a troubled zone. Beneath its smooth skin lie muscles ranging in size from the huge lats (*latissimus dorsi*) that surround the chest area to the little *teres minor* muscles that pull your upper arms toward your shoulder blades. A cat's cradle of tendons and ligaments helps the muscles support the 26 bones of the spine.

The back is complex, efficient and wondrous. But there is a lot that can go wrong. Muscles can pull or tear, and stress can tense them up for easy damage. Ligaments might sprain; tendons can strain. Ill use—poor posture, bad lifting techniques, lack of exercise— can insult our backs. Even when we don't damage them through injury, eventually, age wears down the back's spools of bone, along with the shock-absorbing disks between them.

Relief Happens

So it's no mystery why the back is a mystery. Even the federal government has ac-knowledged that the healing of bad backs is a complex process with no pat system of recovery. When the federal Agency for Health Care Policy and Research reviewed 3,900 studies of treatments for back pain, it found only a few of the treatments to be scientifically valid. Even such established programs as traction, steroid injections and acupuncture don't hold up to rigorous scrutiny.

Getting Adjusted

If you go to a chiropractor for treatment of back pain, you can expect many of the usual doctor things. A chiropractor takes a medical history, does a physical examination, orders lab tests and sometimes does x-rays. (You might not have x-rays right away, however; some doctors and chiropractors say you don't need x-rays unless the symptoms continue for four weeks or more.)

Once the diagnostic part is over, the chiropractor will do a spinal manipulation, making adjustments of your spine on a special table built for that purpose. The goal is to realign your spine so that muscle and bone can move normally and start to heal. It's a hands-on experience.

"Basically, the chiropractor pushes or pulls different parts of the spine to improve muscle and joint function," says Scott Haldeman, M.D., D.C., Ph.D., associate clinical professor of neurology at the University of California, Irvine, and adjunct professor at Los Angeles Chiropractic College in Whittier. "When the chiropractor moves into a spinal adjustment, she usually gives a short thrust to the spine with the heel of her hand. And you commonly hear a click or a pop. That means there's been some movement within a joint."

In fact, the agency's guidelines for health come down to something like this: Take two aspirin and don't call the doctor in the morning. For nine out of ten people, researchers found, back pain—even acute back pain—goes away on its own within a month as mysteriously as it came.

If you're wondering whether you're someone who definitely needs to see a doctor for back pain, "the danger signs are weakness or numbness in the legs or loss of bowel or bladder control," says Jeffrey Susman, M.D., member of the U.S. Public Health Service Agency for Health Care Policy and Research and vice-chairman of family medicine at the University of Nebraska College of Medicine in Omaha. If you don't have these or other uncommon difficulties, however, symptoms usually disappear—and without a clue to their cure.

Does that mean there's nothing you can do? Not at all. According to experts, there are quite a few relief measures that help the majority of bad-back sufferers. The first one probably sounds familiar.

Take two aspirin. Sure, the advice is old. But it's also tried-and-true. "The safest, most effective drug is probably in your medicine chest," says Dr. Susman. "Aspirin proved to work as well as anything stronger—like muscle relaxants. So did acetaminophen and ibuprofen. And they don't have the side effects of strong prescription drugs." If aspirin or ibuprofen, which are both anti-inflammatories, upsets your stomach, you can use acetaminophen.

Get your spine in line. The only other clinical method of treatment offering relief for back pain is the spinal manipulation that chiropractors perform. (Osteopathic doctors also do spinal manipulation.) The federal study found that spinal manipulation works especially well in people who have some level of

The Back Doctors

Although studies show that chiropractors are often consulted for acute back pain, many other medical specialists also treat backs. Though their titles are different, many of their methods are similar. In fact, "at this time, many of the treatments prescribed by different specialists are coming together in agreement," says Edward Hanley, M.D., chairman of the Orthopaedics Department at Carolinas Medical Center in Charlotte, North Carolina. Here are the front-runners for back treatments.

- A chiropractor, or D.C. (Doctor of Chiropractic), focuses on manipulating the spine into proper alignment, relaxing muscles and increasing motion to relieve abnormal pressures in the back. Many also prescribe physical therapy exercises, although they cannot prescribe drugs.
- A neurologist is an M.D. who focuses on the diagnosis of neurological disorders.
- A neurosurgeon specializes in spinal surgery.
- An orthopedic surgeon is a medical doctor (M.D.) or D.O. who has specialized and can treat any problem of the musculoskeletal system and can operate. Some prefer to call themselves orthopedists to highlight the nonsurgical component of their practice.
- An osteopath, or D.O. (Doctor of Osteopathy), can practice spinal manipulation, prescribe drugs and perform surgery, if she has specialized in orthopedics or neurosurgery.
- A physiatrist is also an M.D., one who specializes in rehabilitation medicine and physical therapy.
- A physical therapist, or P.T., is licensed in physical therapy, but she cannot prescribe drugs. Physical therapists are expert at prescribing therapeutic exercises for backs and at checking proper posture.

Get Better with Yoga

Two yoga exercises, the yoga sit-up and the mountain pose, both help relieve back pain, according to Mary Pullig Schatz, M.D., yoga instructor and author of <u>Back Care Basics</u>. Here's how they're done.

<u>Yoga sit-up.</u> Lie on your back with your calves resting on a chair seat as shown in the illustration, bottom left. Your hips as well as your knees should be bent at 90-degree angles. Cross your arms in front of your chest and place your hands on your shoulders.

Inhale and exhale slowly as you press your lower back to the floor and flatten your abdomen. Raise your shoulders six to ten inches off the floor and hold. Lower your left shoulder to touch the floor and then raise it back up as shown in the illustration, bottom right. Then lower your head and shoulders back to the floor. Repeat the sequence, using your right shoulder.

Continue the exercise until your abdominal muscles feel warm, then do one or two more sit-ups and stop. Be sure that you don't hold your breath during the exercise. It's important to inhale and exhale steadily in order to avoid straining.

<u>Mountain pose.</u> Stand barefooted, with your feet five to eight inches apart, placed directly under your hips. While keeping your upper body erect, bend your knees so they move forward over the center of your feet as shown. There's a tendency for the curve of your back to increase in the lumbar area, which is the small of your back between your rib cage and pelvis. Try to keep this curve constant, so your abdomen doesn't "pouch" forward.

Inhale, then exhale, and as you exhale, slowly push your feet into the floor and straighten your knees. (But don't lock your knees in place.) Hold this position for 30 to 60 seconds, breathing normally.

Practice this standing posture as often as you can during the day.

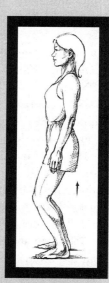

Mountain pose

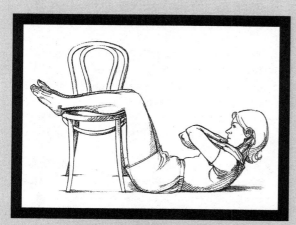

Yoga sit-up—starting position

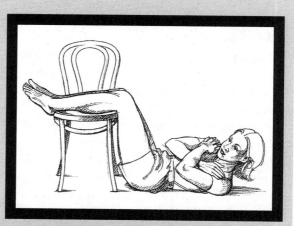

Yoga sit-up—left shoulder lowered

acute back pain—the kind that comes on suddenly and doesn't last very long—notes Scott Haldeman, M.D., D.C., Ph.D., associate clinical professor of neurology at the University of California, Irvine, and adjunct professor at Los Angeles Chiropractic College in Whittier. But he did say that studies are being done that indicate spinal manipulation also helps people with lingering chronic back pain.

Get up and at 'em. One of the traditional treatments for back pain—bed rest—got thoroughly trounced in the federal guidelines. Bed rest that exceeds four days weakens your muscles and bones and impedes your recovery, warns the panel. Most experts advise that you get no more than two days of bed rest—tops.

"Inactivity is bad for the body," says Dr. Loeser. "Don't go home to bed. Resting until you feel better is likely to make you worse. Bed rest is deleterious to your health."

"Get up and get active," says Dr. Susman. "Plan an early return to activity." That means as normal a work schedule as you can manage and low-stress exercise such as walking, swimming or biking.

Make love, not hurt. How to snuggle with your honey when your back hurts is a topic that comes up often with patients, says Dr. Haldeman.

"I remember one patient who used to come in on Mondays with horrendous back pains. They'd improve during the week after an office visit. But every Monday the woman would be back in my office again. It started to get expensive, so her husband got a little angry, and he came in one Monday with her. He turned out to be six-foot-four and about 300 pounds. She's five-foot-two and 110 pounds. And they had sex every Saturday and Sunday night.

"I asked them what position they used,

and they said the standard one. I said, 'Well, it's time to change the position.' No way that woman could handle all that weight.

"As a rule of thumb, the person with back pain should be on top during intercourse and in control of the movement and pressure," he concludes.

Back-ercise

If there's any miracle cure for back pain, it's exercise. But the key is sensible exercise—not Margaret's version of ten aerobics classes a week. "You do need regular aerobic exercise for back health," says Dr. Susman.

Moderate exercise can also help prevent a recurrence of the pain if you do it regularly. As you get fit, your back and abdominal muscles that support your torso grow strong and resistant to injury. Not only do they armor and protect the spine, they also protect tendons and ligaments by absorbing stresses that might irritate those soft tissues.

If your back spasms or cramps easily when you make a sudden move or attempt a long reach, exercise will probably banish that pain, too. Weak, underused muscles (or overused muscles) are the reason for cramps or spasms, as all the fibers in the core of the muscle contract at once. Movement releases the fibers of a cramped muscle, but the fibers of a muscle in spasm stay locked for a while.

Walking Away from Back Trouble

"Walking, swimming or cycling can be excellent exercises for your back," says William Case, P.T., president of Case Physical Therapy in Houston.

An increase in overall physical fitness can decrease occurrences of back injury. Improved physical conditioning increases the postural

Holding the Line on Posture

Mom was right when she told us to sit up. Absolutely correct when she told us not to slouch. On the mark when she said to stand up straight.

Posture may sound old-fashioned, but it's a big back deal. When we slouch, swagger or sprawl, we skew our joints out of alignment. Being pushed out of their natural places stresses and strains them.

"Just sitting round-shouldered puts tremendous mechanical stress on the ligaments, soft tissues and muscles in the back," says Wayne Rath, P.T., co-director of Summit Physical Therapy in Syracuse, New York. "It's been established that there is 300 percent more tension in that position than in sitting up with a normal curve in the back."

The key to perfect posture? According to Mary Pullig Schatz, M.D., yoga instructor and author of <u>Back Care Basics</u>, the rules are straightforward: "As much as possible, keep your ears over your shoulders, your shoulders over your hips and your hips over your knees and feet."

To check out your own alignment, just look at yourself sideways in a mirror. You should be able to draw a straight line all the way from your ears to your feet, as shown above.

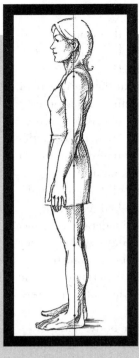

Perfect posture. Note that ear, shoulder, hip and ankle are all aligned.

much less precarious—maneuver: "To become more aware of how to maintain erect posture, sit, stand and walk with a bag of dried beans or rice on your head."

<u>S-T-R-E-T-C-H.</u> If you're trying to break the slouching habit, the stretch shown at right is especially useful for desk-bound workers. "Get up every 15 minutes, place your hands in the small of your back and lean backward," says William Case, P.T., president of Case Physical Therapy in Houston. Hold that position for a few counts—it reverses a slouch. It also reminds you to sit straight in a chair—just like your mother told you to do.

<u>Pinch it.</u> Case also recommends shoulder pinches. Stand up and clasp your hands behind your back near the waist. Lift your hands and stretch backward. Try to pull your shoulder blades together. Hold the stretch for a few seconds.

Practice Makes Posture

Most of us need a few reminders to keep our posture looking good. Here are some simple tricks and cues that can chase out the slouch and get you upright again.

<u>Beanbag it.</u> Remember when growing girls used to practice good posture by walking with books balanced on their heads? Dr. Schatz suggests a similar—but

In Good Standing

Another way to be kind to your back is by paying attention to how you stand. The more erect, the better. Here are some tips for maintaining a good standing posture.

<u>Wear good footgear.</u> Running shoes are best, but of course you can't wear them all the time. So, for work and dress, alternate

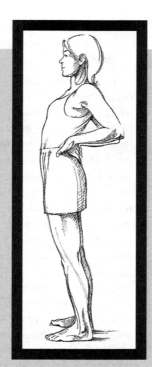

Shoulder pinches. With your hands in the small of your back, lift or push your hands slightly upward and lean backward for a few seconds.

your flats, low pumps and—if you must wear them—high heels. "High heels may aggravate your back—they increase the curvature and affect your gait," says Case.

Raise a foot. If you're standing in one place for a long time, look for something you can put a foot on, just to elevate a leg and change your position. If you're standing by the sink or folding clothes by the dryer, put one foot on a stool. Waiting in line for a movie, find a ledge or curb. If you're in a grocery store, put one foot up on the front rung of the shopping cart when you're waiting at the checkout line.

"You know why there are foot rails at the bottom of bars?" asks Alan Bensman, M.D., medical director of Glenwood Rehabilitation Center in Minneapolis. "Bartenders knew that people would stand at the bar and drink longer if they could put one foot up on the rail and be comfortable."

Don't bend and brush. When you bend from the waist with your legs straight, the tension tugs at your back muscles. It's the typical tooth-brushing position, though. To avoid straining your back while you're brushing your pearly whites, open one door of the cabinet under the sink and rest your foot on the ledge. Or use a footstool.

muscles (in the back, buttocks, abdomen and legs) that you need to maintain peak posture, the foundation of solid backs.

It's best to begin walking within two weeks of the first onset of symptoms, most doctors agree. You don't have to wait until you're totally pain-free, but do start your program slowly. Try ten-minute walks every other day and work your way up to a half-hour or full hour as you feel better, suggests Dr. Loeser. You might even enjoy walking daily.

Working Abs for Your Back

The abdominal muscles in the front of your trunk and the back muscles behind them form a kind of corset that supports your back. That's why back experts recommend strength-training exercises that target both the back muscles and the abdominal muscles that counterbalance them.

"You shouldn't work the back muscles to the exclusion of the abdominal muscles," warns John J. Triano, D.C., staff chiropractor at the Texas Back Institute in Plano. "You need to train in a balanced manner, or you set yourself up for further problems."

The abdominal crunch and the single-arm row (see pages 448 and 446) will help you firm up some fine support.

Back-Smart Living

Life has lots of booby traps for backs. Whether you're raking the yard, vacuuming the carpet, toting a heavy handbag or driving a car, pain can pounce when you least expect it. Before you turn your back on these harmless-looking troublemakers, here's how to prevent pain from starting.

Check your tool technique. When you're working with a rake, vacuum cleaner or broom, stand up straight when you use it. When you're raking, for instance, don't extend the rake out in front of you so that you have to lean over to reach the leaves. When you're sweeping, keep the broom close to your body. When you vacuum, use the long wand of the cleaner—don't bend over the short one.

Put your purse on a diet. If you routinely stuff your handbag full of magazines, makeup, sunscreen, hand lotion, keys and coins, lighten up. It's probably a good idea to use a backpack if the weight of your purse noticeably causes an increase in back pain, says Case.

A backpack may be an alternative to a heavy purse because it balances the weight on your back. With a heavy purse you usually favor one side. (It's not the only factor, however—the way you hold your body and move when walking can also aggravate a weak back.) Without proper body mechanics and good posture when walking, you can still aggravate a weak back. If you do wind up carrying a hefty bag, shift it occasionally to the other side so you don't strain your back, suggests Case.

Bolster your curve. Many people who drive mega-miles carry along a "lumbar support": That's a fancy name for a very simple cushion or roll that supports the small of your back, which is the lumbar area. You can buy the cylindrical support in a medical supply store.

Rolls come in different diameters, so find a chair or take it out to your car and test the support before you buy. You can also make your own lumbar roll by rolling up a towel smoothly and wrapping it with tape. Try out different sizes and different types of towels until you find one that offers support to your lower back when sitting and feels comfortable against the small of your back. The roll should fit in the small of your back, providing

Laid-Back Ways to Sleep

Even sleeping has some rules. When it comes to avoiding back trouble, here's what experts advise.

Sleep on your side. The ideal sleeping position is often the fetal one, with a pillow between your knees and with one or both knees slightly bent, says Alan Bensman, M.D., medical director of Glenwood Rehabilitation Center in Minneapolis. If you do sleep on your back, place a pillow under your knees. Keeping your knees flexed, however, may make your hamstrings tighten.

Stretch before rising. Before you get out of bed in the morning, it helps to get ready. Lying on your back, hug one knee at a time to your chest and hold it that way for five seconds, giving your back a chance to stretch. Then roll onto your side and push yourself up with your arms. Swing your feet onto the floor and greet the morning, says Dr. Bensman. When you get out of bed, attempt to keep your back as straight as possible. Then try arching your back once or twice, holding for five sec-

some pressure on the area and helping you to maintain the natural arch.

Fidget. "The majority of people slouch when they're sitting for long periods of time. That's when the muscles supporting the lower back become tired and weak. A slouched posture puts additional stresses on the ligaments of the spine, which results in pain," says Case. To relieve the stress on the back, all you need to do is stand and move around. If you want to ease the stress while you're sitting, just roll up a towel and place it behind your lower back to provide some support.

When you're on a long trip in a car, try to

onds each time. Also, you can rotate your back to the left side and hold for five seconds, then rotate to the right and hold for five seconds.

Update your mattress. Buy a new mattress and box spring every seven to ten years. They don't always show their wear, but mattresses and box springs exhaust themselves, too, after 20,000 to 30,000 hours of your Zzzs, according to Louis Sportelli, D.C., a chiropractor in Palmerton, Pennsylvania, and director of public affairs for the American Chiropractic Association.

Use a bed board. If your current mattress sags and you're not prepared to invest in a new one, tuck a bed board between the box spring and mattress to firm it up. The Care Catalog Services in Portland, Oregon (1-800-443-7091), offers both regular bed boards for the home and portable bed boards you can take along on trips. You can also put the top mattress on the floor or get a futon for the floor, according to Mary Pullig Schatz, M.D., yoga instructor and author of **Back Care Basics.**

stop every hour or so to exercise your back. Walk around outside your car a little. If you're in a plane or train, shift your rear end from side to side, wiggle your feet and tighten your abdominal muscles to realign good posture and give your back muscles a break.

Fidgeting for better circulation helps when you're in a car, too. The beaded wooden rollers that fit over the seat make it easy to move around a bit even while you're driving. "They're pretty neat," says Case. "They can give your back a massage effect if you move around on them." You can usually buy these roller-bead seat covers at auto supply stores.

Easing Your Sitting

If you're not sitting properly, you're putting increased demands on your lower back. "Bodies were made to move, not sit," says Case. Here are some tips to take the load off when your back is under pressure, according to Mary Pullig Schatz, M.D., yoga instructor and author of *Back Care Basics*.

• When you're flying, ask the flight attendant for two pillows. Put one behind your back and put the other one under your feet. (After takeoff you may want to substitute a briefcase for the foot rest if you're more comfortable that way.)

• On long bus rides try using the foot rest.

• Don't cross your legs. It creates uneven weight on your hips and pelvis and throws your back muscles off balance. If you can't kick the habit, switch legs often.

• Don't sit on soft couches or in deep chairs. Softness may feel like comfort, but your back needs support.

• Try out a rocking chair for back comfort. (President Kennedy always used one to help ease his back pain.) When you're rocking, you're using your legs, and that stimulates circulation.

• Another alternative is the "kneeling" chair, such as the Balans chair, which has one cushion for the knees and a second, firm cushion that supports the buttocks. With no back or arms, it may be hard to get used to, but it's a very good chair for tasks where you tend to lean forward, like microscope work or sewing. The design of the chair helps keep your spine erect.

• Place your keyboard so that you don't have to raise your shoulders to type. Ideally, your elbows should be positioned at a 90-degree angle when you're working.

• For activities where you tend to lean back slightly—such as reading or watching television—use a chair with an adjustable low-back support. Or make sure you use a rolled-up towel or a lumbar roll to support the curve in the small of your back.

Lifting Lessons

Large economy sizes of soap powder and cat litter are thrifty—but not smart if you strain a back muscle lifting them. Buy the smaller size, suggests Dr. Schatz. When you lift the bag, here's how she recommends doing it.

1. Position yourself close to the package.

2. Plant your feet about shoulder-width apart, with one leg slightly forward and alongside the package.

3. Lower your body by bending your knees. Keep your back straight and upright, as shown in the illustration, top right.

4. Hug the load to your body and stand up by pushing down strongly with both feet as you straighten your legs as shown in the illustration, bottom right.

Positioned this way, you lift with your legs, not your back. "Never lean over or bend from the waist to pick up anything," says Dr. Schatz. "If you must lean over, support part of your body weight by pressing one hand down onto your thigh or a sturdy piece of furniture."

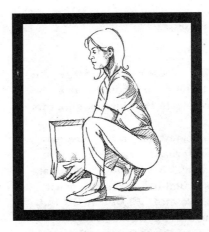

Lifting position. Bend your knees, not your back.

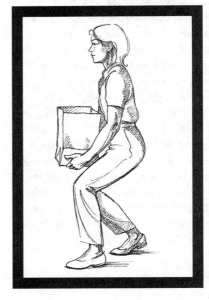

As you lift, keep the package close to your body.

Toddler Transport

Many women don't think about the connection between toting toddlers and the incidence of their backaches. Any baby or toddler over ten pounds should be centered in a carrier on your back, not torqued off to one side on your hip, says Annie Pivarski, orthopedic physician's assistant and supervisor of ergonomics and injury prevention at Saint Francis Memorial Hospital in San Francisco. Look for back slings or carriers in the children's sec-

tions of department stores. For longer hikes, look for child-carrying backpacks made by outdoors outfitters.

When you do pick up a child, make sure you do it properly: Lower one knee to the floor, ask your toddler to put her arms around you, hold her close to your body, then lift her up. Keep your abdominal muscles contracted to provide support as you lift, suggests Pivarski.

See also Muscular System, Nervous System, Skeletal System

Belly Button

IT'S JUST A SCAR IN THE MIDDLE of your lower abdomen, but the belly button sure can get people stirred up. Back in the 1960s actress Barbara Eden alarmed censors when she exposed hers, wearing harem-girl pajamas on *I Dream of Jeannie*. A decade later, Cher drew flack for her navel-baring costumes on *The Sonny and Cher Show*.

Today, the belly button is out in the open. Now that some women are getting their belly buttons pierced for jewelry, it has become all the more fashionable to display this center point on your midriff.

What's now a trendy place for a gold hoop started as the spot where you were attached as a fetus to the placenta in the uterus of your mother. "It's the conduit through which nutrients and oxygen and waste are transmitted between mother and baby," notes John Hratko, M.D., an obstetrician/gynecologist in private practice in Bethlehem, Pennsylvania. Your belly button marks the site of the umbilical cord, made up of two umbilical arteries and one umbilical vein.

But how do some people end up with the sunken innie belly button as opposed to the protruding outie?

The innie is actually the norm, says Dr. Hratko. Any protrusion in that area is considered an umbilical hernia. It might have been that way from the time you were an infant, or some other cause might have turned an innie into an outie later in life—including obesity, heavy lifting or straining or pregnancy.

"Some people have outies in various degrees, from mild to moderate protrusions," he says.

Birth Control

QUESTION: WHAT DO YOU CALL A COUPLE who uses the rhythm method for birth control?

Answer: Parents!

Okay, so the joke's not Seinfeld material. And you realize that the rhythm method is not much of a method at all. But are you up-to-date on current forms of birth control? Do you know as much as you need to know? And is what you *think* you know really accurate?

There's a chance the answer is no.

That's because quite a few myths and misperceptions about birth control persist, doctors say. For example, once women pass age 35, they often think they don't need to worry about birth control as much. The reality is, they do.

Some women view sterilization as the only effective long-term method of birth control. The truth of the matter is, it's not.

Still other women may fear that the Pill is unsafe. Yet for the right women, doctors say it's very safe.

Many women probably think the intrauterine device (IUD) isn't really an option for them. It's one that some women should consider more, doctors say.

When it comes to birth control, clearing up rumors and misconceptions is a full-time job for Mythbusters. Here are some of those myths—and what experts say about them.

Myth #1: I'm Too Old to Get Pregnant

The first myth is the idea that birth control isn't really an issue for women once they pass age 35 or 40, says Andrew Kaunitz, M.D., professor in the Department of Obstetrics and Gynecology at the University of Florida Health Science Center in Jacksonville.

When women reach their late thirties and early forties, they often perceive that their chances of conceiving are less likely, agrees Paul Blumenthal, M.D., assistant professor of obstetrics and gynecology at Johns Hopkins University Medical Center in Baltimore. While that can be true for some women, it's not always true.

While one-third of unintended pregnancies occur in teens, two-thirds of them happen in women over 20 years of age. In other words, unintended pregnancy is not just a teen problem. Yet "older women believe it happens only to teens," says Anita L. Nelson, M.D., associate professor of obstetrics and gynecology at the University of California, Los Angeles, UCLA School of Medicine and director of the women's medical clinic at Harbor-UCLA Medical Center in Torrance.

Thirty- and forty-something women can accidentally get pregnant when their birth control methods fail, when they choose less effective methods with high failure rates and when they forget and don't use anything, says Dr. Blumenthal.

Some forms of contraception are more popular than others—though that doesn't mean that one way is better than another. For women past age 35, sterilization is the most common method of contraception. Among the runners-up: Oral contraceptives, otherwise known as the Pill, rank second. After those top two choices come a host of other methods—the condom, diaphragm, IUD and other hormonal forms such as Norplant and Depo-Provera.

Which method should you use at this point in your life? Here's what doctors recommend.

Start with the kid question. For women over 30, the first question to ask is, "Do I want to preserve my future fertility?" says Margaret Dooley, nurse practitioner at Thomas Jefferson University in Philadelphia, Pennsylvania.

The answer to that question will help you decide between reversible and irreversible methods and between long-term and short-term methods.

If you think that you might want to get pregnant within the next year, for instance, you'll want to go with the methods that can be easily reversed—such as the diaphragm, condoms or the Pill.

If you want to wait between two and five years, you might want to consider Depo-Provera, the birth control shot, says Dr. Blumenthal. And if you decide that you don't want children for five years or more, then the Norplant implant device and IUD are additional options. (For information on Depo-Provera and Norplant, see "Implanting Some Protection" on page 23.)

Talk it over. "The most important thing—for any method—is to talk it over with your partner," says Dr. Blumenthal. Try to arrive at a mutually agreeable decision, he says.

Ask questions. Don't be afraid to ask your doctor for her opinion on what methods might be good for you to consider. If you don't ask questions, your doctor might assume that you are satisfied with your current method and might not offer suggestions.

Myth #2: Only One Method Is Sure

Sterilization is a very popular means of birth control in the United States among women in the 30- to 45-year-old age group, says Dr. Blumenthal. An estimated 14 million women rely on sterilization as their

Sterilization: Should She or Should He?

Suppose you and your husband decide you don't want any more children, and sterilization is your answer to birth control. The next question, then, is who should get sterilized?

Some studies have shown that male sterilization—called vasectomy—is safer and more effective than female sterilization, says Paul Blumenthal, M.D., assistant professor of obstetrics and gynecology at Johns Hopkins University Medical Center in Baltimore.

For one thing, the procedure for female sterilization is often performed under general anesthesia, even though only local anesthesia is usually needed, says Dr. Blumenthal. A vasectomy is performed under local anesthesia. In addition, a vasectomy is cheaper, requires less time to do and generally requires a shorter recovery time.

But despite the advantages of a vasectomy, more women get sterilized than men. Dr. Blumenthal offers several possible reasons. Women often bear the responsibility for birth control, and they visit doctors more than men do—so they may be more likely to have the procedure recommended to them. Also, the majority of tubal sterilizations take place after a woman has given birth to what she has decided will be her last child. While she's in the hospital anyway—generally within two days of the birth—it's a convenient time to have her tubes tied.

means of contraception—but of course it's not just women who request the procedure. About 9.6 million women have been sterilized, which means having the fallopian tubes closed off so sperm can't reach the egg. Another 4.1 million women are relying on their partners' vasectomy—the sterilization procedure for males—to ensure that they don't have children.

For a woman, sterilization requires a surgical procedure under either local or general anesthesia. The fallopian tubes are sealed with either clips or rings, or they're cauterized with a quick application of electrical current in the form of heat. Once you've had the procedure, your chances of getting pregnant during the first year are less than 3 in 1,000. That's lower than the failure rate of most temporary methods.

But . . . should you have it done?

While the procedure is superb for women who have decided that they definitely don't want to have any more children, says Dr. Kaunitz, the idea that it is the *only* effective long-term method is a myth. The IUD, Depo-Provera and Norplant can provide long-term protection and can be just as effective as sterilization, and yet they're reversible, he says.

The only good reason to decide on sterilization, says Dr. Kaunitz, is if you decide that you *never ever* want to be pregnant—or you have children and you know you don't want to get pregnant again. "If any reason prevails other than not wanting more children, the chance that a woman may regret the choice later is very real."

"We do know that the younger a woman is when she chooses sterilization, the higher the rate of regret," adds Alan Rosenfield, M.D., dean of the School of Public Health at Columbia University in New York City. "I tell women to consider this a permanent procedure. There is the misconception that sterilization reversal is easy to do; it's not."

Myth #3: The Pill Isn't Safe

After sterilization, the Pill is the contraception method women choose most. The Pill prevents pregnancy by interfering with ovulation, among other things. It also thickens the cervical mucus—the layer of slippery cells lining the cervix that makes a slick passageway for sperm. Thicker mucus means that sperm have a tougher time swimming their way toward the uterus.

Even though the Pill remains popular, doctors say that misperceptions and myths abound. One prevailing myth, says Dr. Kaunitz, is the assumption that it is too risky to take the Pill after ages 30 or 35. Yet both the Food and Drug Administration and the American College of Obstetricians and Gynecologists have found the Pill to be safe for nonsmoking, healthy women of any age, he says. *Nonsmoking* and *healthy* are the operative words when it comes to the Pill and women over 35.

The concern over the safety of the Pill hails primarily from the days when oral contraceptives contained higher doses of estrogen. Researchers sounded the alarm when they suspected that women taking higher estrogen levels were at higher risk for heart attacks and strokes. Over the 30 years since the Pill was introduced, however, the dosage of estrogen in the Pill has been reduced to one-fourth what it originally was, says Dr. Blumenthal.

The lower dosage of estrogen has not reduced the Pill's effectiveness, yet it's safer, Dr. Blumenthal says. In women who don't smoke, Pill takers have no significant increase in cardiovascular complications over non-Pill takers, agrees Dr. Rosenfield.

In addition to being safe, the Pill has a number of noncontraceptive benefits—but women aren't always aware of them. "Clearly,

one of the biggest fears women have regarding taking hormones is the fear of cancer, particularly breast cancer," says Dr. Kaunitz. "Many women are not aware that by taking oral contraceptives they can substantially reduce the risk of ovarian cancer."

While ovarian cancer is rare, it's the leading cause of gynecological cancer death. A woman who takes the Pill for only a year or so can decrease her risk for the deadly cancer by as much as 50 percent, he says.

If a woman takes the Pill longer than a year, she cuts the risk of ovarian cancer even more. A woman who takes it for a decade or longer can reduce her risk as much as 80 percent, says Dr. Kaunitz. This protective effect persists for years after she stops taking the Pill.

Not only that, the Pill will also slash your risk of getting endometrial cancer—cancer of the lining of the uterus, says Dr. Kaunitz.

But what about the risk of breast cancer? On this topic the message is somewhat less clear, according to Dr. Kaunitz. Studies are contradictory. Some show that the Pill increases breast cancer risk; others indicate a decreased risk. Overall, though, when you look at all the studies on oral contraceptives and breast cancer combined, researchers conclude that the Pill does not increase breast cancer risk.

In addition, the Pill offers protection against ectopic pregnancy, a sometimes life-threatening form of pregnancy in which the fertilized egg implants outside the uterus—usually in the fallopian tubes. The Pill can also help make menstrual periods more regular and relieve menstrual cramping. Dr. Kaunitz says that if you use the Pill regularly, you might lower your chances of eventually needing a hysterectomy—surgical removal of the uterus. You'll be less likely to have the heavy,

Implanting Some Protection

In 1990 the Pill was no longer the only form of hormonal birth control available in the United States. That year, hormonal implants known as Norplant were introduced, and 1992 saw the approval of the birth control shot known as Depo-Provera. Both are currently available to women in this country.

Norplant consists of six matchstick-size capsules that are inserted under the skin on the inside of your upper arm. The capsules contain progestin, a synthetic form of the hormone progesterone, which prevents pregnancy by inhibiting ovulation, thickening the cervical mucus and thinning out the lining of the uterus. This one-two-three combination interferes with egg production, makes it harder for sperm to reach the uterus and—by thinning the uterine lining—makes a less friendly nest for the fertilized egg.

Norplant is a long-term method of birth control that provides protection for five years. And failures are rare. Fewer than 1 out of every 100 women experiences an accidental pregnancy during the first year of use.

But what about getting the Norplant removed? There's been controversy about this surgical procedure, with some women reporting complications. The key, according to experts, is to see a doctor who is trained to do a Norplant removal.

The advantages of Norplant are that it is a long-acting contraceptive, and it's convenient. Once it's in, you don't have to remind yourself to take a pill every day. Furthermore, once the Norplant is removed, protection against pregnancy is gone immediately.

Disadvantages? Some women have experienced disruptions to their menstrual cycles, from lighter bleeding or missed periods to increased days of heavier bleeding after having their Norplant capsules inserted. In fact, this is often the reason for discontinuing Norplant use.

Like Norplant, Depo-Provera, a birth control shot, only contains progesterone—no estrogen—and has effects on your reproductive system similar to those of Norplant. If you opt for Depo-Provera, you'll have to see your doctor for a shot every three months.

During the first year, you might see some spotting, and after that you may stop having periods. A significant advantage of the shot, doctors say, is that it is a totally private method of birth control. If you're getting the quarterly shots, your doctor is the only other person who needs to know about it.

But Depo-Provera is not a good choice for women who are ready to become pregnant right away, cautions Andrew Kaunitz, M.D., professor in the Department of Obstetrics and Gynecology at the University of Florida Health Science Center in Jacksonville. It can take women six months or more to get pregnant after they stop receiving the shot, he says, and it takes some women a year or more.

painful periods that lead some women to opt for the procedure.

Women often believe they need to take a break from the Pill. Some doctors have advised women who have been on the Pill for a number of years that they need to stop taking it and let their bodies "rest" for a while. But it's not necessary, Dr. Rosenfield advises. "If

They Call It Emergency Contraception

Forget something?

If the cold light of day finds you worrying about what happened last night—and the possible consequences—you may still have an option.

"I think one thing women in this country should be aware of is emergency contraception," says Paul Blumenthal, M.D., assistant professor of obstetrics and gynecology at Johns Hopkins University Medical Center in Baltimore. This is a form of contraception that women can access within three days after they've had unprotected intercourse.

If taken within 72 hours of unprotected intercourse, low-dose birth control pills are 97 percent effective in preventing pregnancy, says Dr. Blumenthal. If your doctor recommends this route, you'll get a prescription for eight pills: four to take immediately, with another four 12 hours later.

If conception hasn't occurred yet, the pills will interfere with the movement of sperm toward the egg by thickening the cervical mucus and changing the rate at which the sperm move through the fallopian tube, if they make it that far. Even if a sperm has fertilized an egg, pregnancy might be blocked, because the pills change the lining of the uterus so that the fertilized egg cannot implant.

While birth control pills are not approved by the Food and Drug Administration as emergency contraceptives, doctors are free to prescribe them for this kind of use.

Women who have unprotected sex can also use the intrauterine device, or IUD, as an emergency form of birth control, says Dr. Blumenthal. The device should be inserted within three to five days of unprotected sex, he says. Once in, it prevents a fertilized egg from implanting in the wall of the uterus.

you want to be protected, there's no reason to stop taking the Pill." In fact, when women do come off to "rest," that's often when they get pregnant.

If you're considering the Pill, you should discuss it with your doctor. Here are some considerations.

Look at your medical history. The Pill is appropriate for healthy, nonsmoking women, says Dr. Kaunitz. It might be a less desirable option if you have a history of blood clots, high blood pressure, diabetes or other medical conditions. Also, your doctor might advise against the Pill if you're a regular smoker over age 35.

Look at the calendar. The effects of the Pill can be reversed fairly quickly, says Dr. Kaunitz. While it may take you a little longer to get pregnant when you stop taking the Pill than it would have if you hadn't taken it, the delay appears to be two to three months at most. Nearly 1 out of 50 women, however, will not menstruate for six months or more after coming off the Pill.

Look at your habits. "Sexually active women who miss more than two or three pills in a row will increase their risk of pregnancy," says Dr. Kaunitz. Ask yourself, in all honesty, whether you are a good pill taker. If you aren't, then you may want to consider another method.

Myth #4: The IUD Is Out of the Question

According to doctors, the IUD currently suffers from an identity problem in the United States. "American women need to re-think the IUD," says Dr. Kaunitz.

The IUD is a little plastic device that is inserted by your doctor and sits inside your uterus. A string connected to the IUD hangs down through the cervix and serves as a telltale for detecting if the device is in place properly.

In the 1970s and 1980s the IUD became synonymous with risk and danger. Most of the unfavorable publicity was the result of lawsuits over the Dalkon Shield, an IUD whose use was associated with an increased risk of pelvic infection. "That publicity really killed the IUD in this country," says Dr. Kaunitz.

Studies have shown that the IUD is a safe and effective method of birth control for women who are at low risk for sexually transmitted diseases (STDs), says Dr. Kaunitz. If you have one partner, and you know that your partner is monogamous and disease-free, the IUD can be a very practical form of birth control, offering protection for as long as ten years. So it is a good alternative to sterilization if you're finished with childbearing but have yet to reach menopause.

If you're comparing the IUD with the Pill, the IUD might be preferable if you can't use hormonal methods of birth control—if you're a smoker, for instance, or if you're breastfeeding, says Dr. Blumenthal. But some doctors won't recommend the device unless you've had a child.

There are two types of IUDs currently available. The first is the copper-T 380A, also known as ParaGard in the United States. "While we used to think that this device prevented pregnancy by preventing a fertilized egg from implanting in the uterus, we now have learned more about how it works," says Dr. Blumenthal. Research indicates that the device actually interferes with conception. That is, it appears to interfere with the ability of sperm to navigate up through the uterus and into the fallopian tubes.

The second type of IUD is called the Progestasert, an IUD that is medicated with prog-esterone. Progestasert works by changing the cervical mucus so that sperm have a harder time swimming north, so that if conception occurs, a fertilized egg is less likely to implant in the uterine lining.

Myth #5: Barrier Methods Are Old-Fashioned

If you've dismissed condoms, the cervical cap and the diaphragm as too clumsy, out-of-date and unreliable, maybe you should reconsider. Condoms, for instance, are the most commonly used barrier method. Not only are they effective birth control devices, they're also insurance against sexually transmitted diseases, including HIV/AIDS. So if you're not in a monogamous relationship, or you're sleeping with someone who you're not absolutely positive is disease-free, it makes sense to use condoms.

In fact, Dr. Kaunitz says that women who are not in monogamous relationships should use condoms even if they're already using an effective birth control method such as the Pill or sterilization. "Some physicians call this the 'belt and suspenders' approach," adds Dr. Kaunitz. Other barrier methods such as the diaphragm and cervical cap also help prevent some kinds of STDs, especially when they're used in conjunction with spermicidal jellies and foam.

See also Reproductive System, Sexually Transmitted Diseases

Birthmarks

Bladder

A CUTE BROWN BIRTHMARK shaped like the state of Iowa near your belly button is one thing. But having a noticeable birthmark on your face can affect your confidence and self-esteem, says Barry Resnik, M.D., clinical instructor of dermatology at the University of Miami School of Medicine.

Actually, the most common birthmarks are moles or freckles, which are simply malformed pigmentation cells. Since nearly everyone has these, they're rarely a big deal.

More noticeable is the purple-red port-wine stain, which affects about 3 out of every 1,000 children born. It's composed of networks of blood vessels in the skin that lie just under the epidermis, the outermost layer of skin cells. Unfortunately, these birthmarks don't fade, but darken with age.

No one knows what causes these visible patterns. But thanks to laser technology, there's now a ray of hope, says Dr. Resnik.

Lasers emit a pinpoint of light that's absorbed selectively by specific target cells. Since a port-wine stain is composed of red blood cells in vessels, that's where the light is targeted. Port-wine stains can be erased—either in one session or in a number of treatments—and usually without scarring.

Another common birthmark is the strawberry mark, which looks like a flattened version of an actual strawberry. About 90 percent of these bright red, protruding areas disappear by the time a child is nine years old.

WE'VE ALL BEEN THERE: legs clamped together tightly at the knees, trying to think of dry desert sand and arid valleys—anything to keep our minds off waterfalls and streams.

Mind over urgent matters, you might call it. But as hard as you try to ignore the biological need to urinate, you just can't. And that's a good thing. After all, it's how the body disposes of liquid waste products such as urea, uric acid and creatinine, which are waste products of metabolism.

The main storehouse in the urination process is the bladder, a balloonlike structure made of a thin layer of muscle, located at the back of your pelvic cavity. Before you get the urge to void, this balloon conducts an efficient collection process. Every day, about two to three pints of urine pass from the kidneys, which filter the blood and remove waste products, to the bladder. The bladder is essentially a collection sac that holds the urine until you're ready to let go. When you do, a ring-shaped sphincter muscle relaxes, the bladder muscle contracts and the urine is forced out through the urethra, the tube leading from the bladder to the outside world.

Unfortunately, Ma Nature wasn't logical when she placed some of the equipment. Because your urethra is only 1½ inches long and located near your vagina and anus—where unfriendly bacteria run rampant—it's easy for this normally germ-free area to become infected. Each year, in fact, 10 percent of all women will develop urinary tract infections (UTIs). About 20 percent of women will get a UTI at least once in their lives. And if you have one once, there's about an 80 percent chance that you'll get one again within the next two years.

A Better Bladder

While bladder infections, or cystitis, are the most common kind of UTIs, you can also get kidney infections and urethritis—an inflammation in the urethra, the tube leading out of the bladder. With a bladder infection you'll probably feel like your bladder is full even when it isn't. Other symptoms: you might get a burning sensation when you urinate, feel some pain above your pubic bone or, sometimes, see blood in your urine.

"Lots of women are frustrated by these recurrent infections," says David Uehling, M.D., professor of urology at the University of Wisconsin Medical School in Madison. "It makes them miserable."

If you go to your doctor at the first sign of symptoms, she'll test your urine for bacteria and will prescribe a short-term course of antibiotics. But before your bladder has a chance to get fouled up, here are some ways to prevent UTIs.

Catch a cranberry. For years, doctors have recommended sipping cranberry juice to ward off UTIs, observes Mark Monane, M.D., instructor of medicine at Harvard Medical School who specializes in internal medicine, geriatrics and clinical pharmacology. Evidence shows that the remedy can work. "There seems to be something in cranberry juice that stops the bacteria from sticking to the urethra and bladder." In several studies on bacterial growth in the bladder, Dr. Monane has had successful results using Ocean Spray Cranberry Juice Cocktail. Although they are not pure cranberry juice, the cranberry drinks do the job of keeping your bladder clean.

Opportunities for Infections

Although many women will get urinary tract infections (UTIs) sometime in their lives, there are a few groups of women who have special reason to worry about repeat performances. They are:

Postmenopausal women. These women lose estrogen, which helps give the bladder's inner coating a protective layer. When the layer isn't as smooth as it should be, there are more places for bacteria to hide.

Pregnant women. During the later months of pregnancy, the baby is pushing down on your bladder and urethra, which means that leftover urine collects in the bladder. Bacteria grow easily in stagnant urine, setting the stage for a UTI.

Women who have diabetes. Diabetes compromises the immune system, which opens the door to more UTIs. Also, people with diabetes have more sugar in their urine, which gives bacteria a more hospitable place to grow.

After sex, head for the toilet. Since intercourse can drive bacteria from the area around the rectum and vagina into the urethra, urinating afterwards gives you a chance to flush it away, says Alice Stollenwerk Petrulis, M.D., director of clinical nephrology at Metrohealth Medical Center and associate professor of medicine and reproductive biology at Case Western Reserve University, both in Cleveland. It's also a good idea to drink a glass of water before sex, so you'll have the urge to urinate afterward.

Create a flood. Drinking plenty of noncaffeinated liquids—at least six to eight 8-ounce glasses a day—helps keep UTI-causing bacteria away, says Dr. Uehling.

Make sure you're on empty. Don't cut

yourself short while urinating, because the leftover liquid in your bladder can host bacteria, says Irving Fishman, M.D., associate professor of urology at Baylor College of Medicine in Houston. "Some people are very busy and don't take the time to relax and let go."

See what C can do for you. Taking vitamin C can also ward off some UTIs, says Mark Zilkoski, M.D., family practice physician at Trinity Hospital and Listerud Rural Health Clinic in Wolf Point, Montana. Vitamin C lowers the pH, or acidity level, in your urine, says Dr. Zilkoski. This lower pH level creates an environment in which various UTI-causing bacteria cannot survive.

Make a clean swipe. Because UTI-causing bacteria come from the rectum, be diligent about washing that area, says Dr. Fishman. Doctors recommend that you wipe from front to back to avoid dragging bacteria from the rectum to the urethra.

Burning? Maybe It's IC

Another disorder that leaves you burning with discomfort is interstitial cystitis (IC), a painful condition that mimics the symptoms of a bladder infection. This chronic and frustrating disease affects about 450,000 people in the United States every year, 90 percent of whom are women. It is managed with a prescription medicine.

But it helps to follow a low-acid diet as well, says Philip Hanno, M.D., professor and chairman of the Department of Urology at Temple University School of Medicine in Philadelphia. Some of the things to eliminate include caffeine, spicy foods, alcohol and tomato sauce. Long, warm baths can also alleviate some pain by relaxing the muscles, he notes.

See also Urinary System

Blood

IN HOLLYWOOD THEY CALL THE STUFF that splatters on movie and TV screens "reel" blood. Made from corn syrup, red dye and paste, it comes in a variety of shades including fresh, aged and old and dried. A typical horror film may use more than 30 gallons.

Movie blood may be a nifty special effect, but real blood—the sticky serum that life depends on—is far more awesome.

Consider these facts: Of the 50 trillion cells in your body, nearly half are blood. Every second, 2 million red blood corpuscles are destroyed, and 2 million more enter the bloodstream and join a massive transportation system that is responsible for nurturing every cell in your body.

Yet these corpuscles are so tiny that they can squeeze through capillaries thinner than a strand of hair, and they're packed so tightly together that an average woman could drain all four quarts of her blood into a stockpot.

"Blood truly is amazing. It really is the essence of life," says Mercedes Brenneisen, M.D., hematologist at Good Samaritan Hospital in Los Angeles.

How It Works

With each heartbeat, blood rushes life-sustaining oxygen to your cells and sweeps toxic carbon dioxide back to your lungs. At the same time, it helps warm your body and distributes hormones and chemicals that regulate every bodily function, from heart rate to childbirth. In addition, white blood cells and other disease fighters that constitute the im-

What Your Blood Type Really Means

In 1667 doctors attempted to transfuse sheep's blood into a young boy. The procedure failed, but fortunately, the patient lived.

Since that first miserable stab at transfusion, doctors have learned there are several types of blood, and if blood types aren't compatible, a person receiving a transfusion could have an immune reaction and die.

Blood is classified by the type of proteins that coat the cell. You have either type A, B, AB (meaning you have both A and B proteins) or O (meaning you have neither A nor B). People develop antibodies to the proteins that their blood cells don't have. The table below shows who can receive transfusions of what types of red blood cells.

About 46 percent of people have type O, 42 percent have type A, 8 percent have type B and 4 percent have type AB.

Another blood grouping system, the Rhesus (Rh) factor, divides people into Rh positive and Rh negative. About 85 percent of us are Rh positive. Transfusion of Rh positive blood into an Rh negative woman can cause a serious reaction if she has developed antibodies to Rh positive from previous transfusions.

In addition to that, an Rh negative mother can conceive an Rh positive fetus if the father is Rh positive. If that happens, she needs treatment with a blood product called Rh immunoglobulin to prevent the production of antibodies that would destroy the red cells of an Rh positive fetus.

If You Have . . .	You Can Receive . . .			
	A	B	AB	O
A	X			X
B		X		X
AB	X	X	X	X
O				X

mune system diligently circulate in your bloodstream, ready to pounce on any invading organism that might harm you.

Every hour, your body produces up to 10 billion new blood cells in your bone marrow and destroys an equal number of old ones in your spleen and liver. Early in life, your liver, spleen and almost any bone can produce red blood cells, but after you reach age two or three only the breastbone, ribs, skull, thighbones, pelvis and spine continue to create red blood cells and platelets. White blood cells are also manufactured by bone marrow, but some types are produced in the lymph nodes as well.

Keeping It Healthy

Blood is fairly resilient and requires little care or maintenance to do its job. Eating a balanced diet that includes at least five servings of fruits and vegetables a day is the best way to ensure that your blood stays healthy, Dr. Brenneisen says. Here are some important things you can do.

What Can Go Wrong

If you get sick, your blood probably isn't the culprit.

"What's amazing is how well blood works and how uncommon diseases of the blood really are," says John Harlan, M.D., hematologist at the University of Washington School of Medicine in Seattle.

Here are diseases you should be aware of.

Anemia, a lack of red blood cells, is one of the most common blood diseases, mostly because of its everyday form, iron-deficiency anemia. It affects 3 out of every 100 premenopausal women and 2 out of every 100 postmenopausal women.

When you have anemia, your blood has trouble getting enough oxygen to your vital organs and removing carbon dioxide from your body. Symptoms include pale skin, fatigue, weakness, fainting and heart palpitations. Iron-deficiency anemia is caused by lack of iron, but other anemias can be caused by deficiencies of vitamin B_{12} or folate.

Leukemia is a cancer of blood-forming tissues—bone marrow, lymph nodes and spleen—that causes abnormal white blood cells to reproduce at an accelerated rate. These abnormal cells prevent the production of healthy red and white blood cells and platelets.

As the disease progresses, it causes anemia, interferes with blood clotting and impairs the body's ability to fight off infections. Untreated, it can cause death. Leukemia afflicts about 1 in every 1,300 American women. Symptoms include

---

Stoke up on iron. Without iron your body stops making red blood cells, and the red cells you do have have difficulty absorbing oxygen as they pass through your lungs. As a result, you can develop anemia, Dr. Brenneisen says.

Women are at greater risk for iron-deficiency anemia than men, because we lose iron-rich blood whenever we have menstrual bleeding. When our periods are normal and not heavy, we lose an extra one milligram of iron a day. Before menopause about 3 percent of us are likely to develop iron-deficiency anemia, the most common form of the disease in women. After menopause the incidence of iron-deficiency anemia falls to about 2 percent.

Because of increased risk of iron deficiency, it's important to try to get enough iron through your diet. Most women need about 18 milligrams of iron daily. Pregnant women need up to 30 milligrams a day. Good food sources of iron include lean meats, poultry (dark meat is best), clams, oysters, dried apricots and dark green leafy vegetables such as spinach and broccoli.

If you're worried about getting enough iron from your diet, talk to your doctor about taking an iron supplement. But doctors warn that you need to be careful about supplementation, because too much iron could prevent your body from absorbing other nutrients, such as zinc and copper. Excessive iron can also cause liver damage in some people.

Recharge with B_{12}. Low levels of vitamin B_{12} disrupt reproduction of red blood cells and increase your risk of heart disease. B_{12} is found almost exclusively in animal products—fish, beef, poultry and dairy foods such as cheese and yogurt. Because the vitamin is

chronic fatigue, bone pain, weight loss, easy bruising and bleeding and fever.

Polycythemia, too many red blood cells, is usually a sign of an underlying ailment, such as lung or heart disease, that disrupts the flow of oxygen in your body. In response the bone marrow produces more red blood cells than are needed. Because polycythemia thickens the blood, clots are more common, and that increases the risk of heart attack and stroke.

Malaria, caused by a parasite transmitted by mosquito bites, is a common blood disease in tropical regions. Parasites attack red blood cells, causing them to rupture. To prevent it, ask your doctor to prescribe an antimalarial drug before you travel to areas where the disease is prevalent.

Hemophilia, a genetic bleeding disorder that prevents blood from clotting, is passed from mothers to sons. Women merely carry the recessive gene for hemophilia; they do not develop the disease, which affects 1 in 10,000 men in the United States. England's Queen Victoria was a famous carrier of the disorder, and several of her royal descendants, including Alexis, the last crown prince of Russia, developed the affliction.

Sickle cell disease, an ailment that causes abnormal hemoglobin in 1 in every 1,000 African-Americans, is another rare but well-known inherited blood disease. In this disease sickle-shaped cells disrupt blood and oxygen flow to vital tissues.

easily stored in your body, Dr. Brenneisen says, B_{12} deficiencies are rare as long as you're eating some of these foods. If you're a vegetarian, you should discuss with your doctor whether to take a supplement.

Think folate. Folate is another B vitamin that is crucial for the development of healthy red blood cells, Dr. Brenneisen says. Since we don't store folate, we need a daily dose of 400 micrograms. Lentils, wheat germ, oranges and green vegetables such as asparagus are good sources of folate.

A deficiency can cause fatigue, weakness, cramps, depression and other symptoms of anemia. Folate deficiency has also been linked to birth defects, so women of child-bearing age need to be extra careful.

Get an E grade. Vitamin E, an antioxidant, may help protect membranes and keep aging blood cells vigorous, according to Stephen Shohet, M.D., professor of laboratory medicine at the University of California, San Francisco, School of Medicine. Vitamin E is most abundant in oils, nuts and seeds. Unfortunately, these foods are also high in fat. But taking a multiple vitamin daily will usually supply you with the Daily Value of 30 international units—that is, enough vitamin E to maintain your health.

Don't forget the C. Vitamin C, another antioxidant, also might help keep your blood cells healthy, says Joanne Curran-Celentano, R.D., Ph.D., associate professor of nutrition at the University of New Hampshire in Durham and nutrition research coordinator at the Center for Eating Disorders Management in Dover. It's abundant in the diet as long as you eat plenty of fruits and vegetables

A Blood Test Primer

Like any great detective, your doctor is always looking for clues. Your blood is often a good starting point.

Although normal results vary depending on a person's age, sex and the method the laboratory uses to conduct its tests, a typical blood screening can reveal a lot about you. Here's a look at the most common blood tests.

Bilirubin. High levels of this pigment released when old blood cells are destroyed may be an indication of liver disease or anemia. Jaundice, a yellowing of the skin and eyes, also is caused by excessive amounts of bilirubin in the blood.

Blood glucose (blood sugar). High levels could be a warning sign of diabetes.

Carbon dioxide. High levels suggest lung problems such as emphysema or pneumonia.

Chloride. Low levels of this important chemical that helps keep body fluids in balance may point toward infections, intestinal obstruction or severe diabetes.

Complete blood count (CBC). The most basic test, it determines the number and appearance of red cells, white cells and other components present in the blood. A CBC will also tell your doctor how much oxygen your blood cells can carry and how well they can fight disease.

Creatinine and blood urea nitrogen (BUN). Elevated blood levels of either of these two waste products normally excreted in urine may be an indication of a kidney ailment.

Potassium. High levels may be a sign of kidney failure.

Sodium. Excessive amounts in the blood could be a sign of dehydration or congestive heart failure.

---

every day, such as oranges, strawberries, brussels sprouts and red bell peppers. Although 60 milligrams is the Daily Value, she recommends that you get 100 to 500 milligrams daily for healthy blood.

Take an aspirin. Aspirin can reduce the stickiness of blood platelets and reduce your risk of stroke and heart attack. Take one coated 325-milligram aspirin tablet every other day, suggests Dr. Brenneisen. But be sure to check with your doctor before taking aspirin regularly.

Ax the smokes. Smoking increases carbon monoxide levels in your bloodstream and destroys hemoglobin, a protein that helps transport oxygen in blood. Smoking also stimulates the production of extra red blood cells, which can thicken the blood and make you more vulnerable to strokes and heart attacks triggered by clots, says Arthur R. Thompson, M.D., Ph.D., hematologist and professor of medicine at the University of Washington in Seattle.

Limit liquor. Overindulging in alcohol can interfere with absorption of folate. Consume no more than one or two drinks a day, Dr. Brenneisen says.

See also Circulatory System, Lymphatic System

Body Hair

ANY WICKED WITCH WORTH A WHIT has a kettle brewing with eye of newt and toe of frog—and a nose with a hairy nevus. That's the medical term for a mole with hair growing out of it.

But hairy nevi aren't confined to wicked witches. Any woman can sprout mole hair—or hair in other unexpected places, including her upper lip, chin or chest.

Actually, body hair is all over us. But the fine body hairs that cover us from head to toe, called vellus hairs, are barely visible. It's the coarse terminal hairs—which are thicker and darker in color—that make us hair haters. This is the hair that shows up on a toe or a nipple or peeks out the edge of a bathing suit. In fact, the only body hair that most women like is their eyelashes.

Eyelashes at least have a job to do—shield our eyes from the dirt. Nose hair also has a function—to block particles like dust. It's the other kind of body hair that only serves to annoy.

And annoy it does. "It drives women off the old rock and roller," says Victor Newcomer, M.D., professor of dermatology at the University of California, Los Angeles, UCLA School of Medicine.

A Little Shaver

Probably the most annoying, because it's most visible, is facial hair. "It's the mustache area that bothers women the most," says Seth L. Matarasso, M.D., assistant professor of dermatology at the University of California,

San Francisco, School of Medicine.

While you can't cover up a mustache the way you can hide underarm or leg hair, there's nothing to stop you from shaving it off. "Shaving isn't as irritating as waxing," according to Dr. Newcomer. And once you've shaved, the hair doesn't grow back very fast. "You may only need to shave it once every week or two."

Some women, however, find shaving their mustaches a little too masculine for words, says Dr. Newcomer. Or they've bought the myth that shaving makes hair grow in thicker—which it doesn't. "But you will feel rough stubble when it grows in." That's because shaving removes hair at the surface of the skin, where it's thickest. Hair removed by other methods, such as plucking or waxing, comes from deep in the follicle, the cradle of new hair. When new hair grows in, it has a fine, tapered end, compared with the blunt-tipped hair that grows in after shaving.

To shave a mustache, blot it with warm water until it's moist. Then apply a gentle shaving cream. Let the shaving cream soak into your skin for two or three minutes so the hair gets swollen. While that's happening, soak your razor in warm water.

Use a lightweight razor made for women—and be sure to replace it after three to six shaves, before the blade dulls. Shave in the direction the hair grows. Then rinse and blot dry.

Dr. Newcomer recommends following up with a moisturizer.

A Smooth Upper Lip

For mustache removal, waxing is often the method of choice. Big beauty salons often have a waxing section where technicians work on facial and leg hair, underarms and the bikini line. When you go in, the technician

Waxing Elegant

If you don't mind pulling a sticky bandage off your own skin, and if you have too much unwanted body hair but too little time to run out to waxing salons, then you may be the perfect candidate for a home waxing kit.

You can use a home kit to wax your bikini line, legs, underarms or facial hair. But a word of warning: Read the directions on the label and don't use the wax in non-appropriate areas—including the inside of your nose or ears, nipples, eyelashes or on irritated skin, warts, moles and sunburned skin. Also, you should not wax over recent scar tissue or too near the genital area.

The kits run from about $6 for a simple pot of wax that you heat in hot water to a $30 box that contains an electric warmer for heating the beeswax, two disposable roll-on wax-filled applicators for the face or the body (replacement applicators are available) and wax remover strips.

Also, read the label to find out how much time it takes. One kit, for instance, specifies that you do a patch test, then wait 24 hours to check for allergic reactions. If all is well, you can go ahead—but you have to heat the applicator for 30 to 45 minutes in the warmer. If you're waxing your chin or upper lip, you can't use soap or makeup in that area for the next 12 hours.

The actual waxing and hair removal don't take long at all, however. You simply roll the wax-filled applicator along your skin in the direction the hair grows. Then you apply the wax remover strip, rub it four or five times and pull it off your skin.

All you need is the fortitude to rip the strip from your flesh in one swift motion. "The first time I did it, it brought tears to my eyes," says Nancy Miller, an insurance agent from Phoenix who's been waxing at home for eight years. "But your skin gets tougher after four or five times. You get used to it."

For your long-term preparations and short-term pain, you're rewarded with up to six weeks of hair-free skin.

applies hot wax to an area of skin with a wooden spatula. After the wax hardens, the technician yanks it off.

Waxing keeps the mustache area hair-free for about six weeks. The new hair that grows in is usually soft and silky. Some women find waxing painful, though. And it can irritate the tender skin above the lip.

"You can cut down on the irritation if you use a mild topical steroid cream such as West-Cort and a topical antibiotic such as T-Stat before and after you wax," says Anita Cela, M.D., clinical assistant professor of dermatology at Cornell University Medical College in New York City.

The medications should be applied immediately before and just after waxing, according to Dr. Cela. If the irritation continues, the topical steroid cream can be used twice a day for a few more days. Both the steroid cream and the antibiotic are available by prescription.

Lots of Pluck

If you have single little strands that crop up here and there on your face, they're easy to remove. Give these tricks a try.

Snip it. The easy method: Cut off the hair at its base with a pair of fine manicuring scissors, suggests Dr. Newcomer. Be sure that the sharp blades don't slice your skin, though. This technique is fine for any facial hair, and it also works with hair on your nipples or chest—places where plucking might be painful or irritating.

Opt for electrolysis. The only permanent way to remove unwanted body hair is with electrolysis in a salon or hair-removal office. The technician inserts a needle or probe about the width of a hair into each follicle, then turns on a mild current of electricity. That destroys the hair root about 75 percent of the time.

"It's a long and tedious process," says Dr. Matarasso. "You go for half-hour sessions every couple of weeks." Removing an area as large as the bikini line can take a year of treatments, so the method is best for small areas. And you may get problem reactions, such as acne or inflammation of the hair follicles. Electrolysis also carries some risk. There is a remote chance of infection by a transmissible disease such as hepatitis, and it's possible there could be some scarring.

"So you should go to an electrologist who has a lot of experience and does it all the time. It's wise to do a few small areas to see if you can tolerate it without scarring. I've seen women with scars above their lips from electrolysis," says Dr. Newcomer.

Electrolysis is costly and often painful. Fees range from $15 or $20 up to $100 and over, depending on how many visits you need.

The Hardest Hairs

It's not just teeny-weeny yellow polka-dot bikinis that can make our pubic hair public.

Bleach for the Beach

For legs to dye for, try a hair bleach kit available from your local pharmacy. Several highlights of hair bleach make it an appealing choice for some women—it's accessible, quick and, best of all, painless.

For most people, bleaching works well, according to Anita Cela, M.D., clinical assistant professor of dermatology at Cornell University Medical College in New York City. "However, it's best used by women with dark but very fine, not thick or coarse, hair. Especially in the upper lip area. If your hair is too thick, it will still be noticeable after you dye it."

There are hair bleach kits manufactured specifically for facial hair as well as for more general body areas. The cost of each kit varies, depending on how many ounces of cream it contains and whether it is regular or extra strength. Most range between $4.50 and $9.50. To obtain a kit, check the depilatory or shaving needs section of your local drugstore—the kits are most often stocked there, not in the hair dye aisle.

All hair bleach kits come with two essential components: the actual hair bleach mixture, which is most often in cream form, and the activator mixture, which is always in powder form. Follow the instructions to obtain the proper proportion of bleach to activator. Some words of caution, however: Never combine the two until you're ready to begin bleaching, always immediately discard any unused portions and never mix the two together in any kind of a metal bowl or container.

Whatever bleach you get, be sure to do a patch test, says Dr. Cela. Instructions for the patch test come with the kit. If no redness, irritation or eruption occurs, you can proceed with the full application.

Zap Time

If you're considering electrolysis and wondering what the experience is like, here's a firsthand report from <u>Prevention</u> magazine beauty editor Pam Boyer.

"I'd often toyed with the idea of electrolysis—specifically, for getting rid of my excess eyebrow hair for good. But the time and expense required, the incidence of regrowth and the risk of scarring all held me back. Most of all, I was afraid it would hurt.

"I overcame those concerns, though, and began my hunt for an electrologist. I knew that the treatment involved a series of visits, so I wanted somebody local. Surely a doctor could refer me to a qualified practitioner, I thought. But the referrals weren't really recommendations; they didn't come with praise, just 'no complaints.'

"The first electrologist I met hooked me up to an electrolysis machine and gave me damp, felt-covered handles to hold in both hands. They were attached to the machine, so my body was acting as the electrical ground.

"Surprisingly, the part I was most afraid of—the insertion of the needle into the hair follicle—wasn't even uncomfortable. The jolt that would kill the hair root (as long as the follicle was in its growing phase, not its resting phase) did hurt—but not unbearably. It felt like a mosquito bite at some times— at other times, like a hornet sting. Over the next few visits my discomfort increased; the jolts felt like a swarm of stinging hornets. On the third visit I had to ask that the treatment be cut short.

"Later, I found out why it may have hurt so much. Some operators inaccurately zap both follicles and bare skin. Others apply the needle longer to hair roots that didn't die the first time. Some simply get sloppier as treatments continue.

"So I searched for another electrologist and found one whose treatments were less painful. But after four treatments I had more hair regrowth than I'd been led to expect.

"I decided to look for one last electrologist before I gave in to discouragement. A Philadelphia dermatologist recommended an electrology group called Lucy Peters, International. First I visited Lucy Peters herself in her Manhattan office, where she told me about the equipment she helped develop. Instead of a needle, Peters said, they use an insulated bulbous probe that prevents the current from destroying anything but the hair. With this procedure, according to Peters, the skin is protected from damage or discomfort.

"Treatments with the probe caused only occasional, minor discomfort. The job was complete after seven treatments. And there was no regrowth. Insulated probes are available to electrologists nationwide. They are a piece of equipment I would insist upon," says Boyer.

Some white aerobic tights and most bathing suits reveal some telltale signs of pubic hair. And that makes most of us self-conscious and uncomfortable. But getting rid of pubic hair is a very uncomfortable proposition.

It's not the only challenging area of our bodies. If you're one of the majority of American women who shave under their arms, you know that those hairs are equally difficult. Here are the best ways to handle both spots.

Snip it in the bud. If summertime is approaching and you'll soon be wearing a bikini, shaving is the quickest, cheapest, least painful way to draw the line on pubic hairs. Before you get started on a shave of the area, try on your briefest bikini to see exactly where you need to shave. Then soak the area, apply shaving cream and shave it just as you would a mustache.

Pamper the pits. The hair under our arms is so hard to shave that we pull and stretch and scrape the skin raw in the shower to make a level shaving field. We crane our heads like, well, cranes, to get a view through the shower waterfall.

To prevent nicks and scratches, Dr. Matarasso suggests a milder attack with the razor. Even an imperfect shaving job looks and feels better than the damage you do when you're overzealous, he points out.

Another option is an electric shaver, he says. It doesn't shave as closely, but it's kinder to your skin. And you can use it in front of the bathroom mirror—to actually see what you're doing.

The Depilatory Story

Depilatories don't win any awards in the Grammies of hair removal, but some over-the-counter drugstore products are easy to use at home. These are chemical agents that remove hair—and while they do work, you have to be ultra careful. "I don't like them. They're messy, they can have an offensive odor and they can irritate the skin," says Dr. Cela. If you do decide to use a chemical depilatory, here's how to prevent problems.

Hold tryouts. Depilatories not only irritate sensitive skin—a light-haired blond's, for in-

stance—they can also cause allergic reactions: bumps, pimples and itching. So it's best to test a patch of skin first.

Apply a small amount to your inner arm below your elbow—a thin-skinned area that's not too noticeable. Cover that spot with a bandage. Leave the depilatory on the test area for the amount of time recommended in the instructions. If you're sensitive or allergic to the depilatory, the patch of skin will be red or broken out when you remove the bandage.

Count down carefully. You should time the application as closely as a knitter counting stitches. Set the timer when you apply the depilatory, and remove it as soon as the timer goes off.

"Depilatories have strong alkaline-reducing agents to soften the hair and break down the keratin that hair is made from. It's very easy to burn your skin if you leave it on too long," warns Dr. Newcomer. "Every time there is a big ad in the newspaper for Neet or Nair, doctors know we'll see a dozen people who have overused it and burned their skin."

Can a Doc Help?

Some women are more prone to dark-haired excess than others, and hormonal changes can change the body picture, too. Women with a Mediterranean background tend to have thicker body hair. And some women get more body hair when they hit menopause—including mustaches, chin hair, even cheek and chest hair. But sometimes body hair can be a sign of health problems that you might need to check out.

If excess body hair is caused by a medical problem, the reason is most often an excess of hormones, says Dr. Cela. The excess can be related to the ovaries, adrenal glands or thyroid. Problems in any of these areas can cause

us to notice changes in hair growth. Unwanted body hair may become "terminal"—
that is, get darker in color and grow thicker.
Conversely, scalp hair may thin, recede and
fall out.

When you have a problem with the hormones produced by your ovaries, adrenal
glands or thyroid, you're likely to see three
kinds of symptoms: acne, scalp hair thinning
and hirsutism—the medical term for excess
terminal hair on the body—according to
Marty Sawaya, M.D., Ph.D., assistant professor of dermatology at the University of
Florida Health Science Center in Gainesville.
If you develop all three, you should see your
doctor, who will probably refer you to an internist or a specialist for testing. A dermatologist, gynecologist or endocrinologist (a
specialist who studies hormone glands) can
give you a series of blood tests to pinpoint the
cause, he says.

Body Type

IT'S A TERRIBLE TEASE. Three simple words in
green and yellow glow at you from across the
mall. The Body Shop.

Oh, if only it were true—a place where you
could go and actually purchase a different
body. Or order up various parts. You know
exactly what you'd ask for. Longer legs. A
smaller derriere. And oh please, yes, don't
forget the slimmer waist.

But it's a dream, a mirage, a fantasy. While
you can get environmentally friendly bath
beads and potions to soothe your tired self,
you can't order a new body at The Body
Shop.

Maybe it's just as well. After all, is this
body that has served you so well all this time
really all that bad?

If you find yourself blurting out a resound-
ing "YES!" take a minute to reconsider. Before you resign yourself to that conclusion,
let's take a closer look at the type of body you
have. How is it shaped? What impact does
that shape have on your physical health?
Your emotional well-being? Most important,
how can you come to terms with it and learn
to accept it as the wonderful piece of human
architecture that it is?

Body Type-ography

Chances are you think of your body in
terms of short, tall, fat, thin, top-heavy or
bottom-heavy. A lot of us do.

But researchers and health experts have
another way of describing the various shapes
and sizes we come in. One system classifies

our bodies into three categories, called somatotypes.

Women who are long, lean and lanky, with a small, delicate bone structure, narrow hips and a small waist are called ectomorphs. Their legs tend to be longer than their torsos. This body type—most models have it—has become our society's current ideal.

Women who are more heavily boned, carry more fat than muscle and accumulate their fat mainly around their abdomens are called endomorphs. Their legs are generally shorter than their torsos, their breasts tend to be larger than average and they tend to gain weight rather easily. Endomorphs are sometimes referred to as apple-shaped.

In between the tall and skinny ectomorphs and the shorter, plumper endomorphs are bodies called mesomorphs. Mesomorphs tend to be athletic and have broad shoulders and hips, narrow waists and a high percentage of muscle in comparison to fat. These are the "pear-shaped" women.

Where the Fat Lies

Whether you're an endo, meso or ectomorph, you can change the amount of fat on your body by changing your exercise and eating habits. What you can't change are the areas where the fat is located.

Pear-shaped women, or mesomorphs, tend to carry whatever fat they have on their hips and thighs, rather than around their waists, or abdomen. Apple-shaped endomorphs, on the other hand, carry their extra fat around the middle.

Many women get upset because they're carrying fat at their hips and thighs, says Carol Kennedy, assistant director of fitness/wellness at Indiana University Bloomington. But in fact, that may be one of the

better areas to accumulate fat if you're going to accumulate it at all. Extra fat in those areas is less of a health threat than if it's located around your middle, or abdomen.

"People who carry fat around their waists are at highest risk for certain health problems," says Wendy Kohrt, Ph.D., associate professor in the Department of Internal Medicine at Washington University School of Medicine in St. Louis. Among those problems she includes heart disease, diabetes and high blood pressure.

Why does abdominal fat increase your health risks?

The majority of fat is stored just under the skin. In the abdominal area, however, fat can be located deeper, surrounding the internal organs, says Dr. Kohrt. The by-products produced by this fat during the metabolic process (turning nutrients into energy) often spill into a vein that leads to the liver.

"The liver is command central for many metabolic processes," says Dr. Kohrt. So if a lot of the by-products of fat metabolism flood it, theoretically, that can cause a lot of changes that lead to health problems.

But the somatotype system is only one way to look at your body and judge health risks. More often medical professionals are using waist-to-hip ratio measurements and body fat measurements as a means of assessing health.

Your Body, Your Esteem

In addition to affecting your physical health, your body type can often play a significant role in how you feel about yourself.

Research indicates that there are a lot of women who are dissatisfied with their bodies. In a survey of 1,000 women between the ages of 18 and 60, conducted by two researchers at

(continued on page 42)

In Good Shape: How to Dress Your Best

Karen Kaufman, president of Kaufman Professional Image Consultants in Philadelphia, has worked one-on-one with over 150 women a year and has addressed thousands of others over the past 16 years. In all that time, she has not found a woman who is completely happy with her body.

Kaufman pays attention to the shape, color and texture of clothing. She also looks at how clothes are proportioned. The best clothing makes a woman's body look balanced, she points out.

Here is Kaufman's advice.

Long-waisted women should use wider belts rather than narrow ones, because wide belts will help a long waist look more in proportion to the rest of the body. Also, they should wear a different color above the waist than the color below the waist to break up the length of a long torso.

Short-waisted women need to choose narrow belts and wear the same color on top as on bottom. Both strategies will help create the illusion of a longer waist.

Women with broad hips should wear straight trousers or skirts, preferably in solid colors. They should go with flat fabrics such as wool, gabardine or wool crepe, because they won't add bulk. Another option: a flowing pants-skirt or dress.

Women with narrow hips can go with pants and skirts that have gathers at the hip and waist, to bring their hips into proportion with their shoulders. Blouson jackets with elastic that ends at the hip can also add balance to the hip area. Hip belts are also a flattering option for this body type.

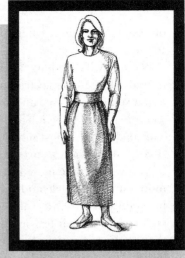

If you're long-waisted, try a wider belt with some outfits.

Large-busted women should be sure to have bras that fit them well—and should steer away from blouses that have pockets on the chest area. They should avoid blouses that have a lot of gathers, tucks or large patterns at the bust.

Small-busted women need well-fitting bras that add shape and shirts with pockets, gathers or tucks at the chest area that

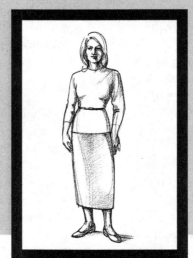

For the short-waisted woman, a narrow belt may be more flattering.

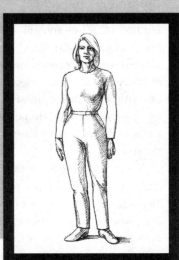

You can de-emphasize broad hips with straight trousers.

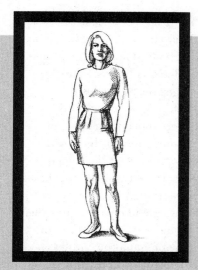

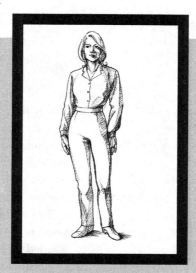

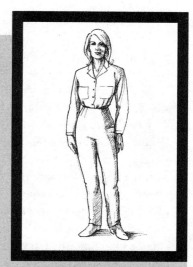

A skirt with a gathered
waist can add dimension to
narrow hips.

To de-emphasize a large
bust, wear blouses without
pockets or gathers.

Or you can emphasize your
bustline with a blouse that
has pockets and a long collar.

can help accent their chests.

If you have a long neck, go with
scarves, turtlenecks or necklaces that end
at the collarbone. All these accessories
will help fill in space.

Women with broad shoulders can discard
the shoulder pads from shirts and jackets.
Also, they should shop for jackets with a
notched collar: that vertical notch helps

draw the eye vertically.

Women with narrow shoulders should
keep a variety of shoulder pads on hand in
various sizes to add to shirts, sweaters
and jackets as necessary. They can also
leave already set-in shoulder pads in place.
In addition, they can make their shoulders
look broader by wearing a large decorative
pin at the shoulder.

Try a turtleneck—either light
or dark—if you're long-necked.

If you're broad-shouldered,
try a lapelled jacket without shoulder pads.

Leave in the shoulder
pads if your shoulders
are narrow.

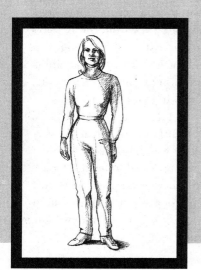

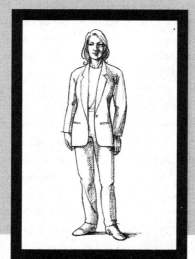

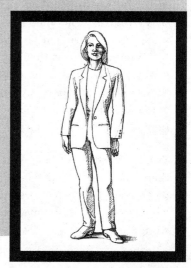

Wesleyan University in Middletown, Connecticut, a whopping 91 percent said they wanted to change their bodies.

Additional research conducted at Yale University shows that the things women wish they could alter are their faces, muscle tone, breast or chest size, overall appearance and weight.

Researchers attribute this dissatisfaction to the cultural messages that are sent to women about appearance. Part of that message comes from the media. Open a glossy magazine or switch on the television, and you're bombarded with images of women who are tall and thin —in other words, with images of ectomorphs. By constantly showing these images—and often *only* these images—the media send the message that the ectomorph body type is the ideal one to have; that it's the body type our society sees as acceptable, worthwhile and desirable. And it seems that some women really take that message to heart.

In a study of 75 women between the ages of 19 and 27 at Stanford University, Debbie Then, Ph.D., social psychologist and lecturer at the Health Improvement Program at Stanford University, found that self-esteem plummeted in two-thirds of the participants after they read through a bunch of glamour model–packed women's magazines.

"What happens is they compare themselves with the photos of models, and then they look in the mirror and say, 'I'm never going to look like this,'" says Dr. Then. "So they feel depressed and worse about themselves."

Even in the world of women's magazines, there are some editors who hope we'll someday see more diverse representation of women's bodies in the media. "My dream would be that we would see a mixture of various women in all of our magazines, including a broader range of body shapes and various ethnicities," says Barbara Harris, editor-in-chief of *Shape* magazine. She notes that *Shape* purposely chooses to photograph women who are more toned than the average woman, but some of the models have wider hips, while others don't. "Well-developed bodies span a range of body types, and that is one message we are trying to convey."

Not all magazines are likely to change their policies soon. As long as the media present you with a long line of glamorous professional-model ectomorphs, you're unlikely to find a flattering view of the real you in ads or articles.

Nice Lines

Your best guide to body shaping really is you. You may be perfectly happy with how you feel and how you look. Or you may decide, whatever your body type, that there are a few areas where you'd like to see some improvement. Whether you decide on change or the status quo, here's what experts recommend.

Believe in your own beauty. "It's important for a woman to own her own body and accept her body and work from there," says Karen Kaufman, president of Kaufman Professional Image Consultants in Philadelphia. "It's all about working from the inside out."

"It's not about what you look like; it's about what you feel like," agrees Harris. "We have so much potential to be perceived as beautiful people, if we first believe that ourselves. If we were supposed to be and look alike, we would. There is a reason why we differ from each other. All of us have unique strengths, and we should focus on developing and experiencing them."

Take a look around. To feel better about your body, one thing you can do is take a look around at some real women, says Dr. Then. Next time you go to the mall or the movies, "do some people watching for about an hour." Chances are you will see very few women who look the way professional models look, and that can help you feel better.

Dump the mags that nag. A number of women in Dr. Then's study chose not to read the women's magazines that made them feel bad about themselves. So if particular magazines make you feel worse about yourself after you read them, consider doing away with them, says Dr. Then. Go for the ones that motivate you to improve yourself but don't make you feel like pulling the covers over your head.

Tone up to feel fine. Both aerobic and strengthening exercises can help us tone our bodies and keep us feeling fit and good about our bodies. If you want to exercise to tone up and feel better about your body, it's often a good idea to start on an exercise program slowly, says Kennedy. One way to do that is to start with a basic walking program, she says.

Find the right gym. If you decide to join a gym to work out, pick one where you are comfortable, says Kennedy. At one gym women may wear spandex and thongs, while at another gym, shorts may be the attire of the day. Research indicates that overweight women tend to drop out of exercise class, not because they aren't having fun, but because they are worried about how they look. So it's important to go to a gym where you feel comfortable with the "dress code."

Give yourself a lift. Strength training can have a positive impact on body image, says Kennedy. When we increase our muscle mass, we feel better and function better. If you haven't done any weight lifting before, start by lifting your own weight with exercises like push-ups, leg lifts and abdominal curl-ups. Once you've started with a basic range of exercises, you may want to start lifting leg weights or arm weights. Or start in with a circuit training program at a gym or fitness club. Be sure to get instruction from a qualified individual—someone who has a certificate in strength training or a degree in exercise physiology, athletic training or physical therapy, Kennedy advises.

Focus on doing. Concentrate on the experience of activities you enjoy, rather than on what you look like, says Harris. Tune in to your working muscles and what they feel like.

See also Skeletal System

Brain

BACK IN THOSE HEADY, science-will-save-the-world days of the Industrial Revolution, inquiring medical minds left little to chance. They studied germs and gerbils, bacteria and birds, mold spores and monkeys—anything they could slice into little pieces and slip under a microscope.

When opportunity presented itself, they even studied each other's inquiring minds. Fun-loving groups like the Mutual Autopsy Society of Paris scoured the Western Hemisphere for the brains of the eminent. When they got hold of one, they weighed it, measured it and compared brain size with intelligence.

This society along with other organizations with similar pursuits found that brains were like zucchini—bigger didn't mean better. Napoleon III, the negligible nephew of Napoleon Bonaparte, weighed in with a 1,500-gram brain—17 percent larger than poet Walt Whitman's 1,282-gram offering. (Poor Walt: After the weigh-in a shaky member of the American Anthropometric Society dropped the great poet's brain on the floor, where it splattered like an egg.)

Crazy King Ludwig II housed a 1,349-gram brain inside his Bavarian skull, besting Albert Einstein, Mr. Theory of Relativity himself, by almost 10 percent. History fails to even record the size of Abraham Lincoln's brain—perhaps, some historians say, because records were lost during the assassination mayhem, or scientists found it shockingly small for such a statesman.

If size doesn't matter, what does? Above all, your brain's care and feeding. Nourish it with the right nutrients, give it enough mental stimulation, get enough physical exercise, and it will probably serve you well—no matter what its size—for decades to come.

"People used to think there was nothing they could do to help their brains," says Douglas Herrmann, Ph.D., memory researcher at the National Center for Health Statistics and author of *Super Memory*. "But that's not true. Nutrition and other factors can improve memory and other brain functions. You can definitely make a difference."

Divvying the Duties

The brain is the business end of the body's central nervous system. It takes electrical impulses from nerve endings all over the body, sorts out what the body is trying to say and then transmits messages back through the nerve network, telling the body what to do. Sweat. Sneeze. Breathe.

Of course, the brain does much more than that. It's responsible for higher functions such as language, creativity and logic. It stores memories. It interprets impulses from our eyes so that we can see. Though it only weighs about three pounds—2 percent of your body weight—the old noodle uses up 70 percent of all the air you breathe and the food you eat.

Brains are divided into a number of interconnected parts, each of which controls different body functions. The cerebrum, the largest chunk of the brain, takes care of distinctly human traits such as reasoning and intellect. Most of our reasoning takes place in the part of the cerebrum called the cortex—the gray, folded layer of skin that looks like a walnut shell and covers the surface of the brain. The cortex takes information from

Five Sure Ways
to Mangle Your Memory

Just as some lifestyle factors such as school, food and exercise can boost your brainpower, so, too, can other behaviors take a serious toll on your mental powers, says Douglas Herrmann, Ph.D., memory researcher at the National Center for Health Statistics and author of <u>Super Memory</u>. Here are five of the brain-numbing factors that Dr. Herrmann has identified.

1. Stress. So many memories, so little time. Stress decreases concentration and short-term memory in many people. If you need to remember something important, set aside a block of time to concentrate— and allow no interruptions.

2. Lack of sleep. Your brain files memories while you sleep. Sleep makes you more alert during the day, so you can concentrate better. Be sure to not deprive yourself of your shut-eye, or you may deprive yourself of memory.

3. High blood pressure. This impairs short-term memory and slows down your mental processing. It also may destroy brain tissue by depriving it of blood and nutrients. Get your blood pressure checked at least once a year.

4. Alcohol. Even a couple of beers will fog your concentration, so you'll be unlikely to retain details of an event where you've been drinking. Booze also kills brain cells. Over time, alcohol abuse impairs your ability to store and recall long-term memories.

5. Caffeine. This reduces concentration and can affect sleep patterns. One cup of coffee a day is probably okay—but anything more than that may hurt memory. Also, avoid stimulant pills that contain caffeine. They keep you awake, but you won't remember much.

nerves in the body and directs voluntary movements, like bending your fingers or walking. It's also where you perceive the senses; the cortex sorts out impulses from your eyes, ears, nose, tongue and skin and figures out colors, sounds, smells, tastes and feeling. The cortex appears to house memories, too, storing many of them in the areas called temporal lobes.

In the Main Brain

Deep under the cortex lies the thalamus. This area serves as a cerebral distribution center, routing information from along sensory pathways to the proper part of the cortex. The thalamus, in fact, seems to be just a dumber version of the cortex. It can sense pain, for example, but it can't tell the difference between pain from a paper cut and pain from a wildcat attack.

Even deeper in the brain is a cluster of structures such as the almond-shaped amygdala that make up the limbic system—the ancient seat of our darkest, most secret emotions. Though limbic means, literally, the peripheral limits of our system, this area controls many of the everyday functions such as digestion, heartbeat and smell as well as many aspects of emotion and behavior.

As for the rest of the brain, it handles run-of-the-mill, any-mammal-can-do-it stuff. The brain stem—which includes sections called the midbrain, pons and medulla oblongata—

Boost Your Creativity:
Storms and Dreams

It's the difference between Einstein and orangutan. Picasso and possum. You and yak. Thanks to our brains, we humans are creative. Thanks to their brains, animals stand around and grunt a lot.

You don't have to be some kind of beret-wearing, poem-writing, angst-riddled slacker to be creative, either. "Everyone has the ability," says William Shephard, director of programs for the Creative Education Foundation in Buffalo, New York. "In fact, creativity is becoming a survival skill in today's workplace. You have to come up with new and better ways to do things, or you and your company will get left behind."

Of course, you can't just sit down at your desk and say, "Okay, brain, be creative." You have to know how to coax your mind into a creative state and learn how to take advantage of its ability to interpret information in unique ways. Shephard offers these tips.

Don't be so critical. A technique called brainstorming can help boost your creativity, either alone or in a group. First define the problem you want to solve, then start thinking up solutions. They don't have to make sense, be practical or even sound good. Just keep kicking out ideas—and write them down. Don't make judgments about how good the ideas are until later. Go off in any direction the thoughts take you, so long as you keep the focus on the problem you're trying to solve.

After a set period of time, maybe 10 or 15 minutes, stop. If you can, put all your notes aside for a day or so, then come back and look at what you've written. You'll probably find the solution to your problem right in front of you.

Change the subject. Sometimes we focus too hard on the task at hand, and our brains don't respond to the pressure. If you feel like you've hit a mental wall, take a break and do something entirely different. If you can't come up with the right

controls activity in the heart, blood vessels and respiratory system. The tiny hypothalamus, located at the base of the cerebrum, controls body metabolism, temperature, blood sugar levels, appetite and sexual arousal. The cerebellum orchestrates muscle action; once your cortex orders a movement, the cerebellum tells which muscles to move and how.

Nourish Your Neurons

The average human brain contains about 100 billion nerve cells, each with several tiny branches of communication called dendrites that allow fellow cells to communicate with each other. The point at which these dendrites meet is called a synapse. Your brain can make 100 billion separate connections with itself— a nearly infinite number of possible combinations.

Sounds like a lot, doesn't it? But brain cells don't replenish themselves like skin cells. Constant stress or alcohol abuse can destroy some of that treasure. Then, late in middle age, we all start to lose neurons—the brain cells that send signals to each other. (Other brain cells, called glials, support and repair the neurons.)

Good food and exercise can fatten our brain cells and lengthen dendrites. These

phrase for a cover letter, for example, go pull some weeds. This gives your brain a chance to mull things over in a more relaxed setting.

Make a dream date—with yourself. Next time the boss catches you daydreaming, tell her you're actually doing some serious semiconscious creativity enhancement. Daydreaming for a few minutes lets you escape the pressure of here and now and allows your brain to work its creative magic.

"Daydreaming should actually be encouraged," Shephard says. "You shouldn't drift away for hours at a time, but taking a little time to toy with an idea, to imagine its applications, can be tremendously helpful." Again, don't make judgments about what you're thinking. Just let the thoughts flow. Worry about the details later.

Make new connections. Most of us think in preprogrammed ways. Table: chair. Salt: pepper. If you want to unleash creativity, compare things that seem to have nothing in common. French fry: jet plane. Fence post: laptop computer. Take a few minutes to list all the similarities you can think of. "This helps you make new associations, to see things in new ways," Shephard says. "It can break up the thought patterns that most of us always fall back into."

Once you're done with that warm-up, move on to the real problem. If you're trying to think of new ways to market your company's candy bar, compare its attributes to those of the Eiffel Tower. Or Bigfoot. Or the paneling in the conference room. Make a list of the similarities—then see if any of them warrant further discussion.

Be ready when lightning strikes. Creative thoughts can pop into your mind anywhere, anytime—in the elevator, at the lunch counter, while changing a diaper—so be ready. Keep a notepad or tape recorder close at hand so you can jot down your idea before you forget it.

branchlike pieces of neuron collect and help process information. But thickening a wig of dendrites isn't the same thing as growing a whole new cell. Actually, most scientists thought building new brain cells was something that ceased at birth. That was before the canary scam.

Bird Clues to Brain Work

Back in the 1930s the so-called canary scam started a chain reaction of neural curiosity in a nest of brain researchers at Rockefeller University and Cornell University Medical College in New York. A pet store owner knew why the caged bird sings: Males sing, females don't. So he injected his female birds with testosterone. They sang. They sold—but they stopped singing as soon as the hormone wore off.

Intrigued by the effect of testosterone, in the early 1980s the scientists at Rockefeller University and Cornell University Medical College found that new neurons lay at the heart of the female's testosterone-stimulated song. In subsequent studies Cornell researchers identified precursor cells—primed to create new neurons—in rat brains and in human brains. Later on, the researchers managed to grow new neurons from those cells in a petri dish.

"We can grow hundreds of neurons at a time that way," says Steven A. Goldman, M.D., Ph.D., associate professor of neurology at Cornell and attending neurologist at New York Hospital in New York City. "But we need to grow tens to hundreds of thousands if we're going to even think about dealing with brains damaged by stroke or degenerative disease," such as Alzheimer's, Parkinson's and multiple sclerosis, he adds. "We don't even know whether they'll be useful in clinical repair. That would be years off, but that's the hope."

After engineering those first neurons, Dr. Goldman and his colleagues found out that the truly creative sex hormone wasn't testosterone but estrogen. "In bird brains and perhaps in human brains, too, right underneath the areas that generate new brain cells—just a few cells away—is an area where testosterone gets converted to estrogen. And the estrogen causes other cells in the immediate vicinity to make a substance that allows the new neurons to survive—in its absence, they die."

"Estrogen also appears to protect neurons in women, too, in a variety of degenerative brain diseases," Dr. Goldman adds. So the brain may be a beneficiary of hormone replacement therapy—the kind described beginning on page 231.

Gender Differences

Hormones aren't the only sex-related discoveries that brain researchers have been making. They know that the fetal brain of the female develops faster than that of the male. And they've found actual scientific data to back up the argument that men and women really are from different planets when it comes to brain function. Among the gender differences: The corpus callosum, which is the bridge connecting the right and left hemispheres of the brain, is bigger in women than it is in men. And brain scans that reveal "thinking" activities show that women tend to use both parts of their brains, while men weigh in more heavily on just one side.

Another difference is that while men's brains are bigger by about 10 percent, women have 11 percent more neurons, densely packed into the layers that allow us to understand language and recognize melodies in music and tones in speech. "Women seem better at verbal memory and fluency," says Ruben Gur, Ph.D., professor in the Department of Psychiatry at the University of Pennsylvania in Philadelphia and director of the University's brain behavior laboratory. "But men do better at almost any spatial task, like reading maps, as long as it doesn't involve memory. They also do better at any motor task, like finger tapping."

Dr. Gur and his wife, Raquel Gur, M.D., Ph.D., professor of psychiatry and neurology and director of the neuropsychiatry section in the Department of Psychiatry at the University of Pennsylvania in Philadelphia, are both neuroscientists, and they started studying sex differences in brains because they were piqued by their own contrasting temperaments. For a while their research didn't reveal many brain differences. In men and women, scans of the cerebrum, cerebellum, cortex and lobe showed mostly similarities.

Differences only showed up when the Gurs probed deeper—into the brain's limbic system, where so many promptings of emotion and behavior arise. In men the most primitive part of that system, which governs action and aggression, was highly active and lit up like a firecracker when imaged with a method that measures how much energy is consumed by brain regions. In women it was the most highly evolved area, the cingulate gyrus, that glowed brightest. In that limbic region an emotion like anger prompts a look or a word, not a punch.

More between the Sexes

Given these brain differences, what can women and men do to connect with each other? Here are some hints from researchers.

Spell it out. In one interesting experiment, the Gurs tested how men and women read facial moods. With groups of each sex, the Gurs displayed photographs of men and women with happy and sad faces. They discovered what every woman knows—men have a hard time reading a woman's sad expression.

The implications? Since men aren't so good at reading signals, such as a frown or pursed lips, the sexes need to talk about disturbances and disagreements. You can't assume a man will automatically understand an expression that—to you—conveys your emotions very clearly.

"If I talk to someone who doesn't answer, I'll think he's rude—but not if I know he's deaf," observes Dr. Ruben Gur. "Men have a very hard time recognizing sadness in women. And now that women know, maybe they won't attribute that lack of response to a lack of caring. Recognizing our differences may help rather than hinder us."

Write down directions. If women excel at the subtleties of emotion, men tend to excel in spatial matters. They may not be able to read faces, but in general, they sure can read maps.

If you tend to be frustrated by maps, it's more likely you'll prefer written directions, especially if they include visual landmarks like: "Turn left at the church on Main Street, then right at the light."

Keep reminding him. Learning faces is a spatial task involving memory that men don't do well, says Dr. Ruben Gur. So if you find you have to keep introducing your husband to your friends, don't get testy. Just help him along: "You remember Meredith—she is the one who lives next to the post office."

Despite these general differences, however, research shows that both men and women can get better at using the less-developed areas of their brains. Those dendrites can be developed. Besides, there are many exceptions to the general observations of gender differences. Some male brains act more like females'—and some women's brains act more like men's.

Pumping Up the Power

While we can't grow new neurons in our lifetime, we can usually promote optimal function of the ones we have. One way is to boost the levels of zinc—the memory mineral found in beef, beans and oysters, says James G. Penland, Ph.D., research psychologist with the U.S. Department of Agriculture's Grand Forks Human Nutrition Research Center in North Dakota. The nutrient boron—in peanuts, raisins and leafy vegetables—appears to be good for memory, too, and also for attention and motor skills. Smart friends are also good food for the brain, since it's been shown that stimulating conversation also stimulates your dendrites to grow.

But the richest Miracle-Gro for the garden of your brain is probably exercise. Studies of people who exercise keep showing links between physical activity and mental ability. These links have been related to substances called nerve growth factors that have been studied by Carl W. Cotman, Ph.D., professor of psychobiology and neurology and director of the Institute for Brain/Aging and Dementia at the University of California, Irvine.

Conducting animal studies, Dr. Cotman put running wheels in rat cages and observed the rodents' behavior. He found that the rats assumed individual exercise routines, just like humans do. Some rodents proved to be couch rats, some were marathon rats and some were runaholics. But many settled down naturally to an hourly run a day.

To study the effects of exercise, Dr. Cotman measured the rats' levels of a particular type of nerve growth factor that makes neurons flourish. The rat racers' levels of nerve growth factor turned out to be higher than levels found in couch-potato rats.

"But the increases didn't show up just in the motor areas of the brain. They showed up in the brain structures for cognition, learning and memory. That was a pretty exciting surprise," he says.

The lesson? "What we think is that—at a minimum—exercise makes brain cells healthier, work better and probably resist minor insults like a minor stroke. My guess is that the activity should be something not terribly long, but consistent—I'm not sure it means every day. Some rats that seem to naturally run about an hour a day show an increase," says Dr. Cotman.

Listen Up—Then Smell the Lemons

The next time you have to work on a budget or balance your checkbook, slip some Mozart in your headphones. Specifically, "Sonata for Two Pianos in D Major, K. 448."

Researchers at the University of California, Irvine, played a recording of that sonata for 36 college students, then gave the students an IQ test measuring abstract reasoning. The students who heard the music scored eight to nine points higher than those who studied in silence. "Listening to a complex and highly

Remember the Alamo (and Everything Else)

Yes, there are specific techniques that have been shown to help people remember things better. Here's what memory experts recommend for starters.

Pick some letters. To remember a short list of names or groceries, make a word out of the first letter of each item. Suppose you just met Wanda, Omar, Rita and Ken. Remember WORK—the first letters of each name—and you have a better chance of recalling your new acquaintances. Or you need to get soap, ham, oranges and pistachios. Remember SHOP. This process is known as mnemonics.

Distract yourself. Learn to concentrate amid chaos. Try reading a book with the radio turned up full blast. Try watching two television sets at once. Then try remembering what you read, saw and heard. This will teach you to tune out what's not important—a key step in improving memory.

Join the group. Your brain remembers items best in groups of 5 through 9. So if you have to recall a long list—say, 30 things—try breaking the items down into

patterned piece of music acts as a 'warm-up' for the mind, which could be good for high-level mathematics," says Frances H. Rauscher, Ph.D., research psychologist at the University of Wisconsin-Oshkosh who specializes in the effects of music on intelligence.

In addition to music, certain fragrances might make it easier for you to think more clearly and help reduce mistakes. "You can change brain frequencies with smell," says Alan Hirsch, M.D., psychiatrist, neurologist and neurological director at the Smell and

six groups of five items each. The process is called chunking.

Group items with common themes. If you have a shopping list, for example, make a vegetable grouping, a canned goods grouping and so on.

<u>**Just imagine.**</u> If you have trouble remembering names, try visualization. Associate the person's name with an object or action, then make a mental picture of the object. To remember Neil, picture a man kneeling.

Rhyming also can solidify the connection. If Larry has a beard, try remembering him as "Hairy Larry." Just don't call him Hairy by accident.

<u>**Store in a drawer.**</u> If you're always losing your keys or misplacing your wallet, create a memory drawer. Make it a point to put easily lost items in this place every day. It doesn't have to be an actual drawer. A closet, countertop or nightstand will do fine. The process will quickly become a habit—and you'll never run around the house checking the pockets of all your pants and coats again.

Taste Treatment and Research Foundation in Chicago.

Japanese researchers have discovered that air scented with a lemon spray decreases errors among workers by 54 percent. Other fragrances also reduced goofs, though not as sharply. Jasmine cut mistakes by 33 percent, lavender by 20 percent. Lavender induces a more relaxed state so you can think more clearly, says Dr. Hirsch. As for jasmine, Dr. Hirsch notes that it has the ability to excite—even in concentrations so low you wouldn't know it's there—resulting in quicker thinking. But Dr. Hirsch found that the odor that has the greatest effect on the speed of learning is a mixed floral scent.

The Wisdom of Age

Does your brain slow down as you age?

Some studies in this fresh area of research indicate that the brain is like a muscle—it seems to get stronger with use. While it may take an older person somewhat longer to learn a new computer system or memorize French idioms, we can keep lots of brain power into our eighties and beyond. You might not make a good computer analyst at age 75, but a superior court judgeship isn't out of the question. Unless you develop a brain disorder such as Alzheimer's or have a serious stroke, your brain can continue to function at a high level right into and through old age, according to Dr. Herrmann.

Here are some tips to keep that gray matter going.

Get your Bs daily. Vitamin B_6 helps your body create neurotransmitters—chemicals that allow brain cells to fire off messages to one another. In 1992 a study of 38 elderly Dutch folks found that a 20-milligram daily supplement of B_6 could help improve long-term storage of memories. That's ten times the federal government's recommended Daily Value of 2 milligrams, so you wouldn't want to take that much regularly without consulting your doctor.

Your best bet, according to Dr. Herrmann, is to eat a balanced diet containing lots of fruits and vegetables. Since freezing and processing vegetables can rob them of 15 to 70 percent of their B_6 content, you definitely want fresh produce whenever possible. Other super sources of B_6 include chicken, fish and lean cuts of pork.

Use it or lose it. Flex your brain as well as your body. Researchers have found that people with college educations who remain mentally active throughout their lives have 40 percent longer dendrites than less-educated, less-challenged people. The longer the dendrites, the more information you can receive and understand.

But you don't really need a diploma to develop those dendrites. Most kinds of mental activity help keep the connections between your brain cells humming, so try continuing education courses at the local college, crossword puzzles or even playing along with television game shows, suggests K. Warner Schaie, Ph.D., professor of human development at Pennsylvania State University in University Park.

Dr. Schaie's research team found only one game that was not too helpful: bingo. Unless you play about 20 cards at once, he says, you're better off guessing along with Vanna on *Wheel of Fortune*.

Keep the pressure down. High blood pressure is a three-prong problem. It's been implicated in 40 percent of brain-busting strokes. It slows down your thought processes and appears to impair short-term memory. Worst of all, a study of 35 people between ages 51 and 80 showed that high blood pressure appears to cause permanent structural changes and tissue loss in the brain. One of the authors of the study, Declan Murphy, M.D., senior lecturer and consultant psychiatrist at Bethlem Royal Hospital in Kent, England, says that this could over time cause problems with memory, language and sense of direction.

Make sure you get your blood pressure checked by a doctor or health professional at least once a year. And then follow your doctor's advice to help keep your blood pressure under control.

The Price We Pay

Complexity hardly ever comes cheap. With billions of neurons buzzing bounteously in your brain, things sometimes go very, very wrong. Even a simple blow to the head can erase your command of the English language and have you fluent in a language you haven't spoken in decades. For example, an 80-year-old woman can suffer severe brain trauma that erases 70 years' worth of English language and begin communicating in the native Italian she spoke as a young girl.

A more common mystery is why you sometimes feel dizzy or faint. That giddy, light-headed, unsteady sensation can be caused by something as simple as a glitch in your sensory network or disturbances in the movement of fluid—you bend over or stand up too quickly, and you haven't given your blood enough time to get to your brain. Severe anemia, high blood pressure, low blood pressure, low blood sugar and side effects from drugs can also dizzy you. When it comes on suddenly and is accompanied by chest pains, rapid heart beat, blurred vision or numbness, dizziness can also be a warning sign for stroke.

Sometimes dizziness precedes fainting—the loss of consciousness that could come from interrupted blood flow to the brain. If that happens often, you should have an evaluation by your doctor or internist. But the more usual causes are circulatory problems.

Actual brain disorders range from infections such as meningitis to genetic breakdowns such as Down's syndrome and mental conditions such as schizophrenia. "The brain is extremely complicated," says Francis Pirozzolo, M.D., neuropsychologist at Baylor College of Medicine in Houston. "We're learning more about it every day, but it con-

The Warning Signs of Stroke

Know the warning signs of stroke, says the American Heart Association. The Association provides a doctor-approved list of the most common warning signs. They include:

- **Sudden weakness or numbness of the face, arm or leg on one side of the body**
- **Sudden dimness or loss of vision, particularly in only one eye**
- **Loss of speech or trouble talking or understanding speech**
- **Sudden, severe headaches with no known cause**
- **Unexplained dizziness, unsteadiness or sudden falls, especially if you get these symptoms with any of the other ones**

If you notice one or more of these signs, don't wait—see a doctor.

tinues to puzzle us and frustrate us. Sometimes things go wrong that we just can't fix."

Age-Old Afflictions

Among the most feared of all brain diseases are Alzheimer's and stroke. About four million Americans have Alzheimer's, including one in ten people over age 65 and nearly half of everyone over 85.

Simply put, Alzheimer's kills brain cells. Millions of them. As the cells die, over the course of months and years, victims begin to suffer severe memory loss, loss of language and reasoning skills, physical deterioration and, eventually, death. The disease can take from 3 to 20 years to run its course, and there's no known cure.

While Alzheimer's is the fourth leading cause of death among adults, we know little about its origins. Victims often show altered levels of neurotransmitters—the elaborate, chemically connected messengers that send impulses between brain cells. High levels of aluminum may also be found in the brain tissue of some people with Alzheimer's. Researchers are studying factors such as head injury, education and gender that pose risks for developing Alzheimer's disease. Other researchers have located and identified genes associated with the disease.

Mental activity may even help fight Alzheimer's disease. Research from Columbia University in New York City shows that people with high education levels and high achievement on the job had just one-third the risk of developing Alzheimer's than others. That may be because people who use their brains build up a reserve of synapses. And that means there is less communication breakdown between brain cells when Alzheimer's embarks on its path of destruction.

As for stroke, it's one of the brain's deadliest enemies as well as the leading cause of serious disability in the United States. Doctors say there are two basic kinds of strokes. The first is usually caused by clots in the arteries leading from your heart to your brain. The clots block blood flow, cutting off oxygen and nutrients and killing brain cells.

The second type of stroke is caused by hemorrhaging in the brain. An aneurysm—a blood-filled pouch ballooning out from a weak spot in an artery—may burst suddenly. Blood flow to the brain is interrupted, and surrounding cells are deprived of blood. While hemorrhages account for one in five strokes, they are usually more deadly than strokes caused by blood clots.

See also Nervous System

Breasts

TO MEN THEY'RE MAINLY EROTIC—the subject of locker-room jokes and goofy nicknames that range from the ridiculous to the more ridiculous—hooters, knockers, jugs, bazooms, boobs, kasabas, ta-tas, coconuts and melons.

Even women can get caught up in the sexualization of mammary glands. In her book *The Female Eunuch*, feminist activist Germain Greer lamented the plight of the busty female as she's viewed by men:

She is never allowed to think that their popping eyes actually see her. Her breasts . . . are not parts of a person but lures slung around her neck, to be kneaded and twisted like magic putty, or mumbled and mouthed like lolly ices.

Jugs? Lures? Putty? It's obvious that breasts represent much more in this society than mere mammary organs. Like it or not, these two mounds of glandular, fatty and fibrous tissue located over the pectoralis muscles of the chest have a lot to do with our identity as women. For many women they're also a source of pleasure. Because their stimulation often causes sensual arousal during sex, the breasts are also secondary sexual organs.

Breast Basics

Breasts begin to emerge during puberty responding to the hormonal changes in the body.

Usually, adult breasts are tear-shaped, with breast tissue running from the collarbone all the way down to the last few ribs, and from the breastbone in the middle of the chest to the back of the armpit. Most of the breast tissue is toward the armpit and upper breast, with fat located in the middle and lower part. Like the rest of the body, breasts also have arteries, veins and nerves.

The areola—or darker area of skin surrounding the nipple—varies in shape, size and color. In blonds it's often pink; in brunettes it's browner and in Blacks, it is black. It also changes colors during sexual arousal or orgasm.

What's in a Lump?

Breast and lump—the two words clash as badly as drinking and driving. With one out of every eight women in the United States getting breast cancer, it's no wonder that new lumps cause consternation. But despite the ominous implications, lumpy breasts are simply a fact of life—like freckles or body hair.

Because most normal breast tissue is lumpy glandular tissue, about 75 percent of women get what could be called fibrocystic changes in their breasts, notes Kerry McGinn, R.N., author of *The Informed Woman's Guide to Breast Health* and certified oncology nurse at the University of California, San Francisco, Mount Zion Home Care.

"Every month, the body has a dress rehearsal for what would happen if a woman has a baby," according to C. H. Baick, M.D., founding director of and breast surgical oncologist at the Breast Health Center in Santa Ana, California. "The body brings in extra fluids the woman might need. As we get older, things get tired on the job, and the cleanup isn't as effective. Fluids are left in the breast."

It's not uncommon for women to have lumpy breasts, says Lydia Komarnicky, M.D., radiation oncologist at Thomas Jefferson Hospital in Philadelphia and co-author of *What to Do If You Get Breast Cancer*. Normal breast tissue often has a lumpy consistency.

Signs of Trouble

Aside from everyday lumpy breast tissue, there are two types of nonmalignant lumps to be aware of. The first are cysts, which are most common in women nearing menopause. These fluid-filled sacs are smooth on the outside and often tender when touched. When you're treated for cysts, the doctor first anesthetizes the skin over the lump and then draws out the fluid with a needle—causing the cyst to collapse.

The other common lump is a fibroadenoma, which is a round lump that feels smooth and rubbery. It can be as small as a pencil eraser or as large as a lemon. To make sure the lump is harmless, a biopsy is often done, during which a piece of tissue is removed and then analyzed. After diagnosis is made, the doctor removes the lump while you're under local anesthesia.

Despite the fact that only 1 in 12 lumps in premenopausal women is malignant, it's still important to have any suspicious lumps checked out by a doctor before you write them off as harmless, notes Dr. Komarnicky.

Smooth Strategies

Although most lumpiness can be blamed on hormonal changes in your body, you can try some strategies to help smooth things out. Here are some doctors' recommendations.

Dry your whistle. It's important to cut back your alcohol intake or stop imbibing altogether, says Susan Lark, M.D., a physician in private practice in Los Altos, California, and author of *The Woman's Health Compan-*

A Fitting Experience

The average woman buys four to six bras a year, but that doesn't mean she'll wear all the ones she buys. Sometimes we just have to keep shopping to find just the right fit.

Before bra shopping, make sure you get the correct measurements, advises Gloria Falla, vice president of design at Playtex Apparel in Stamford, Connecticut. To find out your body size, wrap a measuring tape around your diaphragm while wearing a bra. Add five inches to this measurement to find out your total body size. If it's an uneven number, round up.

Then place a measuring tape around the fullest part of your bust. The difference between this measurement and your total body size decides your cup size. Here's how to calculate.

- If your bust measurement is up to an inch larger than your body size, your cup size is A.
- If your bust measurement is up to 2 inches larger than your body size, you're a B.
- Three inches larger, you're a C.
- Four inches larger is a D.
- Five inches larger is a DD.
- Six inches larger is a DDD.

To make sure the bra fits, you should always try it on before you buy it, Falla advises. Make sure the cup completely contains your breasts, with no bulges at the top or sides of the cups.

The bra should be comfortable enough for you to slip a finger under the band at the base of the cups. If there are wrinkles in the cups, it means the bra is too large.

Also, make sure the bra doesn't ride up in back. If it does, the bra may be too large, or hooked too loosely, or the straps may be adjusted too tightly.

Downsizing

The next time you see Dolly Parton, consider the down side. Think of the backaches she must have! Consider the strap marks imprinted after a day of toting that weight. For every bonus of being over-endowed, there's a drawback.

That's why some 36,000 women opted to have their breasts surgically reduced in 1994—surprisingly, just 3,000 fewer than those who chose augmentation.

There's little wonder that breast reduction, or reduction mammoplasty, is so popular, notes Petra Schneider, M.D., a plastic surgeon in private practice in Melbourne, Florida. Women with large breasts have a lot of medical problems: upper and mid-back pain, headaches, breast pain, shoulder pain, grooving in the shoulders from bra straps, skin rashes under the breasts and numbness of the little fingers caused by nerve pressure.

Mammoplasty usually takes between three and six hours and is more complicated than a breast augmentation procedure, notes Dr. Schneider.

The nipple is usually preserved on a small flap of tissue, and tissue is removed from around this flap and the sides of the breast. The nipple is then elevated and the flaps of tissue brought together, which both uplifts and reduces the breast.

The procedure leaves scars. And there are other possible problems that have to be weighed against the benefits. Only about half of the women who've had reductions can still nurse babies, and some of the sensation in the nipples or even in the breast itself is reduced. There's also the possibility that weight gain or loss will change the cup size once again.

But the surgery can have psychological benefits, especially among teens, notes Sharon Webb, M.D., Ph.D., assistant clinical professor of surgery at Tufts University School of Medicine in Boston.

Many of her patients with larger breasts have a tendency to be overweight, possibly as a result of trying to camouflage the size of their breasts, says Dr. Webb. When patients lose breast size, they often lose weight in other places as well.

"Girls come in to me at first with an extra-large sweatshirt on, all hunched over," she observes. "They come in afterward with cutoffs and a T-shirt, standing up straight and smiling. They've gotten the weight off their chests—literally." Dr. Webb adds that the breasts need to be fully mature and the girl also needs to be fully mature. Some girls are mature enough at age 15 to have the procedure done, but many are not.

ion. "Alcohol elevates levels of estrogen in your system, which makes breast lumpiness worse."

Defat your diet. A low-fat diet that's high in fiber, fruits and veggies is a great way to get excess estrogen out of your system, notes Dr. Lark. A high-fat diet impairs estrogen excretion and raises estrogen levels by promot-ing growth of bacteria. That growth increases the absorption of estrogen back into your body instead of allowing it to be excreted through your intestinal track. "Vegetable-eaters excrete estrogen more effectively." Significant sources of fat are foods such as salad dressing, cheese, margarine, lunchmeats and other fatty meats.

Drink an un-cola. Avoiding caffeine could help cut back on lumpiness, notes Dr. Komarnicky. "Some people do seem to be very sensitive to caffeine. When they stop drinking cola or eating chocolate, their lumps decrease in size or go away, and breast tenderness decreases also." So if you are particularly sensitive, you might consider decreasing your intake of caffeinated products.

Check with your doc for E loading. A good way to smooth out your breasts is with vitamin E, notes Dr. Lark. "You need 400 to 1,600 international units (IU) of vitamin E a day to help combat cystic breast changes." Since this is a high level of vitamin E—which can be toxic in large doses—you should check with your doctor before taking this much. (The Daily Value for vitamin E is 30 IU.)

What a Drag

Gravity is an inexorable force. For the woman with breasts like overpumped volleyballs, the sheer weight makes them hard to support. Unfortunately, even the breasts that fit in A and B cups may succumb to sag. Doctors call it ptosis—which simply means droop. Women call it a pain in the butt.

Like it or not, the droop factor is a fact of life, notes Sharon Webb, M.D., Ph.D., assistant clinical professor of surgery at Tufts University School of Medicine in Boston.

"All soft tissues on the human body respond to gravity—from the ear lobe to the nose to the chest to the rear end," Dr. Webb says. "Since there is no intrinsic support to the breast, the forces of gravity take their toll."

The tissues responsible for holding up breasts are the suspensory ligaments that run underneath them. But they're not very strong, and they lose elasticity when the breasts are

From Checking to Checkup

Say you're doing your monthly self-exam, thinking about nothing in particular, when you suddenly feel a hard growth on your breast that wasn't there before. Your heart races. Your mouth gets dry. Panic sets in.

Where do you go from here? Straight to your doctor, says Kathleen Mayzel, M.D., assistant clinical professor of surgery at Tufts University School of Medicine and director of the Faulkner Breast Center, both in Boston.

"If it's truly a breast lump, a biopsy is the only way to prove that it's not cancer," she says. Anyone with a new lump should have it evaluated. But sometimes your doctor can tell by using painless ultrasound if it's a cyst that's not cancerous.

What happens if your worst nightmare comes true, and your test comes back positive?

"It's a very slow-growing cancer," Dr. Mayzel says. Once it's diagnosed, she advises getting several doctors' opinions before making a decision about treatment.

A common treatment is mastectomy—the goal of which is to surgically remove the breast before the tumor can spread.

Another treatment option is a lumpectomy, followed by 6½ weeks of radiation.

Which is more effective—mastectomy or lumpectomy?

A 1995 study compared ten-year survival rates of women who'd undergone mastectomy for early-stage breast cancer with those who'd had lumpectomy. At ten years relative survival was 75 percent for those who'd had mastectomy and 77 percent for those who'd had lumpectomy and radiation.

large and heavy, notes Dr. Webb.

Lots of other factors add to the drooping dilemma: weight gains and losses, pregnancy and breastfeeding all cause breasts to enlarge. These changes stretch the skin. Later, after childbearing or a period of weight gain, the tissues go back to normal, but the skin doesn't, according to Dr. Webb.

Although some of these changes are unavoidable, you don't have to completely succumb to the sag. Here are some tips to keep your breasts saluting the sun as long as possible.

Push it up. Exercise can't correct a sagging breast, but it can give the illusion of a firmer bust, notes Dr. Lark. Anything that builds up the pectoralis muscles of the chest, such as bench presses or resistance exercises for the arms will help to firm and tone the muscle underneath the breasts.

Get some support. Contrary to the popular thinking of the 1960s, going braless does not foster perky breasts. "It does help to wear a bra," notes Petra Schneider, M.D., a plastic surgeon in private practice in Melbourne, Florida. "It puts less stress on the ligaments. The more you wear one during the day, the more it helps."

Save your skin. Too much sun exposure and smoking both take their toll on the skin's collagen—the fibrous protein that holds skin together, notes Dr. Schneider. "Some people have very elastic skin that holds up well, and others have thin, very fragile skin that doesn't." Whichever kind of skin you have, a lot of sun exposure and smoking damages the skin and its elastic fibers.

If you've tried every trick in the book and still have breasts like deflated balloons, you might even consider a breast lift, called a mastopexy. The surgery involves a doctor moving the nipple by elevating it and trim-

Get in Touch with Your Breasts

If you know the shape and texture of your breasts by sight and touch you're more likely to detect changes. "Some women say their breasts are so lumpy that they just don't know what they're feeling," notes C. H. Baick, M.D., founding director of and breast surgical oncologist at the Breast Health Center in Santa Ana, California. "You have to get to know your breasts. It's the only way you can detect unusual changes." Because the texture of your breasts changes according to your cycle, Dr. Baick recommends doing the exam at the same time each period—seven to ten days after your period begins.

Begin with a visual inspection. Stand before a mirror with your hands at your sides. Raise your hands and clasp them as shown in the illustration below. Then press your hands firmly on your hips with your shoulders and elbows pulled forward as shown in the illustration, above left. Look for any changes in size or shape of your breasts, as well as for nipple discharge,

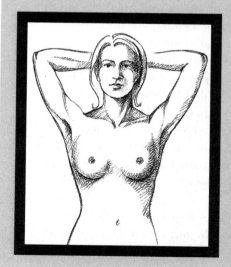

For a visual self-exam, clasp your hands as shown and press forward against the back of your scalp.

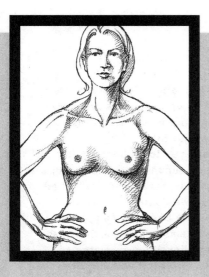

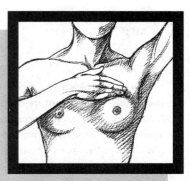

Complete the
visual exam in
this position.

Circular pattern.
First place your
fingers at the
outer edge of
your breast and
slowly compress
the tissue.

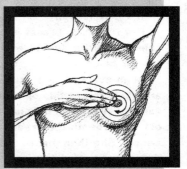

redness, puckering or dimpling.

Following the visual exam, check your
breasts by touch.

It's important to follow a definite pattern—vertical, wedge or circular—to make
sure you examine yourself thoroughly for
any unusual lumps. You can use one of
these methods or all three. You may want
to do it in the shower with soapy water so
your hands slide smoothly.

Circular pattern.
Then move your
fingers in small
circles, working
toward the nipple.

Circular pattern.
As the last step,
check the entire
breast and
underarm,
including the
armpit.

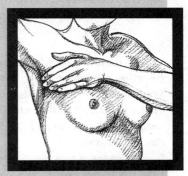

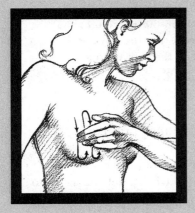

Vertical pattern. Slide the hand
up and down to methodically
examine the entire breast.

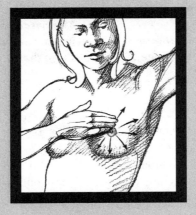

Wedge pattern. From the nipple,
examine outward toward the
edge of the breast as shown.

Making Mountains out of Molehills

When you wish for more than you have, the world seems full of cruel reminders. Bikinis display assets you can only dream about. Strapless evening gowns dare your nonexistent chest to hold them up. And most of the actresses who make it big remind you of the true meaning of big.

It's just not fair.

But thanks to breast implants, medical science can tip the scales—and cup size—in your favor.

In an average year some 40,000 women are likely to get this operation. A plastic surgeon makes an incision around the areola, underneath the breast or through the armpit. She then places the implant under the breast tissue (between the breast and the chest muscle) or underneath the muscle. The whole procedure can be done in approximately two hours on an outpatient basis.

The typical patient is a woman in her twenties who is striving to improve in all aspects of her life, notes Sharon Webb, M.D., Ph.D., assistant clinical professor of surgery at Tufts University School of Medicine in Boston.

Self-esteem is a big issue, regardless of age, Dr. Webb notes. "I'll have someone 35 years old who's otherwise secure who says she hates trying swimsuits on every year. The bottom fits fine, but she can never find a top that fits."

Before you say yes to an implant, it's important to consider the possible health risks and complications. Silicone gel–filled implants have drawn controversy since 1990, when women began to complain about health problems such as arthritis and lupus that they believed were related to silicone gel. In 1992 the Food and Drug Administration banned silicone implants, not because they were known to pose a risk, but because manufacturers hadn't done all they could do to collect data on whether or not they were safe.

While research has not conclusively linked silicone with sickness, some doctors are convinced it's harmful. Frank Vasey, M.D., professor of medicine and chief of rheumatology at the University of South Florida College of Medicine in Tampa, says he believes that the silica in the wall of the implant activates the immune system, causing flulike symptoms. The harder silicone on the outside of the implant breaks down, and the gel bleeds through and spreads through the body.

ming off excess skin. You'll have a scar around the nipple and undersurface of the breast, notes Dr. Webb. "You haven't altered the force of gravity; you're just tightening up the skin envelope." To see if you qualify for this surgery, look at the position of your nipples in relation to your breast fold. If your nipples are at or above it, you're probably not droopy enough to have a breast lift done.

Your Risks of Breast Cancer

If breasts make us uniquely female, then to lose one is almost like being defeminized—to some it's a loss of sexual identity. But breast cancer means much more than possible disfigurement. It's the second most common cause of cancer death among women in the United States.

Currently, saline implants—filled with saltwater solution—are the only types that doctors use, except in the case of breast reconstruction surgery following mastectomy or in replacing a defective silicone implant.

There are a few drawbacks to saline as well, such as the fact that it will eventually leak, notes Petra Schneider, M.D., a plastic surgeon in private practice in Melbourne, Florida. "It's like having a flat tire. The breast goes down in size, and you know you have to get a new one." When that happens, the saline is harmlessly absorbed into the body.

But some doctors have reservations about the wrapping that holds the saline. The envelope containing the saline eventually disintegrates, and there's silica in the envelope, notes Dr. Vasey. "How safe they are, exactly, remains to be seen." If you have the implants removed because of adverse symptoms, Dr. Vasey believes that they should not be replaced with saline.

Dr. Webb disagrees. The silica envelope making up the implant is not an active immunological agent, she says, and is made of a super-hard plastic so safe that it's also used to coat pacemakers and catheters.

Breast cancer can be slow- or fast-growing. The actual cancer cells are microscopic and may take one to five years before the cancerous area grows large enough to be felt as a mass or tumor.

From 70 to 80 percent of all breast cancer develops in the ducts of the mammary glands. It's best to discover cancer while it's still growing in the ducts before the cells have spread outside the duct lining and potentially throughout the body.

Although breast cancer will strike over 180,000 women in the United States each year, that doesn't mean a death sentence—and many times, not even loss of a breast.

These days more and more women are opting for lumpectomies and radiation (called breast conservation therapy) rather than mastectomy—which means only the tissue around the lump is removed rather than the whole breast. Dr. Komarnicky says that more and more physicians are starting to recognize breast conservation as an equal option to mastectomy in early localized breast cancer, so the mastectomy trend is changing.

In addition, mammography and monthly self-exams give women the chance to catch cancer early, says Dr. Komarnicky. "There can be a 95 percent survival rate if it's found in the earliest stage. We can excise the area and then treat the breast with radiation."

Open That Family Album

Another vital step in beating breast cancer is knowing your risk factors. Many factors are linked to conditions that affect hormonal patterns and increase estrogen metabolism in the body, notes Larry Kushi, Sc.D., associate professor of epidemiology at the University of Minnesota School of Public Health in Minneapolis.

You're at higher risk for breast cancer if you've never had children or if your first child was born after you reached the age of 30. Other women with a higher risk factor are those who had their first period early or started menopause late in life. Being on estrogen replacement or supplements may also raise your risk of breast cancer.

"It's often linked with a high constant exposure to estrogen," notes Dr. Kushi. "Before family planning, when women were often pregnant or breastfeeding, the breast cancer rates were low. Now women have fewer children later in life and don't breastfeed as long."

Also, having first-degree maternal relatives like a mother or sisters who got breast cancer raises your risk 1½ to 2 times. If a relative had cancer in both breasts or before menopause, you're 50 percent more likely to get breast cancer than the woman who has no family history of the disease.

Go Looking for Trouble

To spot breast cancer early, doctors recommend both self-examination and mammography. But a number of experts debate the effectiveness of self-exams and question how often the exam should be done.

While many physicians advocate doing self-examination at the same time every month, a growing number, including Susan Love, M.D., author of the best-selling *Dr. Susan Love's Breast Book*, disagree.

In her book Dr. Love says that self-exam "alienates women from their breasts . . . it puts you in a position of examining yourself once a month to see if your breast has betrayed you." Instead, she advocates simply touching and getting to know your entire body without making a monthly "search and destroy" mission out of it.

But Dr. Baick says that's a defeatist attitude. Instead, he's for monthly self-checkups.

"Self-exam should be once a month and no more, because you cannot detect a change in your breast if you're doing it every day," he notes. "The important thing is to get to know your breasts."

Farsighted Screening

The other method of detecting early signs of breast cancer is baseline mammography. Once your breasts are x-rayed, the doctor has a record of normal breast tissue appearance, and later x-rays can be compared for changes. With annual or semiannual screenings, the doctor can detect possible abnormalities.

You should have your first mammogram when you're between ages 35 and 40—the earlier the better if you have a family history of breast cancer, previous biopsies or a record of breast problems. Between 40 and

When Your Breasts Are a Real Sore Spot

It's a couple days before your period, and you're feeling as bloated as the Sta-Puf Marshmallow Man. So, fitness devotee that you are, you decide to take a little jog.

That's when it strikes: the pain in your breasts that makes menstrual cramps seem like a day at Walt Disney World. What's going on here? It's breast tenderness—usually beginning at the time of ovulation and continuing until your period. Caused by hormonal variations, this pain can be so intense during this time that some women can't stand to lie on their stomachs.

"Some researchers believe it's set off by the fluid that accumulates in the breast," notes Kathleen Mayzel, M.D., assistant clinical professor of surgery at Tufts University School of Medicine and director of the Faulkner Breast Center, both in Boston.

50, you should have a mammogram every one to two years. After 50, doctors say, you should have a mammogram done annually, according to Dr. Baick. In his practice, which is predominantly a population of women ages 65 and younger, Dr. Baick estimates that 50 percent of those diagnosed are women between the ages of 45 and 50. "That's a very, very vulnerable age." Among those women, about 50 percent of their cancers were diagnosed by mammography. He has found mammography a very valuable tool in diagnosing breast cancer, even in these younger women.

What can you do when breast pain reigns? Here are a few tips.

Oil up. In her practice Dr. Mayzel and her associates have found that evening primrose oil can work for many patients with breast pain. She recommends taking three capsules a day, spaced out over the course of the day. They are available in health food stores. Women have to take these for about three months before they see a benefit, Dr. Mayzel notes.

Eat a pepper. Bioflavonoids, which are found in foods like buckwheat, alfalfa sprouts, green and red peppers and berries, are great at modulating the body's estrogen, notes Susan Lark, M.D., a physician in private practice in Los Altos, California, and author of The Woman's Health Companion. You can even get bioflavonoids in supplement form. Dr. Lark recommends getting 800 to 2,000 milligrams a day, taken with meals or a snack.

The Breast Defense

Even if you're a childless, postmenopausal woman over 50 whose mother and sister had breast cancer, it's not at all certain that you'll get the disease.

Studies show that a healthy lifestyle—meaning a low-fat diet that's high in fiber and fruits and vegetables, as well as regular exercise—can help make a difference.

"Prevention has to apply to everyone," observes Kim Westerlind, Ph.D., research scientist at the AMC Cancer Research Center in Denver. "Right now, early detection is what we have, along with healthy diet and physical activity."

Though there is a gene that predisposes some women to early onset breast and ovarian cancer, the majority of us can take steps to reduce our risk. Here are some tactics that doctors recommend to improve your chances of staying cancer-free.

Stop chewing the fat. Cutting down on dietary fat has a powerful protective effect on hormones, which are linked with breast cancer, notes Jon Michnovicz, M.D., Ph.D., president of the Foundation for Preventive Oncology in New York City and author of *How to Reduce Your Risk of Breast Cancer*.

"I recommend getting 20 percent of calories or less from fat a day, plus adding more fruits and vegetables," he says. With those simple changes in diet, hundreds of thousands of women could avoid getting cancer. In China and Japan, where the diets are based on low-fat staples such as rice and fish, women get breast cancer at only 10 to 15 percent the rate of women in the United States, he notes.

A 1994 study by researchers at the Stanley S. Scott Cancer Center at Louisiana State University Medical Center in New Orleans supports the view that a low-fat diet is one way to reduce your cancer risk. In that study doctors compared 40 women who had breast cancer with 40 women without breast cancer of the same age, weight and waist size. In the group that had cancer, researchers found, 45 percent had a higher level of deep abdominal fat.

Although some doctors argue that obesity rather than dietary fat affects breast cancer risk, Dr. Michnovicz disagrees. "Diet is an independent protective factor against breast cancer. Dietary fat and body fat are two sides of the same coin. It's the people who eat relatively low-fat and low calories and are thin who have a low cancer rate."

Can those beers. Staying away from alcohol seems to have some benefit, notes Dr. Kushi. "Among all the diet-related things you can do, the evidence is strongest for cutting out alcohol," he says. "If you look at all the studies, even a little bit of alcohol—a few times a week or more—increases the risk."

A 1995 study in a four-state area compared the drinking habits of 6,662 women who had breast cancer with the habits of 9,163 healthy women. Results showed that compared with women who had no alcoholic drinks, those who had one alcoholic drink a day were 1.3 times more likely to get breast cancer. Those who consumed two drinks a day were 1.7 times more likely to get breast cancer. The women who downed three drinks a day were over twice as likely to get the disease.

Load up on wheat bran. Making wheat-bran fiber part of your diet is another way to eat yourself healthy, notes Dr. Michnovicz. When you eat insoluble fiber—the kind that's in wheat bran—estrogen gets bound up in your stool and therefore leaves your body, he notes. Whole-wheat bread or pitas and tabbouleh made of cracked wheat are other good sources of wheat bran.

Top up your total fiber, too. "You need 25 to 35 grams of fiber a day," says Dr. Michnovicz. Some especially good choices for boosting your total fiber are foods like carrots, squash and cantaloupe, notes George Liepa, Ph.D., professor of nutrition and food sciences at Texas Woman's University in Denton. "Carrots have lignin, a food compound that binds to some troublesome hormones and carries them out of the body with the feces." Like some compounds found in wheat bran, complex carbohydrates in carrots have been shown to help reduce some estrogen metabolites in your body.

Get an A. Some studies have shown that vitamin A may be a good tool in the prevention of cancer, notes Dr. Liepa. In food, this vitamin comes in the form of beta-carotene, which is in many orange- and yellow-colored fruits and vegetables and in dark leafy greens. Dr. Liepa recommends eating foods that are rich in the vitamin rather than taking supplements, because you get a lot more than just beta-carotene. "There are many other compounds in that carrot that a vitamin pill doesn't contain." Many of these other carotenoids are also reported to have some cancer-fighting effects. Dried apricots, beet greens, broccoli, kale and spinach are just a few foods that rate an A in the carotenoid department.

Take a hike. Aerobic exercise just might put breast cancer on the run, notes Dr. Westerlind. "The bottom line in all diseases is that physical activity is a good thing." Try to incorporate walking, biking, swimming, aerobics or some other form of activity into your daily life. "Thirty minutes of moderate-intensity physical activity seven days a week is the ideal."

Pass the olive oil. Using olive oil instead of your standard golden cooking liquid could cut your breast cancer risk, says Dimitrios Trichopoulos, M.D., professor of cancer prevention and epidemiology at the Harvard School of Public Health. There is about 40 percent less breast cancer in Mediterranean countries, where olive oil is a dietary staple, than in the West, he says. "Olive oil also contains plenty of vitamin E, an important antioxidant."

In a Harvard study of Mediterranean women, scientists examined the diets and breast cancer rates of 2,368 women in Greece. The study showed that women who used olive oil more than once a day had a 25 percent lower risk of breast cancer than those who used it less often.

Favor fruits. Having a diet rich in vegetables and fruits—several servings a day—is another good idea, notes Dr. Trichopoulos. "Mediterraneans consume three times as many as Americans." Studies show that women who favor a diet rich in vegetables and fruits have a substantially lower breast cancer rate than those who don't eat them. The extent of protection depends on the amount people eat.

Bring in the phytochemicals. Eating vegetables rich in phytochemicals—cancer-fighting plant chemicals—is a potent weapon against breast cancer, notes Dr. Kushi. These chemicals compete with the binding sites in your body where estrogens start the cancer-producing cycle. So the phytochemicals help alter your estrogen metabolism. Soybeans are a rich source of phytoestrogens, as are other legumes and whole grains.

Beware of pesty-cides. You should also try to avoid environmental estrogens that can also increase breast cancer risk, notes Dr. Kushi. These include pesticides, which can come in contact with your food and water supply. "Eat organically grown food and wash off all your fruits and vegetables if you don't. Have your water tested for pesticides and put a water filter on your tap."

Investigate your HRT. If you are considering hormone replacement therapy (HRT), consider the severity of your menopausal symptoms, your breast cancer risk and your risk for heart disease and osteoporosis, says William Dupont, Ph.D., professor of preventive medicine and biostatistics at Vanderbilt University School of Medicine in Nashville. These are powerful hormones that can have an immediate effect on a woman's quality of life. She must consider all the possible benefits and risks to her entire health in making her decision, he observes.

A 1995 Harvard study of 121,700 female nurses showed that women currently on HRT and who have used it for five to nine years had a 46 percent greater risk of getting breast cancer than those who went through menopause without any kind of hormone therapy. Women over age 60 were especially at risk. The combination of progestin with estrogen did not reduce the risk.

Snack on salmon. Eating a serving of cold-water fish twice a week is another good way to stay healthy, says Dr. Liepa. "Fish oil does its bit to improve the immune system. Omega-3 fats, found in oily ocean fish like salmon, are the best. The Japanese eat a lot of that, and they have a significantly lower number of breast cancers than we do." Trout and water-packed tuna are also good sources of omega-3's.

See also Gynecological Exam, Medical Tests, Reproductive System

Cervix

THE CERVIX IS A CRITICAL PART of your reproductive system. It serves as the passageway between your vagina and uterus.

If you simply insert your finger almost to the back of your vagina, you can probably touch it. If you've never had a baby, your cervix will most likely feel like a nose with a small dimple in it. After you've been pregnant and had a child, though, your cervix changes; it may feel more like a chin.

While it may seem like the cervix is part of your vagina, it's actually the very lower portion of your uterus—the hollow, muscular organ that sheds monthly menstrual blood if you're not pregnant and provides a home for a developing fetus if you are. The dimple that you can feel, which extends into the vagina, is actually the opening to the cervical canal.

Normally, the cervical opening and canal are no larger than a very thin straw, so a foreign object like a tampon can't make its way into the uterus. But during childbirth, the opening expands tremendously in order to allow a baby to pass through.

The cervical canal is also responsible for producing cervical mucus. Around the time a woman ovulates, the thin, slippery mucus makes it easier for sperm to enter the uterus. During pregnancy the cells of the canal build a mucus plug, sealing off the uterus and protecting the fetus from any harmful substances.

Flare-ups and Troublemakers

While your cervix can remain healthy throughout your reproductive life, it is suscep-

tible to infection, sexually transmitted diseases (STDs), precancerous changes and cancer.

One common problem that can arise is cervicitis, or inflammation of the cervix. This may be caused by some type of irritation—wearing a tampon too long, for example, or an infection caused by either a virus or bacteria, says Mark Dignan, Ph.D., associate professor in the Department of Family and Community Medicine at the Bowman Gray School of Medicine of Wake Forest University in Winston-Salem, North Carolina. STDs such as trichomonas vaginalis, chlamydia and genital herpes virus can trigger cervicitis. So can having a baby.

The sexually transmitted disease known as the human papillomavirus (HPV), more commonly known as genital warts, can also affect the cervix, says Dr. Dignan. When a woman has HPV, small bumps or warts are likely to grow on the folds of skin around the entrance to the vagina. These warts can also grow directly on the cervix. Certain strains of HPV have been associated with the development of cervical cancer.

Cervical dysplasia can also lead to the development of some cancerous cells, and it's a condition that has to be watched carefully by a doctor. If you have cervical dysplasia, the cells that make up cervical tissue start to change, according to James Davidson, M.D., assistant professor of obstetrics and gynecology at the Truman Medical Center in Kansas City and the University of Missouri-Kansas City. He says that the condition can range from mild to severe, depending on how extensive the cell changes are on the lining of the cervix.

With severe dysplasia cells change throughout the cervix lining. The cells start to look like cancer cells but don't behave like them, says Dr. Davidson.

Cervical cancer is the third most common gynecological cancer. Approximately 16,000 women develop cancer of the cervix every year, and less than one-third that number die from it. Early detection with a Pap smear is critically important, because it can prevent death from cervical cancer. (For more information on what to expect from a Pap test—and how often to have it done—see page 220.)

Meanwhile, here's what you can do to guard your cervical health.

Practice safe sex. Do your best to prevent STDs and cervical cancer by engaging in safe sex, experts say. That means limiting the number of sex partners you have and knowing your partner's history and STD status before you have sex. (Yes, safe sex means really getting to know someone well.)

If you and your partner are not monogamous, or if one of you already has HPV, the best insurance is to make sure he wears a condom and uses it correctly. You can also reduce your risk of STDs by using an effective spermicide—such as nonoxynol 9—and by using a diaphragm. (For more information on protecting yourself against STDs, see page 341.)

Get your Pap test. The Pap smear is the screening test most doctors use to examine the health of the cervix and look for cervical cancer and some of its precursors, as well as STDs and dysplasia. This test is part of routine gynecological care, so if your doctor doesn't tell you she's doing it, you may not be able to tell. The doctor simply takes a sample of tissue from your cervix and stores it on a slide that will be examined at a laboratory.

The test isn't 100 percent accurate all the time, but it catches 60 to 85 percent of abnormalities—giving you the chance to get earlier treatment.

Pay attention to unusual symptoms. If you experience painful intercourse, an un-usual or odd-smelling discharge, bleeding after intercourse, pelvic pain or unexpected bleeding, call your doctor and tell her what's going on. These are all signs that there may be a problem, says Dr. Dignan.

Test for risky strains. If you have genital warts or HPV—one of the most common types of STDs in the United States—there's a test that shows whether you have one of the three strains of HPV that put you at higher risk for cervical cancer. Be sure to ask your doctor if you need this HPV test to determine whether your type of HPV causes cancer.

Go for the fruits and veggies. Research indicates that folic acid, or folate—a B vitamin found in certain fruits and vegetables—may help decrease the risk of cervical cancer.

Women can maintain proper levels of folate by eating yellow and green leafy vegetables, citrus fruits, juices, yeast and liver. Or go for a supplement: The Daily Value is 400 micrograms, which is the amount contained in many multivitamins.

Give up the butts. Cigarette smoking places you at higher risk for dysplasia, so do your best to cut back or cut the habit altogether.

See also Reproductive System, Sexually Transmitted Diseases

Childbirth

■ **REMEMBER YOUR FIRST LOOK AT MOM?**

Okay, so maybe that wasn't so memorable. You may have been somewhat confused, since everything outside the womb was kind of new at that point.

Well, then, how about this? Do you remember whether it was a windowed room with nice curtains or a sterile delivery room with a definite pallor to the decor? Do you remember whether Dad was there—bothered, bewildered and bemused, but present at the bedside? And, say, how about Mom's bed? Was it a comfy-looking Sealy Posturepedic or something more along the lines of a stirruped platform designed for your longitudinal plunge into the cold, cruel world?

Of course, there might not have been so many environmental options when you were born. But there are now. If you're an expectant mother—looking ahead to those none-too-glamorous hours leading up to childbirth—you're likely to hear quite a bit about your delivery options.

Choosing Your Team

What type of health care professional is right for you? To figure that out, you need to know whether yours is considered a high-risk pregnancy.

If you have no preexisting medical problem that is likely to be a problem for you or your baby, you could choose a nurse midwife, says Teresa Marsico, certified nurse midwife and associate professor at the University of Medicine and Dentistry of New Jersey–New

Not all health professionals receive the same medical training or have similar philosophies about pregnancy and childbirth. Here's an overview of the different types of health professionals you can choose from.

Obstetrician. This is a doctor with a medical degree (M.D. or D.O.) who has received special training in taking care of pregnant women and delivering babies. Obstetricians are skilled at surgery, which might be necessary if your pregnancy develops complications. An obstetrician can do a cesarean section, the surgical procedure in which a woman's abdomen and uterus are opened surgically to remove the baby.

Family medical doctor. A family practitioner has a medical degree, but usually not the same additional specialized training of an obstetrician.

Nurse midwife. In the view of nurse midwives, pregnancy and childbirth should be as natural as possible, according to Marion McCartney, a certified nurse midwife who is president of the National Association of Childbirth Centers in Bethesda, Maryland. Nurse midwives use natural methods of pain relief and do not perform cesarean sections. They may either be lay nurse midwives—who have no formal training and certification—or certified registered nurses who have completed a rigorous national certification program and completed national boards in nurse midwifery. Licensed midwives undergo national training programs that can vary in quality from state to state, but they are not necessarily registered nurses.

Any of these health professionals can do an episiotomy—the procedure of making an incision in the perineum—the skin between the vagina and rectum—to create a larger opening for delivering the baby.

Jersey Medical School in Newark.

But high risk is a different matter. If you have medical conditions such as diabetes or high blood pressure that complicate your pregnancy, you really need to have an obstetrician manage your care. And if your prenatal exams show that you're having twins, that's another reason to choose an obstetrician.

During your initial screening for pregnancy, either a medical doctor or a certified nurse midwife can tell you whether you're in the high-risk category, according to Charles S. Mahan, M.D., dean of the College of Public Health and professor of obstetrics and gynecology at the University of South Florida in Tampa. If you are, then you'll be referred to an obstetrician or perinatologist. If you don't fit into the high-risk category, you can choose an obstetrician, family doctor or midwife—depending on which one you feel comfortable with and which agrees with your philosophy and attitude about birth.

Better yet, you may be able to have both. Many doctors and nurse midwives work collaboratively. Most states require that each birthing center be affiliated with a hospital, with obstetricians who can take over the management of complicated pregnancies.

Doctors and midwives may also work together in hospital settings, says David Kliot, M.D., clinical associate professor of obstetrics and gynecology at State University of New York Health Science Center at Brooklyn. A woman who goes to a certified nurse midwife and an obstetrician can have the best of both worlds, agrees Marsico.

Choosing Your Birth Setting

If you do have the birth-center option, it can be attractive. Birth centers are often located in renovated homes, where each birthing room has a bed surrounded by regular furniture. It's a very homelike atmosphere, sometimes with extra amenities like tubs and whirlpools for use during labor.

The Company You Keep

Perhaps you want your husband with you during labor. Or you might want other members of your family there, such as your mother or sister.

There are other options, too, according to Linda Herrick, R.N., co-director and founder of the Academy of Certified Birth Educators in Olathe, Kansas, an organization that trains and certifies professionals who teach childbirth preparation classes. Your support person might be a professional labor support specialist, also known as a doula. The term originated in Greece, where the woman with the highest stature in the household was the doula or caregiver. It was her assignment to attend to the psychological and physical needs of the woman giving birth. Today, women can hire doulas to be with them during labor and delivery.

These support specialists do not take the place of the woman's husband or prime support person, says Herrick. Instead, they are there as an adjunct to attend to the woman's nonmedical needs.

In one study women who had a professional doula present during labor had fewer complications, shorter labors, fewer interventions and fewer epidurals than women who did not have a labor support specialist, says Herrick.

To find a labor support specialist in your area, contact Doulas of North America (DONA) at (500)448-DONA or write to 1100 23rd Avenue E, Seattle, WA 98112.

Your husband and support persons, including children, are allowed to be in the birthing room with you. When you arrive at a birth center in labor, you're usually greeted by the nurse midwife who stays with you throughout the birth process.

The birthing rooms contain very simple equipment. "It's low-tech, high-touch," says Ruth Lubic, Ed.D., certified nurse midwife and general director of the Maternity Center Association in New York City. Midwives don't use electronic fetal monitoring to check the child's position. Instead, they use a stethoscope or a procedure called a noninvasive Doppler ultrasound to monitor the baby's progress. And the mother can use breathing, spend time in a warm tub or get massage for pain relief.

The birth center is arranged so that you can be transferred quickly to a hospital, if necessary. About 12 percent of women who try to give birth in a birth center get transferred to a hospital, says Marsico.

The Hospitable Hospital

Unlike birth centers, hospitals have on hand the equipment and personnel to handle complicated pregnancies or deliveries that go awry. And that's critical when speed is a factor.

"All of us who have practiced obstetrics have seen this happy, wonderful situation turn into a disaster in a matter of seconds," says Edward Linn, M.D., chairman of obstetrics and gynecology at Lutheran General Hospital in Chicago. "It could be your life or your child's life. I'm not saying birthing centers are bad. I'm saying most of us are uncomfortable with their ability to handle these emergency situations."

At a hospital you'll probably be greeted by a nurse or a medical resident whom you

don't know, says Dr. Kliot. Your doctor may check in now and then, but chances are she will not be with you throughout all the stages of labor.

"When a woman calls and says she is starting labor, a midwife goes and stays with her for the entire labor," says Dr. Mahan. "As an obstetrician, I don't do that."

In the hospital electronic fetal monitoring is often used: Sensors are taped to your abdomen, and an electronic device measures your baby's heart rate and vital signs, tracking the readings on a monitor. Your labor can be monitored from the nurses station rather than from your bedside. Recent studies have shown, however, that electronic fetal monitoring is not really helpful in low-risk pregnancies, says Dr. Mahan. Some experts now believe that it is better to have a nurse stay at a woman's bedside to monitor her and the baby during labor.

The old standard—a big sterile operating room with lots of lights—is not the typical hospital experience anymore, says Lawrence Devoe, M.D., professor of obstetrics and gynecology and director of maternal fetal medicine at the Medical College of Georgia in Augusta. "Most hospitals use labor and delivery rooms that look like real rooms. They have attractive decor, tables and beds that look like real furniture."

A Room for You

If you do have a choice of birth settings, what are the factors to consider? Here's what experts say.

Go with what's comfortable. If you're considering a birth center, you should be really comfortable with the center's approach and philosophy, says Dr. Lubic. Emotions can affect the labor, she points out. If you'd feel

Don't Be Query-less

A hospital can be a confusing place, and you'll have enough to do during labor without worrying about what comes next. So if you're going for a hospital delivery, get some questions answered ahead of time. Here are some questions to ask, suggested by David Kliot, M.D., clinical associate professor of obstetrics and gynecology at State University of New York Health Science Center at Brooklyn.

- Who will greet me when I arrive?
- Who will evaluate me and check me in when I am in labor?
- Who will be with me throughout the entire labor?
- How is the labor monitored?
- Can my support person be with me?
- Will I be allowed to eat during labor?
- Will I have an intravenous feeding as a matter of routine? When?
- Can I walk around while in labor?
- Where will I be (the birthing room, the labor room)?
- Who will be making the decisions?
- If I have a lot of pain, will I get medication? Anesthesia? If so, what type?
- Will I get to hold the baby right away?
- How long will I stay in the hospital afterward?
- Are there restrictions on having visitors?

Go for orientation. Birth centers typically require an orientation to let you evaluate the risks, says Dr. Lubic. If you go to the orientation and ask questions, you'll find out if it's right for you.

Check out the hospital. If you decide to have your baby in a hospital, ask questions about how the labor will be handled, says Dr. Kliot. The more information you get beforehand, the better.

Labor Negotiations

Chances are when your grandma had her babies, she didn't take a childbirth preparation class. These classes are a relatively new invention—for the couples who learn about labor and childbirth from books, doctors and TV shows rather than firsthand family experience.

When your mom was pregnant, she probably went off to the hospital and came back a few days later with a baby, notes Dr. Linn. As a result, this generation of women often knows little about the details.

Childbirth preparation classes have differing approaches and philosophies. But the same core material is covered in nearly all classes, according to Linda Herrick, R.N., co-director and founder of the Academy of Certified Birth Educators in Olathe, Kansas, an organization that trains and certifies professionals who teach the classes. In most classes you'll learn about the phases of labor, your options for pain relief and comfort, relaxation techniques you can use to make labor easier and what role your support person can play in your labor, she says.

But the classes often support a basic childbirth philosophy or approach. There are essentially four methods of childbirth preparation—Grantley Dick Read, Bradley,

more secure with a medical team and equipment on hand, then you should probably choose a hospital instead.

Watch the feedback. Recognize that the input and feedback you get from family and friends can have an impact on you, says Marsico. If you are going to a birth center, and your husband says, "I don't know about this," that could build doubt.

Lamaze and Sheila Kitzinger. Many classes either draw on several of these methods or all of them, says Herrick.

Method Acting

Grantley Dick Read was one of the first people to introduce childbirth preparation. In Read's view, labor and birth involve fear, tension and pain. If a woman is afraid, she will tense her muscles, triggering an increase of pain. Read decided that if the fear/tension cycle could be interrupted, pain could be lessened. He used education, relaxation techniques and medication to help break the cycle, says Herrick.

In the early 1950s Robert Bradley, M.D., introduced his method saying, "Let's involve the partner in the labor and delivery process."

"With the Bradley method the husband is brought in as a trained labor coach," says Marjie Hathaway, executive director of the Bradley Method at the American Academy of Husband-Coached Childbirth (AAHCC) in Sherman Oaks, California, and a Bradley instructor for 30 years. "We want men trained in how to help wives give birth. We teach the partner how to rub his wife's back, how to help her find positions that will be comfortable and how to communicate with the birth team. He can be an advocate for her in labor so she can have the birth she wants and needs." Across the country, the Bradley method results in about 87 percent unmedicated births, says Hathaway. Bradley classes emphasize good coaching, relaxation and tuning in to your body as ways to deal with the challenges of labor instead of medication.

With the Lamaze method, a woman uses breathing and relaxation techniques as ways of reducing pain. As a matter of fact, Lamaze advocates say that proper breathing is a key to minimizing labor pain.

Sheila Kitzinger, an English social anthropologist, felt that sexuality is a major factor with a new mother. She added a marriage counseling component to childbirth education.

Choosing Your Prep School

Whatever childbirth preparation classes you choose, doctors and midwives agree that you definitely should sign up for *some* class and go to it. "The prepared individual tends to deal better with childbirth," says Dr. Linn.

Here are some pointers on finding a class and graduating with honors.

Start class early. Seek out your childbirth preparation class very early in your pregnancy, says Herrick. Some women don't seek prenatal or childbirth care until the middle or latter stages of pregnancy.

Match your philosophy. Find a prenatal class that fits with your overall philosophy about pregnancy and childbirth, says Herrick.

Look for variety. Does the class emphasize only one childbirth preparation method? Does the class advocate one method of pain relief or one approach to breastfeeding? It's an advantage to be in a program that offers a variety of choices, says Herrick. To find out, call before the class begins.

Look for flexibility. Flexible class hours could be a factor in your choice, says Herrick. Is it offered only on weeknights, or are there weekend classes, too? Are there classes throughout the entire course of pregnancy or only in the third trimester?

Shop around. Some classes are sponsored by hospitals, others are offered through a provider's practice, while still others are independent. Check out the different options, says Herrick. "We're talking about one of the most important events in your life."

Find out who's teaching the class and what is covered in the curriculum, agrees Dr. Devoe.

Watch out for bias. Some childbirth preparation classes are sponsored by the hospital in which they are held and therefore have a conflict of interest, says Dr. Mahan. You should find out who funds the class and ask whether the teacher presents all options.

Understanding Your Labor

Many women are concerned about whether they will know when they are in labor, says Marsico. "Labor in and of itself is so individual," she says. Even with the same person, labor with one child can be different than it is with another. But even though nobody can predict exactly what your labor and delivery will be like, it usually has three stages, and there are distinct changes that take place during each of those stages. Being familiar with those stages beforehand can help you know what to expect.

Stage one begins at the start of labor and continues until the cervix is completely dilated. During this stage there are two phases, the latent and the active, says Dr. Linn.

In the latent phase the cervix thins out and is taken up into the uterus. This is known as effacement. Contractions at this time are usually mild, occurring every 15 to 20 minutes and lasting about 60 to 90 seconds. Gradually, the contractions become more regular until they're happening about every 5 minutes. The cervix dilates to about four centimeters, which is a little more than an inch.

During the active phase contractions become much stronger and more frequent, coming about every three minutes and lasting about 45 seconds apiece.

Usually, you can tell the difference between the contractions that take place in stage one of labor and the Braxton Hicks contractions that you might get off and on during pregnancy, says Dr. Linn. Braxton Hicks contractions tend to be irregular and, while the uterus may tighten, the contractions are not particularly painful, he says.

The contractions of labor tend to be painful. They build up, go away and then, over a period of time, become regular. When you're in labor, the contractions become more regular, occurring closer together, says Dr. Linn.

The second stage of labor ranges from the time the cervix is completely dilated to when the baby is born. When the cervix dilates, reaching a width of ten centimeters (about three fingers' width), the baby starts to move down the birth canal and out of the mother's body. This movement is urged on with strong contractions that occur about two to five minutes apart, lasting between 60 and 90 seconds. It's also at this time that the mother can begin pushing.

The third and last stage of labor involves the delivery of the afterbirth, or placenta.

Delivering the Goods

Advice varies about when a woman should come into the hospital or birth center. "If it is an uncomplicated pregnancy, and the bag of waters is intact, I tell patients to come in when their contractions are ten minutes apart," Dr. Linn says.

Despite the many differences in the pace of labor, there are some things that every woman can do to be prepared for the coming hours.

Drink up. Many women stop eating and drinking, says Dr. Linn, but it's important to keep hydrated with juices and water. "I tell them 12 ounces every hour, because you keep losing so much water. When you are dehydrated, the contractions can get stronger without it really being true labor."

Reach for energy boosters. Juices that have natural sugars in them (such as orange juice), warm tea with sugar or hot cocoa helps boost your energy. You need that for your body to work, notes Marsico.

Position yourself. Changing positions during labor can make labor easier and less painful, experts say.

Pain, Pain, Go Away

It's no laughing matter having your baby's head and body pass through and out your vagina. That head is about the size of a grapefruit.

One thing to consider beforehand is whether you want any kind of pain relief.

And if so, what kind?

A nurse midwife is likely to encourage pain relief with certain breathing techniques. During labor the midwife might encourage you to walk around, or she might apply warm compresses to help relieve pain. You may have the option of using the showers, tub or whirlpool at the birth center—or perhaps getting a comforting massage.

If your caregiver is a physician and you are delivering in a hospital, one option you'll have is pain relief in the form of a pain-numbing epidural. This medication is injected into the space that surrounds the spinal canal through a tube that is inserted between the vertebrae of the backbone. While an epidural is generally considered a very safe form of anesthesia, some possible risks are involved, says Dr. Linn. If the injection penetrates the covering of the spinal canal (known as the

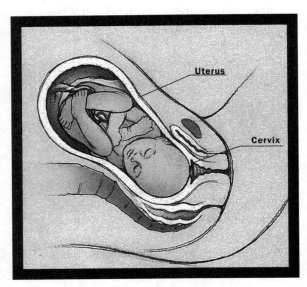

The dilation stage of childbirth begins with the onset of labor. Contractions force the baby's head against the cervix. The cervix softens, becomes thinner and dilates.

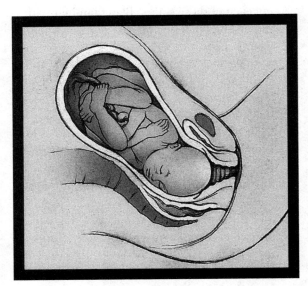

As the dilation stage continues, the baby continues descending down the birth canal. The baby's head rotates as it enters the pelvic outlet.

dura), the patient might experience a postanesthetic headache. The patient's blood pressure may also drop after the epidural is administered. This can usually be controlled, however, by the anesthesiologist without complication.

Having an epidural may also make the second stage of labor more difficult, because it's hard to push effectively if you don't feel anything from the waist down. Dr. Linn points out that this may increase your chance of having a cesarean section or needing the assistance of forceps or vacuum extraction. "Patient selection is critical in the safe and effective use of an epidural," he says.

The Undercut

Should you have an episiotomy? Do you need one?

An episiotomy is a small cut that's made in the skin between the vagina and rectum—the perineum—to allow an easier and less painful delivery. The incision enlarges the vaginal opening so that the baby's head can pass through more easily.

Whether episiotomies are good or bad, necessary or unnecessary, all depends on the health care professional you talk to. Some are adamantly against them, while others think they are okay if that's what a woman wants.

Episiotomies are intended to prevent the vaginal opening from tearing on its own during childbirth. But there is no evidence that the procedure prevents severe tears of the perineum. "Contrary to conventional teaching and beliefs, episiotomies seem to cause the very problems that they are intended to prevent," says Michael C. Klein, M.D., professor of family practice and

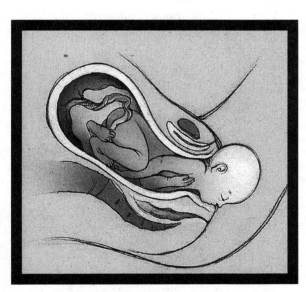

At expulsion stage the cervix is fully dilated and strong contractions occur every two to three minutes, each lasting about one minute.

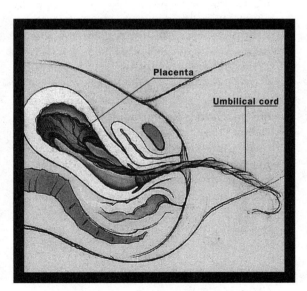

Placenta

Umbilical cord

In the placental stage, the placenta separates from the wall of the uterus as uterine contractions continue. This stage usually happens about 15 minutes after the baby is born.

Too Soon for Sex?

How soon do you want to have sex after childbirth?

Women have all sorts of preferences, says Sharon Dobie, M.D., assistant professor in the Department of Family Medicine at the University of Washington in Seattle. "Some women say they don't have any sex for six weeks."

"It is prudent not to be sexually active while you are still bleeding, because there may be a little bit more risk of infection," says Dr. Dobie. After you have stopped bleeding, however, you can start having sex whenever you want to. Most episiotomies, lacerations or hemorrhoids will be resolved by six weeks postpartum, she says.

"Some women feel like resuming intercourse after three to four weeks if they had no episiotomy or lacerations. As long as a woman's perineum is reasonably healed and it's comfortable—not painful—to be sexually active, then it's okay to be sexually active," Dr. Dobie says. "But my bottom line with patients is, you don't need to be sexually active until you feel like it."

If you're not ready to be sexually active, find ways to maintain a sense of emotional intimacy with your partner, suggests Dr. Dobie. "If you are breastfeeding and not feeling interested in sexual activity, remember that hugs and other kinds of touches and good communication can still keep a couple close during the time of adjustment."

pediatrics at the University of British Columbia in Vancouver.

Dr. Klein and his colleagues studied 697 women in three hospitals shortly after they had given birth and then again three months later. The researchers found that women who'd had episiotomies were more likely to have tears that ran to or through the rectum. "It's much easier to tear a piece of cloth that's already been cut than to tear one that's intact," Dr. Klein explains. "Once the episiotomy is done, the tissue's integrity has been disrupted."

Even if a woman has a spontaneous tear during childbirth, it's preferable to having an episiotomy, according to Dr. Klein. His study showed that the women who had spontaneous tears or who remained intact had less pain, fewer sexual problems and less pelvic floor weakness than the women who had episiotomies.

The Case for Cutting

Some doctors, however, view episiotomies as a means for preventing pain and problems rather than causing them. Years ago, when women had six or more children, all the pushing that went along with that amount of childbirth was believed to traumatize the pelvic wall and cause prolapsed uterus and bladder problems later in life. So doctors started doing the incision as a means to prevent trauma to the pelvic wall, says Dr. Linn.

But women don't have as many children now as they used to, and they are in much better shape, says Dr. Mahan. "Episiotomies should be avoided as much as possible," he concludes. "Even a small tear will be more comfortable when all is said and done than an episiotomy."

Still other doctors think it really is a woman's choice. "Women need to think about what they want," says Sharon Dobie, M.D., assistant professor in the Department of Family Medicine at the University of Washington in Seattle. "My approach is to cut an episiotomy if a woman really wants one, but most of my patients would prefer to not have one." Dr. Dobie says she is able to do most deliveries without cutting episiotomies.

A Checkup on Cesarean Section

While the decision to perform a cesarean is usually not made until labor has begun, your doctor should be able to explain the most likely reasons for doing one, says Dr. Devoe.

You're most likely to need a first-time cesarean if labor has not progressed the way it should or if labor hasn't occurred when it should, says Dr. Devoe. Or a cesarean might be performed if the fetus is in distress, if the doctor thinks the baby can't tolerate prolonged labor or if the baby isn't getting enough oxygen.

But there may be steps you can take to try to lower your chances of needing a cesarean section. Here's what experts suggest.

Check the track record. Make sure you don't choose a doctor who has a high rate of cesarean deliveries, says Dr. Mahan. For some doctors the rate is as high as 50 percent, even though it should be closer to 15 percent, he says. And it's important to find out the doctor's individual rate, not just the hospital's overall rate.

Check other sources. You can check with outside sources to find out your doctor's cesarean rate, according to Dr. Mahan. "I'd refer women to a local childbirth education group or La Leche League," he says. (La Leche League International is a private organization that provides education, information and support to mothers and health care workers interested in breastfeeding. To learn more about their services and publications, you can contact them at 1-800-LA-LECHE.)

These sources will be happy to tell you a doctor's cesarean section rates.

Be sure you can move. One way to lessen your chance of a cesarean is to be sure you will be able to walk and move around during the course of labor, says Dr. Mahan.

Breastfeeding: Giving Nature's Fast Food

For babies the myriad advantages of breastfeeding are well-known: It's cheap, safe, may protect against chronic diseases, helps prevent allergies, and it's more digestible than formula. For moms, breastfeeding not only saves time but also creates a special mother-child bond.

Breastfeeding could even save your life. A survey of 5,878 breast cancer patients and 8,216 healthy women showed that the risk of breast cancer among premenopausal women was 22 percent less for the women who had done breastfeeding. And the risk of breast cancer was lowest for women who had breastfed for the longest cumulative amount of time.

Breastfeeding gained popularity in the 1970s and 1980s, but by 1989 only half of mothers giving birth in hospitals were breastfeeding. One possible reason is that more women are working—and working more hours—so they have less time for breastfeeding. Also, some women complain of sore nipples related to nursing, and others use formula because they fear that the breast milk supply is inadequate.

Betty Crase, director of the Center for Breastfeeding Information at the La Leche League international headquarters in Schaumburg, Illinois, says that mothers should look on the bright side. "The human baby was designed to be breastfed, and the mother was designed to breastfeed. We urge every mother to give serious consideration to what both were designed to do."

Feeding Friendly

If you know you'd like to breastfeed but you're wary of potential problems, here are a few tips from experts to help you and your baby get off to a great start.

Don't worry, be happy. Many new moms believe that their milk supply is inadequate—but that's really because the milk supply declines naturally, according to Jane Anderson, M.D., associate clinical professor of pediatrics at the University of California, San Francisco. "For the first two to three weeks Mom makes enough milk for two babies. Then it goes down to enough for one," she says. "So Mom simply perceives it as less."

How can you tell if Junior's getting enough chow? Monitor that messy diaper activity, suggests Dr. Anderson. If your new infant urinates six times and has four to six bowel movements a day, that's an indication of adequate milk. Talk to your pediatrician if bowel movements and urination are less frequent than that.

You gotta give to get. To ensure plenty of breast milk, you need to provide regular nipple stimulation with suckling or manipulation by hand or pump, says Dr. Anderson.

"Mom needs to sit down and say, 'How many times did I nurse the baby today?'" Crase advises. "Newborns do it anywhere from 8 to 12 times during a 24-hour period. By six weeks, mother and baby are more in sync with each other, and breastfeeding becomes more regular."

Stay off the bottle. Although you can substitute bottle feedings with occasional breastfeedings later on, it's important not to do that for the first two to three weeks, says Dr. Anderson. Otherwise, you could develop an infection in your breast because milk isn't draining properly. Introducing a bottle so early can also confuse the baby, for whom drinking from a bottle is a lot easier than the natural way.

Show good form. Always make sure your baby has latched on to your breast properly, notes Dr. Anderson. The infant should be on her side with her head literally right in front of your nipple and horizontal to the floor, she says. "The legs need to be going straight across, pointed to your other breast. You don't want baby's leg dangling down, or the overall weight will pull on your breast and make it sore."

Check the latch. Another important style tip is to make sure the baby's taking a lot of the nipple into her mouth, says Dr. Anderson. The ducts coming down from the milk glands dilate under the areola, and the baby literally has to massage that area with her tongue and bring milk out to start the milk flow. Some women can feel a tingling sensation in the nipple as the milk comes down, but others don't.

Double-check your birth control. If you're using an oral contraceptive or Norplant while you're breastfeeding, be sure that it doesn't contain estrogen, which can affect the quantity and quality of breast milk. There are progesterone-only versions of the Pill and Norplant that don't affect your milk, so consult with your doctor.

Don't cut calories. Many women want to start shedding those extra pounds as soon as they give birth. But if you're breastfeeding, that's not a good idea, says Bonnie Worthington-Roberts, Ph.D., professor of nutrition at Ohio State University in Columbus. Even moderate calorie restriction can make it difficult for your body to produce adequate milk. It's also important to eat as varied a diet as possible. She suggests waiting six to eight weeks after giving birth to start cutting calories. By then your body is more used to the process of breastfeeding.

Drink plenty. A commonsense rule applies to fluid intake: Drink as much as you want. Since breastfeeding makes you thirstier, you'll probably find that you need to drink more fluids than before, doctors say.

But don't down caffeine. Try to stick with water, juices and other noncaffeinated beverages. Heavy caffeine consumption can cause your baby to be restless and jittery, says Dr. Worthington-Roberts.

Feed before you trot. The research is somewhat contradictory, but some studies indicate that exercise increases the amount of lactic acid in breast milk and that this may make milk taste sour, says Christine Wells, Ph.D., professor of exercise science and physical education at Arizona State University in Tempe and author of *Women, Sport and Performance.* So if you find that your baby has trouble breastfeeding right after you exercise, try switching your exercise session to after you breastfeed, she says.

See also Fertility, Pregnancy, Reproductive System

Chin

YOU MIGHT HAVE a textbook-perfect profile, but the chin can make or break it—depending on how firm the skin beneath it is, says Harold Clavin, M.D., plastic surgeon at the Medical Center of Santa Monica in California.

"People don't realize how important the chin is," says Dr. Clavin. "They don't look at their profiles, but the fact is, other people do."

Here are some ways to keep your chin looking firm.

Avoid neck-stretching exercises. Some cosmeticians recommend neck exercises to reduce sagging skin. If you followed their advice, you'd be craning your chin throughout the day. Overworking the delicate skin under your chin is exactly what you shouldn't do, according to Peter Bela Fodor, M.D., assistant professor of plastic surgery at University of California, Los Angeles. "It's stretching the skin, and it's all wrong."

Don't yo-yo. Repeated weight loss and weight gain stretches out neck skin, Dr. Fodor says. What was once a double chin eventually becomes excess skin if you get on the yo-yo diet merry-go-round. If you want to lose weight for good, the best solution is a regular aerobic exercise program and a low-fat diet. Avoid crash diets, Dr. Fodor advises. Once you take that weight off for good, the better chance you have of losing that sagging skin.

Hands off. Don't habitually tug on the skin under your chin, as ponderous types tend to do, says Dr. Clavin. "Believe me, that can stretch the skin," he notes.

Circulatory System

The circulatory system includes the heart, lungs and blood vessels. Through its network of veins and arteries, it carries life-giving blood loaded with oxygen and nutrients to all the muscles and organs in the body. The heart pumps bright red oxygenated blood out to the body through the arteries. Dark, depleted purplish blood returns to the heart and lungs through the veins, to be refueled with oxygen and sent out again for delivery.

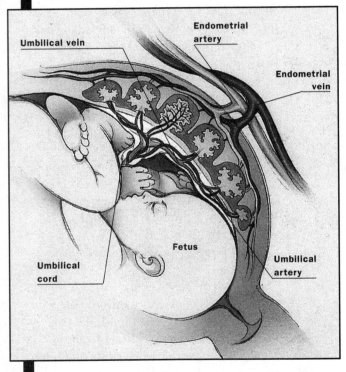

Umbilical vein

Endometrial artery

Endometrial vein

Umbilical artery

Fetus

Umbilical cord

The placenta connects a mother to her growing child by way of the umbilical cord. Through that connection everything a woman eats, drinks or breathes is passed on to the fetus. That's why smoking, drinking and taking some medications are dangerous during pregnancy.

■ The big **carotid arteries** in the neck carry blood to the brain. They're a prime spot for clot-induced stroke. You can lower your chances of stroke with an antioxidant-rich diet of fruits and vegetables. (See "Favor fresh veggies" on page 8.)

■ When the **aorta** narrows with fatty deposits or stiffens with age (or both), it's a principal cause of heart attack. Exercise can keep arteries fit and flexible. (See "Tone up for your arteries" on page 9.)

■ The **heart** is made of muscle. That means use it or lose it. A sedentary lifestyle is one of the risk factors for heart disease. Activity is essential. (For motivation, see "Get up and go" on page 170.)

■ The **veins in the legs** carry blood back to the heart for refueling. Women with varicose veins, though, have veins that get backed up with blood—they can look unsightly and make your legs ache. (To help foil varicose veins, see "Keeping Glorious Gams" on page 433.)

■ **Phlebitis** is an inflamed blood clot on a vein wall. It can be treated easily (see "Pressure to Perform" on page 431).

■ **High blood pressure** beats up the walls of arteries, leading to strokes and heart attacks. (To lower your numbers, see "Eating to Control Your Blood Pressure" on page 174.)

■ To find out what medical experts can read in a **blood test**, see "A Blood Test Primer" on page 32.

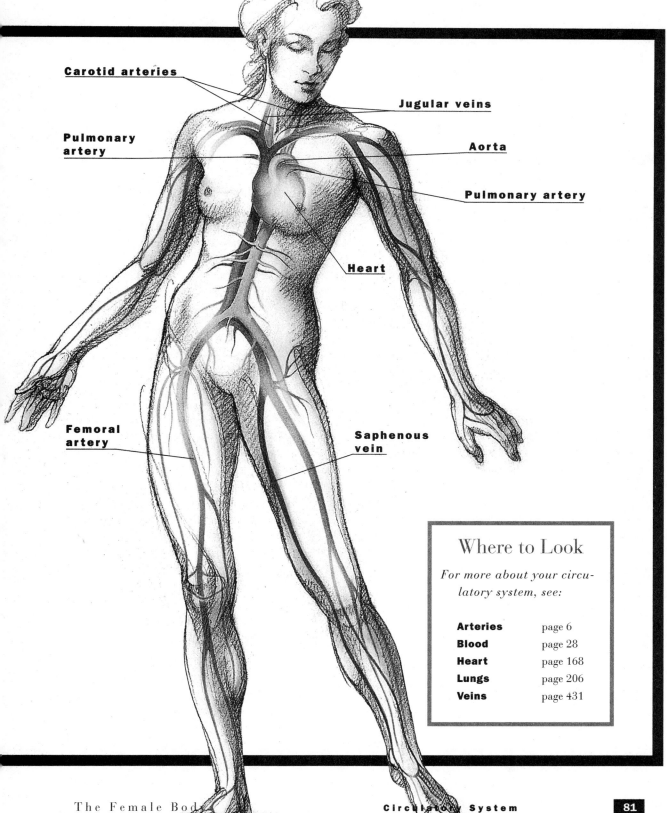

Carotid arteries

Jugular veins

Pulmonary artery

Aorta

Pulmonary artery

Heart

Femoral artery

Saphenous vein

Where to Look

For more about your circulatory system, see:

Arteries	page 6
Blood	page 28
Heart	page 168
Lungs	page 206
Veins	page 431

Clitoris

TRUE, WE DON'T NEED JOCKSTRAPS. But that's only because the female counterpart to the male penis comes much better wrapped than its "hangin'-out-there" male rival.

In other respects the female clitoris has exactly the same component parts as its male counterpart. Not only does it have the same number of nerve endings (researchers *have* counted!), it also has a head, or glans, which is extremely sensitive to the touch.

But back to the obvious difference—size. The clitoris, located at the top of the inside folds where your small and large vulvar lips come together, measures between three-quarters of an inch and two inches. It looks even smaller because it's bent over on itself, with only the head visible. And, unlike the penis, whose purpose is both for sex and urination, the main function of the clitoris is sexual pleasure.

When a woman is sexually aroused, her genital system gets swollen with blood, resulting in the erection of her clitoris. Also, like a man's penis, a woman's clitoris becomes erect about every 90 minutes that she's asleep.

See also Sex

Collarbone

SOME SAY THAT PROTRUDING COLLARBONES on a woman are sexy.

Others think they look sickly.

Whether or not you have prominent collarbones, these S-shaped bones all function the same way. When it comes right down to it, they are designed to hold your shoulders in place.

Your collarbones are located exactly where you'd expect them to be: right where the collar of your shirt fastens. This bony protrusion, the clavicle, extends in a long, S-shaped curve, to the shoulder joint, called the scapula, or shoulder blade. They're held together by ligaments.

People don't often dislocate a collarbone, because the ligaments holding the sternum and scapula are so strong. Fractures are more common. If you start to fall and put out your arm to catch yourself, the jolt gets absorbed all the way through your shoulder to your collarbone.

If you do get a fracture, you'll feel the pain—and your arm will feel like it's gone limp. "One way to tell is if you have direct tenderness over your collarbone," says Bruce Janiak, M.D., director of the Emergency Center at Toledo Hospital in Ohio. "If you have a suspicion, it is best to go get an x-ray."

In the past, fractured collarbones used to be treated by immobilizing the whole upper arm and shoulder area for several weeks. But this practice is changing, according to Dr. Janiak. He believes the collarbone can probably heal just as well on its own. So don't be surprised if the prescription is just "take it easy."

See also Skeletal System

Digestive System

Many interconnected organs digest and absorb the food we eat and rid the body of waste from that process. But problems can arise.

■ **Heartburn** is caused by a too-relaxed muscle at the bottom of the esophagus. (See "Eat small, eat early" on page 107.)

■ **Ulcers** are caused when the lining of the stomach erodes. (See "A Whole Other Matter" on page 390.)

■ You may have **dyspepsia** if a normal dinner makes you feel uncomfortably full. (See "Burn Baby Burn" on page 390.)

■ Sometimes your **bowels** get in an uproar—gas, bloating, diarrhea—and you don't know why. To identify some likely culprits, see "Intestines" on page 183.

■ The **gallbladder** shoots bile into the small intestine to help it break down food. But sometimes bile forms painful gallstones. (See "Scaling Back Your Risk" on page 152.)

■ Your **pancreas** makes the hormone insulin, which helps your body absorb its food. Sometimes the pancreas stops making enough, and the result is adult-onset diabetes. (See "Finding Out Where You Stand" on page 306.)

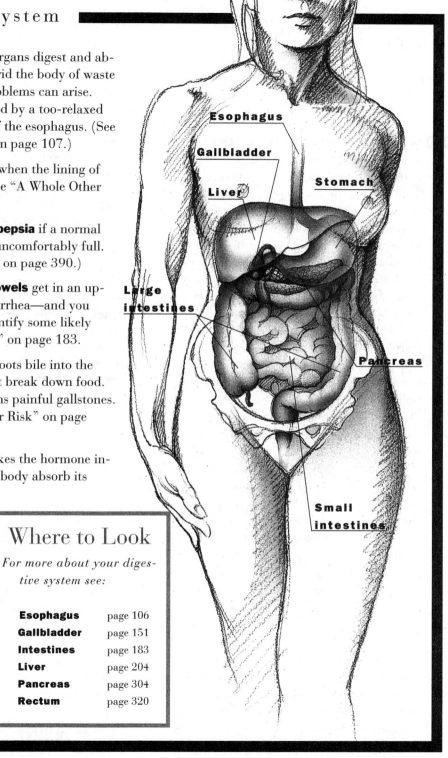

Esophagus

Gallbladder

Liver

Stomach

Large intestines

Pancreas

Small intestines

Where to Look

For more about your digestive system see:

Esophagus	page 106
Gallbladder	page 151
Intestines	page 183
Liver	page 204
Pancreas	page 304
Rectum	page 320

Ears

IN ANCIENT EGYPT MARRIED WOMEN who fooled around often found themselves with nothing from which to hang their earrings. That's right—they were punished for their indiscretions by having their ears hacked off.

It might have looked unsightly, but much worse, they were losing part of their sense of hearing. And most everyone would agree that not being able to wear gold hoops is a stroll along the Nile compared with missing out on music and laughter and conversation.

The wondrous sense of hearing gets its start in the skin and cartilage of the outer ear, which collects sound waves and channels them to the eardrum, a fibrous, circular membrane separating the outer ear from the middle ear. The eardrum vibrates in response to the changes in air pressure that constitute sound.

From there the vibrations go to three small bones, called the malleus (hammer), the incus (anvil) and the stapes (stirrup), which form a chain across the middle ear. The vibrations travel to the inner ear, where the cochlea, a snail-shaped organ that's lined with 20,000 groups of minute sensory hairs, transmits sound to the brain.

Putting the Brakes on Earaches

You might say that ears are like the Carlsbad Caverns of the body. They tunnel into the sides of your head, marked by all kinds of formations, nooks, crannies and passageways.

Like any closed-off area, the ear is susceptible to poor drainage. Stagnant fluid, trapped

Don't Pack the Wax

We poke, prod and probe our ears in an effort to keep them wax-free, but have you ever stopped to ask yourself why?

Ear wax is actually a good thing, notes Steven D. Rauch, M.D., assistant professor of otolaryngology at Harvard Medical School. It serves as a moisturizing agent for the ear, has antibacterial properties and keeps out things such as dust, dirt and bugs, he notes.

In fact, the ear, which produces wax in glands located in the outer quarter of the inch-long ear canal, is a self-cleaning unit.

Though many people use cotton swabs for wax control, Dr. Rauch is against it. "Using one in your ear is like muzzle-loading a cannon. You push all the wax down inside."

But some folks do have more wax or very hard wax. This is especially likely if your ear canal is narrow or if you're on the

in the warm, dark environment of the middle ear, is a good growing place for bacteria and viruses. The result: a middle ear infection and stabbing pain.

Although it's mainly children who get middle ear infections, adults sometimes get them following a cold or as a result of the change of pressure during an airplane flight, notes David Zwillenberg, M.D., otolaryngologist at Thomas Jefferson University Hospital in Philadelphia.

If your ears feel full or if you lose some hearing because of an infection, the problems will generally last from 24 to 48 hours. But if problems persist, you may need to see a doctor about treatment. A bad infection can burst the eardrum. That causes the pain to

phone a lot. Still, you should skip the swab and try this method to prevent build-up: Fill an eyedropper with full-strength hydrogen peroxide (available at pharmacies) and put a few drops in each ear. Repeat about once a week, suggests David Zwillenberg, M.D., otolaryngologist at Thomas Jefferson University Hospital in Philadelphia. "That keeps the wax soft so the ear will drain normally."

Or use this variation of the same method: Soak a small cotton ball in hydrogen peroxide, place it in your ear to cover the opening to the inner ear, but don't stick it into the inner ear. Lie down on your side with your other ear on the pillow. Let the liquid seep into the canal, then turn over and treat the other ear. Wait five minutes and take a shower, cupping your hand to guide the warm water into your ear to rinse the peroxide out.

stop completely, but there's a risk that the perforation will not close, possibly requiring surgery to fix it.

The inch-long ear canal leading from the outer ear to the eardrum can become infected by accumulation of water as well, resulting in an ear canal infection called swimmer's ear. While an outer ear infection usually will go away on its own, a doctor can prescribe antibiotic-corticosteroid eardrops.

How can you tell an outer ear infection from a middle ear infection? Give the earlobe of the offending ear a couple of yanks, notes Anne Simons, M.D., assistant clinical professor of family and community medicine at the University of California, San Francisco, and author of *Before You Call the Doctor.* "If it hurts like crazy, it's an outer ear infection."

If you've been smarting over aching ears lately, here are a few tips from top docs.

Reach for alcohol. Rubbing alcohol is the perfect solution for wet ears, notes Thomas Pasic, M.D., assistant professor of otolaryngology at the University of Wisconsin-Madison. "After you swim take an eardropper, drop in the alcohol, then let it roll out. The alcohol dries up the water."

Blow it dry. Another surefire ear clearer is a blow dryer, notes Dr. Pasic. "Use a low setting—one that's comfortable. Aim the hair dryer at your ear until it's dry." But be sure to hold it far enough away that it just blows gently in your ear.

Deep-six your Q-tips. Cotton swabs have done a lot of ear damage—and Dr. Simons says they're "a common villain in the outer ear ailment. Your ear canal is delicate; you can scrape off the skin deep enough to lose its barrier to infection," she notes. "You also push wax down inside, creating a plug in the canal that can trap water behind it."

Use tissue—with a twist. When you're done swimming or showering, dry out your ears with the twisted end of a disposable tissue, Dr. Simons suggests. "Unlike cotton swabs, the bit of tissue is too soft to push wax back into the ear or cause any damage to the sensitive skin inside the ear canal."

Pass the vinegar. White vinegar is a surefire ear soother, notes Randy Oppenheimer, M.D., clinical instructor of otolaryngology at the University of California, San Diego. "White vinegar has acetic acid, which helps clear up outer ear infections." Try squeezing in a few drops using an eyedropper—and then put cotton in your ear to hold in the vinegar, he suggests. You can remove the cotton after an hour or so. This treatment can be done several times a day.

Airplane Ears: When Flying Leaves You Crying

For some people every airplane flight brings an experience as predictable as the little foil bag containing a teaspoon of roasted peanuts: an annoying, clogged-up feeling that grips your ears during takeoff and landing.

It's not a life and death situation, but it sure is bothersome—especially if you're a white-knuckle flier to begin with. Not only that, it can be searingly painful. And the clogged-up feeling can last for a day or more afterward.

The culprit in airplane ear is the eustachian tube, which connects the back of the throat to the middle ear, notes Anne Simons, M.D., assistant clinical professor of family and community medicine at University of California, San Francisco, and author of Before You Call the Doctor.

To help keep the eustachian tube open, try yawning and chewing gum, suggests Dr. Simons.

If those methods don't work—and you don't have a sinus infection—try this for an ear opener.

Hold your nose closed, open the back of your throat as if you're yawning, bear down, then blow—but very gently. That forces air into the back of your throat and through your eustachian tubes. But you definitely don't want to try this if you have a sinus infection or think you might be getting one: When you bear down, you could force bacteria-laden mucus into your inner ear.

Don't blow it. If you have a cold, blowing your nose too hard is a bad idea, says Dr. Simons. "You can drive bacteria-laden mucus into the middle ear." Try to blow your nose just hard enough to clear the outermost nasal passages. "If you take in a great big deep breath before you blow, you're probably blowing too hard."

Ease your pain. Take acetaminophen or aspirin for the discomfort of an ear infection, notes Dr. Simons. She recommends 650 to 1,000 milligrams every four hours.

Wringing Your Hands over Ringing Ears

You know the annoying, high-pitched tone they play every now and then on television and radio—followed by the announcement that "This is only a test"? Well, think how distracting it would be if that *weren't* only a test. What if that ringing tone were a daily part of your life, even when you slept or listened to Bach or walked by a stream.

That's how it is for people with tinnitus—a ringing, buzzing, whistling, hissing or clicking in the ear. If you have tinnitus, you're liable to hear these sounds whenever the background is quiet.

Tinnitus can be caused by frequent, prolonged exposure to loud noise. It can also accompany hearing loss—or you might get it when the outer ear canal is blocked with ear wax. Auditory nerve tumors, head injuries and certain inner ear disorders such as Ménière's disease can cause it, too. Other culprits are aspirin, some blood pressure medicines and a number of cardiac drugs.

Beginning without warning, and often lasting for years, tinnitus can be extremely upsetting. Because it's related to so many underlying medical conditions, your first step is to have a physician examine your ears, notes Dr. Simons. "It's worthwhile seeing if you have impacted ear wax or an infection," she says. The doctor will also check for hearing loss, since that's another tinnitus-linked condition.

If the racket won't stop, though, here are a few ways doctors say you can make the clicking, ringing or buzzing a bit more bearable.

Wear a white-noise aid. If you have persistent tinnitus, you might want to ask your doctor about getting a white-noise generator the size of a hearing aid, suggests Dr. Simons. The white noise—a tuneless, unvarying hissing—serves as a cover-up. "It masks external sound and makes life more bearable."

Park between stations. Inner ear noise can be most distracting at night when you're trying to fall asleep. You can turn on the radio between stations and let the static drown it out, says Dr. Simons. Or tune in your favorite radio station so it'll distract you until you fall asleep.

Avoid aspirin. High doses of aspirin cause tinnitis, says Dr. Oppenheimer. "Taking a few aspirin doesn't cause it, but if you do have tinnitus, it might be best to take Tylenol."

A Balancing Act

The ear brings us more than melodious harmonics, the honk of a Mack truck and the chatter of a jackhammer. It also contributes a sense of balance.

Without the ear we'd be flopping around like fish on a pier. The semicircular canals located in the back of the inner ear contain hair cells that are bathed in fluid. Some of these cells are sensitive to gravity and acceleration, while others respond to the positions and movements of the head. This information is registered and sent via nerve fibers to the brain so that you always know which end is up.

If you start to feel woozy or queasy when you're riding in the back seat of a car or rolling over the bounding main in a ferryboat, you can blame it—at least partially—on your inner ear.

Motion sickness isn't just the curse of little kids who lose their lunches in the back seat of the car during a trip to the beach. It's a problem for anyone who gets conflicting messages from their body's balance system, says Steven D. Rauch, M.D., assistant professor of otolaryngology at Harvard Medical School.

"The balance system is your navigational system, which gets information from the eyes, inner ear and the bones, joints and muscles of the spine and the neck," he notes. "It all gets processed in the brain, where it's used to help you maintain posture and shift your gaze."

Problems arise when there's a mismatch between the information that comes to your brain through the different sensory channels. When you're belowdecks in a boat, for instance, the scene in front of you doesn't move, but your ears sense movement. That's when the classic motion sickness symptoms crop up: You break into a cold sweat, feel queasy and lightheaded and later progress to vomiting or dry heaves.

There are some tricks to keep your inner ear from pushing you to the outer limits of discomfort. Here's what doctors recommend to help make your travels nausea-free.

Get a front-row seat. While traveling find a seat with a good view of what's happening, notes Dr. Rauch. In a bus or in a car, your best position is the front seat where you can look forward out the window. If you're taking a train, be sure to take a seat that faces forward. On shipboard you may not be able to stay on deck the whole time—but the more, the better.

Make it a pressing matter. Try using an acupressure armband, suggests Dr. Rauch.

Mend Thee Your Ears

When you compose your wish list of body parts that you'd change through plastic surgery, your ears would probably rank just before your feet. Who associates ears with beauty?

Nevertheless, women do have them cosmetically altered. The most common ear plastic surgery is done on protruding ears, notes Darrick Antell, M.D., assistant clinical professor of plastic surgery at Columbia University and attending plastic surgeon at St. Luke's Roosevelt Hospital Center, both in New York City. Most often this type of surgery is done on children when they're over the age of five. But if it doesn't happen then, it's never too late. "I've had young ladies come in who say that they're getting married and want to wear their hair up in a bun for the first time," he notes.

The surgery is done by suturing cartilage from the back of the edge of the ear to the back of the ear—in effect, folding the ear back on itself. The cost starts around $2,500.

Plastic surgeons can also do earlobe repair, which comes in handy if your lobes have been ripped by heavy earrings or when a pierced earring gets caught on something and part of the lobe gets torn off. (Yes, it does happen!) The lobe is sewn back up while you're under local anesthesia—a procedure that can be completed in the span of a lunch hour, notes Dr. Antell.

These devices, available at sporting and boating supply stores, have a plastic button that presses the inside surface of the wrist. "It presses into an acupressure point that reduces nausea," he says. Or you can put pressure on that point by pushing your wrists together with a marble in between. The point you need to press is in the middle of your arm, two finger-widths down from the crease formed by your hand where it meets the wrist.

Go with ginger. Powdered ginger—taken in capsule form—has been shown to help reduce nausea and vomiting during pregnancy, according to a study of women in Denmark. Other research shows that the spice delays the development of motion sickness better than over-the-counter medication. And many people report good luck with ginger ale. Raw ginger has a powerful taste, but either the capsules, ginger ale or other foods such as gingersnaps and crystallized ginger—which you eat like candy—may help settle your stomach.

Go over-the-counter. An over-the-counter medication containing meclizine hydrochloride (such as Dramamine II) is an effective way to avoid the woozies, notes Dr. Oppenheimer. "If you're going on a boat trip, take it about half an hour to an hour beforehand."

Stop the Whirl, I Want to Get Off

If your head is spinning and you haven't just: (a) exited a stomach-churning carnival ride, (b) cartwheeled down Main Street or (c) seen Lucky Vanous's latest workout video, you might just have vertigo, a false sense of motion. Whether it's a bobbing up and down or a floating feeling or a force pushing you to the side or backward, this dizzying disorder can be maddening.

There are various causes of vertigo, often related to damage inside the ear. Sometimes these sensations can be traced to a disorder called labyrinthitis, an inflammation of the whole balance portion of the inner ear. Labyrinthitis is usually caused by a virus or a

Knocked Off Balance—
With Ménière's

Imagine an attack of vertigo so severe that you fall to the ground—your stomach grinding, head spinning, feeling so nauseated that vomiting would be a relief.

That scenario is a fact of life for people with Ménière's disease, a disorder of the inner ear that mainly strikes people over age 50. The onset of Ménière's is a signal that there is too much fluid in the membranous labyrinth, the inner ear canals that control balance. Along with fall-down dizziness, people who have Ménière's disease may also experience abnormal jerky eye movements, tinnitus and deafness. In most cases only one ear is affected.

"About two-thirds of patients have attacks in clusters. It will go into remission for months or for years. Another third have it with no pattern," notes Steven D. Rauch, M.D., assistant professor of otolaryngology at Harvard Medical School in Boston.

Ménière's disease can make you feel helpless. It has no known cure, but there are a few steps you can take on your own. Because the disorder has to do with fluid in your inner ear, the first line of treatment is to alter your body's fluid balance, notes Dr. Rauch. That means no caffeine and no alcohol as well as a strict low-salt diet that allows just 1,000 milligrams of sodium a day. "Buy all fresh foods, do all your own cooking and learn the sodium content of foods," he says.

Also, over-the-counter medications can help people cope with the nausea that comes with an attack. Doctors recommend medications containing dimenhydrinate (such as Dramamine) or meclizine hydrochloride (such as Bonine), nonprescription medications for motion sickness and nausea that are available at most drugstores.

---

middle ear infection and gradually improves as you get over the infection. Far more troublesome than this passing problem is Ménière's disease, which is marked by attacks of vertigo severe enough to cause you to fall to the ground. (See "Knocked Off Balance— With Ménière's.")

Living with vertigo can be a challenge, but there are ways to help ease the unsettling effects. Here are a few well-balanced tips to help keep your feet on the ground.

Be fit. Make sure you exercise, says Dr. Rauch. To keep your muscles working well, you need to work on strength and flexibility. "One of your channels—the inner ear—is wrecked for some reason, so part of the therapy is to learn to compensate by using your

other channels," he notes. Because good nutrition helps you stay fit, you should also eat at least five servings of fruits and vegetables every day.

Light up your life. It's hard to keep your footing when you have vertigo, particularly when you're walking in the dark. So you should keep things well-lit, suggests Dr. Rauch. "Put a night-light in the hallway to the bathroom." Also, try not to drive at night or walk on uneven surfaces that are poorly lighted.

Avoid crowds. If you're looking over a crowd at a shopping center, scanning a sea of bobbing heads, you might aggravate vertigo symptoms, notes Dr. Rauch. That can also happen when you're looking at a wide, unbroken expanse of terrain. "You're depending on your vision to anchor you in space since the inner ear is faulty. Wide-open places or crowded places can make that impossible."

Be a high-top woman. Running shoes might be good for jogging, but their thick rubber soles don't allow you to feel the floor, notes Dr. Rauch. His recommendation is "a hard-soled leather high-top that wraps around the ankle." That kind of shoe gives you a firm, secure feeling of where the floor is.

'Ere's to Hearing Protection

The biggest cause of hearing loss is something you definitely can't avoid. It's old age. In fact, about 30 to 60 percent of people over age 60 have some kind of hearing loss, notes Dr. Oppenheimer.

The second biggest cause of hearing loss is as preventable as a pair of earplugs. Going to rock concerts, hanging around pistol ranges, working with heavy machinery—all these noisy activities take their toll on the delicate hairs of the inner ear, notes Dr. Rauch.

Being assailed by that kind of noise is like walking on the same grass over and over again, according to Dr. Rauch. For a while the grass bounces back, but constant wear kills it eventually. "It destroys the sensory cells in the inner ear. They're brutalized by the intense vibrations of loud noise, and they just wilt."

So how do you know if you're becoming hard-of-hearing? Chances are, someone close to you, such as your husband or best friend, will notice it first. But if you find that you have to keep asking people to repeat themselves, or if you're always the one turning up the stereo or television, or if you think everyone else is mumbling, you've discovered three sure signs that your hearing is slipping.

Holey Earlobes!

Getting your earlobes pierced used to be a rite of passage. Around age 16 you'd pester your mother into letting you get two extra holes in your head—one for each earlobe. But today, piercing has gone north—all the way up into the ear cartilage. This painful-sounding trend has women sporting enough earrings to set off metal detectors—something that doctors such as William Hendricks, M.D., a dermatologist in private practice in Asheboro, North Carolina, do not recommend.

"Don't do it," he notes. "There's a high chance that you can develop problems with the cartilage of the ear. You might get infections that could become very severe." A serious infection of the cartilage can cause collapse of the ear on the site the infection occurs.

Another potential ear splitter is heavy earrings—the ones that resemble hubcaps and over time can tear the earlobes. Often the heavy wire earrings will pull through the lobe and cause a split, notes Dr. Hendricks. Or if you wear heavy post earrings, the back that holds the earring in place can eventually work its way through the front of the ear, he adds. One way you can

If you don't want "What did you say?" to become your catchphrase, follow this prevention advice from doctors.

Know dangerous noise. If an area is so noisy that you can't even hear someone who's standing an arm's length away from you, it's time to put in the earplugs, notes Dr. Pasic. "The chances are that it's too loud, and it's hurting your ears."

Guidelines from the Federal Occupational Safety and Health Administration say that

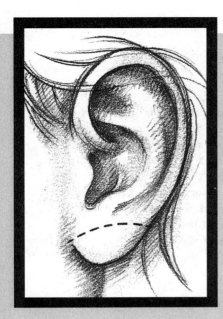

Post holes for earrings should be in the lobe— the "dangling" part of the ear shown below the dashed line.

help prevent this is to make sure that your earring backs also have those round, plastic disks attached.

In the case of a split earlobe, a doctor can sew it back together in her office in about 15 minutes. Dr. Hendricks's advice: "You should wear lightweight earrings that don't put lots of tension on your ears. You have to be careful about how large they are, because you could snag them on sweaters, babies can pull on them and talking on the phone can cause pressure that pulls them down."

you should wear protection if you're exposed to a noise level around 80 decibels for eight hours a day. That's about the level of a symphony concert. According to the same guidelines, you should wear ear protection if you're exposed to 85 decibels for four hours, 90 decibels for two hours or 95 decibels for one hour. Those racket levels are the equivalent of a snowblower, a rock concert or a power saw.

Pick your protection. Both earplugs or bulkier earphones are effective at blocking

out sound, notes Dr. Pasic. Earphones are better at keeping sound out, but earplugs are more convenient and less obtrusive, and they work very well, also, he notes.

There are two types of earplugs: the foam ones you roll up and put in your ears and the rubber ones, which are slightly more effective. "What'll save a person's hearing is if she uses any at all," Dr. Pasic notes. "So use whatever's most convenient for you."

Tone it down. Try to resist blasting your ears with a personal stereo, notes Dr. Rauch. "Keep the level low enough so that others can't hear sound coming from the headset. Otherwise, it's up too loud and could cause damage."

Put yourself in check. Any bothersome ear problems should be seen by a doctor, pronto, notes Dr. Pasic. Symptoms of drainage, blockage, hearing loss, dizziness or ringing of the ears are all reasons to go to the doctor.

See also Nervous System

Elbows

THE ELBOW IS SURROUNDED with misnomers. You don't really laugh when you hit your "funny bone." And tennis elbow isn't always caused by swinging a racket.

But at least they got the name of the joint right. When your arm is bent, it does form the shape of the letter L.

The elbow lets you make an interesting combination of movements. It works like a hinge but also allows some rotation, observes Pekka Mooar, M.D., assistant professor of orthopedic surgery and chief of sports medicine at the Medical College of Pennsylvania and Hahnemann University School of Medicine in

Bumping your elbow on "the funny bone" can cause that strange pins-and-needles tingling sensation through your arm that we're all so familiar with. But the sensation doesn't come from a bone. It's from striking a nerve called the ulnar nerve that runs down the back of the humerus, around the tip of the elbow and along the side of the radius.

Philadelphia. That's why in addition to being able to bend your arm, you can rotate your forearm.

When it comes to elbow injuries, it's possible to fracture it—which would require a doctor's care. And occasionally, people suffer from bursitis in the elbow, which is an inflammation of the bursa, a fluid-filled sac at the joint. If you have bursitis, you'll see some obvious swelling and feel some softness in the flesh around your elbow. (This could also be a sign of arthritis, so you should have a doctor check it out.)

By far the most common elbow injury doctors see is tennis elbow, caused by overuse and repetitive straightening, bending and rotating. Such repetitive use pulls on tendons that attach to an area called the epicondyle, causing irritation and pain. Hence, the medical name for tennis elbow: lateral epicondylitis.

While tennis is one activity that can cause pain, "most tennis elbow I see is not related to playing tennis," says Dr. Mooar. In fact, most people get it from work rather than play. People can get tennis elbow from carpentry work, from pulling files or from doing factory jobs, according to Robert Sallis,

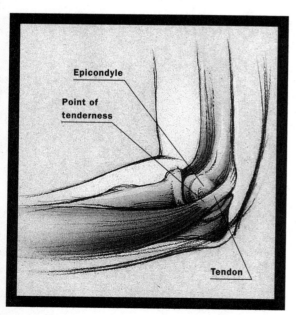

Epicondyle

Point of
tenderness

Tendon

If you have tennis elbow, you'll feel pain or tenderness in the tendon area shown above—near the bony prominence called the epicondyle.

M.D., assistant program director of the family medicine residency program at Kaiser Permanente Medical Center in Fontana, California. Other possible causes include stripping wallpaper, painting or working in the garden.

Whatever the cause, here are some ways to get relief from the pain, whether it's caused by tennis elbow or by bursitis.

Igloo your elbow. "Icing is very helpful, particularly when it is sore," say Dr. Sallis. Wrap a plastic bag of ice in a towel and hold it to your elbow for 10 to 20 minutes. You can repeat this four or five times a day—or whenever your elbow is sore.

Reach over the counter. Nonprescription anti-inflammatory medications such as Motrin or Advil are useful in achieving relief from tennis elbow, says Dr. Sallis. Both contain ibuprofen. Just follow directions on the label.

Give it a break. The best way to prevent tennis elbow is to do your best to minimize activities that involve repetitive bending, straightening and rotation. "The mainstay of treatment, when it does start to bother you, is resting the arm and avoiding the activity that aggravates it," says Dr. Sallis.

Doctor it. If the pain is severe, a doctor might give you a brace or splint to hold your arm steady and prevent motion. "Very frequently, I will put people in a tennis elbow brace, which is sort of a nonelastic strap that fits around the forearm," says Dr. Sallis. "It prevents excessive muscle contraction from pulling on those tendons where they attach to the epicondyle." The brace is available without prescription from most drugstores—or a doctor can supply you with one.

See also Muscular System, Skeletal System

Emotions

WE ALL KNOW THAT HAPPINESS IS GOOD and sadness is bad, right? After all, who would rather be crying in their beer than raising a glass of champagne in celebratory bliss?

But your emotions aren't black and white. In fact, they're quite neutral. Whether an emotion is "good" for you or "bad" for you really depends on how you respond to it.

Because of this, we should welcome all emotions—regardless of their connotation, says Carl Hammerschlag, M.D., a psychiatrist in Tucson, Arizona, and author of *Dancing Healers* and *Theft of the Spirit*. "We can't legislate emotions into submission, because feelings can't be legislated. You have to own your emotions and decide what to do with them."

A Plus of Womanhood

In a way, being female is a bonus when it comes to showing feelings. We're allowed to express joy and get more excited than men. If we cry, we're seen as warm, feeling and expressive. Men are often called unmanly.

The "permission" to be expressive is helpful for women, because reining in emotions can be dangerous business. Holding in feelings is like letting pressure build up inside a balloon. If the pressure soars too high, the balloon will pop. Strong emotions often leak out in physical illnesses or in sarcasm, passive-aggressive behavior, numbness and withdrawal.

So where do all these feelings come from? They're signals that pass from the central areas of the brain to the more peripheral location—the cerebrum—and back again. The endocrine system then releases the appropriate hormones, allowing us to experience the emotions. They're triggered by internal or external stimuli. Basic emotions are short-term but can become long-term, such as when happiness turns into love.

Temper, Temper

Even though women have the advantage when it comes to being able to show the "softer" emotions such as joy and sadness, there's still one taboo for the so-called fairer sex: Anger.

The anger taboo has to do with social learning, notes Scott Vrana, Ph.D., associate professor in the Department of Psychological Sciences at Purdue University in West Lafayette, Indiana. "As they grow up they're taught different things about anger. Boys learn it's appropriate, while girls are taught not only that it isn't appropriate to express anger but also that it's not appropriate to feel it, either."

Anger's original purpose was to stimulate the body to action in the face of danger—to fuel flight and ensure survival. To that end there's a whole cascade of biological changes, otherwise known as the "fight-or-flight response," that accompany angry feelings.

When your body leaps into the fight-or-flight response, your blood pressure shoots up as your heart pumps vast amounts of blood away from your skin and internal organs and directs it toward the large muscles in your legs and arms, enabling you to fend off or to flee. Clot-forming platelets in your blood prepare to repair potential wounds by becoming stickier. Your muscles tense as they prime themselves to run, strike or protect your body from blows. Fat cells release fat into your

bloodstream to be used for emergency energy. And your body suppresses your immune system to prevent it from making antibodies that will attack your own tissues if you're injured in the fray.

"These physiological changes were helpful when we routinely fled the wrath of saber-toothed tigers two million years ago," says Redford Williams, M.D., professor of psychiatry at Duke University in Durham, North Carolina, and coauthor of *Anger Kills*. "But today, the biggest daily threat most of us face is a traffic jam or an unreasonable boss."

The Many Faces of Fury

Anger begins to be harmful to your health when it churns inside of you with no means for escape. It's this double-damaging combination of hostility and suppression that often leads to anger-induced illness and disease, doctors say.

"Our studies show that women who generally perceive the world as unfair and who suppress their hostile feelings experience the greatest and most prolonged physical responses to anger," says Kathleen Lawler, Ph.D., professor of psychology at the University of Tennessee, Knoxville. "And their anger comes back to haunt them. In fact, just remembering what upset them in the first place pushes up their blood pressure."

To keep your blood pressure low—and your body free of *all* of anger's damaging effects—you can adopt a healthy dose of optimism and assertiveness by using the following techniques for managing your angry emotions.

Analyze your feelings. Dr. Williams suggests asking yourself the following three questions when trying to cope with hostile feelings.

1. Is the situation worth my continued attention? You might ask yourself, for instance, whether a rude comment from a crabby waitress will affect your life in ten years—or even tomorrow. If your answer is yes, move on to question 2. If your answer is no, make a conscious effort to let go of your anger. Laugh off the comment. Change the subject. Your current feelings are ultimately inconsequential, so why suffer needlessly?

2. Am I justified? In other words, maybe you misunderstood your brother-in-law's remark; maybe you didn't. Carefully contemplate the other person's side, and if you still feel justified in getting angry, move on to question 3. If you don't, consciously force yourself to release your resentment.

3. Do I have an effective response? Think hard. Will complaining to your boss about a co-worker, for instance, reap positive results? If your answer is yes, your response is a productive one. Proceed in a solution-oriented manner.

If your answer to any one of these questions is no, you have two alternatives, according to Dr. Williams: (1) You can let go of the anger because there's nothing you can do about it. (This would be appropriate in, say, a traffic jam, where you obviously have good reason to be aggravated, but you don't have any real means of effecting change.) And (2) You can brainstorm. Ask a friend, your partner or a trusted co-worker for help in developing an effective strategy for handling your sticky situation.

Assert yourself. On the other hand, if you answer yes to all three questions, then you have a signal to act, says Dr. Williams. But be sure to act effectively by being assertive, not by exploding in rage—which can be equally harmful to your health as suppression.

Using assertiveness rather than anger, you may be able to confront your selfish sibling or

(continued on page 98)

Unmasking Your Anger

During an argument with a man, you might <u>think</u> he can tell that you're about to pop your cork—but guess again. While you might wear your other emotions on your sleeve, anger could be the one you keep <u>up</u> your sleeve—sometimes until it's too late.

When you're in an argument, try to carefully verbalize the things that make you angry early on. You want to do that before the argument builds to a level where it explodes, says Naomi Rotter, Ph.D., industrial psychologist and professor of management at the School of Industrial Management at the New Jersey Institute of Technology in Newark. "Don't assume that someone is reading your angry looks, or assume that people are face readers—especially men," she notes.

Dr. Rotter knows of what she speaks. In a 1988 study of how men and women can read facial expressions, 1,100 undergraduates were shown 120 head shots of men and women who displayed expressions of anger, fear, sadness and disgust.

While women proved better at expressing and identifying emotions, anger was the hardest for people of both sexes to identify. This was especially true when men and women were trying to interpret the expression being shown by a woman.

"Men can identify anger in men much better than in women," Dr. Rotter says.

What are the implications of these findings? In some social situations a woman might try to communicate anger to a man with her expression, assuming that's the only appropriate way to convey her anger. So you flash a look. "But if you flash a look and men can't understand it, imagine how the frustration will start to build," says Dr. Rotter.

Depression

When writer William Styron fell into a devastating depression in 1985, death seemed his only escape from the darkness.

"Death by heart attack seemed particularly inviting, absolving me as it would of active responsibility, and I had toyed with the idea of self-induced pneumonia—a long, frigid, shirt-sleeved hike through the rainy woods," Styron wrote in his 1990 memoir, <u>Darkness Visible</u>.

"Such hideous fantasies, which cause well people to shudder," he explained, "are to the deeply depressed mind what lascivious daydreams are to persons of robust sexuality."

Luckily for Styron, his suicidal thoughts stayed just that—thoughts. He checked himself into a hospital for a seven-week stay that eventually led him out of his crippling emotional state.

It Can Get Depressing

Although Styron's bout with depression was more torturous than many, he's not alone in wrestling with the demons. One in 20 Americans now suffers from a depression severe enough to require medical treatment, and 1 in 5 will have depression at some time in their lives.

So how do you know if you're depressed or just blue? After all, feelings of sadness, pessimism and hopelessness affect everyone sometime in their lives. But if depression occurs without any apparent trigger, then deepens and persists—affecting behavior and your physical being—it becomes part of a true depressive illness.

According to the guidelines that psychiatrists and psychologists use, if you've had five or more of the following symptoms for more than two weeks—and if any of these symptoms are interfering with work or family life, you should see a doctor to be evaluated for depression.

- Persistent sad or empty mood
- Loss of interest or pleasure in ordinary activities, including sex
- Decreased energy, fatigue, being slowed down
- Sleep disturbances such as insomnia, early-morning wakening or oversleeping
- Eating disturbances such as loss of appetite, loss of weight or weight gain
- Difficulty concentrating, remembering or making decisions
- Feelings of guilt, worthlessness or helplessness
- Thoughts of death or suicide, suicide attempts (This is always a signal to see a doctor, even if it is not accompanied by other symptoms.)
- Irritability
- Excessive crying
- Chronic aches and pains that don't respond to treatment

Turning Lemons into Lemonade

The possible treatments for depression range from therapy to medication and often include a combination of both. But many people have developed practical techniques for those times when they're just feeling blue. And studies have shown that it's not life's hard knocks themselves that make you sad or worried or angry. It's more the way you interpret an event than the event itself that affects your mood.

"In all situations, it's what you're <u>telling</u> yourself that created your emotions," says

David D. Burns, M.D., clinical associate professor of psychiatry at the Presbyterian Medical Center of Philadelphia and author of Ten Days to Self-Esteem. That's good news, he says, because we have the ability to change how we look at the events in our lives.

Research by Dr. Burns and his colleague, clinical psychologist Jacqueline Persons, Ph.D., indicate that when it comes to looking at the world, it doesn't matter if you're rich or poor, brilliant or average, old or young, well-educated or not.

Looking at Things Another Way

Changing your thoughts has a huge impact on how you feel. Here are some strategies to help you change your thoughts and find some shortcuts to the brighter side.

Examine the evidence. Let's say you're responsible for planning an event, and it doesn't go well. Afterward, you might think, "I never do anything right." If that's the kind of thought running through your head, examine the evidence, suggests Dr. Burns. "Aren't there some things you actually do quite well? It may be that this event didn't go well, and you can learn from the experience."

Think in shades of gray. Many of us think in absolute terms, says Dr. Burns—a total failure or an absolute disaster. But in fact, there are always shades of gray. "Events are always a mixture of good and bad—never just one or the other," he notes.

Don't apply the old double standard. Consider the negative things you may be telling yourself. Would you be saying these things to dear friends when they're feeling down? asks Dr. Burns. Of course not!

"So talk to yourself the way you talk to others," he notes. "I've found that most people who are depressed are a lot more reasonable and generous toward someone else than themselves."

Tune in to radio station K-R-A-Z-Y. "There's a radio station playing in your head," says Hal Stone, Ph.D., and Sidra Stone, Ph.D., co-authors of Embracing Your Inner Critic: Turning Self-Criticism into a Creative Asset. We call it radio station K-R-A-Z-Y, and it broadcasts a running monologue of self-critical statements. If we're constantly putting ourselves down, many of us aren't even consciously aware of that critical litany running in our heads. So the first step is to pay attention to the things you say about yourself.

Catch yourself when you look disapprovingly at your face in the mirror. Take note when you start reviewing your day in the car on the way home from work and cataloguing your mistakes, they say. It may be easier if you record your inner critic's comments in a notebook. When you start to hear those comments next time, you can recognize them and switch channels to look forward to something coming up or getting into some activity you enjoy.

Talk to a friend. When you talk about your worries, it deflates those worries. "The cat is out of the bag, and thank goodness, it is just a cat, not some horrible monster," says Daniel Wegner, Ph.D., professor of psychology at the University of Virginia in Charlottesville.

back-stabbing colleague with great results. Just make sure that you communicate your frustration as positively and constructively as possible, says Dr. Lawler, so that the confrontation doesn't deteriorate into diatribes, blaming or stony silence.

Exert control. Feeling frustrated, powerless and angry in one area of your life? Dr. Lawler suggests defusing your feelings by creating another arena in which you have control and are successful. Audit a course, learn a craft, compete in a sport, take on a part-time job. You'll feel surprisingly empowered—and less vexed.

Exercise. Research suggests that people who are aerobically fit have a diminished fight-or-flight response and an enhanced calming response. The exercise or combination of exercises you choose is immaterial as long as you put your body through its paces for 30 minutes at a time, at least three days a week.

Keep a cool head. Count to ten before you yell back during heated arguments. Try to visualize positive outcomes to a situation that's turning confrontational and then try to act so you get to a satisfying conclusion, suggests Dr. Lawler.

Good Foods for Blue Moods

Well, you know how it gets sometimes. You have the blahs or the blues. You wish you had some get-up-and-go, but everything seems like too much trouble. You pick up a book and put it down—not interesting. You turn on the TV and turn it off—nothing good is on. Then you open the fridge and reach for that leftover slice of chocolate cake—and begin to eat.

If this sounds like you, you're not alone. Lots of people turn to food when they have "the blahs." Too often, though, all that food indulgence leads to even more "bumming out," say experts.

"It happens all the time," says Larry Christensen, Ph.D., chairman of the Department of Psychiatry at the University of South Alabama in Mobile. "You lose your job, you feel depressed and you start eating. Pretty soon, you're still feeling bad long after the depression about the job has passed. And you're still overeating."

"People who are depressed tend to eat large amounts of refined, processed sweet foods," explains Peter Manu, M.D., director of the Medical Services Department of Psychiatry at Long Island Jewish Medical Center and associate professor of medicine and psychiatry at Albert Einstein College of Medicine in Glen Oaks, New York. "What they don't realize is that by eating all of these foods, they're creating a nutritional deficit. Refined processed flours and sugars not only have limited nutritional value but they also require vitamins and minerals to process them."

The foods we reach for during these blue-mood moments are likely to be high in carbohydrates. These come in two forms: simple—like table sugar, candy bars and chocolate cake—and complex, like pasta and whole-grain bread. Simple carbohydrates act like crumpled up newspapers in your body's furnace. They burn fast and furious, and then they're gone. Complex carbohydrates are like seasoned logs; they burn for hours.

Since carbohydrates increase soothing serotonin levels in your brain, it makes sense that you would crave carbohydrates in times of woe. For most of us, a candy bar sounds better than a bowl of pasta when the weight of the world becomes burdensome. But if you want to rise out of the depression doldrums, it's better to reach for the pasta instead of the candy bar, say experts.

Taming the Green-Eyed Monster

It's often unjustified and leaves you feeling insecure. It's negative and can tear a relationship apart. The green-eyed-monster emotion we're talking about is, of course, jealousy—and it's bad news all around, right?

Well, usually. But believe it or not, the brand of jealousy that's more often called envy can be healthy, says Herbert Fensterheim, Ph.D., clinical professor of psychology in psychiatry at Cornell University Medical College in New York City and author of *Stop Running Scared*. "Envy can be a motivator. You can think, 'I really like his car—what could I do to get one?' and it could spur you on to do well." But Dr. Fensterheim does draw a distinction between envy and jealousy. "Jealousy is destructive."

The difference? Jealousy always comes from uncertainty about yourself, says Dr. Hammerschlag. "It's that you're insecure. It's a part of you that says, 'As much as I want to believe I'm effective, part of me is unsure.'"

You don't have to let the monster get the upper claw. Here's what you can do to tame it.

Catch that thought. Before a thought can lead to jealousy, calmly but firmly tell yourself to stop, notes Dr. Fensterheim. "Relax five to six seconds and think of something else. If the thought comes back in half a second or in a minute or a day, continue to stop, relax and divert the thought."

Love thyself. The better you feel about who you are, the sooner the jealousy will disappear, notes Dr. Hammerschlag. "Don't become crippled by ego. The ego is never convinced it's perfect—it's an absolute pig. The more you feed it, the bigger it gets."

Let yourself go. Whenever you have negative thoughts and feelings, concentrate instead on relaxing, notes Dr. Fensterheim. Try to relax your shoulder muscles by rolling them forward. Take a deep breath, hold it seven seconds and let it out while thinking of a pleasant scene. Do it twice an hour—once on the hour and once on the half hour. Dr. Fensterheim believes that it's possible to train yourself to do it so that it's not obvious to those around you. "I once did it on live TV, and the interviewer never even knew I was doing it."

Accentuate the positive. Focus on making time to do the things you enjoy doing, says Dr. Fensterheim. Devote time to the connections that give you a sense of joy. If you're into in-line skating, then while you're doing it, for that moment, it suspends you from your preoccupation, he notes.

Anticipate inadequacy. Don't let life's setbacks make you feel inferior. That's a feeling that definitely leads to jealousy, says Dr. Hammerschlag.

"Life is like tennis," he notes. "When someone serves an ace, do you stand there saying, 'I can't believe it,' over and over again? No. You walk over to the other side of the court and the game continues. Yeah, there are going to be problems and disappointments, but there's always joy, too."

Endocrine System

The endocrine system is the thermostat of the body, coordinating a complex weather station of glands and hormones. The endocrine glands, scattered throughout the body, include the two adrenal glands; the pancreas; the pituitary, parathyroid and thyroid glands; and the ovaries. All these glands work to regulate vital body functions such as height, weight, growth, metabolism, sexual development and fertility.

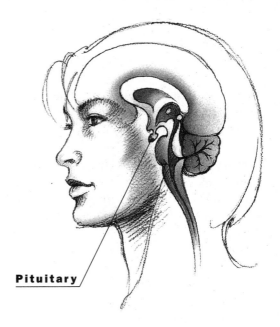

Pituitary

■ The two **adrenal glands**, which sit like small pyramids on top of the kidneys, are famous for making the "fight or flight" hormone, adrenaline. They also influence blood sugar, blood volume and sexual development. One malfunction, Cushing's syndrome, can cause you to gain weight. (See "Adrenal Glands" on page 3.)

■ The **adrenal cortex** produces a hormone called cortisol when you're under stress—and cortisol raises your blood pressure. (To chill out stress, see "Winding Down a Bit" on page 392.)

■ The **pancreas** sits just behind the stomach, linked to the small intestine. It produces the hormone insulin—the chief wizard that turns our food molecules into invigorating fuel. When the pancreas falters, diabetes can be the result. (To lower your chances of adult-onset diabetes, see "Playing the Prevention Game" on page 307.)

■ The four **parathyroid** glands, flanking your throat, control calcium balance in your blood. If your calcium levels fall, the glands release parathyroid hormone, which burglarizes your bones for the mineral. (For one more reason to get enough calcium, see "Hormones" on page 182.)

■ The **thyroid** gland at the base of your neck releases the hormone thyroxine. It tells your body how fast to burn calories. If you're losing weight without really trying, your thyroid may be gushing out too much thyroxine. (See "Thyroid" on page 408.)

■ The two almond-sized **ovaries** on either side of your womb secrete the Earth Mother sex hormone, estrogen. Among its many duties is protecting the bones from calcium loss. So when the ovaries retire at menopause, many women are faced with decisions about hormone replacement therapy. (To help you with your questions, read "The Big Decision" on page 231.)

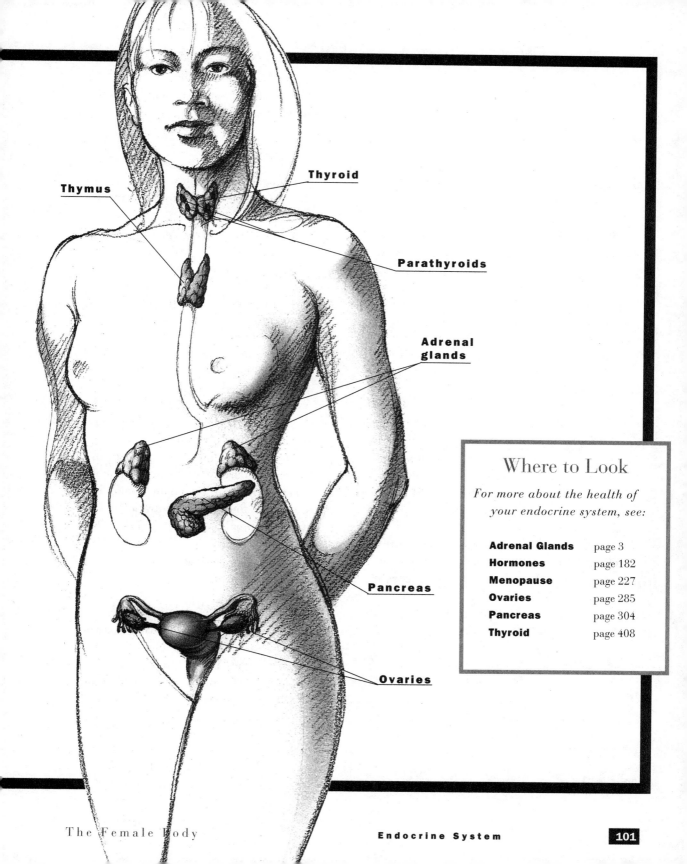

Thymus

Thyroid

Parathyroids

Adrenal glands

Pancreas

Ovaries

Where to Look

*For more about the health of
your endocrine system, see:*

Adrenal Glands   page 3
Hormones   page 182
Menopause   page 227
Ovaries   page 285
Pancreas   page 304
Thyroid   page 408

Energy

NOT MANY PEOPLE KEEP JUMP ROPES in their offices for quick energy breaks. But Ann McGee-Cooper, Ph.D., creativity consultant in Dallas and co-author of *You Don't Have to Go Home from Work Exhausted*, says she always does. In fact, for her, having a jump rope is all part of business. As a consultant to big corporations where executives need all the breaks they can get from long business meetings, Dr. McGee-Cooper has tried just about everything to help her clients renew their energy levels.

So it's no wonder that when the energy expert met legendary anthropologist Margaret Mead 23 years ago, she wanted to know one big thing: "What's the secret of your energy?"

After all, famed anthropologist Mead regularly traipsed off to places such as Bali, Samoa and New Guinea. Mead would zoom from one remote spot to another to study native cultures on their own ground.

Not content limiting her studies to anthropology, Mead readily expressed her views on women's rights, child rearing, sexual morality, nuclear proliferation, race relations, drug abuse, population control, environmental pollution and world hunger.

She was a curator at the American Museum of Natural History in New York City for 52 years.

And, oh yes, she wrote 23 books.

Confronted with Dr. McGee-Cooper's question, Mead stopped and thought a minute. Then she replied, "I suppose it's that I never grew up—while fooling most people into believing that I have."

Bingo. Dr. McGee-Cooper decided that Margaret Mead was dead-on. Who has more energy than children?

It's Child's Play

Think about it. Children never get tired of play. They look forward to recess like no other time of the day.

As Dr. McGee-Cooper points out, we can learn from our kids. Play is stress relief—and stress can be an energy sapper. The light and oxygen outside our doors are energy midwives; they deliver that urge to run through green grass on glorious days. As for recess, it's an energy break—exactly what Dr. McGee-Cooper urges business folk to get every day.

Here's another factor that helps breed energy—the fuel you feed your energy generator. "The body is a sophisticated biological machine, and it needs fuel for the energy to do all the work that goes on in its cells," says Dan Hamner, M.D., a fellow in the American College of Sports Medicine and author of *Peak Energy*. "But what's the right amount of fuel? And what's the right concentration of nutrients in it? What makes you feel the best? You don't want to flood the carburetor—your pancreas. You want to inject a steady stream of gas."

Getting the Octane You Need

Obviously, you can't run your body on empty. Researchers have found that three big meals a day aren't ideal, though. Eating smaller meals and snacks five or six times a day provides you with the most constant energy flow, says Dr. Hamner.

And you have to eat smart. The food that you choose should be low in fat (ideally, 10 to 15 percent, according to Dr. Hamner). It should also be high in complex carbohydrates

Savvy Snacks

If you want to marshal and maintain your zest, practice defensive snacking, says Elizabeth Somer, R.D., author of <u>Food and Mood</u>. By shrewdly spacing an energy-charging snack between breakfast and lunch and between lunch and dinner, you're sure to up your vim and vigor.

For these in-between snacks, complex carbohydrates should be your food of choice. "They're like nutrient-packed, time-released capsules," says Somer. Contained in legumes, vegetables and grains, the organic compounds known as complex carbohydrates are long chains of molecules that unravel slowly, releasing a stream of fuel to feed your energy for several hours.

Here are some sample snacks that Somer and other nutritionists recommend.

Portable Snacks

- **Bagels**
- **Apples**
- **Low-fat or nonfat crackers**
- **Rice cakes**
- **Lightly salted whole-wheat pretzels**
- **Small boxes of raisins**

Refrigerator-Access Snacks

- **Nonfat yogurt**
- **Dill pickles**
- **Frozen yogurt**
- **Grapes**
- **Frozen bananas**

---

that come from sources such as fruits, grains and vegetables. As for protein, you get enough from moderate amounts of lean meat, beans and low-fat dairy products, according to Dr. Hamner. It's also important to limit your calories.

Here are some basics that will help you power up for more energy.

Get your wake-up cals. "Breakfast is critical," says Elizabeth Somer, R.D., author of *Food and Mood*, "and you should eat it within the first couple hours of awakening. If you wait until 11:30 or 12:00 to eat, you'll never regain the energy that breakfast could have given you. It's also the right way to start the day's distribution of calories and nutrients."

For the best breakfast, Somer believes in a mix of complex carbohydrates and protein. "If you eat all carbohydrates at a meal, you'll feel sleepy in an hour or so." That's why you

don't want to eat a bowl of fruit and nothing else for breakfast. Although the fruit is certainly healthful, it should be combined with a little protein, such as yogurt or nuts.

A favorite power breakfast of Somer's is quick and easy: a tortilla with low-fat cheese, plus an orange. Or try this: Have a bowl of whole-grain cereal, milk and a banana.

Eat meat in the morning. If you're a meat-eater, make it the second of your five to six meals a day—and have it by about 10:00 A.M. But take the lean route. To limit fat, have very lean meat, fish or turkey.

"Animal protein takes longer to digest," says Dr. Hamner. "When you eat meat early, your body has time to break it down, and its energy is fed into your system slowly throughout the day. Why eat that hard-to-digest food at night, just before your body is about to switch into its rest pattern?"

Forbidden Foods

When you're fueling up for energy, the foods you avoid can be as important as the ones you favor. Here are some basic rules to help you skip the energy drainers.

Never eat sugar on an empty stomach. It's 3:00 p.m., and your eyelids feel like mattresses. Instant energy—you need it now. And you know how to get it—eat a candy bar.

Bad idea, says Somer. You do get a burst of energy from sugar, she notes, but you pay for it soon after. The pancreas squirts out a burst of insulin to carry that excess sugar out of the bloodstream and into your cells. But the insulin works overtime and . . . thud, now you have low blood sugar accompanied by fatigue, according to Dr. Hamner.

There's a way to guard against plummeting blood sugar, says Peter M. Miller, Ph.D., executive director of the Hilton Head Health Institute in South Carolina. "It's okay if you eat something like a turkey sandwich first. That way the candy bar doesn't undermine your energy level."

Stuff not, slump not. "Large meals—more than 1,000 calories—make you tired no matter when you eat them," says Somer. That's because more blood goes to your stomach area to begin a massive transport operation.

That means the rest of your body is a bit short of oxygen-rich fuel, says Dr. Hamner. All the more reason to nibble and nosh rather than gorge. Have smaller meals subsidized by snacks such as fruits, vegetables and small amounts of other low-fat and no-fat foods. And drink eight 8-ounce glasses of water a day.

Energy Walks

Oxygen is the other element in the energy equation. When the cells in your body don't get enough good air, they burn their fuel fitfully and inefficiently. That makes you feel sluggish and sleepy—as if you've been sitting in a stuffy office all day, says Dr. Hamner. For more ready energy you can't beat a whiff of fresh air. Here are some ways to get it.

Pant like a puppy. Dr. Hamner suggests this exercise to get a quick oxygen rush to the brain. Take 20 quick breaths, rapidly tightening your stomach muscles as if you were panting. (By contracting your stomach area, you pant from the diaphragm rather than the upper lung area.) Follow these panting breaths by taking one very deep breath filling air to the top of your lungs. Then exhale this breath, as if you're emptying your lungs to their very bottom.

Go for a thermal. At the Hilton Head Health Institute in South Carolina, where clients follow a daily regimen for weight loss and better health, everyone takes a 10- to 20-minute walk after lunch—and often after dinner, too, according to Dr. Miller. "It's a way to energize yourself. We call it a thermal walk."

According to Dr. Hamner, the reason that you get tired after meals is that blood and oxygen are diverted to your stomach and intestines for digestion. "A brisk walk will send some blood and oxygen to your brain and tissues, too. That revitalizes you and prevents that postmeal slump."

Stroll in the morning sun. Our bodies are still primitive beasts in some ways. On their own, without our civilized behavior to command them, our bodies would prompt us to rise with the dawn and bed down as soon as darkness falls. Our so-called body clocks, the internal prompts that regulate biological rhythms—put us in sync with light and dark. It's not surprising, then, that a 20-minute walk in the bright sun jump-starts your day better than any cup of coffee. Your whole body responds to the sun's rise-and-shine message.

Iron Woman

Many women are expert jugglers of work, family and multiple responsibilities. "So women think it's only natural that they should be tired," says Somer.

But maybe it isn't just juggler's fatigue. In part, women's exhaustion may be caused by a simple lack of enough iron in their diets, Dr. Hamner says. About 40 percent of all women—especially adolescent girls, athletes and pregnant and premenopausal women—have iron stores that are too low. They're not low enough to show up on routine blood tests. But you can have another simple measurement done—a serum ferritin test—that will identify whether your levels of iron are low enough to make you feel tired.

The iron is for your red blood cells. It helps them haul oxygen from your lungs to your brain and muscles. If your cells don't get enough of this mineral, they'll pull some of the stored iron out of your bone marrow, muscles and other tissues. And the cells in those tissues will slowly collapse, according to Dr. Hamner.

Most premenopausal women should be getting 18 milligrams of iron a day—the Daily Value—to help keep their tissues strong, says Dr. Hamner. Preferably, that iron should come from your food. If your diet is lacking in iron, get it with the help of a supplement, he suggests.

Here are some tasty ways to eat your iron.

Put some stable in your diet. Many women have cut out or cut back on the beef, pork and lamb they used to eat. For the most part, that's healthy. "But the first and best source of iron is red meat—extra, extra, extra

lean," says Somer. She points to research showing that our bodies can absorb up to 30 percent of the iron in meat but only about 2 to 10 percent of the iron in vegetables, fruits, legumes and grains. "You can have just a

---

Energize with Joy Breaks

Are you a fader? Does your energy peak early in the day, then disappear?

You have plenty of company. In fact, the term faders has actually been used by doctors to describe high-speed greyhounds who start off strong but can't maintain their top speed for very long, says Dan Hamner, M.D., a fellow in the American College of Sports Medicine and author of Peak Energy.

A poor diet can cause fading, but so can stress. "The mind and the body are both hooked together," says Dr. Hamner. "Stress releases adrenaline—the fight-or-flight hormone. You can get a kind of adrenal-gland burnout from stress."

You can fight fading with a joy break. It's one of the energy techniques that Ann McGee-Cooper, Ph.D., creativity consultant in Dallas and co-author of You Don't Have to Go Home from Work Exhausted, teaches to people in corporations and in health organizations such as the Cooper Aerobics Center in Dallas. A joy break is simply "two to five minutes of an activity that you enjoy," she explains.

Some of her examples:
- Turn on the radio and invite a friendly colleague to jitterbug for a couple of minutes.
- Call a friend and make a date for lunch.
- Practice a few tricks with a yo-yo.
- Enjoy a pleasant daydream.

---

couple of ounces of meat a day. Mix it into chili and stir-fries," she suggests.

Cook a hill of beans. The next best iron sources, says Somer, are beans and peas. A cup of cooked kidney beans has five milligrams of iron, for instance. And it's so easy. Just add some beans and peas to soups, stews and salads, she suggests. They add iron, fiber, vitamins, minerals, taste and texture.

Chase it with C. Combinations of some vitamins and minerals enhance iron absorption. If you pair iron with vitamin C, for instance, your body will drink in more of that mandatory mineral. It's easy to do, too. Drink orange juice, which is very high in vitamin C, when you have hot oatmeal, which is a respectable source of iron. Or add high-C tomatoes to your iron-rich rice and beans, suggests Dr. Hamner.

Temper your tannin intake. Other substances actually reduce your body's absorption of iron. Both coffee and tea contain compounds called tannins that can reduce iron absorption by 80 percent. So drink your hot brews between meals, not with them, says Dr. Hamner.

Space out some supplements. If you're taking an iron supplement, be aware that calcium or zinc supplements can interfere with iron absorption, too. Rather than taking all those supplements together, space them out during the day, says Dr. Hamner. Take a multivitamin with water before 10:00 A.M. Other supplements and their timing will depend on your activity level, age and general health.

See also Nutrition

Esophagus

THE ESOPHAGUS IS A SIMPLE TUBE that functions like a laundry chute. Put in food at the top, and it plummets about ten inches down through the esophagus to the stomach.

There's one catch—or, rather, hatch. At the juncture with the stomach, the esophagus has a circular muscle—the lower esophageal sphincter (LES). When food needs to get into the stomach, the sphincter opens. Then it squeezes shut. No exit!

Splish-Splash, It's an Acid Bath

If the LES opens when it shouldn't, however, stomach acid can leak back up into the esophagus. This may cause a burning chest pain called heartburn.

Sometimes the sphincter is weak, and if someone strains to lift weights or go to the bathroom, that can cause it to open, says Malcolm Robinson, M.D., gastroenterologist at the University of Oklahoma Health Sciences Center in Oklahoma City. Other times, the sphincter just relaxes. Extra body weight can exert force on it. Some medications can cause LES pressure to drop, he says, so read the labels on any over-the-counter medications that you're taking or check with your doctor about side effects if you're getting a prescription.

Pregnant women tend to get heartburn more often, and that's because of hormonal changes, according to Dr. Robinson. "Increased levels of progesterone have been shown to weaken the muscle." This can also be a problem for women who take oral con-

Heartburn or Heart Attack?

If you experience chest pain that is unusual, lasts longer than 15 minutes and doesn't respond to an antacid, go to a doctor or emergency room within three hours, says Frank Hamilton, M.D., director of the Gastrointestinal Disease Program Branch at the National Institutes of Health in Bethesda, Maryland. It could be a heart-related condition rather than just heartburn. Doctors are seeing a greater incidence of heart disease in women as young as 30, he notes.

traceptives high in progesterone, or progesterone-only forms of birth control such as Norplant or Depo-Provera.

Whatever is aggravating your heartburn, here's what doctors recommend to fend off the fire.

Eat small, eat early. Instead of two or three large meals a day, eat five or six smaller ones, says Frank Hamilton, M.D., director of the Gastrointestinal Disease Program Branch at the National Institutes of Health in Bethesda, Maryland. Your stomach will secrete less acid. "We also find that people get more heartburn when they eat late at night, so eat earlier and wait a few hours before going to bed."

Dine selectively. High-fat foods can trigger heartburn, because your stomach doesn't empty out as fast when you've eaten these foods. "The worst food of all is the onion," says Dr. Robinson, because it provokes multiple LES relaxations. Other trouble foods include orange juice, tomatoes, spicy foods and coffee, both caffeinated and decaffeinated.

Shed some weight. If you're overweight, losing a few pounds may help relieve your heartburn, says Dr. Hamilton.

Give your bed a tilt. When you lie down, you're more susceptible to heartburn, because it's easier for acid to roll into your esophagus. It can help to elevate your chest higher than your abdomen, says Dr. Robinson. Put blocks of wood under the head of your bed to prop it up five or six inches, he suggests. Or lie on a wedge-shaped pillow.

Check your medications. If you take asthma or anti-hypertensive medication and get heartburn, ask your doctor whether the medications could be causing the problem, Dr. Hamilton suggests.

Try an antacid. If you know your chest pain is just heartburn, use an antacid, doctors say. Dr. Robinson recommends tablet antacids, because they mix with your saliva and create a gummy substance that coats your esophagus—which may give you longer relief.

See also Digestive System

Eyes

IT'S EASY TO TAKE YOUR VISION for granted. After all, seeing is as simple as opening your eyes.

Or is it? In reality, just glancing at your watch involves your personal set of complex lens-adjusting, light-transmitting, image-focusing equipment—all within orbs that are about the size of a couple of golf balls.

Talk about Grand Central Station. These busy globes register 36,000 visual messages each hour—about 864,000 each day. With that kind of input, it's no surprise that a full 80 percent of what you learn in life comes through your eyes. In fact, you might say that the eyes aren't just windows on the world; they're your super sensors.

Seeing Is Receiving

The vision process starts with light, which enters the eye by passing through the cornea, the transparent membrane that curves around the front of the eyeball. Just behind the pupil—the black circle at the center of the iris—the eye muscles make minute adjustments in the shape of a tiny lens. With these adjustments a clear image is splashed like an upside-down movie on the retina inside the back of the eye. The pupil reacts to light intensity by expanding or contracting, adjusted by the iris that surrounds it.

The retina, which lies along the back wall inside your eyeball, is the big screen in this whole high-tech operation. It's a light-sensitive layer of membrane with two kinds of specialized nerve cells, rods and cones. Rods are sensitive to the dimmest light. The cones detect color and detail. Both the rods and cones convert light intensity, color and form into nerve impulses, which are conveyed back along the optic nerve—the cable hookup that leads to your brain.

Fast Frame

This whole process occurs at a speed that makes the blink of an eye seem like slow motion. When light hits the rods and cones, the visual impulse—in the form of nerve energy—zooms from the eye into the brain at a speed equivalent to 423 miles per hour. That impulse first reaches the back part of the brain, where the shapes of objects and spatial organization of a scene are interpreted. Other parts of the brain do some further visual processing—and voilà—what you see is what you get.

While all this nerve action is going on, the eyeballs are being tweaked, rolled and adjusted by a set of outside muscles that aim your orbs at whatever attracts your attention. The muscles are attached to the outer coat of each eye and to the cuplike bone that forms each eye socket. They're built to last, too: Each is 100 times as strong as it needs to be to move an eyeball. Coordination of these mighty orb rollers is entirely controlled by the brain.

When the Eyes Don't Have It

Some women never have problems with vision—staying eyeglass-free and contact lens–free into their forties or even later. For many of us, however, nearsightedness (myopia) and farsightedness (hyperopia) come calling at a fairly early age. These eye conditions are especially prevalent in the high-tech

Check Out the Lens Lineup

We've all heard the saying about men not making passes at women who wear glasses, and maybe we've taken that negative press about spectacles to heart. An ever-growing number of Americans are choosing contact lenses over frames.

Doctors pretty much agree that choosing to wear contacts or glasses is a personal decision—based on whatever you feel most comfortable with. If you do go with contact lenses, you should know about the types available, since you do have a range of choices. Here's an overview.

Soft lenses are the most popular type, primarily because they're so comfortable to wear. Some types of soft lenses are designated for daily wear, while others, for extended wear, can be left in overnight.

But even though you can wear some soft contacts overnight doesn't mean that your doctor will advise you to do so. Eye doctors warn that there's a tenfold increase in infection if you leave in your contacts while you sleep.

A 1994 study done at Johns Hopkins University in Baltimore showed that 49 to 74 percent of cases of contact lens–associated ulcers of the cornea (ulcerative keratitis) could be prevented by taking out contacts before bedtime. Consult with your own eye doctor before you decide whether to leave in your contacts or take them out at night.

Rigid gas-permeable lenses give crisper vision, especially if you have astigmatism, an eye condition caused by an irregularly shaped cornea. While these lenses are also for daily or extended wear, they aren't as comfortable as soft lenses. And the same caution applies: Even the extended wear lenses should not be left in overnight.

Disposable lenses are designed to be replaced every week or two. They feel like soft lenses, with one advantage: The coating of body protein from the eye doesn't build up on the lenses, and they feel more comfortable, says Eric Donnenfeld, M.D., associate professor of ophthalmology at North Shore University in Manhasset, New York, and co-chairman of external diseases at the Manhattan Eye, Ear and Throat Hospital. Trouble is, every time you toss out the disposables, you're throwing away $4 or more. If you're ditching them once every week or so, it starts to add up.

Tinted lenses can help a brown-eyed Susan become a violet-eyed Susan. Among other top-selling colors are baby blue, emerald green and hazel hues.

"It's just like the color of your nail polish—you can change it from day to day, depending on your wardrobe," notes Karen Bator, a color contact lens consultant at Wesley-Jessen, a contact lens manufacturer in Chicago. The colored contacts aren't just popular with those who need corrective lenses. About 30 percent of the tinted lenses sold at Wesley-Jessen are nonprescription, bought for purely cosmetic reasons.

1990s, where our days are spent doing paperwork, assembling small parts in factories or staring into a glowing computer screen for hours on end.

"Our eyes weren't intended for hours of close-up work," says Jeffrey Anshel, O.D., an optometrist in Carlsbad, California, and author of *Healthy Eyes, Better Vision*. "For cen-

Toss Out Your Glasses for Good

Thanks to a revolutionary operation called radial keratotomy, contact lenses and glasses aren't the only answer for folks with faltering eyesight.

Since nearsightedness occurs when the eye is too long, the cornea is too steep or the lens can't relax enough to focus distant images, glasses or contacts don't correct the underlying cause of nearsightedness. But surgery can actually correct the shape of the eye. A surgeon cuts into the periphery of the cornea, which changes the focus by flattening it out a bit.

Ninety percent of those who have the surgery don't need glasses most of the time, says Herbert Kaufmann, M.D., chief **of Louisiana State University Eye Center in New Orleans. "There might be some glare at night, but it's a very satisfactory procedure." Some 150,000 radial keratotomies are performed in the United States every year.**

This operation can also be done with the excimer laser, a laser that can cost up to $1 million but is so precise that it can cut a cell in half.

"Twenty seconds, and most people will never need glasses again," notes Dr. Kaufmann. "It removes a little tissue from the top of the dome of the cornea and changes the shape—like grinding a lens in the front of your eye."

turies our eyes were used for hunting and scanning the horizon for enemies. Now, electricity makes it possible for people to work their eyes all day and then read all night. We're feeling the effects of the modern age."

Approximately 105 million Americans need to wear glasses or contact lenses for nearsightedness or farsightedness. The nearsighted crowd is slightly in the majority, and for unexplained reasons, more women than men are nearsighted.

There's a definite genetic link, says Eric Donnenfeld, M.D., associate professor of ophthalmology at North Shore University in Manhasset, New York, and co-chairman of external diseases at the Manhattan Eye, Ear and Throat Hospital. If both your parents were wearing glasses by their teens, you'll probably wear them, too. If you get through your twenties without donning corrective lenses, however, you're likely to be home free until later years.

Aging Eyes

Whether or not you start out with perfect vision, there is one sure enemy of crystal-clear vision: time. After all, the peak of your focusing ability is at about five years of age—which leaves a lot of decades for focusing efficiency to go downhill.

When you look at something up close, the lens in your eye gets thicker to bring the object into focus, says Mary Gilbert Lawrence, M.D., ophthalmologist at Yale University School of Medicine and instructor of ophthalmology at the Manhattan Eye, Ear and Throat Hospital. "As you get older, the ability of the lens to change shape diminishes. It doesn't get quite thick enough to focus up close." Therefore, near vision starts to blur.

This is the condition called presbyopia, which is caused by the hardening of the lens. It's a natural part of aging. Whether or not you wore glasses earlier in your life, you're

Getting Framed

If the eyes are the first thing you notice when you meet someone, their glasses are a close second.

While shopping for specs, you should look long and hard for the pair that complements your face, says Jeffrey Anshel, O.D., an optometrist in Carlsbad, California, and author of <u>Healthy Eyes, Better Vision</u>.

You may think that you have a good idea of your face shape, but here's a way to get a true outline. Pull back your hair, look in a mirror and then use some lipstick to outline your face on the mirror. You'll quickly find out whether your silhouette is oval, round, heart-shaped, rectangular, triangular, square or diamond-shaped. Use the illustrations on this page to determine what shape frames are best suited to your face shape.

In addition Dr. Anshel recommends that you get glasses with a thick, darkly colored bridge that rests low on your nose if you want to de-emphasize wide-set eyes or a long nose. And if your eyes are close-set, choose glasses with a high, thin, lightly colored frame.

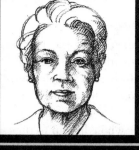

For a rectangular face, try on glasses with a strong top bar and round bottom lines.

If your face is triangular, try heart-shaped frames, square frames, aviator frames with a straight top or wire frames that are rimless on the bottom.

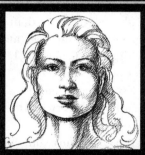

A square face is usually complemented with round or oval frames.

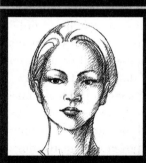

For a diamond-shaped face, try a butterfly-shaped or square frame.

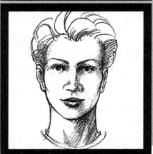

If you have a heart-shaped face, try a frame with straight top lines and rounded sides.

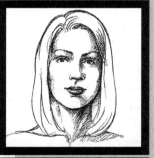

If your face is oval, you can wear just about any well-proportioned frame.

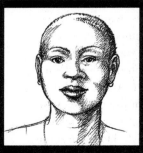

For a round face, try on frames that have an angular shape or geometric angles.

just as likely to become presbyopic later on, according to Dr. Donnenfeld.

As you ease gracefully into your forties, the chances are good that you'll need reading glasses—even if you had normal vision (20/20 vision)—your whole life up to then. The classic sign of presbyopia is when you start holding reading material farther and farther away from your eyes to be able to focus on it. "Patients come in and say, 'Doctor, my arms aren't long enough anymore,'" says Dr. Lawrence.

If you find yourself squinting at the fine print more and more, here are a few tips.

Treat yourself to a spectacle. Try not to let fear of "looking old" keep you from buying a pair of reading glasses, says Jonathan Trobe, M.D., professor of ophthalmology at the University of Michigan Medical School in Ann Arbor and author of *The Physician's Guide to Eye Care.* "Everyone will need glasses by their mid-forties; it's very hard to escape."

Buy off the rack. You won't hurt your eyes one bit if a pair of off-the-rack magnifying glasses works for you—and you'll certainly save some money. Most drugstores carry magnifying glasses marked with different powers, measured in units of diopters. "Take in a newspaper, hold it at a comfortable distance and try on glasses until you get the right focus," suggests Dr. Lawrence. Most people need to increase the power of their reading glasses by a quarter diopter every five years.

Try the focals. If you wear glasses for nearsightedness and then develop presbyopia, your optometrist or ophthalmologist will probably recommend bifocals, which are glasses with two powers: one for distance viewing and one for very close work like reading, says Dr. Trobe.

There are other alternatives, including tri-focals. With these lenses the upper part is for distance viewing, the lower for close-up viewing—with a middle area of the lens that eases the transition from near to far. Both bifocals and trifocals take some getting used to, and you'll need to have your vision checked every year or so as presbyopia advances.

Make some good contacts. If you're comfortable with contact lenses, you might want to stick with them as you enter the bifocal years, says Dr. Anshel. While bifocal contacts aren't 100 percent effective with everyone, the rigid types currently have a 70 percent chance of correcting your vision, while the soft ones are successful about 40 to 50 percent of the time.

Do eye-robics. Although some experts pooh-pooh the notion of eye exercises, others recommend the exercises as a way to improve vision. Dr. Anshel suggests the following exercise to maintain flexibility in the lens: Focus on something at a 16-inch reading distance, then shift your focus to something at least 20 feet away, and then back again. Do this several times a day to keep the lens muscle in working order.

High-Tech Headaches

Sure, they're great time-savers, but computers can also be a big pain—literally. Nearly anyone who works in an office ends up staring into a bright computer screen for a good part of the day. The result: eyestrain, which can mean headaches, watery, red eyes and blurry vision at a distance or up close.

"I rarely have a service station attendant complaining of eyestrain on the job—it's not visually intensive," says Dr. Anshel. "But computers are very demanding on the eyes."

Luckily, there are enough ways to avoid eyestrain to fill a floppy disk. Here are some of the eye doctor's recommendations.

Dim the lights. Bright fluorescent light bounces off the computer screen in the form of glare, says Dr. Anshel. To see if the lighting in your office is too harsh, try this test: Shade your eyes with a hand as if looking over the horizon and look at your screen. Or, if you sit by a window, shade your eyes along the side of your face to block the light. If your eyes feel better being shielded, the light's too bright.

Remember that paperwork reflects light, so you need brighter illumination when doing that than computer work, which gives off light. Dr. Anshel recommends a task light on your desk for paperwork—that is, an ordinary desk lamp with an incandescent bulb.

Leave a couple of feet. The best distance from the screen to your eyes is between 20 and 28 inches, says James Sheedy, O.D., Ph.D, clinical professor of optometry at the University of California at Berkeley.

Peer down. "The eyes work most efficiently looking downward," notes Dr. Sheedy. The center of the screen should be four to nine inches below your eyes, so there's a 10- to 20-degree downward viewing angle when you're looking at the screen. "Anything higher than that is too high."

Take a quick vacation. Look away from the screen for a second or two every five or ten minutes, says Dr. Lawrence. She suggests hanging a picture of an outdoor scene on the wall of your office—ideally, a scene that shows a distant horizon or a body of water such as an ocean or lake. "Look at it every now and then. This helps relax your eyes when they're doing a lot of prolonged near-work."

Change colors. It's better to have black print on a white background than vice versa, notes Dr. Sheedy. "With white on black you're looking into a black hole that doesn't blend." Also, be sure to adjust the screen for brightness so that it matches the overall brightness of the room.

Be a blinker. Blinking is an act that normally helps keep the eyes moist and refreshed—but you may have to remind yourself to do it when you're working on a computer. You normally blink up to 22 times a minute, Dr. Anshel notes. When you're reading, your blink rate drops to 12 times a minute, and in front of a computer, you blink just 7 times a minute. "Blinking helps rest the eye even for a fraction of a second by rewetting it and cleaning its surface."

Sore Eyes

If you look in the mirror some morning and wonder, "Where'd that pink-eyed Gila monster come from?," you may be staring at a case of conjunctivitis, or pinkeye. This problem is usually caused by viral or bacterial infections or allergies. If you have it, there will be redness, discharge and a gritty feeling in your eye. Bacterial conjunctivitis is treated with antibiotic eyedrops. Allergic conjunctivitis is treated with antihistamines and other anti-inflammatory eyedrops. If your eyes are pink and runny, see your doctor, and she'll prescribe the eyedrops if you need them.

Better yet, try these doctor-advised measures to avoid getting it in the first place.

Get all washed up. Conjunctivitis is spread by contact, notes Dr. Donnenfeld. If you touch the hands of a child who has pinkeye, for instance, you can easily pick up the infection, because children rub their eyes, and their hands carry the virus or bacteria. "Or they touch a doorknob and you touch it, then rub your eyes and give it to yourself."

To make sure you avoid carrying it to your

own eyes, wash your hands with soap and water three times a day and after you're near someone with red eyes, Dr. Donnenfeld suggests. The average virus lasts about a week, so you should continue the washing routine up to a week after the last signs of infection have showed up.

Invest in new cosmetics. Get a new tube of mascara about every six to eight weeks, says Dr. Lawrence. "Your eyelashes are colonized with many bacteria. After you've had conjunctivitis, throw away all your eye makeup—it may be contaminated with the virus."

Clean your contacts. Some of the worst eye infections can come from contact lenses, notes Herbert Kaufmann, M.D., chief of Louisiana State University Eye Center in New Orleans. So make sure that you clean them with sterile solution, he notes. And remember: Although extended-wear lenses are comfortable and convenient, the risk of infections goes up when you wear them overnight. Contacts block the oxygen that reaches the surface of the eye. The closed eyelid rubs the lens against the eyeball, and infection can flourish in this sheltered under-the-lens environment.

How to Stymie Sties

Sties are painful, red, swollen bumps that sometimes pop up at the base of eyelash follicles. They usually go away by themselves after a while—but the faster, the better. So here are a few steps you can take to keep away these ugly bumps—or make them get lost.

Compress the issue. Because a sty is like a pimple—caused by a clogged-up oil gland—you should try to bring it to a head with a warm washcloth, notes Dr. Trobe. Hold a warm washcloth against the sty for a few minutes three times a day.

Sideline the eyeliner. Some women put eyeliner on the inside inner margin of the eyelashes—a practice that breeds sties and inflammation of the eyelids, notes Dr. Lawrence. The meibomian glands, or tiny black holes that produce the oily part of the tear film, open up on that part of the eyelid. "If you put eye makeup along that area, it may plug those glands." When you do use cosmetics in that general area, use an eye makeup remover to take off every bit of it. Then wash with baby soap.

General Orb Work

Sometimes the problem isn't what's going on behind your eye, it's what's *in* your eye. When rubbing against the nerve-covered corneas, something as trivial as a hair or a piece of lint can feel like a needle-sharp pain.

If you're pestered by eye debris, it's best to do the following:

Hose off. Using lukewarm water, you can rinse out the object by either getting in the shower or placing your face under the faucet and carefully pulling your eyelid away from your eye. Let the gentle flow of lukewarm water run directly in your eye. Or irrigate your eye with a clean eye syringe or a general-purpose bulb aspirator. Fill the syringe with lukewarm water. Pull your eyelid carefully away from your eye and apply the contents to the surface of your eyeball.

Refill the syringe and repeat several times. Just be sure you put in the drops gently, without squeezing the syringe, since a hard squirt can actually hurt the eyeball, says Thomas Gossel, R.Ph., Ph.D., professor of pharmacology and toxicology and dean of the College of Pharmacy at Ohio Northern University in Ada. It would be wise to purchase a syringe before you need it so you'll have it on hand.

Don't knuckle under. Remember, the cornea is extremely sensitive, says Dr. Gossel. So trying to rub your eyelid with your knuckle is just what you shouldn't do. "The cornea can scratch very easily."

Thieves of Sight

Going blind—it's a fear that most people rank higher than that of death and cancer. No one wants to hear her doctor say "glaucoma." Unfortunately, the eye disease glaucoma strikes 2 percent of the over-40 population.

People who have glaucoma often show no symptoms at all until significant vision has been lost. In fact, half of the three million Americans who have it don't know it.

The most common form of glaucoma is the chronic simple form, which usually hits after age 40 and tends to run in families. It's actually a case of clogged pipes. Inside the eye there's a fluid called aqueous humor that maintains a constant pressure, pumping up the eyeball to its natural shape. Over a period of years, the microscopic pores that carry the fluid may start to get blocked—and the resulting buildup of eye pressure eventually affects the optic nerve that transmits images to the brain. The optic nerve, under pressure, can't interpret images as it used to, and it goes on the fritz.

Because this sly buildup of pressure rarely causes dramatic symptoms at first, it's usually detected only through a routine eye exam. The doctor will check your eye pressure, and if it's high, she'll probably recommend regular, continuous treatment with eyedrops to bring the pressure down. Once the treatment is prescribed, you have to keep it up to control the glaucoma condition.

In addition to treatment, there are some simple tips that you can follow to help prevent glaucoma's progression.

Dry up. Drinking lots of fluids in a short period of time can increase pressure in an already fluid-filled eye, notes Jay Cohen, M.D., associate professor at the State University of New York College of Optometry in New York City. "Don't drink more than eight ounces in one hour," he cautions. Drink liquids at various times throughout the day—not all at once.

Drain it with a vitamin. Vitamin C has been shown to pull some of the moisture from the eyes, says Dr. Cohen. "One thousand to 2,000 milligrams a day can help lower pressure in the eye by one or two millimeters." Since this is far higher than the Daily Value of 60 milligrams—and vitamin C can be toxic in some people if they take more than 1,200 milligrams a day—you should consult a doctor before going on a large dose to relieve eye pressure.

Break a sweat. Regular aerobic exercise such as walking or running—which allows muscles to work at a steady rate with a constant supply of oxygen-carrying blood—can help reduce eye pressure in people with glaucoma, says Dr. Cohen. "There are prolonged drops in pressure from it. Even after you stop, the effects last a few weeks." He recommends 40 minutes of brisk walking five times a week.

Get a checkup. Regular eye exams after age 40 are a must—especially if you have a family history of glaucoma and if you're in a high-risk group. Among those who have a higher-than-average risk of glaucoma are African-Americans and people who have diabetes, says Ivan Schwab, M.D., professor of ophthalmology at the University of California, Davis.

According to experts, if you aren't experiencing vision problems, you should see your

Be a Shaded Character

The same sun rays that damage your skin can also do a number on your eyes. Ultraviolet A (UVA) rays and ultraviolet B (UVB) rays are two forms of high-frequency light that may increase your risk of cataracts, according to Richard Bensinger, M.D., a Seattle-area ophthalmologist and spokesman for the American Academy of Ophthalmology. Visible blue light may be another culprit, too.

Protection? Wear sunglasses whenever possible, Dr. Bensinger advises—the wrap-around kind that say "blocks UV" are best, since they block incoming rays from the side, as well. Then add an extra measure of protection by wearing a hat or a visor.

eye doctor every three to five years if you're age 20 to 39. Women ages 40 to 64 need an exam every two to four years. If you're 65 or older, get an exam every one or two years. If you are having vision problems, see your eye doctor right away.

Not Every Cloud Has a Silver Lining

Another potential sight stealer is the cataract, which is a partial or complete clouding of the lens of the eye. Between the ages of 65 and 74, about 23 percent of the population will develop one. After the age of 75, nearly half of us will have cataracts.

Fortunately, cataract removal has come a long way. In addition to standard surgery, there is the option of phacoemulsification surgery, in which the nucleus of the cloudy lens is broken up and liquefied by ultrasound.

In most cases people can live with cataracts for a while, but at a certain point, it makes sense to have them removed. Doctors say that when vision is reduced to levels of 20/70 or 20/100—where you can't drive a car or easily read a newspaper—it's a good idea to go ahead with surgery. If both eyes are affected, surgery is usually performed on the worse eye.

There is also plenty that you can do when you're younger to help prevent them or at least slow their development.

Don't smoke. The pernicious weed that's behind so many other health problems also contributes to cataract development, notes William Christen, Sc.D., instructor at Harvard Medical School and Brigham and Women's Hospital in Boston. "It's not clear exactly why, but one possibility is that cigarettes decrease blood levels of nutrients that help maintain lens transparency."

Dr. Christen points to the results of a 1992 study that involved over 17,000 participants in the Physicians Health Study. The study showed that people who smoked 20 or more cigarettes per day had about twice the risk of cataracts as people who had never smoked.

Wear shades. Because years of unprotected exposure to ultraviolet (UV) light has been linked to the development of cataracts, it's a good idea to wear sunglasses outside, says Dr. Lawrence. "All you need are lenses that will protect you from UV light. You can buy the $8 bargains—as long as it says 'blocks UV' somewhere on the glasses." Gray is the least color-distorting lens, she notes.

Peel an orange. Eating fruits and vegetables containing antioxidants like vitamins C and E and beta-carotene may help slow cataract development, says Dr. Christen. Fruits such as strawberries and cantaloupe are rich in vitamin C. Orange and yellow vegetables and fruits are good sources of beta-carotene. Almonds, peanut butter and shrimp are high in vitamin E.

The Art of Plucking

Well-plucked brows help to flatter your eyes—and eyebrow plucking can be quick and painless, if you follow the rules of the game. Here are some suggestions from a New York City theatrical makeup expert, Joseph Anthony.

Before you begin, says Anthony, you should clean the skin under and between your eyebrows with witch hazel or skin toner to remove oil. Make sure you are in a well-ventilated area so that these va-porish products won't irritate your eyes. If you wear contacts, remove them. Then brush translucent powder onto your brows to highlight the lighter hairs. For the actual plucking, Anthony recom-mends using an eyebrow tweezer that has a slanted tip rather than one that's pointed or blunt. Here's how.

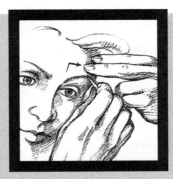

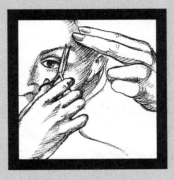

2. With the tweezer, pull the hair gently back in the direction it grows, then up and out.

3. Trim very long eyebrow hairs with a small scissors. (Don't pluck out the long hairs, as this could leave a gap in your brow.)

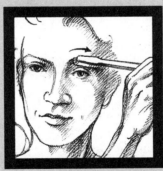

4. To hold coarse eyebrows in place, spritz a toothbrush with hair spray. Then brush your eyebrows smooth with it. Again, make sure that you are in a well-ventilated area.

1. With the index and middle fingers of your left hand, hold your eyebrow slightly taut by the hairline.

Although studies regarding antioxidants and cataracts show conflicting results, Dr. Christen says a healthy diet is always a safe bet. "The best advice is to have a diet high in fruits and vegetables," he notes.

See also Nervous System

Fallopian Tubes

PICTURE A NARROW PASSAGEWAY that's open to two-way traffic and ready for a lot of wild action, and you have the portrait of a healthy fallopian tube.

A pair of these tubes, each about three to four inches long, link the uterus and the ovaries and provide an environment where sperm and egg are welcome to meet. At the far end of each fallopian tube is a bunch of fingerlike projections called the fimbria that is draped over the ovary. When the ovary releases an egg, the egg is caught by the fimbria and then transported within the tube. The contractions of the tube and the tiny whipping projections of the tubal lining propel the egg on its downward journey. If that egg meets a sperm coming the other way—usually near the middle of the tube—well, that's where the action begins.

What happens after that depends on whether the egg is fertilized. If it is, the egg will travel from the tube into the uterus, where it implants into the uterine lining. But if the egg proceeds through the tube without encountering a sperm, it will disintegrate.

Dodging Damage

The health of the fallopian tubes—named in honor of the sixteenth-century Italian anatomist Gabriele Fallopio—is central to a woman's fertility. Damage to the fallopian tubes can interfere with this process. Most problems fall into the category of tubal occlusion next to or around the fimbria. Only 10 to 20 percent of tubal obstruction occurs within the fallopian tubes and next to the uterus, says Edmond Confino, M.D., associate professor and director of the In Vitro Fertilization Program at Northwestern University in Evanston, Illinois.

One type of obstruction is caused by pelvic adhesions. Bands of connective tissue attach to the surface of the ovary or form a barrier between the ovary and the fallopian tubes. These adhesions are sometimes the result of endometriosis, a disease where tissue similar to the lining of the uterus is located outside the uterus. Another cause of the adhesions is pelvic inflammatory disease (PID), a condition of the female pelvic organs that's often caused by sexually transmitted diseases (STDs) such as gonorrhea and chlamydia. Both endometriosis and infections like PID can also block tubes at their connection to the uterus.

The fallopian tubes can become obstructed if the fimbriae are damaged, says Dr. Confino. Occasionally, a blockage within the tube is created by microplugs—small masses of proteinlike tissue that form inside the tubes.

Keeping Them Clear

How can you protect your fallopian tubes and safeguard your fertility? Here's what experts recommend.

Give the red light to PID. Since significant tubal damage is caused by PID, and PID is often transmitted sexually, you should take every precaution to practice safe sex. In other words, be sure to use a condom—and use it the right way—if there's any chance that your partner could have a sexually transmitted disease.

Think twice about douching. Studies indicate that women who douche may increase their risk of PID. In fact, douching may actually cause infection to travel into the upper

Out-of-Place Pregnancies

Ectopic pregnancies are on the rise. But there's still good news: Treatment is improving all the time.

An ectopic pregnancy, such as a tubal pregnancy, occurs when a fertilized egg implants itself somewhere other than in the uterus. While ectopic pregnancies can occur on the ovary, cervix or even in the abdomen, nearly all occur in the fallopian tubes.

Fewer than 2 out of every 100 pregnancies are ectopic. But experts estimate that the incidence has increased two-to three-fold over the past 20 years.

In a tubal pregnancy—because of damage to the fallopian tubes or other reasons—the fertilized egg doesn't migrate to the uterus. Instead, it remains trapped in the fallopian tube. When this happens, a woman usually shows some of the signs of pregnancy—including a delayed or abnormal menstrual period—and she may experience abdominal pain, says Edmond Confino, M.D., associate professor and director of the In Vitro Fertilization Program at Northwestern University in Evanston, Illinois. Any woman with these signs should see her doctor immediately, he says.

The best way to help prevent an ectopic pregnancy is to avoid sexually transmitted diseases and pelvic inflamatory disease by practicing safe sex: Avoid multiple partners and use barrier contraceptive methods, experts say. But if you do have an ectopic pregnancy, you should be seen as soon as possible by a gynecologist, says Dr. Confino. Left untreated, an ectopic pregnancy can be potentially dangerous.

Abdominal surgery used to be necessary to open the fallopian tubes and remove the pregnancy. Now, doctors can often do it with laparoscopy, a less invasive surgery. Women can also be treated with medications that dissolve the ectopic pregnancy in some patients, according to Dr. Confino.

In a tubal ectopic pregnancy, the embryo is implanted in the wall of a fallopian tube rather than the uterus.

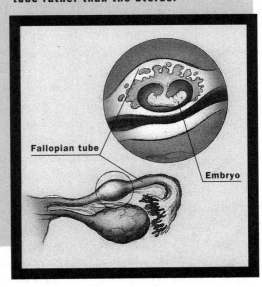

Fallopian tube

Embryo

reproductive tract and fallopian tubes. So experts advise against the practice.

Pay attention to changes. If you experience pelvic pain, with or without a fever, see your doctor. It may be a sign of either PID or endometriosis.

Quit smoking. There appears to be some connection between smoking and the development of PID and premature menopause, studies show. If you're a smoker now, it's just one more reason why you should try to kick the habit.

See also Fertility, Ovaries, Pregnancy, Reproductive System, Sexually Transmitted Diseases

Fat

IN MANY REMOTE CULTURES, EVEN TODAY, fat is beautiful. In some societies women put on pounds in order to make themselves more attractive. They're happy to see excessive fat on their buttocks, a condition called steatopygia. Some tribes and villages reserve the best foods for girls who are approaching marrying age. The biggest in girth make the most desirable brides.

It was like that in primitive times, too. Back before farms and supermarkets, food was hunted and gathered, not raised. Famines were bad then and fat was good. Body fat kept our ancient ancestors alive—the equivalent of carrying their own personal grocery store.

Fat is the body's in-house hoard of food. It's pure stored energy. But most women deplore that extra bonus, especially when they're confronted in the media with supermodels Cindy, Christie and Kate. Seeing their clothes-hanger bodies promoted as "ideal," too often we succumb to the fashion world's very narrow definition of beauty.

"Living organisms have been around a lot longer than the fashion industry," says Phillip Sinaikin, M.D., author of *Fat Madness* and a psychiatrist in Longwood, Florida, who specializes in addiction and dieting. "Our bodies say that survival still outweighs looks. Biology is reality."

Fat-Fertile Fields

Compared with men, women bear an extra burden of body fat. On average we have about 8 percent more body fat than most men, which makes sense since we're designed to carry reserves for childbearing. So we pack an extra 120,000 calories—stored as fat—to see us through any situation.

There's a relationship between fat and hormones. A woman needs to tote at least 16 percent body fat to produce estrogen, the hormone that's essential for conception.

It works the other way, too, with some hormones promoting fat storage—others discouraging the process. "Estrogen promotes body fat storage," says Richard S. Surwit, Ph.D., professor and vice-chairman of the Department of Psychiatry at Duke University Medical Center in Durham, North Carolina, "and testosterone promotes lean muscle mass."

What Are the Risk Raisers?

The fat that women carry—generally on their hips, thighs, breasts and buttocks—is fairly innocent stuff, says Joanne Curran-Celentano, R.D., Ph.D., associate professor of nutrition at the University of New Hampshire in Durham and nutrition research coordinator at the Center for Eating Disorders Management in Dover. "It's subcutaneous fat—right under the skin." For the average woman this body fat makes up 20 to 25 percent of body weight. (Men's subcutaneous fat averages 15 to 20 percent of their weight.)

There is another kind of fat that puts us at risk of all sorts of health complications: abdominal fat. It doesn't feel soft and flabby like subcutaneous fat does. It's hard and unyielding, formed by deep, visceral fat packed around internal organs.

"Visceral fat is associated with blood sugar problems, adult diabetes, high blood pressure, high cholesterol and heart disease," says Dr.

Curran-Celentano. We know what visceral fat looks like on men. They tend to put on weight in the abdomen in the form of the classic pot-belly. Women tend that way, too, once they reach menopause.

Although abdominal fat is associated with increased health risks, it has one advantage. It's known to be more metabolically active than fat on the hips and thighs, which means that abdominal fat is somewhat easier to take off than fat in the other areas. "It accumulates faster, but it also breaks down faster than fat on the thigh or butt," says Jill Kanaley, Ph.D., assistant professor of exercise physiology at Syracuse University in New York.

"Activity—exercise—can turn it all around," says Dr. Curran-Celentano.

Why It's So Hard

Man or woman, beer belly or thunder thighs, 1 out of every 3 Americans is over-weight. And more than 50 million people are on diets. They all know how hard it is to get rid of fat. But why?

Let's take a look at a fat cell—an adiposite, as researchers call it. That fat cell is just 1 of 30 or so billion that you have in your body. Together all these cells make up the adipose tissue. Because adipose tissue is such a health threat, molecular scientists and researchers have looked hard at the behavior of the fat cell to find out how we can shed our high-risk fat easier and faster.

"A fat cell looks like a little bag full of oil," says Dr. Sinaikin. In that bag is both fat that's produced by our bodies and fat that we eat in our diets. (Both kinds of fat are called lipids.)

Scientists have learned that even though we're all born with a certain number of fat cells, that number increases during infancy and again right before puberty. After that,

most of us won't make any more fat cells unless we gain more than 160 percent of our ideal weight. If your ideal weight is 130 pounds, for instance, you wouldn't be adding any more fat cells until you reached 208 pounds.

The Abdominal Slow Man

A fat cell is like a balloon—it can expand and contract. If we overeat and underexercise, the energy we store as fat makes us (surprise!) fat. And sluggish. When fat cells fill up, they don't do their work well. When they should be thinning excess blood sugar out of the bloodstream and escorting dietary fat toward the nearest exits, they lumber along, barely doing their jobs. The worse they perform, the more vulnerable we become to problems such as diabetes and heart disease.

When we diet, says Dr. Sinaikin, the body calls on those stored reserves of fat for fuel and empties out those swollen fat cells. "Your fat cells can shrink a thousandfold, and as they get smaller, you get smaller."

But your body isn't crazy about either diets or starvation. "Dieting goes against all the trends in evolution," Dr. Sinaikin says. "All those cells cry, 'Oh my God, we've run out of food. I have to motivate this mechanism to survive.' So they create the state called hunger."

Yes, but what about our skinny sisters and slim friends—those lucky ducks whose fat cells never expand? They can eat till the cows come home—then eat the cow, too. How come?

Jeans and Genes

Researchers at Rockefeller University in New York City and Duke University are look-ing at the genetic stitching that helps decide the size of our jeans and the span of our thighs. They've found a gene that tells us when we're full, a hormone that makes us burn excess fat and a metabolic defect that tampers with our ability to burn fat. Dr. Sinaikin and Dr. Surwit are intrigued by the role a substance called brown fat plays in the fat picture, too.

So far, most of what we know about brown fat comes from animal studies at Duke. When a mouse mom leaves her nest to forage for food, her babies burn brown fat for heat while she's gone. In other words, it's the fat that's quickly consumed for survival rather than stored.

As in mice, brown fat in humans is made up of fat cells that burn fat rather than store it. Those adults who seem to be able to eat a lot without gaining weight may have a larger-than-usual proportion of brown fat. So your fortunate friends who "have a high metabolism" or "burn up everything they eat" may in fact be walking storehouses of brown fat.

Dr. Surwit speculates that people are born with a genetic tendency to store certain amounts of fat. "It's clear as day that it's passed on from parent to child," he says. "There are thin families and fat families."

Sometimes the genetic factor is clear in a whole ethnic group, Dr. Surwit observes. "Native Americans probably have the greatest problem with obesity of any group, and also with diabetes. Seventy years ago, though, they had no problem. They may have developed genes to deal with repeated famines, which allowed them to store fat easily when food was available. What was an advantage to them in a time of scarcity is now a disadvantage in a time of plenty."

Dr. Sinaikin thinks that heredity carves about 30 percent of our body shape. And it's heredity that probably sticks us with a set point—the weight that we tend to maintain, through thick and thin and diet and exercise.

But the other factors that control size and shape are more likely to be within our control. "Genes do not determine what you're going to have for dinner tonight or how much you're going to exercise," says John P. Foreyt, Ph.D., director of the Nutrition Research Clinic at Baylor College of Medicine in Houston and author of *Living without Dieting*. Only you can regulate that, of course. What you decide to eat or do will influence every fat cell in your body.

Measuring Up—And Out

How much body fat is too much? Probably anything over 30 percent of your total weight is unhealthy and needs to be reduced, says Bryant Stamford, Ph.D., professor and director of the Health Promotion Center at the University of Louisville.

Trouble is, you can't drop a quarter in a body fat scale and get an instant readout—because such a handy-dandy device doesn't exit. The most reliable method—underwater measurement—is not widely available. More often a doctor will use calipers to pinch an area of skin and measure the adipose tissue in that area. Or she might measure by a method called bioelectrical impedance to find out how long it takes a painless current to go through the fat of your entire body. Electrodes are placed on your toes and fingertips. The more fat you have on your body, the slower the current. But neither the calipers nor electrical impedance methods are entirely accurate.

A pair of measurements that you can take at home, though, can give you a reliable figure for percent of body fat. These measurements are your weight and your height—

Finding Body Mass Index

To find your body mass index (BMI), locate your height in the left column. (If you've lost inches over the years, use your peak adult height.) Move across the chart until you hit your approximate weight. Then follow that column down to the corresponding BMI number at the bottom of the chart.

Height	Body Weight (lb.)													
4'10"	91	96	100	105	110	115	119	124	129	134	138	143	148	153
4'11"	94	99	104	109	114	119	124	128	133	138	143	148	153	158
5'0"	97	102	107	112	118	123	128	133	138	143	148	153	158	163
5'1"	100	106	111	116	122	127	132	137	143	148	153	158	164	169
5'2"	104	109	115	120	126	131	136	142	147	153	158	164	169	174
5'3"	107	113	118	124	130	135	141	146	152	158	163	169	175	180
5'4"	110	116	122	128	134	140	145	151	157	163	169	174	180	186
5'5"	114	120	126	132	138	144	150	156	162	168	174	180	186	192
5'6"	118	124	130	136	142	148	155	161	167	173	179	186	192	198
5'7"	121	127	134	140	146	153	159	166	172	178	185	191	197	204
5'8"	125	131	138	144	151	158	164	171	177	184	190	197	203	210
5'9"	128	135	142	149	155	162	169	176	182	189	196	203	209	216
5'10"	132	139	146	153	160	167	174	181	188	195	202	207	215	222
5'11"	136	143	150	157	165	172	179	186	193	200	208	215	222	229
6'0"	140	147	154	162	169	177	184	191	199	206	213	221	228	235
BMI	**19**	**20**	**21**	**22**	**23**	**24**	**25**	**26**	**27**	**28**	**29**	**30**	**31**	**32**

which you can use to chart your body mass index, or BMI.

The BMI, a ratio of height to weight, is determined by a mathematical formula: Divide your weight (in pounds) by your height squared (using inches). Multiply the resulting number by 705. (If you would rather short-cut the math, see "Finding Body Mass Index."

Your BMI, doctors say, should be somewhere between 19 and 30. One large-scale study—the Nurses' Health study, based at Harvard University and Brigham and Women's Hospital in Boston and involving 115,886 women—points to a BMI below 21 as ideal for preventing heart disease in women. The study showed that there was no elevated risk of heart disease among women whose BMIs were under 21. But for women whose BMIs were 21 to 25, the risk was 30 percent higher. Also, the risk of heart disease soared 80 percent higher for women having a BMI of 25 to 29.

In the same study, researchers found that the weight-related risk of cancer begins to rise among women whose BMI was 26, 27 or higher.

What's Your Ratio?

While BMI is one good measure of fat-related risk, it doesn't tell the whole story. The fat most associated with health risks is on

Liposuction: Fat Be Gone

While diet and exercise can shrink and shrivel them, fat cells are forever. So if you've inherited the family droopy chin or your mother's thunder thighs, you can only diminish them and tighten them up. You can't get rid of them for good, even if you exercise hard and always eat lean.

The surgical procedure called liposuction can siphon out the family fat cells. Though the procedure is no cakewalk, "liposuction methods have evolved over the years," says John E. Sherman, M.D., assistant clinical professor of surgery at New York Hospital–Cornell University Medical Center in New York City. The method that Dr. Sherman uses is called tumescent liposuction. It's a technique that produces less discomfort and blood loss and a quicker recovery than older methods.

Thigh reduction is the most popular plastic surgery for women, says Dr. Sherman. If you decide you want to shed your saddlebags and you sign up for tumescent liposuction, you'll first get a mild sedative and then a local anesthetic—to relax you and numb your legs. Then, the plastic surgeon will inject your thighs with a combination of lidocaine (a diluted local anesthetic), adrenaline (which constricts the blood vessels) and a buffer (to lessen the pain of injection). "That pumps up the area," he says.

Plumped up like a pillow, the fat is less dense and easier to reach, break up and suck out with a small tube called a cannula. The blood vessels don't bleed much because of their constriction, and the thighs show little bruising.

"With traditional methods of liposuction, a surgeon might have to perform a revision—a second round of surgery—to touch up a bump or take more fat out," according to Dr. Sherman. The rate of revision for regular liposuction is 10 to 15 percent of surgeries, but less if you have tumescent liposuction.

Recovery time varies, but with a tumescent procedure, you can be back to work in several days and completely recovered in a month or two.

"Having liposuction done doesn't mean that you can't gain weight," Dr. Sherman says. But the new fat won't go to the area where the procedure was done, because those fat cells have been dismantled and taken away. Most likely, the fat will go to established fat cells in your breasts or, less often, to fat cells around your knees.

---

the upper body—from the abdomen upward. You can judge whether you have too much of it by comparing your waist measurement to your hip size.

• First measure your waist. The place to measure is at the midpoint between your bottom rib and hipbone.

• Measure your hips at their widest point. When you have these two numbers, divide the waist measurement by the hip measurement.

The resulting number is your waist-to-hip ratio (WHR). Although scientists can't agree on the exact numbers to target, most doctors agree that any number below 0.80 is optimal.

Note: WHR isn't very reliable for women who are very thin or very overweight.

With one number for your BMI and a second for the waist-to-hip ratio, you can then use the "Healthy Weight Target" to help you evaluate your fat-related health risk.

Being a Smart Goalie

While fashion styles come and go, our bodies aren't meant to shed fat at the blink of an eye.

Whatever your weight-loss goal, it should be reasonable. "People with moderate weight problems will never be as lean as some of their friends," observes Dr. Surwit. "But they can keep themselves reasonably lean—and healthy—with low-fat diet and exercise." (For tips on how to do that, see "Insights on Successful Slimming" on page 282.)

Meanwhile, to get started on slimming, here are some guidelines to keep in mind.

Get real. A 10 percent loss of body weight is enough to improve a health risk profile. No matter what you weigh, "you can lose about 10 percent without a whole lot of difficulty," says Dr. Foreyt. Then, if you keep that off for a year, set another 10 percent goal. "Focus on feeling good rather than looking good. Ask yourself how your exercise and diet program feels in day-to-day functioning."

Make like a tortoise. Weight control is a long haul. "There isn't any magic solution," says Dr. Curran-Celentano. "It takes a lot of hard work and strong will to be able to reverse the condition that led to excess weight gain."

Weight should come off slowly. Any loss over two pounds a week is probably the result of an untenable program, she notes, so be patient with yourself.

Commit to ten weeks. It takes time to break old patterns and establish new ones. "Habits are incredibly powerful," says Dr. Sinaikin. If you've been having three butter pats on your toast every morning, and you switch to a teaspoon of all-fruit jam instead, it will take weeks before you're used to the new routine.

You should pledge your body to ten weeks of effort, experts advise. When you get past

Healthy Weight Target

To find out whether your body weight is on target or whether it's too high (increasing your disease risk), find your body mass index (BMI) on the vertical column and your waist/hip ratio (WHR) on the horizontal line. Locate the point at which they meet to find out whether you may need to trim some pounds or inches.

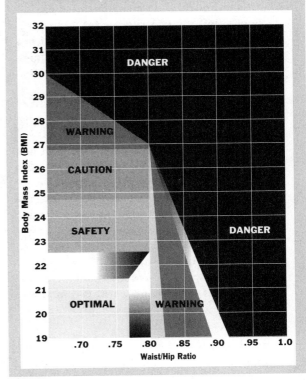

three months and you're still eating low-fat, you've probably established the healthy new behavior, says Wayne C. Miller, Ph.D., professor of exercise science at George Washington University Medical School in Washington, D.C.

The Key to the Kingdom

Fasting, starvation and measuring out your food with coffee spoons is not the way to shed

The Trouble with Cellulite

Dimples are cute on babies but not on buttocks, thighs or hips. So how come so many of us suffer the curse of very un-cute cellulite in those below-the-waist areas?

What is this maddening fat that hits us below the belt, making pleasantly plump skin look like an orange peel from hell? "It's not covered in many dermatology books, but it's just regular fat," says Diana Bihova, M.D., clinical assistant professor of dermatology at New York University Medical Center in New York City. That's regular fat with a lattice of fibrous, elastic connective tissue over it, though.

Blame that lattice of tissue for cellulite's bad looks. Over time that tight net relaxes, and the fat underneath practically herniates through, Dr. Bihova says. Because it is pushing through the lattice, the fat looks pitted and dimpled and pocked.

Smoothing that bumpy skin is no easy matter. "Nothing is 100 percent successful," says Dr. Bihova.

Theoretically, liposuction—the surgical removal of fat—should work. But in practice it's dicey, says John E. Sherman, M.D., assistant clinical professor of surgery at New York Hospital–Cornell University Medical Center in New York City. "That's because liposuction is not as exact an operation as a procedure like rhinoplasty (nose surgery) is."

So it's all too easy for a woman to wind up with uneven patches of cellulite after she's spent the time and money required to have liposuction done.

There are also cellulite creams that may reduce your lumpy fat a little. "But the reduction is very minute," says Dr. Bihova. And beauty salon treatments like seaweed wraps achieve their small reductions mainly through water loss. After the procedure the water quickly returns, and so does the cellulite.

"Really, the most effective treatment for cellulite is reducing the layer of fat underneath. You very rarely see cellulite on the toned body of a dancer, for instance," says Dr. Bihova. Tightening up your body by body shaping (also called strength training or weight training) is the closest thing we have to a cellulite cure.

---

and keep off fat. Besides, "It's not overeating that's the biggest problem," says Dr. Curran-Celentano. It's a well-documented fact that the number of calories an overweight woman eats isn't much greater than the number on a skinny person's plate. "It's underexercise—underactivity—that's the problem. And we do know that sedentary people are fatter than active people."

Movement, exercise, or even fidgeting burns calories. Your level of activity may explain almost entirely why you have more or less body fat than your next-door neighbor,

according to William J. Evans, Ph.D., director of the Noll Physiological Research Center at Pennsylvania State University in University Park. Researchers have learned that some people are natural-born fidgeters and movers, and those movers are almost always leaner than their calmer sisters, says Dr. Evans.

Whatever our natural tendencies, we can all increase our movement by adding more exercise. As soon as we burn more calories in activity than we consume in food, we shed fat: Once we've burned the calories we eat in our daily meals (when we don't eat too many of them), we begin to tap the stored energy in our fat cells, too.

Exercise can also build muscle. That muscle tissue, once built, burns 30 to 50 more calories than fatty tissue. So, the more muscle you have, the higher your calorie burn. In fact, folks who exercise an hour a day use up about 8 percent more calories than the average couch potato—even when the exerciser is at rest.

Taking Steps toward Tummy Taming

The best news of all is that exercise can move you to the lowest rung of your set point—the weight your body tries to maintain. Round women don't turn wiry, but with exercise their curves can be sleek, taut and trimmer.

"Exercise greatly improves a person's ability to maintain weight loss, too," says Dr. Evans. "No other method has been shown to be more effective in weight maintenance."

If you're wondering how, here are some tips from experts.

Return to your childhood. First you have to pick a likely sport or activity. No clue? Well, what did you do as a kid? If you were a roller skater extraordinaire, try today's new, grown-up version: in-line skates. Some sports stores offer clinics where you can try out the skates with the guidance of a certified fitness instructor.

If tricycling was your childhood choice of sport, the increasingly popular pastime of mountain biking might be right up your valley, says Joan Price, certified fitness instructor, author of *Yes, You CAN Get in Shape* and owner-director of Unconventional Moves in Sebastopol, California. (See "The Calories You Burn Having Fun" on page 128 for more ideas.)

Do what you like. "Make exercise a treat, not a treatment," says Price. If you try in-line skating and don't take to it, toss the notion away.

"We know the real key to exercising regularly is whether you like the activity. That's why you should choose the one that grabs your fancy," says James O. Hill, Ph.D., associate director of the Center for Human Nutrition at the University of Colorado Health Sciences Center in Denver.

Master machines. The shiny machines in a nearby gym might turn you on to a convenient, easy-to-measure exercise routine. The high-tech gleamers that burn the most calories are the machines that work both arms and legs. A cross-country ski machine is number one, because it works your torso, too, says Dr. Stamford. You'll also get a good workout from stationary bikes with arms to push and pull. And you can paddle your whole body to better health on a rowing machine with a sliding seat that makes you push your legs while you pull the oars.

Moderate or Maniac?

Some exercise experts swear by aerobic exercise for fat loss. The first choice of others is weight training (also called strength training, resistance training or body shaping). There are many who favor a combination of both.

Actually, it may not matter what brand of exercise you pursue—at least not at the beginning of a weight-loss program, according to Dr. Miller. "We've been studying the effects of different programs—weight training, a combination of weight training and aerobics and aerobics alone—on weight loss in overweight people. At least over a ten-week period they all lost the same amount of body fat no matter what kind of exercise they did."

The Calories You Burn Having Fun

The following chart shows how many calories you'll use up during an hour of exercise. The first group includes mild to moderate activities. Or step up the pace (and calories burned) with the activities in the moderate to intense category.

Mild to Moderate Exercise	Calories Burned per Hour*
Tennis	425
Bicycling or stationary cycling (10 mph)	415
Hiking with a 20-lb. backpack (3 mph)	400
Aerobic exercise, moderate intensity	350
Horseback riding	350
Roller skating	350
Square dancing	350
Treadmill walking (4 mph)	345
Ballroom dancing	300
Calisthenics	300
Rowing machine, low intensity	300
Strength training	300
Table tennis	300
Aerobic exercise, low impact	275
Golf, walking with clubs	270
Bicycling or stationary cycling (5.5 mph)	245
Walking, mild (2–2.5 mph)	185–255

Moderate to Intense Exercise	
Martial arts	790
Running (7.2 mph)	700
Stair-climbing machine	680
Rope-jumping	660
Bicycling or stationary cycling (13 mph)	655
Rowing machine, moderate intensity	655
Running/jogging (5.5 mph)	655
Step aerobics, moderate intensity	610
Cross-country skiing (5 mph)	600
Handball	600
Walking, vigorous (5 mph)	555
Polka dancing	540
Swimming	540

*The caloric listings for all of the activities above are estimates based on what a 150-pound person might burn over one hour's time.

Then there's the question of whether to take a long walk or a short run. Or should you simply accumulate 30 minutes of daily activity as you garden, work in the house or climb up and down office stairs? (That's one recommendation of the American College of Sports Medicine.) "To lose fat, you have to burn more calories than you take in," says Dr. Curran-Celentano. "So your objective should be to do whatever you can to burn calories. No matter what they do, people should just start moving."

Here's how to put your weight-loss notion into motion.

March it off. If you prefer a fairly mellow activity like walking, don't automatically assume that your calorie burn is a mere bushfire next to the fat-consuming bonfires of your running friends.

"The best exercise seems to be anything aerobic that you can do at moderate intensity for a longer amount of time," says Dr. Kanaley. "We promote a 45-minute to one-hour walk. You can walk longer than you can do intense aerobics." Whether you're walking, biking or in-line skating, you shouldn't do it too slowly. "A handy rule of thumb is that you should be a little winded but still able to converse."

Be smart, use dumbbells. It's true, aerobic exercise burns the most calories, which burns up the most body fat. On the other hand, while weight training is a lower burn, it builds muscle. Muscles eat up more calories than body fat whether those muscles are at work, at play or at rest. So a woman who strength-trains cranks her metabolism up a few notches.

Worried about fitting both aerobics and strength training into your strained schedule? The American College of Sports Medicine says you can get by with just two sessions of strength training a week.

The quick, total-body workout on page 443

can help you get started. "By adding strength training to aerobics, you burn more calories every day," says Rebecca Gorrell, certified fitness instructor and wellness education director at Canyon Ranch in Tucson, Arizona. "When you add muscle, you boost your metabolism, which ultimately leads to fat loss. You feel stronger; you can do aerobics for a longer period of time. Even if you have to cut down on your aerobic time to do it, you'll still get better results if you add strength training."

Step deeply. If rows of cardiovascular machines are your workout tools of choice, here's something every gym fan should know about popular stair-climbers. A study of 18 exercisers found that deep, slow, ten-inch steps required 5 percent more energy than short, fast five-inch steps. So you burn more calories with slower but deeper steps. The turtle wins again.

Work out after eating. Some research suggests that doing moderate exercise after a meal burns more calories than doing the same routine on an empty stomach—about 15 percent more, according to Dr. Stamford.

"Exercise after eating seems to give your system a double boost—it hypes your metabolism," he says. But he emphasizes that exercise should be moderate—a walk rather than a run, for instance. Otherwise, your muscles and your digestive system will be competing for blood flow to do their respective jobs. If you channel blood flow toward the muscles and away from the intestines, the digestive process gets disrupted, and your stomach may become upset.

The Fuel to Burn

Both Dr. Sinaikin and Dr. Curran-Celentano caution newcomers to exercise not to fall into the reward trap. "People exercise so hard that they think they can reward themselves, and they start eating more," says Dr. Curran-Celentano. "But most people only exercise three or four days a week, and eating is seven days a week."

So even when you pay attention to your exercise first, don't ignore your diet or, above all, the fat in your diet. While your body breaks food down into carbohydrates, protein and fat, a gram of fat carries more calories than the other two, and it's about twice as easy for your body to store. Net result: The fat in food quickly and easily becomes fat in your body.

As you may have discovered, you can't turn the tide just by switching to low-fat or no-fat foods. Carbohydrates still have calories. Eating healthy while eating to lose weight means that you take in fewer calories than you expend, says Dr. Curran-Celentano. Any time you take a bite or sip of anything (except water), you're taking in calories.

Healthy eating, however, isn't a two-lettuce-leaves-a-day menu. Here are some ways to make a weight-loss diet a matter of habit.

Cut down, not out. You don't have to ban any of your favorite dishes or desserts, say nutrition experts. Just cut down on their frequency; then cut their size in half. "It's not as difficult as cutting out all cake, for instance, or all meat," says Robin Kanarek, Ph.D., physiological psychologist and professor at Tufts University in Medford, Massachusetts.

You can even eat dessert occasionally—but share that triple-chocolate brownie with your most loved friend. The half-portion technique is a good way to tackle the briers of restaurant eating, too. Take the other half home for another meal.

Be a sub sister. Substituting low-fat or nonfat items for their fully fatted cousins is another effective and easy technique, says Alan Kristal, Dr.PH., assistant professor of epidemiology at the University of Washington in Seattle. Nonfat mayonnaise and salad dressings cut out substantial numbers of calories. A couple of tablespoons of salad dressing can have well over 100 calories, for instance, but the same amount of its nonfat version can have as few as 32.

If you consistently substitute low-fat for high, you're sure to get used to the low-fat life. It took 2,000 women at the Fred Hutchinson Cancer Research Center in Seattle six months or less to lose their taste for fat, researchers found. Dr. Sinaikin says that it takes his patients about a year to get rid of their fat tooth.

Graze. Wise grazing—eating five or six times a day—will keep the wolf of hunger from your door. When you go longer than four hours without food, your blood sugar drops, and you're likely to get famished. Add a healthy snack such as fruit, raw vegetables or nonfat yogurt between meals, and you'll quell the urge to pig out. Just make sure that you cut down portions at your main meals to compensate for the calories from snacks you've been eating, says Elizabeth Somer, R.D., author of *Food and Mood*.

Banish buffets. Stay away from all-you-can-eat buffets, where the urge to splurge can be overpowering, says Dr. Sinaikin. "We don't pay enough attention to how we feel after we eat. Often we have to recover from a meal. We get so uncomfortable that we have to loosen our belts and lie down on the couch. Then we say it was a great meal."

See also Nutrition, Toning Your Body

Feet

DURING A LIFETIME of trekking upstairs and down, outdoors and in, over hill and down dale, we tread the equivalent of four times around the earth.

Given that our feet get that kind of workout, we ought to show some respect. But in practice women squish them more than they care for them.

Consider Cinderella's story. Prince Charming rediscovers Cinderella because she has the daintiest feet in town. The evil stepsisters seem all the uglier just because they have—oh no!—big feet. This is just the kind of story that gives perfectly normal foot size a bad name—and makes a virtue of dainty little toes stuffed in triple-petites.

As if fairy tales weren't bad enough, consider the time-honored tradition of foot binding. In China, where minuscule feet (called Golden Lotuses) were considered wonderful, the most prized bound feet were just three inches long. To achieve these pedestals of perfection, a girl's toes were bent under and bandaged to her foot. Only the big toe was left free. The little girl grew up with bones that were permanently deformed. But at least she had tiny feet.

That was then; this is now. Nobody seriously believes that small feet are the signs of perfect prettiness. Do they?

Well, if not, how come "the fashion shoe is a slowly deforming device?" according to S. W. Balkin, D.P.M., attending assistant professor of podiatry, podiatry section, in the Department of Orthopedics at Los Angeles County–University of Southern California

Medical Center. Over a lifetime of wearing high heels and tight shoes, each set of five toes assumes the triangular shape of pointed toe boxes. "It's analogous to foot binding," he says.

The fact is, women pay dearly for fashion. Ninety percent of the surgery on common foot problems such as bunions and hammertoes is done on women, notes Carol Frey, M.D., director of the Orthopedic Hospital of Los Angeles Foot and Ankle Clinic and a researcher on the Women's Shoewear Council of the American Orthopaedic Foot and Ankle Society.

Also, women are much more likely than men to suffer from neuroma, an inflammation and thickening of nerves between the toes. In fact, more than 90 percent of people with neuroma are women. "The modern fashion shoe is to blame. Not weight, work or heredity," says Dr. Balkin. "The sad fact is that these conditions are nearly 100 percent preventable, yet once they have gotten severe enough, they require lifetime care or surgery."

Many women over age 65 have worn pointy-toed pumps for much of their lives, and their feet pay the price: These women have 3½ times more corns and calluses and 13 times more bunions than men.

But maybe that will change.

These days, females are wearing more sensible foot gear, at least some of the time, according to James McGuire, D.P.M., director of physical therapy and instructor in the Department of Orthopedics at the Foot and Ankle Institute of Pennsylvania College of Podiatric Medicine in Philadelphia.

In roomier shoes feet spread more comfortably, and fewer bones are scrunched. Not surprisingly, the roomier footwear is resulting in the foot assuming a more natural size.

"The average size of women's shoes has

grown from 6½ to 8½ in the past 25 years," says Carl Barone, owner of Carl's Shoes in Moorestown, New Jersey, and a shoe salesman for some 50 years. But you can still have problems if the shoe doesn't fit right.

If the Shoe Doesn't Fit

"My feet are killing me" is a common expression—but it's usually the shoes that are doing the damage, especially for women.

Orthopedic experts estimate that ill-fitting shoes provoke 75 percent of our foot problems, including bunions, hammertoes, neuromas, corns and calluses and blisters. Here's how they happen.

Bunions. A bunion is a bony growth that forms on the joint at the base of the big toe. An inflammation begins on the side of the toe joint, and gradually the metatarsal bone moves outward as the big toe starts to move inward. That lumpy side growth of bone, combined with the dislocaton of the joint, creates the problem.

Hammertoes. When a pointed shoe squeezes the big toe and the smallest toe toward the middle, the toe in the middle may get forced upward, resulting in a hammertoe.

Neuromas. If you wear high heels, the foot position pressures the toes into the toe box of the shoe. If the toe box is pointed and tight, a bone at the base of each toe (usually at the base of the third and fourth toes) sometimes rubs. It's the rubbing action that eventually inflames and thickens the nerve between them, causing a neuroma. Irritated neuromas cause burning and cramping.

Corns and calluses. These are created where an ill-fitting shoe rubs the foot too much. They're thickened nubs or clumps of dead skin cells—more protection than a problem when they start, but they become

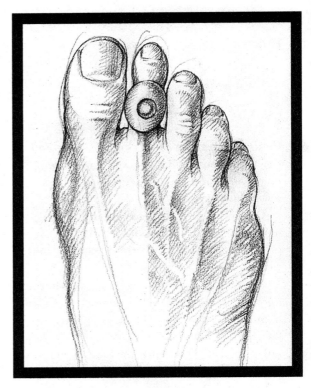

To protect a corn from pain and friction, buy a small oval pad and cut a hole in the center that's the size of the corn. Position the pad to protect the corn as shown and attach with self-adhesive or surgical tape.

painful when they get too big. Corns are smaller and usually form on top of the toe or in between toes. Calluses are bigger and usually form on the bottom of the foot. They can be caused by shoes that have inadequate padding under the foot.

Blisters. Usually a temporary problem, blisters are caused by rubbing between the toes or between the foot and shoe.

What's Good for the Sole

There are ways to assuage almost any foot complaint. Here's what foot care specialists recommend.

Stretch this little piggie. "In a way, hammertoes are part of being human," says

Melanie Sanders, M.D., chairwoman of the Women's Shoewear Council and an orthopedist in Indianapolis. "To walk upright, you roll across your foot from heel to toe. That pushes your toes upwards, pulling the normal padding upward with them. High heels worsen that tendency," she says. "But you can counterbalance that movement you do all day long."

Dr. Sanders suggests stretching your toes. First, sit down on a low stool or a pillow on the floor and place one foot flat on the floor. Then, "put your finger right where the hair on your toes tends to grow and push each toe down firmly, so that you feel the stretch on top of your foot. Hold it down for 30 seconds. Do each toe. Then go back and do them again. You can do it while you're watching the news. It takes four or five minutes."

"Do it daily if your feet are bothering you," Dr. Sanders says. "For maintenance you just need to do it two or three times a week."

Sleep with a splint. After a day under pressure from shoes, bunions often ache. If you have a bunion that's kicking up, try using a foot care product called a night splint. It works while you sleep. You can get a night splint from an orthopedist or podiatrist, according to Dr. Sanders.

The night splint is a small apparatus with a plastic piece that fits the big toe. An elastic strap pulls the big toe into a straighter, more normal position. "The new position helps relieve the pressure and takes the strain off the area around the bunion," he says.

Check your seams. Athletic shoes are generally good for your feet. But women who have bunions should double-check the construction of their cross-trainers and step or aerobic shoes, according to Dr. Sanders. "Some sneakers have a little fashion seam that goes right across the top of a bunion."

Because the seam doesn't stretch, you get an area of high pressure over the bunion.

Prick a blister. Blisters happen when you break in a new pair of shoes or when you do too much walking in the wrong shoes. A blister can make you miserable.

You probably won't want to walk or work out very much until the blister heals. In the meantime, though, "you don't need to wait for it to get big. You can drain it as soon as you see it," says Rodney S. W. Basler, M.D., assistant professor of internal medicine (dermatology) at the University of Nebraska Medical Center in Omaha.

Sterilize a needle with the flame of a match or rubbing alcohol. Then pierce the blister at its edge. Press it to drain as much fluid as you can, but don't remove the blister's roof.

"Drain it every 12 hours," says Dr. Basler. "That appears to bring about the fastest healing."

Size Things Up

Though choosing the proper shoe would clear up most kinds of foot pain, choice is never easy. One foot is generally bigger than the other. In fact, when the Women's Shoewear Council surveyed 356 women from around the country, they found that 66 percent of them had one foot larger than the other.

Despite the imprecise nature of foot size, you can make a well-considered shoe selection if you're prepared. Here's how.

Make yourself a shoe sizer. "The main issue in shoes is their width," says Dr. Sanders. Eighty-eight percent of women wear shoes that are one or two sizes too narrow, the Women's Shoewear Council found. To prevent this, make a handy shoe sizer at home, then bring it to the shoe store.

How to Make a Sizer

To make a handy shoe sizer, all you need are a pencil, plain cardboard (shirt cardboard is fine) and scissors. Here's how it's done.

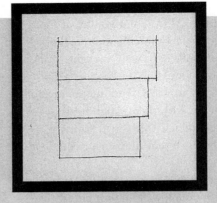

Adjoining the first rectangle, measure a second rectangle that equals your widest measurement minus ¼ inch. So if the first rectangle is 3½ inches by 1 inch, the one next to it will be 3¼ inches by 1 inch. Then, right next to that, draw another rectangle that equals your first measurement minus ½ inch. (So this would be 3 inches by 1 inch.)

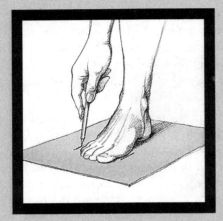

To measure the sizer, stand normally, with one foot on a sheet of plain cardboard, so the ball of your foot is spread to its full width. Then mark the dimensions on either side of your foot. Measure both feet this way and use the widest measurement for your shoe sizer.

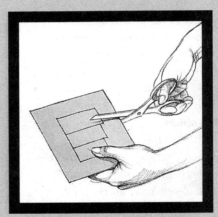

After you've finished measuring, cut out the shoe sizer with a pair of scissors.

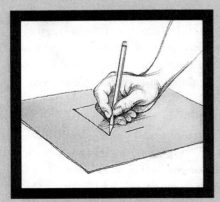

Measure a rectangle that's as wide as your foot by 1 inch. If your foot measures 3½ inches wide, for example, draw a long rectangle that is 3½ inches by 1 inch.

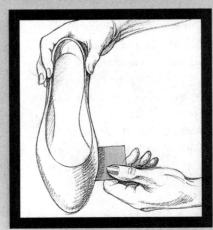

Take along all three sizers the next time you go shoe shopping. Measure the shoe width as shown—using the largest sizer for athletic shoes and either of the smaller ones for dress shoes.

The Best Device

Orthotics are just pieces of plastic, foam, rubber or fabric that resemble lightly sculptured innersoles. By redistributing the pressure on your foot when you walk or run, they can help relieve a host of foot problems. Simple though they are, these shoe inserts can resolve or relieve foot problems about 90 percent of the time, says David Alper, D.P.M., visiting professor of podiatry at Northeastern University in Boston.

Orthotics are especially beneficial to people who have flat feet that turn (pronate) inward, helping prevent inflamed ligaments and heel spurs. Orthotics can also subdue the nerve pain of neuromas and throttle troublesome corns and calluses.

"Most foot problems are mechanical ones," says John B. Redford, M.D., professor of rehabilitation medicine at the University of Kansas School of Medicine in Kansas City. "There's some deficiency in the way your foot strikes the ground—the muscles are weak or the bones aren't formed right."

"What an orthotic does is shift the pressure into the proper place," explains Rodney S. W. Basler, M.D., assistant professor of internal medicine (dermatology) at the University of Nebraska Medical Center in Omaha. Some standard orthotics are available over-the-counter in pharmacies and sporting goods stores. But they can also be custom-designed from casts of your feet made in podiatrists' offices.

Before you invest $200 or more in custom-made orthotics, though, try an over-the-counter pair that will cost you about one-tenth that price, suggests Dr. Alper. "They usually don't have to be custom-made."

Account for swelling. Since your feet swell during the day, you should measure for your shoe sizer in the afternoon. Late in the day, after you've been walking around, is also the best time to shop for shoes, since that's when your feet are largest.

Shop with your sizer. Take along the sizer whenever you go shopping for any kind of shoes, says Francesca M. Thompson, M.D., assistant clinical professor of orthopedic surgery at Columbia University College of Physicians and Surgeons in New York City and a member of the Women's Shoewear Council.

Your athletic shoes should be as wide as the widest measurement on the sizer. For dress shoes use either of the two smaller measurements. Don't go any narrower than the smallest width, she cautions.

Check the nation. Shoe sizes are inconsistent today because 88 percent of American shoes are made outside the country, says Barone. Each country makes shoes according to its own standards of size. That means you always need to try shoes on. A size eight from Brazil, for instance, is not necessarily the same size as an eight from Italy.

Remeasure as you age. Once you have reached adulthood, your feet don't grow, but they do change. By the time you're in your thirties, changes in the ligaments—bands of tissue that join the bones in the sole of your

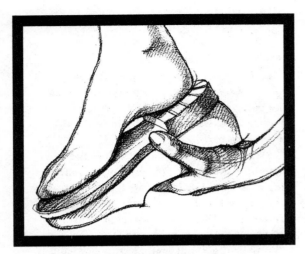

To make sure there's ample room in your shoes, try this measurement test. If the sole of your right foot overlaps the sole of your left shoe at any point, the shoes are too small.

foot and raise the arch—allow your foot to collapse. And your foot begins to spread, or "splay."

"That spread is often responsible for an increase in shoe size of one to two sizes during your lifetime," says Dr. McGuire. In general, your feet are likely to increase in size during and after a pregnancy, because of the body's response to increasing demands. In addition, there's a hormone called relaxin that causes the ligaments to relax in the last month of pregnancy—and as the ligaments in your feet relax, your feet may get larger.

Exercise can also make a difference. "Aggressive exercise may make your foot meatier and bigger," he says.

To monitor your changing feet, measure them every three years, suggests Dr. Sanders. And revise your shoe sizer accordingly.

Styling Sensibly

Despite the bonanza of comfortable athletic shoes—and even some comfortable

pumps—it's still all too easy to stray into Sore Foot Gulch. Here are some pointers to keep you safe from painful shoes.

Round it off. Whether you buy a flat or a heel, look for shoes with a rounded toe box instead of a deforming pointed toe box. There's a simple test to see whether a shoe is rounded enough. Hold the bottom of the left shoe against the sole of your right foot as shown in the illustration at left. Then hold the bottom of the right shoe against the sole of your left foot. If either shoe fails to cover your foot's sole, the shoes are undersize. Pick a larger size or another style and test again.

Strap your heel. In order to get a shoe wide enough for your foot, you may have to buy one with a little too much heel room. "The heel doesn't spread with age the way the balls of your feet do," says Dr. Sanders.

Try a shoe with an adjustable heel strap. That way, you can get one with ample toe room, then cinch in the strap to prevent slippage.

Or pad it. If you have a favorite pump with the right size toe box, but it's a little too slippery on your heel, try a heel pad, suggests Dr. Sanders. It has done the trick for many of her patients, she says.

Healing Your Heel Pain

In terms of body parts, "the heels are the first things to hit the ground," says William Case, P.T., president of Case Physical Therapy in Houston, Texas.

Heel pain most often comes from an inflammation of the plantar fascia, the main ligament that stretches across the bottom of the foot from heel to toe. When you overuse your foot or pronate (turn the foot inward when you walk), you may irritate and inflame the ligament. If you do that often enough, a

Pamper Your Feet

A pedicure won't cure any foot problems, but it will make your feet look better. And you don't have to make a beauty salon appointment to treat your toes. Here's how to give yourself a pedicure.

- Assemble your instruments. You'll need a foot or wash basin, foot-soak powder (which helps moisten toenails and calluses), a bath towel, a metal manicuring pusher, moisturizing cream, a pumice stone or pumice pedicuring tool, toenail clippers, an emery board and nail polish. These supplies can be purchased at drug or beauty supply stores.

- Add the foot-soak powder to the basin and run warm—not hot—water, into it. Soak your feet for ten minutes.

- Towel your feet dry. Then, with the straight edge of the manicuring pusher (not the pointed edge), gently push down your toenail cuticles and scrape off any debris that accumulates. Gently cleanout any dirt underneath your toenails.

- Rub moisturizer into your feet and give yourself a foot massage.

- With a pumice stone or tool, sand some of the dead skin off your calluses. You don't need to be too aggressive—you can work on your calluses whenever your skin is soft from a bath. (You can also apply sloughing lotion, which allows you to rub away dry skin.)

- Cut your toenails straight across with toenail clippers.

- With an emery board, file your toenails smooth and straight across.

- Clean off any remaining moisturizing oil from your toenails with nail polish remover. (This is only necessary if you want to use nail polish.)

- Apply one or two coats of clear or colored nail polish.

- Let the polish dry for 15 minutes to let it set. If you can stay barefooted for a while, let your toes dry longer—preferably one hour. Nail polish is especially slow to dry on toenails that have been soaking. To prevent smearing the polish as it dries, you can buy reusable, inexpensive toe separators in the drugstore. (They look like a set of spongy rubber bumpers.) Relax, watch television or read a book while you're waiting.

---

bony growth called a heel spur sometimes develops at the point of injury.

Pain from an inflamed ligament or a heel spur feels worst in the morning and diminishes as the day goes on. But the correct shoe insert can cure most heel pain, according to David Alper, D.P.M., visiting professor of podiatry at Northeastern University in Boston. So it's worth shopping in the foot products section of a drugstore or sport supply store.

Here are some foot soothers to look for.

Lift with a cup. You can get a heel cup that goes under the back of your foot to relieve some of the pressure on the ligament. Or find a foam insole that cushions the entire foot. Either one may relieve heel pain.

You might also get relief from inserts called orthotics, which cushion your heel and align

Aaaaahhhh!

Nothing feels better when your feet are sore or tired than a foot massage. Here's one you can do yourself, as recommended by Edith Malin, a shiatsu practitioner and a teacher at the International School of Shiatsu in Doylestown, Pennsylvania. Perform the full routine on your right foot and then switch to your left, instructs Malin. Here are the steps to follow to give yourself a complete foot massage.

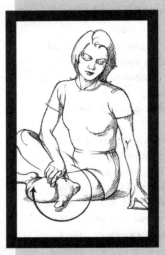

1. Sitting on the floor on a mat or pillow, grasp your right foot above the ankle with your right hand. Circle your foot five times to the right, using a full range of motion, then five times to the left.

2. Pull back the five toes of your right foot with the five fingers of the right hand—just enough to make the sole feel a little tighter. With

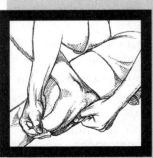

your right foot in this position, lightly pound the bottom with your left fist. Hold your fist as if you were knocking on a door. Lightly pound up and down your foot three times.

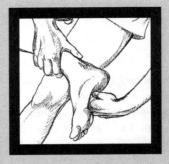

3. With your left hand knead the bottom of your right foot. Use a rocking motion and go up your foot from the heel to the top of the ball.

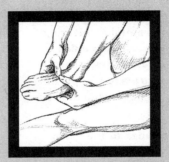

4. Place both thumbs on the top of your right foot. Clasp the underside of your foot with your fingers. Starting in the center of the bottom of your foot, press and hold your foot with your fingers for several seconds. Then slide your fingers a couple of inches up the center and hold the press again for several seconds. If the spot feels tender, hold it a little longer. Continue until you reach the base of your toes. Repeat the motion along both sides of the same foot, one side at a time.

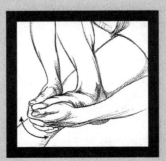

5. Put your hands together, palms facing each other, and lace your fingers. Place your right foot between both hands, with the bottom of your foot on your left palm and your right palm on top of your foot. The tips of your toes are in the laced part of your fingers. Stabilize the top of your foot along your big toe with your thumbs. Using your hands, quickly bend your toes back and forth across the widest part of your foot about 12 times. Then squeeze your toes in between both of your hands.

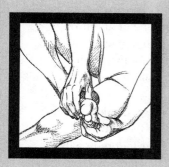

6. Press your finger-tips in between the bones on the top of your right foot. You can stabilize the bottom of your foot with your thumbs. Rub gently and deeply all around the top of your foot. Do this massage slowly and thoroughly.

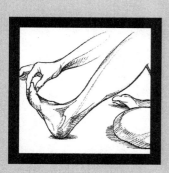

7. With your right thumb and index finger grasp your right big toe and rotate it around its joint. Squeeze your big toe at its base, then pull it gently but firmly from the base to the tip, sliding your fingers off the end. Repeat with the next toe until you've done all the toes of your right foot.

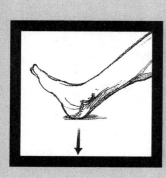

8. Lifting and dropping your right leg quickly, pound the floor lightly with the back of your heel 12 times. Now repeat steps 1 through 8 with your left foot.

and control your foot when you walk. Unfortunately, orthotics don't work in pumps or high heels because of the way the shoes are designed.

Flex your leather. Before you toss out a too-tight shoe, try using a shoe stretcher, suggests Dr. Sanders. It's a device you can buy in a full-service shoe store or a shoe repair shop starting at around $11.

The stretcher looks like the front part of a shoe tree. Some have round, ball-like attachments that allow you to stretch specific sites—where the shoe presses against a bunion or corn, for instance.

You can use the shoe stretcher alone or maximize its effectiveness with a liquid lubricant available at the shoe repair shop or a drugstore. It works best on leather shoes, because they have greater give than most vinyl and are less likely to be damaged by the product. (In fact, some experts say you shouldn't use the product on vinyl at all, because you'll ruin the shoes—despite what the product label says.) Apply the shoe-stretching liquid to the inside of your shoe. Then position the shoe stretcher and gently tighten it to press against the inside of the shoe. Let the shoe stretch overnight or longer.

Steps toward Prevention

If you don't want to turn into one of the 43.1 million Americans with feet that hurt, here are some basic all-purpose guidelines to follow.

Wear running shoes. You don't have to run to wear running shoes. Many experts tout them as the best all-around shoes for foot support, because the heel is so thick and stable. "It's better than any other kind of athletic shoe," says Bruce Lebowitz, D.P.M., director of the podiatric clinic of the Johns

Eau de Toe

With 250,000 or so sweat glands in our feet, it's a wonder they don't stink all the time. Women don't put out quite as much scent from those glands as men do, but they also suffer from toxic sock syndrome.

"That's what we call it," says Rodney S. W. Basler, M.D., assistant professor of internal medicine (dermatology) at the University of Nebraska Medical Center in Omaha. "The odor is caused by the bacteria that invade your foot when you sweat. And the bacterium that causes odor is related to the bacterium that causes acne. So acne medication, like 10 percent benzoyl peroxide, works well for foot odor, although it can take the color out of your socks."

Keeping your feet dry and sweat-free also foils odoriferous organic life. Here are some tips.

- **After each use, give sneakers a full day to dry out.**
- **Apply antiperspirant to your feet.**
- **Try anti-odor shoe inserts.**

shoes, though. Just note the date of each new pair you buy. If you run 25 miles or more a week, replace them every 2½ to 3 months, says Gary M. Gordon, D.P.M., director of the running and walking clinic at the Joseph Torg Center for Sports Medicine at Hahnemann University Hospital in Philadelphia. If you take three or more aerobics classes a week, you're wearing out the padding at about the same rate. So you should also replace those sneakers every two to three months. With a lighter aerobics schedule, replace them every four to six months.

That may seem like a heavy sneaker toll, but it's worth it for pain-free feet. "If you wear worn-out sneakers, your foot pain will come back," warns Dr. Lebowitz.

See also Skeletal System

Hopkins Bayview Medical Center in Baltimore.

Even if your workplace forbids sneakers on the job, you can do what many businesswomen do—wear them to and from work and at home and play.

Date your sneakers. As the padding in your athletic shoes ages and wears down, your feet start to do double duty in the shock-absorption department. Worn-out shoes sneak up on you; they get old before you know it, and the once-comfortable athletic sneaker may cause real foot problems.

You can keep track of your own athletic

Fertility

    WHAT DOES AN AMERICAN WOMAN in the 1990s do for a fertility rite? Well, she probably starts playing the numbers.

We're not talking lottery, here. No, the name of this "game" should be Calendo.

It involves using a yearly planner and a red pen. Circles get drawn around certain days, a particular month or a landmark year. Then a few whispered words or silent prayers are made for the circled dates to be the lucky pick.

Women who are actively trying to get pregnant focus on the days of the week: They count out 14 days since their last period and schedule sex. We have to do it on Thursday, they insist. Don't be late!

Others—waiting as long as possible before getting pregnant—find themselves counting the years. How many left before I turn 35? they ask. How much longer after that can I push it before my time runs out?

Either way, it can all feel like a gamble.

Conception Concepts

Fertility basically refers to our ability to conceive. That ability generally begins shortly after we get our first period—which on the average happens around the age of 12. Fertility lasts until our periods cease at menopause, which usually occurs around age 51.

While that makes it sound like we have 40 years of time to get pregnant, we actually have less. That's because women are not fertile on every day of the month, every month of the year. Instead, an egg can be fertilized 12 to 72 hours after it's released. That really adds up to about 4 years of fertility.

When are those fertile days? It all has to do with your menstrual cycle. In the first half of your cycle, your brain signals your body to release hormones, triggering eggs in your ovaries to start growing. One egg will go on to develop fully and be released by the ovary in the process known as ovulation. Some theories suggest that when this egg is released—usually midway through your cycle, about 14 days after the start of your last period—that's when you are fertile.

There are other theories, however, that suggest your fertile time ends with ovulation. One study found that pregnancies occurred when intercourse took place—within six days prior to ovulation. "The data indicates that sperm can live in the reproductive tract three to five days prior to conception," says Allen Wilcox, M.D., Ph.D., chief of epidemiology at the National Institute of Environmental Health Sciences in Research Triangle Park, North Carolina, and investigator in this study. He found that after ovulation there's a drop in the probability of pregnancy. According to Dr. Wilcox, this may be because the egg lives for a short time after ovulation, or because a change in the cervical mucus after ovulation prevents the passage of new sperm.

For conception to occur, the egg must be released, but it also must travel into the fallopian tube. If the egg encounters a sperm there while the egg is still alive, and if the sperm is able to penetrate the egg, conception takes place. Then the fertilized egg has to travel down the fallopian tubes and into the uterus, where it implants in the uterine lining.

So fertility basically requires several things: Your ovaries must produce healthy eggs, your partner's sperm must be healthy and able to reach and fertilize an egg, the fallopian tubes must be clear so that sperm can reach an egg and the sperm must reach an egg in time.

The Big Threats

Given the intricate timing involved in making babies, the last thing you want to do is throw anything into the equation that's going to make it harder for you to get pregnant.

Every woman should be aware of the significant threat to fertility posed by sexually transmitted diseases (STDs), says Randall Barnes, M.D., chief of reproductive endocrinology and fertility at the University of Chicago. He points to chlamydia and gonorrhea as major threats—both diseases that can migrate into the upper reproductive tract to cause damage.

Time (read "aging") can pose another challenge to your fertility. Basically, the older you get, the less fertile you become. This is true more so for women than men because, as we all know, our fertility tapers off more dramatically at an earlier age. What many women don't realize, however, is how sharply fertility can decline before menopause.

In women there is a slight decline in fertility between the ages of 25 and 35. "The decline is sharper after 35 and then falls off precipitously after 40," says Dr. Barnes. About a decade later (for most women), menopause puts an end to menstrual cycles and with them, our fertility.

While on the average women go through menopause at age 51, some women have premature menopause putting an unexpected halt to their childbearing years. Premature menopause can occur as early as the late twenties or early thirties.

Spare the Stress and Start the Child

We've all heard the stories. A woman tries over and over—unsuccessfully—to get pregnant. Then she quits her job. Bam! Child on the way.

What's going on here?

"Scientifically and medically, it has been demonstrated beyond doubt that stress can be a cause of infertility," says Reed Moskowitz, M.D., medical director of the Stress Disorders Services at New York University Medical Center in New York City.

Studies show that high levels of emotional stress can contribute to infertility through several mechanisms, says Dr. Moskowitz. In addition to causing hormonal changes and irregular ovulation, stress can cause fallopian tubes to spasm as well as disrupt the implantation process of a fertilized egg, he says.

Doctors can't find a specific medical cause for infertility in about 10 percent of women who have it, says Dr. Moskowitz. But between one-third and one-half of the women with "unexplained infertility" will be able to get pregnant if the stress in their lives is removed.

Some simple and effective techniques that women can use help decrease their stress, says Dr. Moskowitz. Here's what he recommends.

Recognize it. The first step is to become aware of your stress, says Dr. Moskowitz. First, heighten your awareness physically

Here's what you can do to safeguard your fertility.

Fend off invaders. One of the main things you can do to preserve fertility is purely preventive. Avoid getting sexually transmitted

by doing a body scan. With your mental focus move down your body and ask yourself, "Where do I feel tension? In my neck? In my abdomen?" Once you've identified the physical area, focus on "letting go" there to release the built-up tension.

Then think back, reviewing the nature of the emotions you felt throughout the day. Are they negative or positive? If they are negative, what triggers them? When you've identified the triggers, it then becomes easier to deal with them.

Relax your body. You can work on physical relaxation by doing some deep-breathing exercises or yoga, says Dr. Moskowitz. For deep breathing, simply lie down on a couch, rest one hand on your abdomen and begin breathing slowly and deeply in and out, he says. You should see your hand rise and fall.

Visualize the calm. Try using visualization, says Dr. Moskowitz. Take a few minutes each day to visualize a calm scene—maybe the beach, the mountains or the countryside. Visualize a scene that is relaxing and try to get into it with all your senses.

See a mind-body specialist. "If a woman gets diagnosed as having unexplained infertility, then that should cause a lightbulb to go off: This might be a stress-related problem," says Dr. Moskowitz. You should ask your doctor to refer you to a stress specialist.

Don't wait too long. While women certainly shouldn't rush to conceive before they're ready to take on the demands of parenthood, doctors urge us not to wait too long. If you know that you want to get pregnant and have a baby, it's probably best to get started before the age of 35, says Dr. Barnes. Certainly try to do it before 40, he advises.

Talk to Mom. To figure out when you're likely to go through menopause, check with your mother. Women tend to go through menopause around the same age that their moms did, says Dr. Barnes.

If your mother went through menopause early, then you may be at greater risk of doing that too, he says. If she's in her mid or late forties and still hasn't gone through menopause, or if she had it around the average age of 51, then you're less likely to have premature menopause.

Don't fear the Pill. "Taking the Pill does not make you infertile," says Dr. Barnes. It may take a few months for you to start ovulating again after you stop Pill use, but generally, ovulation will resume, and you'll be able to get pregnant.

Understand the IUD. While doctors deem the intrauterine device (IUD) safe and effective for women in disease-free, monogamous relationships, the method can be risky for women who are at risk for sexually transmitted diseases.

If you are exposed to an STD, the IUD may help bacteria travel up into the uterus and fallopian tubes where they can cause damage, says Dr. Barnes.

Go clean. Give up those cigarettes, experts say. Kicking the cigarette habit is really important, because nicotine can be poisonous to sperm, and high quantities of it have been found in the cervical mucus of women who smoke.

diseases, advises Dr. Barnes. Being monogamous, using condoms and having yourself and your partner tested for STDs are all things you can do to keep STDs from taking a toll.

How They Inject Some New Life

A time may come when your doctor recommends moving on to high-tech assisted reproduction methods. Here are some of the options.

In vitro fertilization (IVF). Eggs and sperm are united in a petri dish and incubated until fertilization takes place. The fertilized egg is then transferred into the uterus for implantation.

Zygote intrafallopian transfer (ZIFT). Again, the eggs and sperm go into a petri dish. Once an egg is fertilized, it's moved into the fallopian tube. From there it travels down to the uterus. This technique may enhance the chances of implantation.

Gamete intrafallopian transfer (GIFT). Eggs are removed from the woman, sperm from the man and the doctor places them directly in the fallopian tube. If the sperm penetrates the egg in the tube, the fertilized egg will then move down to implant in the uterus.

Subzonal sperm injection. Doctors use a thin needle to inject a single sperm just under the outer layer of the egg. This procedure begins in a petri dish, and the fertilized egg is then transferred into the uterus.

Introcytoplasmic sperm injection (ICSI). This is the same as subzonal sperm injection, except the sperm is injected deeper— into the middle of the egg cell, rather than just beneath the surface.

When Trouble Strikes

Maybe you've been trying to get pregnant but haven't been having any luck. Does that mean you're infertile?

If you've been having unprotected intercourse for over a year and haven't conceived, doctors would say that the answer is yes, as a couple, the two of you are infertile. That doesn't necessarily mean that you won't or can't get pregnant, but if you want that to happen, you'll probably have to identify the cause of infertility. Often tests can determine whether the cause lies with you, with your partner or with both of you. But sometimes the cause remains unknown, even after medical testing.

Doctors estimate that 30 percent of infertility cases are attributed to the woman, 30 percent are attributed to the man, and 30 percent are from some combination of the two. The remaining 10 percent are unexplainable.

Helping the Hormones

If you're having trouble getting pregnant, maybe it's because you're not ovulating. That happens in about 30 percent of infertile women. Producing and releasing a mature egg requires signals from the brain to the ovaries to produce estrogen and progesterone hormones. Insufficient amounts of these hormones can cause a breakdown in the chain of command, and ovulation can be foiled.

Your doctor can test to see if you are ovulating by giving you a basal body temperature (BBT) test and thorough blood tests. During the BBT test you track your body temperature across your menstrual cycle. The blood tests help your doctor assess whether or not your body has the hormone levels necessary to trigger ovulation.

If you're not ovulating because of inadequate hormone levels, most likely your doctor will try treating you with some drugs—such as clomiphene citrate (Serophene)—that help induce ovulation. The drugs basically trick your body into producing more of the hormones needed to stimulate the ovaries. If those drugs don't work, your doctor will probably recommend some other, stronger drugs aimed at inducing ovulation.

Fallopian Troubles?

Another trouble spot could be your fallopian tubes. They might be damaged or blocked, which appears to be the cause in about 50 percent of infertile women.

Damage can be the result of pelvic inflammatory disease that developed when STDs such as gonorrhea and chlamydia migrated up into the fallopian tubes, says Cheryl Walker, M.D., assistant professor of obstetrics and gynecology at the University of California, Irvine. When this type of infection invades, the tubes become damaged or blocked, making it impossible for a sperm to reach an egg and fertilize it or for a fertilized egg to travel down into the uterus and implant.

Fallopian tubes can also be affected by endometriosis, a disease in which tissue similar to the lining of the uterus is located outside the uterus. This growth can cause infertility by interfering with the natural movement of the ovaries and fallopian tubes, says Paula Bernstein, M.D., Ph.D., attending physician at Cedars Sinai Medical Center in Los Angeles.

Your doctor can check out the condition of your fallopian tubes with a test called hysterosalpingography, says Dr. Barnes. Dye is injected through the cervix, and from there it travels up into the uterus and fallopian tubes. The doctor then takes an x-ray of the fallopian tubes, enabling her to see whether the tubes are blocked or free. Sometimes surgery can clear the tubes.

Occasionally, there's trouble in the uterus. Some women can have fibroids—benign tumors that poke into the cavity of the uterus,

says Dr. Barnes. Or infertility could be associated with an infection of the uterus called endometritis, or even endometrial cancer. All of these uterine conditions can interfere with a fertilized egg's ability to implant in the uterine wall. For some women, doctors recommend surgery to correct the problem.

Or the culprit behind infertility could be the immune system. By mistake, the bodies of some women react to sperm as if they were unwelcome invaders. If your body produces antibodies to attack the sperm, they obviously don't have much of a chance. Your doctor can tell if you are producing these antibodies through blood tests and may recommend some other conception method if this is what's going on.

Sometimes the reason you can't get pregnant has to do with your partner's sperm rather than your own reproductive system. Most infertile men have a low sperm count, says Dr. Barnes. If your man has enough sperm, the problem may be that the sperm aren't shaped properly or that they don't swim fast enough to reach the egg in time.

What You Two Can Do

If you think that you or your husband may be infertile, here's what you can do.

See a specialist. If you've been trying unsuccessfully for a year to get pregnant, it may be time to see an infertility specialist. Look for a doctor who is board certified in obstetrics and gynecology, reproductive endocrinology or urology. You can also ask if the doctor specializes in fertility and is a member of the American Fertility Society.

Other things to find out are the doctor's hospital affiliation, how many infertile couples she has treated and what her overall success rate is for live births. If you're to the point where you are considering using high-tech methods to conceive, look for a center or institution that is registered in the Society of Assisted Reproductive Technology, says Dr. Barnes. For a list of registered clinics in your area, write to the American Society for Reproductive Medicine, 1209 Montgomery Highway, Birmingham, AL, 35216.

Don't go it alone. "I encourage people to use support groups," says Dr. Barnes. For some women and men the groups can be very helpful. To locate an infertility support group in your area, contact RESOLVE at the RESOLVE National Office, 1310 Broadway, Somerville, MA 02144-1731.

See also Menopause, Reproductive System, Sexually Transmitted Diseases

Fingernails

LIKE MOST BODY PARTS, our fingernails rarely measure up to perfection. Those tapered, precisely filed pink frosted nails you see in magazines obviously don't belong to women who toil at work or at home. But the wear and tear of daily living doesn't have to mean worn and torn nails. There is hope for those "hopeless" nails.

Few of us have the nails we'd like to have, says Paul Kechijian, M.D., associate clinical professor of dermatology and chief of the nail section at New York University Medical Center in New York City. "Some people were just born with weak, brittle nails."

Tough Cells

A fingernail is a hard, curved plate made of keratin, a tough protein that's also the main constituent of skin and hair. At the bottom of the nail is an area called the matrix, which is the nail manufacturing area of the finger. In the matrix the cells get tightly packed to form keratin. The pink color of the nails is caused by a bed of blood vessels that lies underneath them.

If it seems your nails grow at a snail's pace, it's because they do: they creep along at the rate of 0.1 millimeter a day. Start a new nail on Labor Day, and by Christmas it will be nearing the tip of your finger. And, by the way, if you're right-handed, the nails on that hand grow faster, but for lefties the left nails are the quicker growers.

It's unlikely that you'll have nail illnesses, but they can signal problems elsewhere in

When There's a Fungus among Us

No matter how diligent you are about nail care, your filed and polished prizes could still fall victim to nail fungus, which causes discoloration, thickening and even shedding of the nail.

While toenails are affected by nail fungi about four times more often than fingernails, once fungus finds a foothold, it can spread from nail to nail, from foot to foot and then to your hands.

Sometimes a doctor treats fungus by trimming back the infected nail and prescribing a topical antifungal cream or liquid for daily use. Here are steps you can take to prevent further spread of fungus, as recommended by Paul Kechijian, M.D., associate clinical professor of dermatology and chief of the nail section at New York University Medical Center in New York City.

- Keep your nails clipped or filed back so they don't extend beyond the tips of your fingers. (The same goes for toenails.)
- Use separate sets of clippers for infected nails and for healthy nails to avoid spreading the fungus.
- Disinfect manicure and pedicure tools after each use. Wipe them with gauze or cotton balls saturated with alcohol. Pay special attention to the jaws of the clippers, where infected debris tends to accumulate.
- Keep your hands clean and dry. Wash your hands and nails with soap and water every day and dry well.
- Wear cotton-lined work gloves when you submerge your hands in water or soil. Change cotton gloves frequently.
- Don't let your cuticles get so dry that they crack—leaving openings for infection. Keep cuticles moisturized with petroleum jelly or hand cream.

your body. Problems such as psoriasis—the skin condition that causes itching and inflammation—may lead to fragile nails. Hyperthyroidism, or an overactive thyroid gland, can also lead to fragility. Brittle, ridged, concave nails are a sign of iron-deficiency anemia. Fiberlike growths on the nails are a sign of tuberous sclerosis, an inherited disorder affecting the nervous system and the skin. But most nail problems are caused by injury or lack of tender loving care.

Making More of Your Nails

With all the day-to-day beating that injures our nails—not to mention nail-biting episodes that some of us have—you may be looking somewhat sadly at the ragged nubs, wondering how to make them presentable nails. There's always the expensive manicure, of course. But apart from that there are plenty of things you can do on your own to help make your nails the crowning glory of your hands. Here's how.

Let the moisture in. "The first step toward healthier nails is to apply moisturizer to your hands every time you wash them—or any other time they've been in water," says Dr. Kechijian. Rub it in well and apply it frequently during the day.

In healthy nails a cell "adhesive" holds the tightly packed pancake-shaped cells of the nails together. When something damages this adhesive, you're likely to get weak, brittle nails. Many elements—from cold, dry winter weather to repeated soakings in water—can damage this intercellular substance, resulting in nails that chip, peel or break easily.

"If you apply a lotion to your hands as soon as you've lightly dried them, while they're still a bit damp, the lubricant helps to better seal the moisture in your skin and nails. A moisturizer prevents the rapid evaporation of water from the nail plate and prevents the contraction that can cause the nail to crack or peel," Dr. Kechijian says.

There are so many hand creams, cuticle creams and lotions on the shelves that choosing one may seem daunting. The best cream is the one that rubs in well and whose consistency feels best. Some of the newer extra-moisture-enhancing ingredients include alpha hydroxy acids, such as lactic acid, glycolic acid and urea.

Cover up. To prevent future dehydration, start protecting your hands when they're exposed to environmental hazards such as detergents, household cleansers or dry, moisture-robbing winter air, says Dr. Kechijian. For indoor jobs use lined rubber gloves with separate cotton gloves inside that can be removed as your hands become sweaty. Don't forget to wear warm gloves outdoors, even when you're out for a short time. If it's cold enough for a jacket, it's cold enough for gloves, says Dr. Kechijian.

Get the most from your moisturizer. When you apply your hand cream or cuticle cream, take a minute to massage the cream into your skin and nails. Not only is this relaxing but it also stimulates the skin and helps it absorb the cream. Massage your hands every night as well as during the day when you find that it's necessary to keep the cuticles from becoming brittle and dry.

Tickle the ivories (or computer keys). While so many things we do affect nail-plate growth negatively, a certain amount of trauma seems to help those nails a bit.

"Certain people, such as computer programmers or pianists, subject their nails to chronic, low-grade trauma when they hit the keys," says Dr. Kechijian. "This has been shown to actually stimulate nails to grow a little faster and stronger than they otherwise would." So any time at the keyboard is good for the nails—and even drumming your fingers on your desk might help them grow stronger.

Don't bully your nails. Most of us know when we're sabotaging our nails. Nail biting, for instance. Cuticle biting. Picking off polish. Pulling at the cuticle. An inventory of damaging nail habits reads like a list of deadly sins—at least to anyone who values nail appearance.

"Many children bite their nails, and most just grow out of the habit," says Dr. Kechijian. "If you're still biting them as an adult, the easiest thing to try is a nasty-tasting liquid you simply paint on your nails. Nail biting can be a reaction to stress, so if you really want to stop and can't, it might even be worth your time to work with a psychologist to find another way of coping."

Keep your cuticles cute. Healthy cuticles are vital to healthy nails. A common mistake people make is either to remove cuticles by cutting or to push them back, both of which impair the cuticle's ability to protect the finger, says Dr. Kechijian. Any damage to the cuticle affects the nail's healthy growth pattern—and a torn cuticle can open the way to infection.

Shower first, nails second. If your nails are thin or weak, you stand a chance of causing further damage when you groom them. "To lessen the possibility of this happening, cut or trim your nails only after bathing, because the nails will be softer," says Dr. Kechijian. "If you cut the nail when it's dry, it will

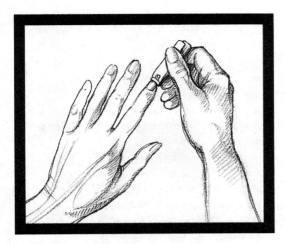

When trimming your nails, use clippers to cut straight across, leaving the corners square.

be a lot more brittle and crack more easily."

File them away. Carry an emery board with you, and at the first sign of an uneven tip, gently smooth it, always filing in the same direction. "You can be doing everything right and still get a little chip in your nail," says Dr. Kechijian. "If you deal with it at

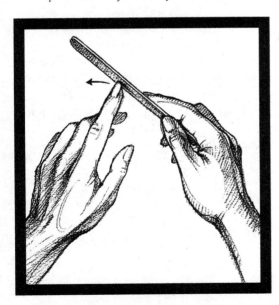

You'll prevent damaged nails if you always carry an emery board and smooth out any un-evenness as soon as possible.

once, you can prevent further damage."

Square them up. Fingernails can be rounded at the tip but should be left square at the corners, which maximizes nail strength and helps avoid ingrown nails, says David M. Stoll, M.D., a Beverly Hills dermatologist and author of *A Woman's Skin*. Clippers are better than scissors for squaring the edges.

Keep them short. Fragile nails look their best if they're kept on the short side, says Dr. Kechijian. "The less the nail extends beyond the end of the finger, the less likely it will be to incur more damage and break."

Polish with care. When you apply polish, brush it over the top of your nail behind the tip, notes Mona Winograd, owner of Dyanna Body and Nail Salon in New York City. This provides a protective cushion. And when it comes to colors, clear or light polish is actually the best, because it usually lasts longer and shows wear less, she notes.

Reduce remover use. All nail polish removers can be rough on nails, so try not to use them more than once a week. If your polish chips before then, just do a touch-up with your nail polish rather than using the polish remover and starting over, suggests Dr. Kechijian.

Building Them Better

Your nails shouldn't be as hard as nails, but there are things you can do to make them stronger.

"What you're really aiming for are healthy nails that are tough, not hard," says Doug Schoon, polymer chemist in Vista, California, and consultant to the Nail Manufacturing Council in Chicago. "Healthy nails are tough enough to withstand daily abuse and bend without breaking."

To improve your nails' ability to tough it

What Your Nails Say about the Rest of You

Feeling under the weather? Check out your fingernails.

Revealing a great deal about your general health, your nails could even help you detect undiagnosed illnesses. Here's a breakdown of conditions and what they could mean.

- Thick, yellow nails can indicate diseases of the thyroid, lymph system and respiratory system. Long-term use of the antibiotic tetracycline could also be the culprit.
- Blue nails can mean a circulatory problem caused by heart disease or Raynaud's disease, a condition that impairs circulation in the hands.
- White marks can signal cirrhosis of the liver.
- Horizontal grooves, also known as Beau's lines, are furrows that can be caused by malnutrition, certain toxic substances or a number of illnesses.
- Horizontal lines, also called Mees' lines, are white stripes that can be caused by heart attacks, kidney failure, Hodgkin's disease or sickle-cell disease. Red streaks can mean high blood pressure or heart valve disease.
- Pitting in the nails can indicate psoriasis or eczema.
- Spooning—the appearance of large indentations in the nails—may indicate anemia.
- Clubbing is the term for curled nails. These may signal diseases of the liver, colon, lung or heart.

---

out, here are some tips.

Get creamed. The cuticle cream that moisturizes also protects the nail's matrix. Creams or oils that you rub into your cuticles and nails help strengthen your nails while helping to retain moisture, says Schoon.

Don't dry them to death. If you have brittle or weak nails that you want to improve, steer clear of nail hardeners that contain formaldehyde, says Richard K. Scher, M.D., professor of dermatology and head of the nail section at Columbia Presbyterian Medical Center in New York City.

"Formaldehyde-based products do make your nails hard, but they do it by drying them out. That is the last thing you want to do to brittle or even soft nails; it just makes them crack more," says Dr. Scher. "In addition, many people are allergic to formaldehyde."

Try a resin. There are hardeners that contain resins as hardening top coats or base coats, but you have to read the labels. These products reinforce nails with a stiff outer covering, but they don't help the nail itself become healthier or sturdier, says Dr. Kechijian.

See also Hands

Gallbladder

"YOU HAVE A LOT OF GALL!"

Well, if anybody ever says that to you, tell them that you only have a couple of table-spoons. And tell them that gall is a good thing.

Gall is an old word for bile. And bile helps us digest the fat in our food. The liver, not the gallbladder, actually makes gall—out of a soup of cholesterol, salts and pigments. But the gallbladder simmers the soup down to a concentrate and then stores the greenish brown bile. It is either stored or released internally when we eat.

The gallbladder resembles a piece of food, specifically fruit—a three-inch-long green pear. Snuggled under the right lobe of the liver, it's muscular but thin-walled. It uses its strength to spit a wad of stored bile into the small intestine after a meal, teaming up with the deconstruction gang that turns our food into fuel.

Unlike the stomach or the liver or the small intestine, though, the gallbladder is a disposable worker. Take it out, and the liver and small intestine fill in for the missing organ. "The gallbladder isn't that important. It just concentrates the bile for digestion," says Thomas Nolan, M.D., associate professor of obstetrics and gynecology and internal medicine at Louisiana State University in New Orleans.

Lucky for us we can live without it, because cholecystectomy—as gallbladder removal is called—constitutes a large chunk of the surgical docket. Roughly half a million of us will give up our gallbladders this year,

mostly because of gallstones. And women are three times as likely as men to be "chole" patients.

Gallstones happen because bile is a tricky liquid. If the liver puts too much cholesterol into the basic mix, or not enough of the bile salts and detergents that keep cholesterol floating free, then bits of the cholesterol can solidify in the gallbladder. They begin to grow like grit in an oyster. About half of the 20 million people who walk around carrying gallstones have "silent stones"—pearls that produce no symptoms.

The opposite of silent stones is more than just noisy stones—they're also painful.

Throwing Stones

When gallstones start to move, they can get stuck in the cystic ducts that lead out of the gallbladder. That causes nasty bouts of biliary colic: The gallbladder clamps and contracts, trying to spit out the bad seed.

Before the organ gives up and rests, our right sides may ache. Or we may have abdominal pain that moves around to the back. Nausea and vomiting are other symptoms. If the stone doesn't fall back into the gallbladder and unplug the duct, then inflammation or infection can occur in the gallbladder.

A stone could also get caught in the main bile duct leading from the liver—the same duct that catches whatever leaves the gallbladder. When the stone gets trapped there, it causes bile pigments to build up, turning the skin a pale shade of yellow, which is a condition called jaundice. Other problems could result from this type of buildup, including pain, fever, infection and inflammation of the pancreas.

Researchers aren't sure why women get so many more gallstones than men, but they do.

Not only that, the more children a woman has, the more likely she is to get gallstones.

Doctors can also name some factors that just seem to complicate the puzzle. Certain racial and genetic groups—among them, Mexican-Americans, Native Americans and Swedes—are at higher risk of getting gallstones. But since women in all groups get more gallstones than men, experts conclude that hormones definitely figure in the gender phenomenon.

Even pregnancy and childbirth can precipitate gallstones, Dr. Nolan says. "And I hate to say it, but hormone replacement therapy (HRT) increases the incidence of stone formation. It's two times greater with the lower doses of estrogen and four times greater with the higher doses."

This doesn't mean that you should avoid HRT just to avoid gallstones. "The benefit-to-risk ratio of HRT is still extremely high," Dr. Nolan adds. "I wouldn't advise anybody to go off HRT because of the risk of gallstones."

What is it with hormones, anyway? "One possible explanation is that hormones tend to relax smooth muscle—and the gallbladder is a smooth muscle organ. So if the gallbladder is sluggish, cholesterol crystals can grow and grow. When the organ is vigorous, it can contract and squirt small crystals out into the small intestine when we eat meals and get rid of them," says Roger Gebhard, M.D., professor of medicine at the University of Minnesota in Minneapolis.

Scaling Back Your Risk

While we can't do anything about being born female, Mexican-American, Native American or Swedish, we can tackle our weight.

"Obesity is the single biggest risk factor for gallstones," says Dr. Gebhard. "Obesity is associated with increased secretion of cholesterol in the bile. This allows supersaturation, which causes cholesterol crystals to precipitate out and become stones."

One landmark study of 88,837 women done by researchers at the Harvard School of Public Health found that slightly overweight women had almost twice the chance of developing gallstones as women of normal weight. Obese women were six times more likely to form stones.

But the way we lose weight is important, too. So doctors give this advice to help women dodge stone problems.

Don't crash and burn. "Rapid weight loss has been associated with gallstone formation," says Janice Rothschild, M.D., general surgeon and assistant professor of surgery at Tufts University School of Medicine in Boston. "Some of the diet programs have been implicated, but I don't think it's a matter of a specific diet program. Any alteration of the concentrations in bile can start stone formation."

If you're out to lose weight, take it slow and continue to eat regular, healthy meals. Maximum weight-loss velocity shouldn't be more than two pounds a week. If you're losing less than that, be satisfied, as long as the progress is slow and steady.

Don't go too low. While low-fat diets are recommended for weight loss, a diet that contains very low fat, such as a less-than-two-grams-a-day diet, may not be fatty enough for some women. When dietary fat goes that low, you may potentially run into gallbladder problems.

"You may benefit from having some fat in your diet to empty the gallbladder and preserve its function," says Dr. Gebhard.

Don't smoke it off. Reaching for a cigarette instead of a cheeseburger never was a good weight-loss strategy. Now here's one more brick to hurl at the butts.

"Smoking has recently been implicated in gallstone formation," says Dr. Gebhard. "We don't know why. The studies are just epidemiological—they only associate smoking and gallstones. But we think it's a factor. So avoiding smoking is something you can do for your gallbladder."

When Good Gallbladders Go Bad

Maybe you had one heck of an upset stomach last night. Or it seems like you burp and pass gas too often. Or it could be that you can't eat fatty foods anymore without paying the fat tax—a grumbling gut.

If you mention those symptoms to your doctor, she may send you for an x-ray or an ultrasound to test for gallstones. Then, if she finds one, she'll roll out some options. Oral drugs can dissolve gallstones, but they take a year or two to do it. Lithotripsy uses sound waves to pulverize gallstones, but few hospitals use lithotripsy machines for anything but kidney stones. In any case, the success rate is low for both techniques. Gallbladders can always produce more stones, so most often gallstones are cured by removing the gallbladder.

Gallbladder surgery used to be a big deal—major surgery that left fair-size scars and cost weeks of recovery time. Then, in the late 1980s, Nintendo surgery came along. That's a popular term for laparoscopic surgery, which involves high-tech miniature scalpels and forceps and a kind of periscope equipped with a tiny camera that transmits blown-up pictures of your insides to a TV screen. With Nintendo surgery you could have your gallbladder out on Monday—through a dime-size hole in your belly button—and go home on Tuesday. You could be back at work in a week.

"Laparoscopy just swept the world, and it seems to make a substantial difference. People can be out of the hospital and back to work in a couple of days," marvels Dr. Gebhard.

By 1990, thanks to "lap choles" (laparoscopy cholecystectomies), doctors reported that surgery rates for gallbladder removal had jumped almost 60 percent. Meanwhile, the use of ultrasound in diagnosis made spotting gallstones a snap—even when they weren't the problem in question. So, if you or your doctor knew that you had a gallstone, the temptation would be to remove it, whether it was silent or not.

But it's so easy now that some doctors are skeptical about how many operations are being done.

"There's a real controversy about who needs to have her gallbladder out," says Dr. Nolan. "Who do you operate on? And when? It should be the patient with symptoms. The controversy is ongoing."

Even if you've had what you and your doctor think may be a gallbladder attack, "Be cautious," says Dr. Gebhard. "It could be an isolated gastrointestinal attack. So it's important to work with your physician to make certain that your symptoms are actually related to a gallstone."

See also Digestive System

Gums

BENEATH EVERY GREAT GRIN is a good set of gums. They're the scarcely seen tissues that combine efforts with the underlying bone to provide pillar and posthole for a snug-fitting set of strong teeth.

When they're in good health, your gums are either pink or grayish brown depending on the color of your skin. Gingiva—as gums are called in medical language—both cover and protect the hidden roots of your teeth. They have important tie-down tissues called periodontal ligaments that tightly lash each tooth to the bony sockets in your jaw.

Each tooth is held in a kind of cradle. "It's suspended like a swing in the bone socket, and the ligaments look like little whiskers that attach the tooth root to the bone," says Ray C. Williams, D.M.D., professor and chairman of the Department of Periodontics at the University of North Carolina School of Dentistry at Chapel Hill.

Unhealthy gums look shiny, red and swollen. They bleed easily, even when you're brushing gently. What pushes our gums across the line from lusty pink or brown to angry red is advancing plaque. That's the soft, sticky web that bacteria weave over our teeth and gum line.

Some of us produce more plaque than others, and dentists have found that this tends to run in families. But if we carefully brush and floss away plaque daily, our gums should always be in the pink of health.

What you need to watch out for—especially if your family has always had gum problems—is plaque that builds up and seeps below the gum line. As plaque irritates the gums, the gums swell and lose their grip on the teeth. A moat starts to form between the gum line and the teeth, growing ever deeper as gum disease develops.

Mild gum disease—gingivitis—is "generally reversible if you brush and floss and remove the plaque," says Dr. Williams. "Your gums will revert back to healthy tissue."

No More Loose Teeth

Leave gingivitis untreated, however, and dire things start to happen. Eventually, you'll get hard, yellowish brown crusts of tartar—calculus—which is formed when minerals in your saliva bond with plaque. Tartar is so hard that it takes professional cleaning to remove it—you can't do it at home. Once you have it, tartar starts to trap even more plaque.

When plaque and tartar continue their inexorable march down to the roots of your teeth, you have the beginnings of serious gum disease, called periodontitis. Bacteria in the plaque start eating away the whiskery ligaments that connect tooth to bone. Eventually, teeth loosen. Then bacteria bully their way down to naked bone, where they undermine the last connection. Untethered to gum or bone, the tooth can fall out.

That's the extreme—the very worst. Still, Americans do lose more teeth to gum disease than to tooth decay. The best way to nip gum disease in the bud—besides routine flossing and brushing—is to visit your dentist regularly. That way you'll spot gum disease when you can easily treat it.

Either a dentist or periodontist (a gum specialist) can treat gum disease by cleaning out the plaque, tartar and bacteria from the gums. Maybe a good cleaning is all that's necessary—the gum will heal right up and hug a tooth.

Other times, surgery is necessary to remove the diseased tissue and fix the damage. If the tooth is loose, a periodontist can often graft gum tissue to correct areas of recession. Periodontists have new techniques to regenerate gum tissue, too.

Another innovation: The periodontist tucks a tetracycline-treated string, such as Acticipe R, between the tooth and gum to get rid of bacteria. Usually, the string is removed after ten days. There are also antibiotic gels being developed.

It's much easier to brush and floss, of course, than to endure a periodontist's attention and go through the treatments. There are times in a woman's life, however, when she may need even more than the usual brush-and-floss routine to guarantee gum health.

Hormonal Heck to Pay

"Women have to know there are certain times in their lives when hormones make them more susceptible to gum disease," says Barbara J. Steinberg, D.D.S., professor of dental medicine at the Medical College of Pennsylvania in Philadelphia.

Our gums contain hormone receptors. High levels of female hormones make the gum membranes permeable, thus causing an increase in fluids in the gum tissue, which makes the tissue swell and redden.

Hormone increases exaggerate the way gum tissues react to irritants in plaque, mak-

Your Personal Floss-ophy

Today's choice of flosses runs the gamut from thick to thin, flavored to plain, waxed to unwaxed.

So . . . what'll it be?

"Picking out floss is like picking out carpenter's tools," says Jeffrey M. Shubach, D.M.D., a family dentist in private practice in Voorhees, New Jersey. "You have to find what works best in your hands. It's more important that you use it than that it be any special kind."

Here's a quartet of floss choices—all available at most drugstores.

Unwaxed or waxed. "There's a theory that unwaxed dental floss is better than waxed floss because the waxed leaves a small wax residue," says Dr. Shubach. "If you can use unwaxed just as easily as waxed, you might as well use it. But if your teeth rip it to shreds, go to waxed floss."

Extra-fine. This is the thinnest floss, for people whose teeth shred even waxed floss.

Precision. The last resort for intransigent shredders, single-strand Precision brand floss slides through tight teeth with great ease. It costs twice as much as regular floss. "It's a godsend, though, if your teeth shred everything else," says Richard H. Price, D.M.D., clinical instructor of dentistry at Boston University Henry Goldman School of Dentistry.

Super. Super Floss comes in packets of single strands that look like regular floss, but has a stiffened end made for threading under and around braces. This kind of floss also maneuvers around fixed bridges—teeth that are connected to neighboring teeth with little or no space between.

ing gums more sensitive to even small amounts of plaque. Gums get puffy from plaque when hormone levels are high, especially during puberty, before menstruation and during pregnancy. Since birth control pills mimic some of the hormonal changes that happen at pregnancy, they too can cause gum changes. But then the puffiness goes down when hormone levels return to normal.

Other health factors that can raise your risks for gum disease include diabetes and epilepsy as well as smoking—which impairs the bacteria-fighting cells in your mouth.

Battling Bacteria

More than 40 different kinds of bacteria are rambling around your mouth on any given day. So keeping an eye on them—and stopping them in their tracks—takes vigilance.

Here's how to stay on your guard.

Get full disclosure. Colorful and revealing, disclosing tablets give you a visual report card on your brushing and flossing technique. You can get the tablets from your pharmacy or dentist.

First, floss and brush your teeth as usual. Then chew a tablet and swish the particles around your mouth, says Richard H. Price, D.M.D., clinical instructor of dentistry at Boston University Henry Goldman School of Dentistry. Rinse with water, then examine your teeth in a mirror. Wherever you see a red stain, that's plaque. Those are places where you need to brush more enthusiastically and floss more thoroughly next time.

Flood the lowlife. "Even the most valiant patients may sometimes need extra assistance to combat bacteria and plaque," says Kenneth Burrell, D.D.S., senior director of the Council on Scientific Affairs for the American Dental

Deep Pockets

Deep pockets are fine things to have in a coat or a jacket. In your mouth, though, deep pockets between your teeth and gums are a sign of trouble.

Healthy gums have a little space that dentists call a sulcus, lying between the gum line and the tooth. When plaque inflames the gum, though, the gum swells, then moves away from the tooth. The sulcus turns into a large, unhealthy space between gum, tooth and bone that dentists then call a pocket. They start tracking its depth with a slim periodontal probe, inserting the probe to measure the pocket's depth in millimeters. The deeper the pocket, the harder it is to get the area below the gum line properly clean, says Jeffrey M. Shubach, D.M.D., a family dentist in private practice in Voorhees, New Jersey.

If plaque spreads unchecked, it turns into tartar; the gums may recede and the pockets may deepen. Then bacteria in the plaque can erode the roots and the bone that supports them. This condition, called periodontitis, requires tedious ongoing care and maintenance.

Association. For reinforcement when hormone levels are high, your dentist may prescribe an antibacterial mouth rinse that contains the ingredient chlorhexidine. To get it, you'll need a prescription from your dentist.

Over-the-counter mouthwashes such as Listerine have been shown to fight bacteria, too, so they're good substitutes if you don't have a prescription for chlorhexidine.

Break up the bugs. With an oral irrigator such as a Water Pik, you aim a stream of

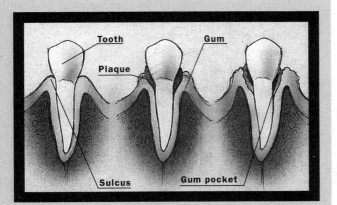

Tooth

Gum

Plaque

Sulcus

Gum pocket

When gums are healthy, they fit snugly around the base of the tooth, as shown in this cut-away illustration.

If plaque builds up around the edge of the tooth, it can cause painful inflamma-tion—the be-ginnings of gum disease.

Bacteria in the plaque can damage the bone and the fibers that anchor the tooth. A gum pocket devel-ops between the gum and tooth.

creates a little firehose action that could jam bacteria deeper into the gum." So make sure you set the device on medium or low.

When to Get Finicky

When hormones are running high, brush-ing twice a day may not be enough; you'll probably need to remove plaque after every meal or snack. Here are some other steps to help your gums stay healthy.

De-gunk the spaces. Some dentists recom-mend using wooden dental sticks, such as Stim-U-Dent, in addition to flossing. A Stim-U-Dent, which you can find in most drug-stores, is shaped like a large toothpick that's three-sided, so it looks triangular in cross sec-tion. The pointed end is like the narrow tip of a pyramid. Here's how to use it.

Moisten the pointed end in your mouth. "Then push that end in and out three times between each tooth. That will squeeze out all the gunk there," says Dr. Williams.

After that, place the base of the triangle against the gum between two teeth. "Gently rotate and vibrate the stick from side to side as you lift the gum and clean out the debris. Use a light, gentle pressure," advises Jeffrey M. Shubach, D.M.D., a family dentist in pri-vate practice in Voorhees, New Jersey.

"Stim-U-Dents are clean, lovely, cheap, simple little things," says Dr. Williams. The dental sticks are also portable and more dis-creet than floss—perfect for a quick tooth-cleaning session at the office after lunch.

Don't be blood shy. Bleeding gums may be an early sign of gum disease—a signal that you'd better pay a visit to your dentist. In the meantime, however, don't let bleeding stop you from flossing and brushing, warns Dr. Steinberg. Early care can stop and even re-verse any damage.

water at the gum line to hose off the bacteria. "The irrigator interrupts bacteria formation. Your purpose is to disrupt its ecological niche," says Dr. Price.

Instead of using water, you can fill an irriga-tor with an antibacterial mouth rinse such as Listerine, or a prescription mouth rinse such as Peridex or Periogard. "They have been shown to decrease plaque buildup," he says.

But don't drive 'em deeper. "Don't turn the Water Pik on high," warns Dr. Price. "That

Look up. Most of us bend our heads and stare down into the sink when we brush our teeth. Instead, look in the mirror over the sink to watch yourself brush.

"The mirror is a great tool to use for tooth brushing," says David F. Halpern, D.M.D., a dentist in Columbia, Maryland, and a spokes-dentist for the Academy of General Dentistry and the state of Maryland. "You can watch the bristles penetrate into the gum area. If your gums bleed, you can see where the trouble spots are."

Enlist Listerine. In addition to using toothpaste, you can lend your mouth a helping hand if you brush with Listerine—or any other mouthwash that says "antibacterial" on the label and has the approval of the American Dental Association. Brush between your teeth and gums with it, suggests Dr. Halpern.

"Fill the cap from a large bottle with the mouthwash, then dip your toothbrush in it," he suggests. "Hold your toothbrush at a 45-degree angle where the gum meets the tooth. Then press the bristles gently against your teeth so they spread into the gum crevice. Use a small circular motion to dislodge food and bacteria from beneath the gum."

To make sure that you get below the gum line, you can look in the mirror. "The mouthwash will start to kill off the bacteria. It's like an antiseptic," he says. When you're done, use whatever is left in the cap to rinse out your mouth.

Paste the tartar. Tartar-control toothpaste is another weapon to add to your hygiene arsenal. "It contains sodium pyrophosphates, which interfere with tartar formation," says Dr. Price.

The anti-tartar formulation can irritate the gums, though. "If your gums feel raw or if you have any burning sensations, you may be allergic to the toothpaste," he warns, noting

that more women than men seem to have these allergies. If your gums clear up when you switch to a nontartar toothpaste, then you'll know that it's not your gums, it's your toothpaste.

Mention the Pill. If you end up needing dental treatment for your gums, and you're also taking birth control pills, "let your dentist know," says Dr. Price. "Antibiotics that are prescribed for dental work can weaken the effects of the Pill. You may need another form of birth control until you're finished with the antibiotics."

A Pregnant Pause

It's downright odd how folktales tangle up teeth and pregnancy. One myth says that a fetus leaches calcium from the mother's teeth for its growth. Not true: It's your diet that provides calcium for the growing baby.

Another tale says that you lose a tooth for every child. But if you're fastidious about your gums, your teeth are secure.

It's not a folktale, however, that women may tend to neglect their gums during pregnancy. That's because it can hurt to brush them, according to Dr. Steinberg. "Then the gums get even more sensitive."

Sixty to 75 percent of all pregnant women develop gum disease that ranges from mild to severe, says Dr. Steinberg. It even has a name: pregnancy gingivitis. "It's marked by increased redness and swelling and bleeding in response to very small amounts of plaque," she says.

Because of these gum changes, dentists target pregnant women for particular attention, says Dr. Price.

If you're pregnant, here are some special tips for gum care.

Go to a pro every 90 days. The key to

healthy gums during pregnancy is the removal of *all* plaque. That's why many dentists recommend a professional cleaning every trimester in addition to persnickety home care.

"Serious gum disease doesn't go away like morning sickness does. If you don't take care of your teeth, your gums won't be as good as new after the baby, when hormones rebound," says Dr. Price.

Use the safe zone. There are two stages of pregnancy when dentists may want to avoid any dental treatment besides cleaning: during the first and third trimesters. The first trimester is a delicate time because the fetus is forming; during the third trimester pregnant women are often uncomfortable.

"Schedule elective dental treatment during the second trimester, when the fetus is less vulnerable," says Dr. Steinberg. "And be aware that if you do need x-rays for the dentist to diagnose and treat your problems, there's no danger from the low doses of radiation, especially when you're wearing a lead apron, which will insulate the baby."

See also Mouth, Teeth

Gynecological Exam

WHEN GENE AUTRY SANG "Back in the Saddle Again," he seemed like a real happy guy. So happy that you're sure he never rested his bum on a gynecological exam table. If he'd put his feet in *those* stirrups, you know he'd be singing a different tune.

Yeah, the annual trip to the gynecologist isn't one we tend to praise in song. Instead, mere mention of the words "pelvic exam" is enough to elicit moans of dread from most women. Some of us put off scheduling the event indefinitely. Others manage to actually get it into the appointment book, but when the day is upon them, every other activity under the sun suddenly starts looking more attractive. Even those three-o'clock meetings suddenly seem like can't-miss events.

If you think it's no big deal to skip your annual exam, think again. This is the time when your doctor can perform several important exams that are crucial in monitoring your health. It's also the time when you can talk to your doctor and ask questions about birth control, sexually transmitted diseases (STDs), prepregnancy planning, prenatal care or any other issues on your mind.

Just Checking—Everything

Your annual exam with your gynecologist should begin with an interview with your doctor, says Eddie Sollie, M.D., associate clinical professor of obstetrics and gynecology at the University of Texas Southwestern Medical Center at Dallas and author of *Straight Talk with Your Gynecologist.* This should take place while you are fully clothed and before any exams are done. It's a chance to discuss what's happened since your last exam, he explains. If you aren't offered an interview but want one, don't be afraid to ask, says Dr. Sollie.

Following the interview a nurse might weigh you, ask for a urine sample and do a blood test. As usual, you'll be shown to the exam room and asked to get undressed and put on a cloth or paper exam robe.

Your doctor should start the examination at the top of your body and move downward from there, says Dr. Sollie. Your doctor may examine your eyes and ears, feel your throat to see if your thyroid is enlarged and listen to your heart and lungs with a stethoscope. Then she'll move on to the four central components of the annual gynecological exam— a breast exam, a pelvic exam, a Pap test and a digital rectal exam.

The breast examination is the time when your doctor can visually inspect and manually examine your breasts to search for any lumps or discharge. This should also be a time when your doctor instructs you on how to do a proper breast self-exam. (To make sure you're getting the whole story on this, see "Get in Touch with Your Breasts" on page 58.

Your doctor will also examine your abdomen and groin area, gently pressing the area to check for any masses that might mean tumors.

Here's Looking at You

When your doctor starts the pelvic exam, she'll generally begin by examining your vulva (or external genitalia), the area that begins at your pubic hair and extends to your anus. She's looking for any discharge, sores or bumps that may indicate an STD,

a cancer or other skin changes.

During this part of the gynecological exam, ask for a mirror that you can hold while your doctor's having a look, suggests says Anita L. Nelson, M.D., associate professor of obstetrics and gynecology at the University of California, Los Angeles, UCLA School of Medicine and director of the women's medical clinic at the Harbor UCLA Medical Center in Torrance.

Be sure to tell the doctor about any changes that you've noticed in your genital area. Holding the mirror, you can follow the doctor's exam. This also helps the doctor point out any condition that you should monitor at home.

Then the doctor will do the speculum exam. First, she'll gently insert a warm, lubricated speculum—which is simply a sterile examination tool—into the opening of your vagina. While the speculum is in place, your doctor will look at the vaginal walls, looking for any abnormal discharge or lesions.

The Pap test—which most doctors recommend having annually—begins with a gentle cleansing of the cervix. The doctor then takes a sample of cells from your cervix and places them on a slide.

The cells are sent to a laboratory for analysis, primarily to detect precancerous changes and cervical cancer.

If early changes are detected, they can usually be treated to prevent a progression to cancer. Occasionally, the Pap test can also indicate the presence of other infections, some of which are STDs.

Following the Pap test your doctor should do a bimanual pelvic exam, which just means the doctor uses two hands to check your uterus and ovaries. After removing the speculum, your doctor will insert several fingers into your vagina and feel the top of your ab-

Can You Trust Your Pap Test?

There's a certain percentage of error in every medical test, and to some degree, that's unavoidable. Here are some things that you can do to reduce the margin of error.

Check the lab. The lab doing the work should be certified by the College of American Pathologists or the American Society of Cytologists, says Eddie Sollie, M.D., associate clinical professor of obstetrics and gynecology at the University of Texas Southwestern Medical Center at Dallas and author of *Straight Talk with Your Gynecologist*. Be sure to ask, even though you might feel uncomfortable. No question is a bad question.

During your period, skip it. The test won't be trustworthy if it's done during your period, according to Dr. Sollie. So if you're having your period when you're supposed to go in for the test, call and postpone it.

Clear the area. If you've been having a discharge from an infection, you should first treat the infection. Later, after it's cleared up, return to the doctor for your Pap test, says Dr. Sollie.

Don't douche. If you douche before the exam, the Pap test won't be accurate, says Dr. Sollie.

Go for doctor detection. If some abnormality has been reported from a previous Pap test, you may want to ask that your test be read by a pathologist, says Dr. Sol-lie. An abnormal Pap test is usually the result of some cellular changes in the cervix, and a pathologist may be more skilled at interpreting and monitoring those changes.

Check it yourself. While not all doctors advocate this, Dr. Sollie strongly urges you to request a copy of their Pap test lab reports. This allows you to check the name and social security number on the report and make sure that it's yours. You can also check to see if the Pap test was of adequate quality. Look specifically for one or two statements that will give you a clue. The report should say "endocervical cells are present" (unless you have had a hysterectomy) or "smear quality: satisfactory or optimal specimen."

If you don't see these terms, your physician should repeat the test at no cost to you, Dr. Sollie says. Or if the test says "inadequate specimen" or "endocervical cells not present," you should get a second test done.

Don't accept classes. The up-to-date system for analyzing Pap tests is the Bethesda system. Your lab report should list a descriptive term—"normal," "atypia" or "dysplasia"—in the section reporting cell examination, called cytological diagnosis. If your results come back to you listing a class—Class I, Class II and so on—don't accept that, says Dr. Sollie. That indicates that an outmoded method was used to analyze your Pap test.

domen with the other hand. By doing this she can detect whether your ovaries are enlarged or have cysts and can feel any fibroids or other tumors growing in the uterus.

Finally comes the digital rectal examination. Placing a finger in your rectum, the doctor feels for tumors in that area. Your pelvic exam is not really complete unless your doctor does a rectal exam, says Dr. Sollie.

How You Can Ace the Exam

Here's what doctors recommend that you do to get the most out of your annual exam.

Time it right. Schedule your annual exam at the right time in your menstrual cycle, says Dr. Nelson. The best time is 10 to 14 days after the first day of your period. At this time in your cycle, your breasts won't be as lumpy and tender as they can be in the latter half of your cycle. This is also the time to get the best Pap test results; your cervix is more open at this time of the month, allowing your doctor to get a better sample.

If planning your exam that precisely is difficult for you, just be sure you do not have your period at the time of your exam and have been finished with it for at least a few days, so your vagina is free from any discharge.

Fend off interference. A number of things—including douching, medications and spermicides—can interfere with your Pap test results, says Dr. Nelson. Many doctors warn against douching at any time, since it can contribute to the spread of some infections in the reproductive tract.

Bring your script. If you have questions for your doctor, write them down and bring them with you to the office. That way you'll be less likely to forget something.

Bring a friend. One of the most important things is to have a chaperon present, says Dr. Sollie. This could be your doctor's nurse, a friend, or husband, he says.

Speak up. Just because your doctor has done a bimanual pelvic exam doesn't mean that a Pap test has been done. So be sure to ask whether it has. Also, if you have a new sexual partner or are concerned about STDs, you should specifically ask to be tested for STDs, says Dr. Sollie.

See also Reproductive System

Hair

"RAPUNZEL, RAPUNZEL, let down your hair!" the prince hollered.

Rapunzel, in the Brothers Grimm fairy tale, did as she was told. From the top of the tower, she unwound her crowning glory. The prince grabbed hold and—

Right there, the story might have taken a bizarre turn. Did Rapunzel ask the prince how much he weighed? Did she pause to consider what would happen if all her stressed tresses suddenly snapped?

Fortunately, hair is strong enough to support even a heavy date. Theoretically, a fullback-size prince really could climb a dangling hank of hair, since each hair on our heads can support almost three ounces, and we have 100,000 or so. Very theoretically, an 18,000-pound prince—or a whole platoon of princes—could have inched up Rapunzel's braid.

Hair is more often praised for its beauty than its strength, however. "Hair is very important psychologically. It displays femininity or masculinity, and it can be a sign of one's individuality and image," says Susan Detwiler, M.D., dermatopathology fellow at Stanford University School of Medicine.

The fact is, when your hair looks damaged and lifeless, you might start to feel the same way. When a glimpse of your hair in the mirror gives you that "Oh no!" feeling, it's probably time to do something about it. Fortunately, there's a lot that can be done.

Raising the Dead

Hair is just hard, dead protein. Even so, a healthy head of hair looks vibrantly alive,

Trim Your Own Bangs

Why trek out to the hair salon when it's only your bangs that need trimming? You can do it yourself. Here are some tips from hairstylist Louis Gignac, owner of Louis-Guy D Salon in New York City and author of *Everything You Need to Know to Have Great-Looking Hair*.

- Use a good pair of sharp hairdresser's scissors. They're available at beauty supply shops for a wide range of prices.
- Make sure your hair is dry. If your hair is wet, it will dry an inch shorter.
- Avoid frowning while you cut—it changes the bang length.

Gignac recommends that you use a piece of plastic wrap as an aid in trimming your bangs. Cut a piece that's long enough to fit across your forehead and tuck above each ear. Then follow these steps.

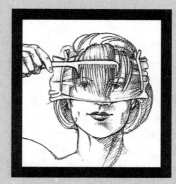

2. Starting one inch forward from the center of your scalp, comb your bangs forward in a triangle effect.

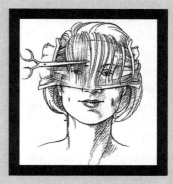

3. Start trimming your bangs from a point one-quarter inch below your eyebrow line. "Always start below your eyebrows, never above," Gignac says. That's because movement can make the bangs appear shorter. If you decide you want them shorter, trim the bangs again following the same line.

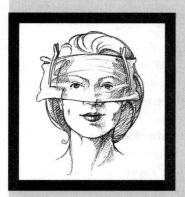

1. Comb your hair back and center the strip of plastic wrap across your forehead, securing it behind each ear with hair clips.

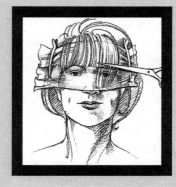

4. Follow the slight arch of your eyebrows as you trim. Gignac advises against cutting your bangs straight across—which could give you a dowdy look.

says Diana Bihova, M.D., clinical assistant professor of dermatology at New York University Medical Center in New York City. "That's the interesting thing. It's smooth. It shines. You almost want to touch it."

The outer layer of each hair is made up of

overlapping shingles of keratin cells called the cuticle. When our hair is clean, and when we don't torture it with perms and dyes, those shingles lie flat and reflect light—so hair is shiny. Dirt and damage from hair dyes or permanents can rough up those shingles. That's when our hair looks dull or lifeless.

For healthier, gleaming tresses, gentle washing and gentle conditioning are the keys. That's why shampoos get so much attention in the hair-coddling world. Here's what experts say about using them.

Brush up your technique. The first step to a good shampoo is a good brushing. "This loosens excess grooming products, dirt and natural oil as well as stimulates your scalp," says Damien Miano, top hairstylist and co-owner of New York's Miano/Viél Salon and Spa. Begin by brushing just the ends of your hair to detangle it. Then gradually work your brush in toward your scalp. If you brush in one stroke from the scalp out to the ends, the force of brushing can damage the oldest part of your hair—especially if you have long hair—and cause split ends.

Don't brush too long or too strong. "You'll traumatize the hair if you brush it 100 times, like the old adage says," warns Dr. Bihova.

Select a smart one. Shampoos are becoming more and more select, with many new products targeted to treat specific hair types. For example, blonds with fine hair can pick thickening shampoos to add body. The label may say "thickening," "volumizing," "re-moisturizing" or "body-building." Other shampoos are custom-made for processed hair that's been dyed, bleached or permed.

Hair isn't predictable, and you can't go entirely by the label. Even baby shampoos aren't as gentle as they're touted to be, says Marty Sawaya, M.D, Ph.D., assistant professor of dermatology at the University of Florida Health Science Center in Gainesville.

So how do you test them out? Dr. Bihova recommends that you audition shampoos. Buy sample sizes until you find ones that you like.

Do the ol' switcheroo. "Don't get stuck with one shampoo; keep switching them often," says Dr. Bihova. "This is especially important for people with scalp problems like dandruff, psoriasis or dermatitis." You'll know that it's time to switch when the shampoo is less effective than it was when you first started using it. This doesn't mean that you have to buy a new brand every week. "Keep two main brands around and interchange them. For normal hair, switching gets rid of buildup."

Wash out a myth. The old saw that washing your hair every day dries it out is untrue, says Philip Kingsley, owner and founder of Trichological Centers in London and New York and author of *Hair*. "If you get the correct shampoo, it does just the opposite. And it's a misconception that daily washing dulls your hair. It makes those cuticles lie down flat and tight and shiny."

The more frequently you wash your hair, the less shampoo you'll need at each washing, experts say. A nickel-size dab is the maximum amount for a daily shampoo, and one application will do the job.

Condition hair into shape. After shampooing keep the water running and work in a conditioner. Many conditioners are targeted for your hair type just like shampoos are. Use a lightweight conditioner on fine, thin hair and a heavier conditioner on coarser or curly hair, Kingsley advises. (Using a heavy conditioner on fine hair could make it limp and greasy, and a light conditioner on heavy or curly hair won't condition sufficiently.)

If your hair is chemically treated or damaged, look for a deep conditioner to apply once or twice a week. Some deep conditioners are applied before you shampoo, allowed to set, then shampooed out. Others are leave-in versions. You work them into your hair after you shampoo, while it's still wet. As for how much you should use, that's a matter of trial and error, according to Kingsley.

The Thin, Gray Line

Most women don't change their hair as dramatically as Madonna does. One-third of American women do color their hair, however, especially as they start to go gray.

If you're happy with gray hair, there's no reason to dye it. But hair dyes can not only add color, they can also fluff and roughen hair cuticles, which makes thin hair appear fuller. That can be an advantage. Even luxuriant hair can start thinning around the time you're age 40—or earlier. So there may be a time when you want to try dye. (But remember, while dye can make your tresses appear fuller, the coloring also damages your hair.)

Once you've decided to color your hair, what's the best way? It helps to consult a good hair pro. She not only can tell whether you should color your hair, she can also actually look at your hair and tell you the percentage of gray in it. That number can help you make some decisions.

"If you're more than 50 percent gray, you'll need permanent hair color to cover it," says John Corbett, Ph.D., vice president of scientific and technical affairs for Clairol in Stamford, Connecticut. If you're just 30 percent gray, you can use semipermanent hair dye. Semipermanent color is gentler on your hair. It's easy to use at home, too. Semipermanent dyes only last through 6 to 12 washings—but that's a plus if you're undecided about color choice.

Hands

YOU HAVE TO HAND IT TO THE HAND: This body part can really grab your attention. Whether it's flagging down a taxi, waving to a friend or flipping someone the proverbial bird after he cuts you off in traffic, the hand simply cannot—and *will* not—be ignored.

It's no wonder that Captain Hook was so bad-tempered. Think of the problems he encountered, lacking this most versatile of body parts. The hand brings many of life's basics within reach—allowing us to write, drive a car, hold a baby, feed and groom ourselves and perform a handful of other activities.

The hand is made up of the wrist, palm and fingers. The tendons that attach the muscles of the forearm to the bones of the hand are mainly what make movement possible. These tendons are surrounded by sheaths containing a lubricating fluid that prevents friction. Other movements are controlled by short muscles in the palm of the hand.

Some 90 percent of healthy adults use the right hand for writing, and two-thirds prefer it for activities requiring coordination. Just what makes a righty or a lefty isn't known, although heredity is probably the biggest factor.

Looking Younger, Hands Down

The weight- and age-guessing guy at the carnival knows the secret. Whenever he takes a stab at guessing how old people are, he has them hold their hands out in front of them. The aging result of a lifetime of dishwashing and sunbathing is right there—from the top of your middle finger to the top of your wrist.

Go Ahead—Snap, Crackle and Pop

Despite Mom's warnings about permanent damage, popping your joints doesn't cause arthritis, mutate your knuckles or separate your head from your spine. It only makes noise and, in a very few cases, relieves joint tension, says Mary Ann E. Keenan, M.D., chair of the Department of Orthopaedic Surgery at Albert Einstein Medical Center and orthopaedic director at Moss Rehabilitation Hospital, both in Philadelphia.

For most people, cracking knuckles is a habit born of a need for distraction. Though you may think you're rearranging your bones, the noise is really created by shifting joint fluid and escaping gas. If nothing else, popping your joints is a great way to clear a crowded room.

Here are a few ways to help perk up your hands by turning back the hands of time.

Wax therapeutic. Having your hands dipped in paraffin wax is a sure way to smoother, less-dry skin, says Mona Winograd, owner of Dyanna Body and Nail Salon in New York City. Paraffin wax traps moisture and stimulates the blood supply, leaving hands feeling soft and healthy, says Winograd.

A manicurist dips your hands in warm paraffin several times and covers them with plastic gloves. Then, warmer mitts are put on for 15 minutes, says Winograd. "That way, moisture from the skin cannot escape." The treatment is usually every other week.

Cover up. To prevent snags and splits, use gloves whenever you do anything around the house—even light housework such as dusting, says Winograd. Wear plastic gloves when you're washing dishes and cloth or rubber gloves for all other household chores, she suggests. Gloves protect hands from harsh household cleaners.

Moisten your mitts. Don't forget the benefit of good old moisturizer, says Lisa Siegle, esthetician (a specialist in skin treatments) at Aveda Esthetique in Los Angeles. "If you wash your hands a lot during the day, keep moisturizer by the sink and reapply lotion each time." Even better, don't dry your hands completely. Apply the lotion while the skin is still damp, which helps to lock in moisture.

Siegle advises her clients not to use petroleum-based products such as mineral oil. She prefers naturally derived substances such as botanical oils.

See spot fade. Doctors say that liver spots are mainly caused by sun exposure. To keep spots from recurring, however, it's vital to use sunscreen on your hands first thing in the morning, says John E. Wolf, Jr., M.D., professor and chairman of the dermatology department at Baylor College of Medicine in Houston.

The Drying Game

Sweaty palms don't make a great first impression—and many women are self-conscious about palm perspiration that seems to pop up when they least want it. You don't need to worry, since lots of people get that sweaty palm feeling. But if your palms sweat like a soda can on a hot day when you're nervous, you may want to do something about it.

Here are some quick fixes.

Bag it. Hold a wet tea bag in your palm for 10 to 15 minutes each day for a week or two. The tannin in regular tea is an astringent; it decreases sweating and shrinks pores, says Karen Burke, M.D., Ph.D., a research scien-

Unwrapping a Sticky Situation

A ring may be a symbol of wedded bliss, but it can pose real danger when it's stuck on a swelling finger. Injury to the hand—as well as the finger—can cause your ring finger to swell. Because that ring can cut off blood circulation just as surely as a tourniquet, that band of gold has to come off—the sooner, the better, if your finger starts to swell for any reason.

If your knuckle has swollen and is already too big to slip the ring over, try this trick using dental floss—or better yet, waxed dental tape. This technique, used by emergency medical technicians, is recommended by John C. Johnson, M.D., past president of the American College of Emergency Physicians and director of Emergency Medical Services at Porter Memorial Hospital in Valparaiso, Indiana.

To make the procedure even easier, grease the finger with petroleum jelly from the stuck ring up to the fingernail before you remove the ring. Then try the following steps.

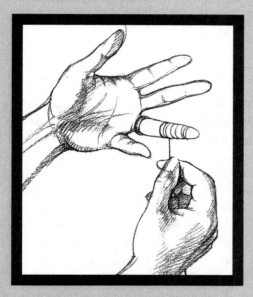

Take a *long* piece of floss—as much as two to three feet—and begin wrapping at the tip of your finger, closely wrapping the floss around the finger and spiraling down toward the ring as shown. Keep the encirclements an eighth-inch apart or less.

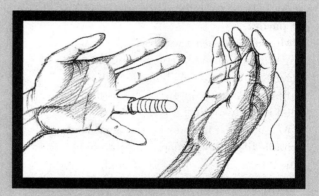

When you get to the ring, slip the end of the floss under the ring and pull that end toward your palm. Then lift the end of the floss over the top of the ring and pull up toward the tip of your finger. As the floss unwinds, it will ease the ring up and off your finger.

---

tist and dermatologist in private practice in New York City.

Give them a clean swipe. If you rub witch hazel or medical alcohol over your palms before you have to shake hands, you may have a drier grip. These astringents shrink pores a bit and help diminish sweating, says Dr. Burke.

Apply an antiperspirant. The same spray that keeps armpits dry can work on palms, says Dr. Burke. Just choose the invisible kind, rather than powder sprays that leave a white coating.

See also Skeletal System

Heart

REALLY, ALL THIS ROMANTICIZING has to stop. Hearts aren't achy or breaky, they don't cheat or catch on fire with desire. No, the Tin Man couldn't have been dancing, singing and witch-busting without one, despite what he told the wizard.

They're not instruments, so forget about plucking the old heartstrings. They're thief-proof, so stealing someone's is out. And for goodness sake, know that wearing your heart on your sleeve could be *really* messy at dinner parties.

Although the heart was mythologized in song, literature, and language long before Edgar Allan Poe wrote about the telltale one that kept beating from beyond, this fist-size organ is really all business.

Weighing just ten ounces, the heart is a veritable life-support machine—pumping some 2,000 gallons of blood through 60,000 miles of blood vessels every day. Your heart beats 100,000 times a day, forcing the blood through a complex system beginning with the heart's four chambers.

First, blood is collected from the body's veins and sent to the two chambers on the right side of the heart. The blood first enters the right atrium, which churns it into the right ventricle. The right ventricle then pumps blood into the lungs, where carbon dioxide is removed and replaced with oxygen. The oxygen-filled blood is pumped to the left side of the heart, where it's delivered through two more chambers: the left atrium and the left ventricle.

After it leaves the left ventricle the blood enters the body's largest artery, the aorta. Then the arteries divide into successively smaller vessels, finally bringing blood to the tissues. Here's where the real work begins, with the circulatory system providing oxygen and nutrients to the tissues while also collecting carbon dioxide and waste products.

That's a lot of work, but if you take good care of your heart—which means eating right, exercising regularly and not smoking—it should be good for 2.5 billion contractions over the course of a long and healthy lifetime.

Heart Disease: Not for Men Only

True or false: Heart attacks are something that usually happens to hefty middle-aged men who chain-smoke and eat lots of salads—taco salads, that is.

While it's true that men between ages 25 and 35 have three times as much heart disease as women, and that men between ages 36 and 49 have 1.7 times the incidence, cardiovascular disease is an insidious killer of women. Although we don't get it as often early on, after the age of 75 we do. Remember: Most women don't show symptoms until at least ten years later than men.

Still, most of us are in the dark when it comes to understanding our potential for heart disease later in life, says Joseph Alpert, M.D., head of the Department of Medicine at the University of Arizona Health Science Center in Tucson. "Women are somewhat protected as long as they're still menstruating," he says. "Some people say that it's not a disease women get. Ask ten women the most common killer of women, and they'll say breast cancer, but that's a complete myth. You're five to ten times more likely to die of heart disease."

Impediments to Heart Health

Just what is this much talked–about disease that kills 400,000 women in the United States annually?

The major culprit is atherosclerosis, which causes the heart or the vessels to get clogged. The arteries can get clogged with fat deposits, or plaques, which build over time on the inner portion of the arteries, impeding the flow of blood.

The arteries can grow stiff with age or disease, making them less effective. All this puts a woman at an increased risk of heart attack. A heart attack might not cause death, but it is the death of a portion of the heart—taking place when one or more coronary arteries to the heart becomes clogged or damaged and closes off. If this happens to part of the left ventricle—the heart's major pump—blood flow is stopped to the rest of the body.

Heart attacks are just as serious as they sound. Each year, 300,000 Americans who have suffered one die before they can even get to a hospital, with 10 percent of all patients who are hospitalized dying within three days.

That's the bad news. But the good news is great: Heart disease truly is something you can head off at the pass, says Howard Hodis, M.D., assistant professor of medicine and preventive medicine and director of the atherosclerosis research unit at the University of Southern California School of Medicine in Los Angeles.

"It's a very preventable disease. Simple exercise and dietary adjustment can cut your risk by 50 percent," notes Dr. Hodis. "This is just by lifestyle modification. While cholesterol plays a very important part, it's enhanced and sometimes overshadowed by lifestyle."

A Balance of Good and Bad

Call it a tale of two cholesterols. Both are from the lipid family, but one is an evil ne'er-do-well called low-density lipoprotein (LDL). Then there's high-density lipoprotein (HDL), the good guy and hero of our story.

Both types of cholesterol are found in the blood, but too much bad, or LDL, cholesterol, and you could be a prime candidate for heart disease. Anything over 160 milligrams per deciliter (mg/dl) is considered too much. Ideally, your LDLs should be below 130 mg/dl. Your protective HDL cholesterol, on the other hand, should be above 35 mg/dl and preferably above 60 mg/dl to truly be considered your knight in shining armor.

Although the U.S. Public Health Service recommends a reading below 200 mg/dl as

Do You Measure Up?

You have a total cholesterol level of 220 milligrams per deciliter (mg/dl). That's higher than you'd like. But your good cholesterol (high-density lipoprotein, or HDL) is a very healthy 110 mg/dl. With those two numbers you can figure out where you stand.

This is the formula: Take your total cholesterol and divide it by your HDL. The result is what your risk ratio is. Using this table, dividing 220 by 110, you can figure that your ratio is 2—a *very* low risk, indeed.

Ratio	Risk
6.0	High
5.0	Higher than average
4.5	Average
4.0	Lower than average
3.0	Low

the desired cholesterol level, that's misleading. The most important thing is your risk ratio when your good cholesterol is compared with your overall cholesterol.

So what can you do if your LDL looks more like the national debt than a healthy 100 or so? Plenty! From eating veggies to taking vitamins, here are just a few of the tips experts give to keep your numbers out of the danger zone.

Get up and go. Exercise is probably the best way of conditioning your heart, because it may also raise your HDL level, notes Sidney Alexander, M.D., cardiologist and former director of the cardiovascular division at Lahey Hitchcock Medical Center in Burlington, Massachusetts.

Although doctors recommend working out at least three times a week for 30 minutes in order to increase fitness, Dr. Alexander says that any kind of movement is a boon to your body. "Go out for a walk. That'll improve your fitness. For the person who's daunted by jogging or swimming or riding a bike, it's great," he notes. "Taking a brisk walk an hour a day uses up lots of calories, and you

Walk to Your Heart's Content

Heart disease is a problem that comes with aging—right?

Well, not quite. Problems can start at any age. But no matter whether you have heart disease or not, a walking program is one of the best things you can do for yourself, says Howard Hodis, M.D., assistant professor of medicine and preventive medicine and director of the atherosclerosis research unit at the University of Southern California School of Medicine in Los Angeles.

When you walk regularly, the conditioning effect enhances the pumping ability of your heart, which means that you can do more work before your heart gets overtaxed. In addition, a regular walking program may lower your blood pressure, improve your cholesterol profile by raising HDL levels and short-circuit depression.

If you have heart disease, you can't afford to presume that regular walking is enough, but if you combine your walking regimen with a low-fat, low-sodium diet, don't smoke and learn to deal effectively with stress, you can expect to see results and feel measurably better. In addition, of course, there are certain precautions you should take. A doctor should help you determine what level of exercise you can perform safely and how fast your heart can beat before you begin to have chest pain, says Dr. Hodis. The doctor can also determine when you might have silent ischemia, dangerous changes in blood flow that might precipitate a heart attack.

By tracking your heart with an electrocardiogram, or EKG, during an exercise stress test on a treadmill, your doctor can find out how hard you can work before you get into trouble. She can then tell you how hard you can exercise without exceeding your danger level.

The challenge then is to have a good time walking—but stay within the safety zone. Generally, if you have heart disease or not, your minimum exercise prescription for conditioning is 30 to 40 minutes of comfortable walking, three times a week. Of course, you should work up to this level slowly, with your physician's approval.

don't hurt yourself."

Little bits of daily exercise also count. "I never take an elevator, and I climb several flights of stairs a day. You could park in the parking space farthest from your building and make yourself walk," he adds.

Any time you exercise for more than a few minutes, you're burning a combination of carbohydrates and fat. And 95 percent of your stored energy is fat.

Go mono-a-mono. If you're going to use oil, olive or canola oil is the way to go, says Dr. Alexander. They're monounsaturated fats, which are easier on the heart than animal fats and tropical oils such as palm and coconut oil, which raise cholesterol levels. "But remember not to use a lot of it just because it's not as bad for you. It has lots of calories, so be careful."

A fat rule of thumb: Saturated fats differ from unsaturated ones in that they're white, oily substances that are solid at room temperature and are found in meats, butter and cheese. Unsaturated fats are clear, oily substances that are liquid at room temperature.

Let's Es-chew the fat. A low-fat diet is the way to go, notes Dr. Alexander. That means getting just 20 to 30 percent or less of your daily calories from fat. "I think if everyone exercised vigorously and was a vegetarian, they would live a lot longer."

Half of all Americans have high cholesterol because of the way they eat—dietary cholesterol is found only in animal food sources such as meat and dairy products, but not in plant food such as fruits, vegetables and beans.

Have your finned and feathered friends for dinner. Fish offers special heart benefits. A number of studies suggest that the omega-3 fatty acids it contains may help your heart, says Dr. Alpert. White-meat turkey and chicken (without the skin) should be second

Win or Draw? Butter versus Margarine

Which slippery character is worse for blood cholesterol levels—the saturated fat found in butter, cheese, whole milk, ice cream and meat or the trans-fatty acids (trans fats) used in margarines, commercially baked goods and french fries?

The American Heart Association says that the worst offender by far is the saturated fat (and cholesterol) in butter. But two scientists at the Harvard School of Public Health made news by tagging trans fat (created when food processors add hydrogen to vegetable oil) as the nastier of the two. The main point is there's evidence that too much of *either* fat helps choke arteries with plaque.

Currently, food producers aren't required to reveal the amount of trans fats that they add to products, so there's no way to know exactly how much is hidden in food you buy. Check out the ingredients list. If any partially hydrogenated vegetable oil is listed in the first few ingredients—especially in a food high in total fat—chances are there's more than a trickle of trans.

on your list, because they're low in total fat and, more important, artery-clogging saturated fat. Choose only the leanest cuts of pork and beef and trim them well before cooking.

Get your fill of fiber. Fiber helps reduce serum cholesterol levels, so you can effectively lower cholesterol by as much as 10 to 20 percent in certain people, says Dr. Hodis. It also helps in that you feel fuller when you munch lots of fiber—therefore leaving less room for things like Snickers bars and ice cream. You can get the fiber you need from food if you eat whole grains, oatmeal, fruits

Nature's Best Cholesterol Crunchers

Believe it or not, there's a natural prescription to lower your cholesterol that you don't have to go to a pharmacy to fill. If you know where to look, this powerful remedy is available right on the shelves of your supermarket. Just load your cart with fabulous foods that are high in soluble fiber, and you'll be stocking up on the safest, healthiest and tastiest cholesterol-crunching substance there is!

Scores of studies by James Anderson, M.D., professor of medicine and clinical nutrition at the University of Kentucky in Lexington, and others now have settled earlier questions about whether soluble fiber really does lower cholesterol.

Today, most heart experts, including those at the government's National Cholesterol Education Program, agree: It works!

Though not everyone responds the same, Dr. Anderson's research shows that for some people, combining soluble fiber with a low-fat diet can mean cholesterol reductions of 50 points or more. Adding soluble fiber to an already low-fat diet could knock cholesterol down to a safe count and make cholesterol-lowering drugs unnecessary. (See the tips for getting more fiber in your diet in "Nutrition" on page 266.

Artichokes, dried apricots and cereals high in oat bran are all fabulous sources of soluble fiber, as are sweet potatoes, brussels sprouts and celery root. Many legumes as well as oat cereals have two grams or more of soluble fiber per serving. Among fruits, oranges and apples are the top sources, but other fruits—such as mangoes, figs, plums, and kiwifruit—are soluble superstars, too. High-fiber wheat-bran cereals are best known as major sources of insoluble fiber, but even they have a very respectable one gram of fiber per serving.

and vegetables. The Daily Value for dietary fiber is 25 grams.

Employ that soy. Replacing cheeseburgers with tofu burgers could be a heart saver, says Bryan Johnstone, Ph.D., assistant professor at the University of Kentucky College of Medicine in Lexington. The key is soy protein, which contains estrogens that may lower LDL cholesterol. Another theory is that soy's amino acid pattern has an impact on the oxidation rate of cholesterol, he notes.

In a 1995 study at the University of Kentucky in Lexington that combined the results of 38 clinical trials, researchers found that a diet with soy protein intake of 47 grams per day lowered total cholesterol by 9.3 percent over a minimum of a month's time. "We're talking about soy substitution, not soy addition," says Dr. Johnstone, one of the researchers. "So if an average diet recommends 70 grams of protein, then we suggest at least 25 grams of soy being incorporated into the diet in lieu of that." This means that somewhere between one-third and one-half of your average daily protein intake would come from soy.

It's a snap adding soy to your diet. Soy concentrate is a tasteless powder you can sprinkle on your foods; one ounce added to pasta gives you 24 grams of soy protein. One eight-ounce glass of soy milk contains 4 to 10 grams, adds Dr. Johnstone. "One of the potential implications is that this is why the Chinese have lower levels of cholesterol and heart disease than we do."

E does it. Taking 100 to 400 international units (IUs) of vitamin E a day might be one way to ditch that bad cholesterol, says Dr. Hodis.

In a study of 156 men with heart disease at the University of Southern California in Los Angeles, Dr. Hodis and researchers found that taking daily doses of vitamin E for two years was associated with a reduction in the development of fatty deposits, or plaque, in heart arteries.

Why is E so heart-smart? Antioxidants prevent the oxidation of LDL cholesterol. When there is less oxidation, the LDL cholesterol loses some of its artery-clogging power. The amount taken—100 to 400 IUs—was higher than the Daily Value of 30 IUs, but the higher dosages are safe, Dr. Hodis says.

Replace hormones with hormones. After you've reached menopause, going on estrogen replacement therapy is an effective way of lowering your bad cholesterol while boosting your good, notes Valery Miller, M.D., research professor of medicine at the George Washington University Medical Center in Washington D.C. "Estrogen might have an antioxidant effect—if the LDL is oxidized, it's more likely to go into the walls of the arteries, where it causes hardening."

According to Dr. Miller, the estrogen causes smooth muscle in the artery walls to relax, and it may prevent spasms. The National Cholesterol Education Program has issued adult treatment guidelines that say that after diet and exercise, estrogen therapy should be considered next in postmenopausal women, and recommend it before drug therapy for high cholesterol.

In a study of 875 healthy postmenopausal women ages 45 to 64, the women were given either estrogen therapy or a placebo and followed for three years. The estrogen-treated women developed significantly lower LDL cholesterol and much higher HDL cholesterol. Also, estrogen takers had a stable level of fibrinogen, a blood protein that's been linked to heart disease, while the nontakers showed an increase.

Although some women are nervous about hormone replacement therapy because of a possible link with increased breast cancer risk, Dr. Miller says the pros definitely outweigh the cons. "They haven't conclusively

Depressurize with Potassium

Potassium works as a blood vessel dilator, and when the vessels dilate, your pressure goes down. But this doesn't mean that huge amounts of potassium are needed to lower blood pressure.

The Daily Value for potassium is 3,500 milligrams, "but it's safe to consume substantially more than that," says Harvey Simon, M.D., associate professor of medicine at Harvard Medical School, founding member of the Harvard Cardiovascular Health Center and author of *Conquering Heart Disease*. The trick is getting enough potassium in your daily menu without going on the chimpanzee diet. Actually, bananas are not the highest source of potassium, which can be found in a wide assortment of fruits and vegetables.

One caution: If you're taking a potassium-sparing diuretic, which causes the kidneys to hoard the mineral, you should not increase your potassium intake without discussing with your doctor any changes you'd like to make.

Eating to Control
Your Blood Pressure

If you have high blood pressure (defined as a reading of 140/90 and above), you want powerful medicine to control it. And—as study after study has shown—diet is powerful medicine.

A healthy diet can't always replace pills and other medical means when blood pressure is elevated, but it often does. Frequently, it can either boost the effect of medication or allow for a lower dose. More good news: Those who are most helped by good eating are the ones who most need help. The higher your blood pressure, the more it is likely to fall if you use your head when you fill your belly.

Diet therapy to reduce high blood pressure calls for the following:

- An eating plan geared to weight control.

For those people who are overweight a low-fat diet (made up of less than 25 percent of calories) high in unrefined complex carbohydrates is ideal.

- Limiting sodium intake to the Daily Value of 2,400 milligrams a day (the amount in a level teaspoon of table salt). Discuss with your physician whether it would be wise to limit your sodium intake even more.
- Including in your diet a variety of fruits and vegetables that together provide at least 3,500 milligrams of potassium a day.
- Getting your Daily Value for magnesium and calcium—400 milligrams of magnesium and 1,000 milligrams of calcium per day for women.

proven the breast cancer relationship, and we know about the benefits, because the data is so consistent and strong."

Take it off. Taking off weight is great, but keeping it off might be the key to lowering your cholesterol, says Rena Wing, Ph.D., professor of psychiatry, epidemiology and psychology at the University of Pittsburgh School of Medicine.

In a University of Pittsburgh study of how dropping pounds affects cardiovascular risk, and the differences between men and women, Dr. Wing found that men are the initial winners in the weight-loss game. Looking at 159 moderately overweight subjects over 18 months, the researchers found that men who lost weight experienced greater decreases in blood pressure, triglycerides and waist-to-hip ratio and had greater increases in HDL cho-

lesterol than women. But modest weight losses (10 to 15 percent of initial body weight) maintained over time resulted in sustained improvements in heart disease risk factors for women as well.

"Women experience an initial decrease in HDL cholesterol with weight loss, then gradually an increase, while men have increases in HDL all along," Dr. Wing notes. "So it is particularly important for women to adhere to weight-loss programs and maintain their weight loss to see the improvement in risk factors."

Even if you haven't reached your ideal weight, keeping off the pounds you've managed to lose—25 was the average in the Pittsburgh study—can increase HDL cholesterol and improve other cardiovascular risk factors.

Other Ways to Be Heart-Smart

Even if your cholesterol levels are a dream, you could still be sabotaging your heart health with the little things you do. You know the no-no's: smoking, stressing out and not controlling high blood pressure. These all take their toll on your ticker, notes Dr. Hodis. "Folks can have a relatively low LDL and still have heart disease. That may be a result of a poor lifestyle."

Sure, there are factors you have little control over. Diabetes, a disorder of the pancreas that affects the body's insulin production, puts women at a higher risk for heart disease than it does men. But watching your weight and also watching out for high blood pressure can ease that risk considerably. You can also control the disease with diet, exercise and medication.

These preventive measures are especially important to African-American women, a very vulnerable group. Up until about age 75, they have higher rates of death caused by heart disease than do women of any other racial groups.

Another factor is simply who your parents are, notes Dr. Alexander. "People who have long-lived parents and grandparents often have the healthiest hearts. Particularly, if they do nothing to jeopardize those good genes by risky behavior."

Studies of families in which heart disease is common before age 55 indicate that if one of your relatives got it early, you're at risk of an early heart attack, too. So it's even more essential to take advantage of the measures that are known to help reduce your risks.

A Plan of No Attack

Whatever your risks, there are many lifestyle changes that you can make to pre-vent heart disease. Here are a few doctors' tips.

Don't be a teetotaler. A glass of red wine a day can't hurt you, and it might raise your HDL level, notes Dr. Alpert. "If you like taking a glass in the evening, do it. It has an antiplatelet effect."

Low-dose alcohol is associated with a 30 to 50 percent reduction in heart attacks—a result that compares favorably with the protection of aspirin, stopping smoking, maintaining ideal body weight and reducing cholesterol. In a Harvard study of 85,709 women ages 34 to 59, researchers found that women who drank one to three drinks a week had a lower total mortality from heart disease. The group benefiting most were the women who reported one or more coronary risk factors. Being moderate is the key, researchers say: When drinking exceeds this level, health risks start to rise sharply.

Don't smoke. Stop smoking, and you'll thank yourself from the bottom of your . . . well, you know, notes Dr. Alexander. Heart problems caused by smoking are twofold: Over the long term smoking predisposes you to hardening of the arteries and puts you at an increased risk of sudden death.

The good news is, if you stop, no matter how much you've smoked in your life, your risk is reduced over time until it's nearly as low as the risk for someone who's never smoked. (For tips on how to stop smoking, see "Lungs" on page 206.)

Big leaguers, reach out. Although women generally deal better with stress than men do, women in higher-level jobs, such as CEOs of companies, have higher blood pressure than other working women. One solution is for them to find support groups and try to network more, notes Kathleen Light, Ph.D., professor of psychology in the Department of

Psychiatry at the University of North Carolina at Chapel Hill.

Studies have shown that women in high-level jobs are more likely to have stress problems than white males in equivalent jobs. In a University of North Carolina study of 72 men and 71 women working full-time outside the home, it was found that 71 percent of women in high-status jobs had high-effort coping, which leads to short-term rises in blood pressure. By comparison, just 36 percent of white men with status jobs had that kind of stress.

"I assume the workplace is more stressful for women and African-American men in part because they're more isolated, and they don't have the same amount of support from colleagues," Dr. Light says. "If a woman could find a peer group of other women in high-status jobs, the others could be supportive and serve as much-needed confidantes."

Let some things go. For women who have a lot of stress, the advice is, learn to let go and cut yourself some slack, says Dr. Light. "If you want to remain at a high-intensity level at work, you should allow yourself to have a dirty house, and to not be the perfect homemaker as well."

Run down blood pressure. Moderate exercise is a great way to put high blood pressure on the run, notes Dr. Light.

Studies show that two groups of sedentary men and women with high blood pressure who rode stationary bicycles at a moderate pace for 20 minutes saw a decrease in their blood pressure for the next five hours. "There's data suggesting that you have to get into an exercise regimen that takes weeks to see benefits from," she says. "This shows that you actually get benefits from day one."

Pop an aspirin. Taking an aspirin a day is a great way of keeping the veins clot-free, says Dr. Alpert. "It's cheap, it's easy and it's

The Hostile Heart

You're in the express line of the super-market, and the inconsiderate person ahead of you has 15 items—in clear view of a sign that announces "10 items or less." If you get so mad that your half-gallon of Häagen-Dazs turns to mush in your sweaty palms, you just might be hostile—a trait that Redford Williams, M.D., professor of psychiatry at Duke University in Durham, North Carolina, and co-author of *Anger Kills*, says can put you at increased risk of heart attack.

"All the hostility studies we've done show that heart patients who have no social support (a common trait of hostile people) have a threefold higher five-year mortality rate," Dr. Williams notes. "Even healthy people with hostile personalities are four to seven times more likely to die from heart attacks and other serious illnesses."

Just what is hostility? It's a potent combination of cynicism, anger and aggression that can mess up your mind and your health.

So what can you do about it?

One way of controlling hostility is to shout "Stop!"—either out loud or to yourself—when you feel anger coming on, depending on the situation. To get started, you could ask someone else to help you, with the friend crying "Stop!" when you start getting mad. Then you could think about a favorite person or hobby in place of the hostile thought.

important. Aspirin is a very good idea even if you don't have heart disease yet. One a day knocks out the platelets—the little clots in the blood." Just be sure to check with your own doctor before starting a regular routine of taking medication.

See also Circulatory System

Hips

TO KIDS ON THE GO, hips are just another body part to wiggle, wriggle and jiggle. From skateboarding to boogying, youthful gyrations require superb hip mobility. It's only as the years pass and girths grow that many of us start to worry more about the dimensions than the swivel of our hips.

Instead of focusing so much on the size of their hips, women need to get hip about the health of that region of their bodies, doctors say. In their thirties and forties there are a number of problems that women can experience in the hip region, including arthritis and bursitis.

Yet the big threat to women is a disease that doesn't actually strike until years later when they reach menopause. Osteoporosis, a disease in which bone density declines, places women at risk for disabling and even life-threatening hip fractures.

Now, not later—particularly when it comes to osteoporosis—is when you can take steps to safeguard the health of your hips, experts say.

Why We Sway

"The hip is what is referred to as a ball-and-socket joint," says Ira H. Kirschenbaum, M.D., arthritis and joint replacement surgeon at Westchester Bone and Joint Associates in White Plains, New York. It has a socket cup that is formed by the bones of the pelvis. The joint also has a ball at the top end of the thigh bone.

The ball fits securely into the cuplike cavity and is attached to the pelvic bone by a se-ries of strong ligaments. This ball-and-socket design makes the hip joint both flexible and stable.

In terms of how the hip joint is constructed, there appears to be little difference between men's and women's hip joints, says Susan Larson, Ph.D., associate professor of anatomy at the State University of New York at Stony Brook. In women, however, hips tend to be wider, because they have a wider pelvis (which is needed to deliver babies). That extra dimension can contribute to knee problems, and it's the reason many women have a walking gait distinctly different from men's.

When we walk, we swing one hip forward. And as we take a step, that hip tends to drop a little lower than the hip of the supporting leg, explains Dr. Larson. Because a woman's pelvis is wider, that hip drop is more pronounced than it is in men. The result is that our hips tend to sway more when we walk.

Building a Better Hip Future

Even if you've been sashaying gracefully through adult life with little or no hip pain, you should start to think about the future state of your hipbones. Every woman needs to, according to Dr. Kirschenbaum. Here's why.

Bone is a dynamic structure that's continually remodeling itself. Old bone goes through a breakdown process called resorption while new bone is building up. When new bone is building up faster than old bone is being resorbed, bones get stronger. But if bone is being resorbed faster than it's being built up, bone is lost.

As we age, both men and women experience age-related bone loss, says Dr. Kirschenbaum. That's because the bone-building process doesn't quite keep pace with the breakdown process.

But women have it worse. In pre-menopausal years, it appears, the hormone estrogen plays a role in inhibiting bone resorption. Once estrogen levels decline, however, its protective action against bone resorption is gone, and women start to lose bone a lot faster than men do.

When women reach menopause and their estrogen levels drop, bone loss increases dramatically. The hips are one of the most vulnerable spots (the wrist and spine are also susceptible).

It's this rapid bone loss that can lead to osteoporosis. The very structure of the bone—the internal scaffolding—starts to thin out. Bone density declines and the bone grows weaker. When that happens, the bone is susceptible to fracture.

Some women are at greater risk for osteoporosis than others, observes Avrum Froimson, M.D., director of orthopedic surgery at Mount Sinai Medical Center in Cleveland. "If you're blond, blue-eyed and thin, then you are at higher risk than if you are dark-haired, dark-eyed and heavier." And if you have a family history of the disease—if your mother or your grandmother had a hip fracture—then you're probably at increased risk for the disease.

An estimated 20 million adults develop osteoporosis each year, and an estimated 250,000 postmenopausal women will suffer hip fractures each year because of the disease. A woman who lives to be 90 years old has a one in three chance of fracturing her hip.

Compared with heart disease or breast cancer, osteoporosis may seem less alarming. But the fact is, a hip fracture from osteoporosis can be difficult to recover from—so difficult, in fact, that many women never do. Some die from complications, while others are left disabled.

Where the Hip Breaks

When a woman breaks her hip, the break usually occurs in a portion of bone called the femoral neck, according to Avrum Froimson, M.D., director of orthopedic surgery at Mount Sinai Medical Center in Cleveland. The femoral neck is located between two larger, chunkier pieces of bone—the ball-shaped head of the femur and the femur bone. Since the femoral neck is the thinnest bone in the area, when something gives, it's usually there.

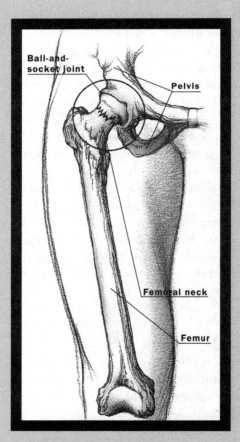

The circled area is the thin femoral neck of the hip joint—where a fracture is most likely to occur.

Amassing More Bone

You can't stop some loss of bone mass; it's an inevitable part of aging. But if you're in your thirties or forties, you can take many steps to help avoid the onset of osteoporosis. Here's what experts recommend.

Walk away from it. A regular program of weight-bearing exercise can help build your bone strength and fend off osteoporosis, says Dr. Kirschenbaum. Impact exercises such as walking, running or step aerobics are very effective. Women should aim for 20 to 30 minutes of continuous impact exercise a day, he says.

Consume calcium. Calcium is one of the building blocks that bone needs to replenish itself. So women need to make sure they have enough calcium in their diets, says Dr. Froimson.

The amount of calcium for premenopausal women is 1,000 milligrams a day, according to recommendations of the National Institutes of Health Consensus Panel. For postmenopausal women not undergoing hormone replacement therapy, the recommended amount jumps to 1,500 milligrams.

It's possible to get all that calcium from food sources—but make sure that the sources are low-fat or nonfat, so you don't put on extra weight while you're getting more calcium. Each one-cup serving of low-fat yogurt and each cup of skim milk has about 300 milligrams of calcium. So you can get the recommended level if you get four or five servings of those low-fat dairy foods every day. Other foods such as low-fat cheese, which contains about 170 milligrams of calcium, can also contribute.

Pop some extra. The calcium you get from food is the best kind, says Dr. Froimson, since it's more readily absorbed by your body than the calcium you get through supplements. But if you can't get all the calcium you need from food sources, ask your doctor about supplements. Many doctors recommend calcium supplements containing calcium carbonate.

Don't smoke bone away. Smoking can have a negative effect on bone density and aggravate your risk for the disease, says Gerald Eisenberg, M.D., director of the arthritis treatment program at Lutheran General Hospital in Park Ridge, Illinois. Do your best to cut back or give up the habit.

Know your medication. A number of medications, including antiseizure medications, anti-anxiety drugs and corticosteroids, have a thinning effect on bone. Women who take these medications may be at increased risk for hip fracture in their thirties and forties as well as in their later years, says Dr. Kirschenbaum. Ask your doctor about any medications that you're taking, and if they could cause bone-loss problems, find out if there are alternatives.

Get tested. If you suspect that you may be at increased risk for osteoporosis because the disease runs in your family, ask your doctor to perform a bone density test. There are a number of different methods for assessing bone density, so ask your doctor about them.

Consider HRT. For women who have entered menopause, hormone replacement therapy (HRT) could be a way to prevent osteoporosis, experts say. That's because HRT formulations include estrogen to replenish the levels of natural estrogen that drop off at menopause—and with more estrogen in the system, there's less bone loss. Experts estimate that starting HRT at the onset of menopause can decrease your risk for osteoporosis by approximately 50 percent. But while HRT can benefit your bone strength,

Replacement Surgery: What You Need to Know

While the average age for hip replacement surgery is in the late sixties or early seventies, some women may need the surgery as early as their thirties or forties, says Ira H. Kirschenbaum, M.D., arthritis and joint replacement surgeon at Westchester Bone and Joint Associates in White Plains, New York. Among younger women who may need the procedure are those who had some type of hip disease when they were children and women with rheumatoid arthritis.

The first question to ask, according to Dr. Kirschenbaum, is, "Do I really need the operation?"

"There is clearly a limited life to hip replacement surgery," he says. If you have the surgery when you're relatively young, you may need what's known as revision surgery again in 10 to 15 years. Revision surgery is associated with more complications than the original hip replacements, he says. So the decision to have surgery should be very carefully considered.

If you do need to have your surgery early, it's most important to decide who your surgeon will be, says Dr. Kirschenbaum. That person should be a hip specialist with advanced training and advanced experience.

there are some risks associated with the treatment. Be sure to discuss all the risks and benefits of it with your doctor.

Joint at the Hip

While all women need to be concerned about osteoporosis, there are some women who are at high risk for two kinds of arthritis that can affect the hips: rheumatoid arthritis and osteoarthritis. Rheumatoid arthritis is a disease in which the bones and cartilage in the joints start to deteriorate, and the joints become inflamed and painful, says Dr. Eisenberg.

With osteoarthritis, stress, strain and damage to the joint cause it to shift out of alignment, which in turn causes added wear and tear. The joint begins to deteriorate.

Hip osteoarthritis "is definitely more frequent in people who are overweight," says Dr. Eisenberg. If you're 25 percent or more over your ideal body weight, that could lead to arthritis trouble, he says.

Anti-arthritis Advice

There are some steps that you can take to lower your chances for osteoarthritis. Even though you can't prevent rheumatoid arthritis, some of these same measures can also be useful for relieving rheumatoid arthritis pain in your hips. Here's what doctors suggest.

Lighten up. "Weight control is very important," says Dr. Eisenberg. By maintaining a healthy weight, you can help fend off osteoarthritis and decrease the pain of rheumatoid arthritis, doctors say. Stick to a low-fat eating plan and exercise regularly.

Wear flats. High-heeled shoes are death to the hips, says Dr. Kirschenbaum. That's because the ball-and-socket joint can be destroyed by anything that increases the force across the hip, and high-heeled shoes do just that. With your foot in a high-heel, too much force is transmitted to the hip joint, and that can wear out the joint, he says. "I tell my patients to wear Rockports, wear sneakers to work, wear oxfords or wear one-inch heels and nothing more. Wear soft-soled shoes your whole life."

Don't jar those joints. If you have either type of arthritis, you're better off with moderate exercise than with no exercise at all, according to Dr. Eisenberg. Try to avoid forms of exercise that are more jarring to the joints—jogging and aerobics—and aim for the gentler modes of sport, such as walking and swimming.

Bursa Woes

A source of hip pain for active women can be hip bursitis, says Dr. Kirschenbaum. That's an inflammation of the tiny fluid-filled sacs that act as a cushion where tendons attach to bone. "Generally, the number one cause of bursitis in the hip joint is overuse." Overenthusiastic aerobics can start bursa trouble—or walking 20 city blocks in high-heeled shoes. Or the bursa might start to swell after you take a bad fall.

If you have soreness or pain that your doctor says is caused by bursitis, here are some things you can do to ease the discomfort.

Pack it up. An ice pack can come to the rescue if you begin to feel hip pain. You should aim to ice the area for 20 minutes three times a day, says Dr. Kirschenbaum. "Also, every time you play sports—tennis, racquetball, aerobics—ice it down for 20 minutes after every event." Ice helps provide pain relief and facilitate healing by reducing inflammation and swelling. "I honestly believe that ice is going to win the war."

To effectively ice the hip, Dr. Kirschenbaum recommends freezing a Styrofoam cup filled with water. Once the water is frozen, cut one inch of Styrofoam off the bottom of the cup and rub the exposed ice over your hip. However, it is important not to overdo it. "Don't freeze the area. The key is the frequency, not the strength, of the ice treatments," he warns.

Pay attention to pain. "Any pain in your hip could be hip bursitis, so don't wait too long to attend to it," says Dr. Kirschenbaum. "If you can get in early with ice and natural treatment, you can win." If you wait too long, he warns, you might have to go to other levels of treatment, such as the use of anti-inflammatory drugs and cortisone injections.

Quench the flame. "The second thing that I tell people is that they can take some anti-inflammatory medications," says Dr. Kirschenbaum. Over-the-counter anti-inflammatory medications include aspirin, ibuprofen and naproxen (Aleve). "Acetaminophen is not an anti-inflammatory; it's just for pain relief."

Go gradual. If you are just starting out on an exercise program, it's important to take it easy. Don't overdo it at the beginning—and stop if you feel pain. "Build up gradually," suggests Dr. Eisenberg.

How do you tell if you're going too fast? If you feel sore or have pain for more than 24 hours after an exercise session, you're probably overdoing it, he says.

Consider a single shot. If you have serious hip bursitis, your doctor may want to give you an injection of cortisone, says Dr. Kirschenbaum. Almost 70 to 85 percent of hip bursitis cases are cured with one injection.

See also Pelvis, Skeletal System

Hormones

A SULLEN TEENAGER, an extra pound, a grumpy mood. "It's all hormonal," you sigh.

And you're right. Almost all our human ups and downs are hormonal. Hormones are powerful chemicals that tell us to grow up, to turn our food into fuel, to continue the human race. They prepare us to fight for our lives or our children's. They're the soldiers in the endocrine system, an army commanded by organs called glands.

"A hormone is formed within one gland in the body and then carried in the bloodstream to other organs and tissues, where it influences their functions and activities. For instance, estrogen is made in the ovaries. Then it goes to a large number of organs, including breast tissue, the lining of the uterus, the lining of the arteries, the liver and the bones," says JoAnn E. Manson, M.D., associate professor of medicine at Harvard Medical School and co-director of Women's Health at Brigham and Women's Hospital in Boston.

Nobody knows how many hormones the body makes. The adrenal gland alone spits out more than 25. But the most telling chemicals can be divided into three categories: sex, food and stress hormones.

After puberty the ovaries begin producing increased levels of sex hormones that prepare the uterus, ovaries and fallopian tubes for ovulation, fertilization or menstruation.

Probably the best known of these sex hormones, estrogen, does double duty, affecting sex and fertility as well as the way our bodies process food. It also helps prevent the bone loss of osteoporosis.

Besides estrogen, there are a number of other hormones that play a big role in food processing:

• Insulin guides blood sugar through the bloodstream and helps regulate the way it's absorbed by cells.

• Parathyroid hormone (PTH) is important in controlling the calcium balance of the blood. The calcium balance is necessary for chemical reactions and muscular contractions needed for voluntary movement and even heartbeat.

• Thyroxine from the thyroid gland helps regulate the way that we burn up calories.

Other hormones come into play when you deal with stress.

• Adrenaline makes your muscles clench. It speeds up your heart, slows your digestion and accelerates blood clotting if you're injured.

• Cortisol, another stress-related hormone, helps reduce swelling around wounds. But because it also pumps up blood pressure, having too much cortisol in your system can lead to high blood pressure.

The best way to keep all your hormones balanced and happy is to eat a healthy diet, get a good night's sleep and exercise, says Jerilynn C. Prior, M.D., professor of endocrinology at the University of British Columbia in Vancouver.

On the nutritional front, it's particularly important for women to eat plenty of food rich in calcium. If you don't, the hormone PTH could start to plunder this crucial mineral from your bones.

Weight control also helps balance hormones. "Obesity alters the way hormones are made and function. So it's important to maintain a healthy weight," says Dr. Manson.

See also Endocrine System, Reproductive System

Intestines

WHEN YOU TELL SOMEONE you hate his guts, it's not a very nice thing to say. But then again, guts are a pretty gross concept. Several yards of pink innards coiled just below your stomach and liver like a giant worm—they could hardly be described as cute.

But the small and large intestines are integral parts of your digestive system. While some of the chow you consume is digested in the stomach, it's the small intestine that adds more digestive enzymes and completes the job. There the digested food is absorbed through the intestinal walls and enters the blood.

The large intestine, just below the small intestine, takes the indigestible parts of the food and gradually absorbs the liquid from it. The semisolid waste is then formed into feces and pushed down into the rectum for evacuation.

Despite its name, the small intestine is actually longer—measuring in at a whopping 20 feet. The large intestine, although wider in diameter, is just 5 feet long.

Keeping Your Pipes in Order

Having intestinal fortitude means that you can suffer the slings and arrows of outrageous fortune without even breaking a nail. But intestinal health is another matter.

To keep your intestines in the pink—and your body free of gas and diarrhea—follow these tips from top docs.

Avoid too much of a good thing. Fresh fruits and fruit juices are important in a healthy diet, but in rare cases, they can bring on intestinal distress. Fruits, honey and especially fruit juices are high in a type of sugar called fructose. Normally, enzymes in the intestinal wall break down fructose so it can be absorbed, but sometimes, when too much of the sugar is ingested at one time, some may escape through the small intestine into the colon, says Charlene Prather, M.D., a gastroenterologist and director of the Motility Clinic at the Mayo Clinic in Rochester, Minnesota.

Fructose that arrives at the colon undigested is readily fermented by the bacteria that live there. Their feast may result in gas, bloating and sometimes diarrhea. Fruits also contain soluble fiber and can cause a lot of bacterial fermentation and gas when it reaches the colon.

Including plenty of fruit in your diet is still a good idea, but limit the amount of fruits and fruit juices you consume at any one time. Fruit juice can be more of a problem than fruit, so eat your fruit instead of drinking it, adds Dr. Prather. The recommended amount is two to four servings per day, says William B. Ruderman, M.D., practicing physician at Gastroenterology Associates of Central Florida in Orlando. But that doesn't mean all at one sitting. Have a piece of fruit now and a glass of fruit juice later—or make fruit a regular part of your meals.

Skip the sugarless chew. Some sugar-free gums contain sorbitol, which is used as a sweetener. Our bodies are not really designed to handle the relatively large amounts of sorbitol that are present in sugarless chewing gum—and it doesn't take much to cause gas and diarrhea, advises Dr. Prather. A single stick of sugarless gum may contain 2 grams of sorbitol—and 5 grams is enough to cause trouble—so by the time you're chewing your third stick, you could be headed for gastric grief. That doesn't apply to everyone, however: Some people can take 20 to 50 grams before their intestines act up.

The reason? "Although we don't absorb sorbitol well, the bacteria that live in our colons absolutely love it," says Dr. Prather. They break it down (in a process called fermentation) and produce large amounts of gas. This gas causes swelling of the colon and pain, which can be compounded by sharp contractions of the muscle in the colon wall. This you feel as cramps. The by-products of fermentation also cause water to flow into the digestive tract, loosening stools and causing diarrhea.

Sorbitol is also found in many "dietetic" candies and is used as a sweetener in some medications. Two other sweeteners—xylitol and mannitol—may have effects similar to those of sorbitol. Any of them may masquerade under the name "sugar alcohol" on gum wrappers and elsewhere.

Juggle your antacids. Antacids offer relief from heartburn, but that immediate relief may mean misery later. Depending on the amount you take, antacids containing magnesium can cause loose stools or diarrhea. That's because magnesium pulls water from the body into the intestines. On the other hand, antacids containing aluminum can cause constipation. In either case, you're not likely to make the connection, because the symptoms can be very delayed.

So what's the solution? First, try adjusting your dose. Generally speaking, the more antacid you take, the more likely you'll experience diarrhea or constipation, says Kenneth Lem, Pharm.D., lecturer in clinical pharmacy and associate dean for educational affairs at the University of California School of Pharmacy in San Francisco. If you take antacids often, switch between a magnesium-based one and an aluminum-based one, he says. If you use antacids only occasionally, he recommends using a balanced antacid with both magnesium and aluminum.

"Every time we swallow food or drink, we're also swallowing air," says Dr. Prather. "Though much of this swallowed air is burped up, swallowing can still add significantly to the amount of gas in the digestive tract, increasing the likelihood of gas discomfort."

Chewing gum, stress-induced swallowing and drinking carbonated beverages are also major sources of gas.

Beware that time of the month. "Many women may not be aware that gut disturbances can come with their monthly periods," says gastroenterologist Marvin Schuster, M.D., director of the Division of Digestive Diseases at Johns Hopkins Bayview Medical Center and professor of medicine at Johns Hopkins University School of Medicine in Baltimore. "Diarrhea is the most common symptom, usually occurring the first two days of the period. It may also occur right before the period."

This gut disturbance may be directly related to increased levels of the female hormones estrogen and progesterone—both of which relax the colon muscles. "Most of the contractions of the colon are involved in halting the movement of the stool," says Dr. Schuster, "so if you obliterate this braking action of the colon, then you get diarrhea."

Women who have these symptoms can treat them with an over-the-counter antidiarrheal drug containing loperamide hydrochloride, such as Imodium A-D. Or, if you have abdominal cramps without diarrhea, your doctor might prescribe an antispasmodic drug such as dicyclomine hydrochloride, as in Bentyl, says Dr. Ruderman.

See also Digestive System

Jaw

NOSHING CHEWY FAVORITES like caramel apples or thick, juicy steaks. Giving your mate a heartfelt, passionate kiss. Laughing it up with old friends. None of these pleasures would be possible without the jaw.

But that hard-working joint can also be the focal point of pain—even if the jaw itself doesn't hurt one bit. It's the culprit behind temporomandibular joint disorder (TMD), a malfunction in the jaw mechanism that can lead to many other kinds of pain around the head, neck and shoulders.

The temporomandibular joint, which connects the jawbone to the skull, allows the jaw to open, close and move from side to side and backward and forward. But occasionally, the jaw gets out of alignment. The result is an upset in the meshing of the upper and lower teeth that can eventually lead to a spasm of the jaw muscles, says Neil Gottehrer, D.D.S., director of the Craniofacial Pain Center in Abington, Pennsylvania. That sets off a chain reaction of other disorders, he notes. "I'd say that fewer than a quarter of my patients come in with a complaint of an aching jaw. They call TMD the great imposter, because it mimics many other symptoms. Some people have headaches, neck pain, shoulder pain, earaches, sore throat or dizziness."

You might also have clicking or popping sounds while opening or closing your jaw, fullness in your sinuses and pain while chewing, according to Dr. Gottehrer.

It's a frustrating disorder that affects about 20 percent of the population, although it's been estimated that only 5 percent of those people are actually being treated.

One problem is the extreme range and severity of symptoms, says A. Richard Goldman, D.D.S., director of the Institute for the Treatment and Study of Headaches and Facial Pain in Chicago. "TMD is a field pregnant with knowledge and misknowledge. The pain can be so mild as not to be noticed or so severe as to render the patient suicidal."

What causes temporomandibular joint disorders? Often it's major trauma, of which there are two kinds, says Gerald J. Murphy, D.D.S., president of the American Academy of Head, Neck and Facial Pain and a dentist in Grand Island, Nebraska. The first kind, known as direct trauma, includes blows to the jaw produced by mishaps during sporting events, by car accidents or by fistfights. The second, referred to as indirect trauma, involves whiplash injuries. These can be related either to neck injuries or to jaw injuries. A significant percentage of jaw-related whiplash injuries involve both the temporomandibular joint and its associated muscles, ligaments and tendons, he notes.

But sometimes it's the result of more subtle factors. Some people have developmental problems of the jaw or temporomandibular joints, such as a deep underbite—a condition where the bottom jaw protrudes. Others may develop temporomandibular disorders when they lose their back teeth and don't have them replaced—resulting in a bite change. In addition, tooth grinding, also known as bruxism or jaw clenching, may over a period of time result in a temporomandibular disorder, notes Dr. Murphy.

TMD can be a maddening ailment, but it doesn't have to make you feel helpless. There are many ways to prevent this painful intruder from becoming a pain.

Keep your chin up. A person with a

Where's That Pain From?

Despite its mysterious nature, temporomandibular joint disorder (TMD) is actually fairly easy for a dentist to diagnose. If you report symptoms that sound like they might be TMD, your dentist will probably ask you for a thorough history to find out what makes the pain worse, when it came on and from where the pain emanates, says Gerald J. Murphy, D.D.S., president of the American Academy of Head, Neck and Facial Pain and a dentist in Grand Island, Nebraska.

One way to check for TMD is by finding out how widely you can open your mouth, according to Charles Longenecker, D.M.D., a dentist in private practice in Emmaus, Pennsylvania. Your mouth opening is measured between the biting edges of your incissors. It is normally 50 millimeters—almost two inches—but it's difficult to open your mouth that wide if you have TMD.

A physical exam also tells a story. "When the doctor pushes in front of your ear, you may feel discomfort," says Dr. Longenecker. "If you press on the muscles inside and outside your mouth that support your jaw, there may be tenderness."

The doctor might take x-rays to check for deformities in your jaw joint. If those don't show the problem, an MRI (magnetic resonance imaging) or CAT (computerized axial tomography) scan might be needed, Dr. Murphy notes. While a standard x-ray only shows a front or side view of your jaw joint, an MRI shows soft tissue and can be used to determine whether or not your jaw disk is out of position. A CAT scan is an even more detailed evaluation of the joint, allowing the doctor to view different sections of your jaw.

How do you know if the doctor has given you a correct diagnosis? Usually, time will tell. "If the patient doesn't see a reduction in symptoms in three to five weeks, the doctor should reassess the diagnosis," says Dr. Murphy. "If it's a habit-related problem, the habit that's causing the condition will have to be modified."

---

whiplash injury has heavy stresses on the neck muscle, says Dr. Murphy. This may cause the head to automatically come forward, which can put heavier stress on the muscles of the jaw. You should concentrate on not habitually jutting your head forward—a posture often acquired by those who work at computers all day. "Changing your head posture changes your jaw position," he says. "Over the course of time, that relates to developing TMD."

Get out of the clench. Constant tooth grinding makes a person's jaw muscles tighten up and become spastic. That jaw action pulls the joint slightly out of place, ac-cording to Charles Longenecker, D.M.D., a dentist in private practice in Emmaus, Pennsylvania.

Grinding your teeth while you sleep—a major aggravator of the temporomandibular joint—can be remedied with a mouth guard. In some cases medication (usually tranquilizers) also reduces the muscle spasms, says Dr. Longenecker. "We put a hard plastic appliance over the upper teeth that keeps the teeth separated. So the lower teeth can glide over smooth plastic instead of biting into the upper teeth."

A hard plastic day splint that fits over the lower teeth is available for people who habitually clench their teeth during the day, he adds. See your dentist about getting one.

Jack up your jaw. Doing daily isometric exercises is a great way to stretch and contract the jaw muscles affected by TMD, says Dr. Gottehrer. One recommendation: Put your finger under your chin and try to open your mouth against slight resistance. Open your mouth about a half-inch with your finger still pressed against the chin—then close. Repeat 10 to 15 times twice a day. This relieves facial pain by stretching facial muscles that may be in spasm.

Exercises like that pay off, according to a six-month study of young adults with TMD conducted at the University of Sydney in Surry Hills, Australia. The study involved 44 people who had clicking in their jaws. One group of 22 did jaw exercises; the other didn't. Researchers found that 18 of the 22 who did jaw exercises were able to banish the clicking. In the other group there was no change.

Avoid steak. Whenever your TMD acts up, go on a soft diet, says Dr. Murphy. Eat things such as well-cooked vegetables, pudding, gelatin desserts, soup, finely chopped ground beef—foods that don't require heavy chewing—for three to four weeks.

Fight inflammation. Take ibuprofen regularly to ease pain and swelling, says Dr. Murphy. To calculate how much you need to take, consult your physician or follow the label directions, recommends Dr. Murphy.

Stay on your back. Lying on your stomach while you sleep is "the worst thing in the world," says Dr. Gottehrer. "It's not a normal body posture and puts stress on the jaw. I recommend sleeping on the side or back if possible."

See also Skeletal System

Joints

REMEMBER THAT LITTLE DITTY you and your friends used to sing when you were learning the parts of the body?

> *The foot bone connected*
> *to the—leg bone.*
> *The leg bone connected*
> *to the—kneebone.*

And onward up the skeleton.

Well, there's just one problem with that song. It leaves out all the important intersections—namely, our joints.

Without joints nothing would hold the skeleton together, and we wouldn't be able to move. If we didn't have joints, what else would we complain about at night after a day of lifting, climbing stairs or walking?

Joints by Group

You actually have several kinds of joints in your body. The ones that are joined by fibrous tissue, called fibrous joints, allow for little or no movement. There are three types of fibrous joints. One type of fibrous joint is in the skull, where the seams are connected by fiber that fuses together during adulthood.

Another kind of fibrous joint is bound with ligaments—cords of fibrous tissue that come in varying lengths. The shorter the ligament, the less movement in the joint. In your lower leg, for example, you have narrow, thick bones—the tibia and fibula—connected with fibrous joints, allowing a little "give" but no real movement between the ends of the two bones.

Still another kind of fibrous joint works like

a peg in a socket. The only example is in your jaw, where your teeth fit into bony sockets.

You also have cartilaginous joints, where the bones are separated or cushioned with a protective material called cartilage. These are the kinds of joints you have in your pelvis, between your first rib and sternum and in your spine. Sometimes the cartilage takes the form of a pad—called a meniscus—that acts as a shock absorber between bones.

At your knees, shoulders, hips and other limb connections, you have yet a third kind of joint, called synovia. Synovial joints have cavities filled with a slippery fluid, called synovial fluid, that's about the consistency of egg white. The synovial fluid allows for flexibility, lubrication and generally easy movement.

The Many Aches of Eves

If women have more joint problems than men, there's a good reason for it: Studies show that we're at greater risk for a lot of joint problems, including the most common kinds of arthritis as well as osteoporosis. We're even at greater risk of getting less-common joint diseases, such as lupus, an autoimmune disease that involves joint degeneration. (Nearly 90 percent of those who get lupus are women.)

Arthritis is a catchall term that refers to pain and stiffness in the joint. While there are many kinds of arthritis, osteoarthritis and the rheumatoid forms are the most prevalent. Osteoarthritis, the most common form, is frequently called degenerative joint disease or "wear-and-tear arthritis." The wear and tear occurs when cartilage—the padding between the bones—begins to fray, turning that ample cushion into a worn-down rag rug. Without their shock absorbers, the bone ends begin to rub against each other, causing irritation, sometimes swelling and eventually the devel-

opment of growths or spurs. You'll feel stiffness and occasional pain—and arthritis can eventually restrict your movements.

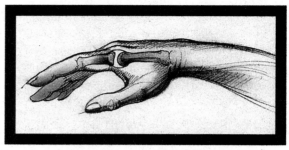
In a normal joint there's ample cartilage between the bones—which prevents wear-and-tear.

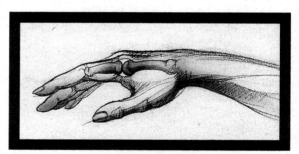
With osteoarthritis the cartilage is worn away, allowing the bones to rub together.

Joints of the body commonly affected by osteoarthritis include the knee, hip, fingers and spine. It usually starts as bumps in the fingers, according to Emil Pascarelli, M.D., professor of clinical medicine at Columbia Presbyterian Medical Center in New York City. Women often get symptoms of osteoarthritis after menopause.

Another kind of arthritis is rheumatoid—a disease in which the immune system actually attacks tissue in the body. Researchers aren't clear what causes the disease, but they suspect it may develop after someone's been infected with bacteria or a virus. This kind of arthritis typically strikes when a woman is in her thirties, but it can occur at any age.

At the onset of rheumatoid arthritis, membrane lining the joints becomes inflamed. Eventually, the disease can progress to the point where abnormal tissue as well as scar tissue forms inside the joint, and sometimes the bone ends actually fuse together.

What Joint Health Hinges On

If you're already getting mild complaints from the joints around your body, you can take measures to ease the discomfort. Here's what doctors recommend.

Take to the high road. It's good for your joints to have weight-bearing, low-impact exercise at least three times a week, according to Dr. Pascarelli. Translated, this means that you should take a good long walk at least several times a week or use that time for step aerobics or a low-impact exercise routine, he adds.

There is no evidence that running is bad for the joints, says Angela Smith, M.D., assistant professor of orthopedics at Case Western Reserve University School of Medicine in Cleveland. If you have an injury already, running may aggravate it. Also, errors in training (for example, increasing distance or speed too rapidly for the body to adapt properly) can cause injury in any sport—even swimming, she adds.

Stretch for the future. Stretching is excellent for the joints, says Dr. Pascarelli, since tight muscles put unnecessary pressure on them. Any kind of stretching is good as long as you don't bounce, which can pull a muscle. Hold a slow, steady stretch for 15 to 20 seconds, then relax and repeat. (For starters, try out the stretches on page 196.)

Chomp on some bone builder. Calcium is an essential building block for maintaining

Pregnant? Baby Your Ligaments

You need to be careful about some kinds of stretching if you're pregnant, doctors say. That's because your ligaments may be more lax than usual, and you could stretch farther than you should.

When a woman is pregnant, her body releases special hormones that tend to loosen up her ligaments, says Steven Stuchin, M.D., director of the Arthritis Center at the Hospital for Joint Diseases Orthopedic Institute in New York City. While the extra stretch in the pelvic girdle ligament helpfully makes way for childbirth, other ligaments throughout the body are affected at the same time. So if you're pregnant, you should talk to your doctor about how much stretching you can do without harming yourself.

strong bones. It also helps prevent osteoporosis or bone loss, which takes its toll when the bone around a joint begins to crack or deteriorate.

Aim to get between 1,000 milligrams and 1,500 milligrams of calcium a day, says Dr. Smith. (For a list of the best food sources, see "Calcium Champs" on page 269.) Many doctors will advise you to take supplements if you don't get all the calcium you need from food.

Don't block the bone builder. Both caffeine and nicotine are believed to interfere with calcium absorption, says Dr. Pascarelli. So do your best to give up smoking and cut back on caffeinated beverages such as tea, coffee and colas. Chocolate also contains caffeine, so sometimes it's advisable to have something else for dessert.

See also Ankles, Elbows, Hips, Knees, Shoulders, Skeletal System, Spine

Kidneys

SURE, THERE ARE MORE GLAMOROUS ORGANS. After all, "I Left My Kidney in San Francisco" or "Kidney and Soul" just don't have the same panache. But when it comes to producing results, kidneys are a top-notch team.

This pair of bean-shaped organs, which weigh six ounces each, are tucked in your abdominal cavity on either side of the spinal column. They work hard, filtering your body's entire blood volume about 40 times a day and converting the waste matter to about one quart of urine. They also control the body's acid-base balance. When blood and body fluids become too acid or too alkaline, kidneys help restore the balance of urine acidity. The key to this is water control—excreting water when there is an excess and conserving it when the body loses too much.

Despite their tough workaholic style, your kidneys are susceptible to infection and disease. The symptoms are more serious and harder to ignore than the burning and frequent urination of urinary tract infections (UTIs). With kidney infection you might have fever, chills, severe pain in either side (depending on which kidney is infected) and blood in your urine.

Women who get kidney infections are often the ones who have recurrent bacteria in their bladders, says Gopal Krishna, M.D., attending physician at Central Coast Nephrology in Salinas, California. So treating the UTI is a step toward preventing the bacteria from getting to the kidneys. If you do develop a kidney infection, the answer is usually antibiotics—most likely a course of ampicillin (Principen)—depending on how serious the infection is.

As with UTIs, Dr. Krishna advises keeping the urinary tract flushed by drinking lots of water. "That can prevent whatever is sitting in the bladder from eventually moving to the kidneys."

Pebble Passing

The pain of passing a kidney stone has been compared with childbirth, so it's only fitting that three times as many men as women will have to "give birth" to kidney stones. But that doesn't mean this nasty little crystal of salt and minerals won't make a guest appearance in your life. (Or maybe even two or three appearances: About 60 percent of all patients treated for a stone develop another within seven years.)

The majority of kidney stones are made of calcium oxalate, which is the end product of body metabolism and is naturally present in urine. The burning pain that occurs in the lower abdomen is a result of a usually pea-size rock traveling through the kidney and then down the ureter, which is a tube connecting the kidney to the bladder. As it travels, the stone gouges the tender ureter, and you feel that passing pebble in a big way.

Although most stones are eventually passed in the urine, sometimes stones larger than one centimeter—about one-third inch—are broken up through ultrasonic lithotripsy. This procedure may be done with an external probe or with a probe that is inserted into the body to break the stones.

Despite the pain they cause, kidney stones are rarely serious themselves, but they can lead to infections and inflammations. They can sometimes be prevented with a few easy steps.

Polycystic Kidney Disease

It's possible for some people to have polycystic kidney disease—an inherited kidney condition that causes gradual deterioration of the organ—and show no symptoms until they're 70 years old, says Gopal Krishna, M.D., attending physician at Central Coast Nephrology in Salinas, California. This inherited disease can be detected by age 25, however, and is usually diagnosed by middle age. If one parent in a couple has it, their children have a 25 percent chance of inheriting the disease.

Although many people with polycystic kidney disease will eventually need dialysis or kidney transplants, it's possible to slow the growth of cysts by getting less protein in the diet, carefully monitoring blood pressure and sticking to a low-fat diet.

Become a drinker. The best prevention is drinking plenty of water to help dilute your urine, says Dr. Krishna.

Especially, make sure that you drink a glass of water before going to bed at night. "Nighttime is when urine is the most concentrated, with the most substances and the least amount of volume," notes Alice Stollenwerk Petrulis, M.D., director of clinical nephrology at Metrohealth Medical Center and associate professor of medicine and reproductive biology at Case Western Reserve University in Cleveland.

Pump potassium, expel oxalates. Found in fruits such as bananas and apricots, potassium has been linked with a lower incidence of kidney stones, says Dr. Krishna. Stay away from foods such as beets, spinach, peanuts and chocolate, which contain stone-forming chemicals called oxalates.

Helping Your Kidneys Succeed

Kidney failure can have many causes, ranging from severe injury to sudden illness. Slow damage to the kidneys can be the long-term result of high blood pressure, diabetes or an inherited degenerative condition known as polycystic kidney disease. There are several steps to help ensure that you won't fail your kidneys and they won't fail you. Here are some keys to kidney success.

Watch your blood pressure. Because uncontrolled high blood pressure can cause kidney damage, "have it checked every time you go in for a pelvic exam," says Dr. Petrulis.

The best way to keep blood pressure low is to watch your weight and get aerobic exercise at least three times a week for about 30 minutes. "Both independently lower blood pressure, and exercise has the added benefit of lowering the weight," she notes.

Quell your pain. Over-the-counter pain-relief drugs containing ibuprofen or acetaminophen can further damage kidneys that already are damaged, warns Dr. Krishna. Such analgesics—also known as nonsteroidal anti-inflammatory drugs—can prevent the kidneys from producing some vital hormones that they need to keep them going despite some damage. So be sure to read the labels on any pain-relief medications. Although aspirin has not been found to increase the risk of kidney failure, "The bottom line is to always be aware of how many over-the-counter medications you take. Take the minimal dose needed," says Dr. Krishna.

Eat to beat failure. Stick to an eating plan that's low in salt and rich in fruits and vegetables, Dr. Krishna advises. This diet is beneficial, because it helps prevent and control high blood pressure.

See also Urinary System

Knees

WHEN SUZANNE DELANEY attended liturgy at the Carmelite Monastery in Towson, Maryland, she was pleased to find something missing: Many of the old, knee-crunching prayer benches were gone. In the newly redesigned chapel at the women's monastery, Sister Delaney found that the women were standing and sitting for worship.

"Kneeling is not necessarily the only posture for prayer," concedes Sister Delaney, a member of the Congregation of Sisters Servants of the Immaculate Heart of Mary.

That's a bonus for the nun's knees. With all the things that can go wrong with these crucial joints, long hours of weight-bearing worship are the last thing knees need.

In fact, anyone's knees are susceptible to a host of problems, including kneecap pain, bursitis, tendinitis, arthritis and ligament and cartilage tears. Any of these problems can cause discomfort and interfere with your ability to get around. But if you start taking care of your knees early, you'll never have to say your prayers for them.

A Pivotal Joint

The knee carries the honor of being the largest and most complex joint in your body. In addition to supporting your weight, it allows your leg to bend, straighten and twist and turn a little bit. Because of this wide range of motion, the knee has been dubbed a modified hinge joint.

The joint is basically the juncture where the femur, or thighbone, and tibia, or shin-bone, meet. Another small piece of bone, the patella, sits in a groove at the lower end of your leg. As you bend, your patella slides back and forth in this groove. In fact, if you put your hand on the front of your knee, you can feel the patella move. It's that roundish piece of bone generally called the kneecap.

Women's knees are made of the same components as men's knees, but they are constructed slightly differently. Because women generally have wider hips than men, the upper legs slant inward at an angle to meet the knee joints instead of extending straight down. That angle is what doctors call the Q angle, and the larger Q angle in women can translate into knee problems. "The more the knees bow inward, the more vulnerable they are to injury," says John Feagin, M.D., associate professor of orthopedics at Duke University Medical Center in Durham, North Carolina.

A Cap of Pain

Do you sometimes feel a sharp pain right under your kneecap? Could be your kneecap is literally offtrack a little bit—like a train car that's about to derail.

Doctors say that pain under the kneecap is a common symptom of women in their thirties and forties. Often this is caused by increased Q angle. Normally, the kneecap tracks back and forth in a groove as the quadriceps muscle on the front of the thigh contracts (straightening the knee) and relaxes (bending the knee). Since the top of the kneecap is connected to the quadriceps by a tendon, an increased Q angle makes the quadriceps pull sideways on the patella, throwing it out of its groove. This irritates the underside of the kneecap, causing pain in that area.

Not all cases of kneecap pain are caused by

Equipped for Knee Needs

Using a treadmill, riding a stationary bike and doing step-ups on an exercise step are some of the knee-strengthening exercises recommended by experts. Here are tips for using that equipment.

Step up to it. Repeatedly stepping up and then back down again can help strengthen the muscles that support your knees, according to Jeff Coilek, P.T., athletic trainer in the sports medicine division at the Cleveland Clinic in Ohio. Put one foot on the exercise step as shown in the illustration. Step up, then slowly lower back down again. Repeat 15 to 30 times on each leg. Start off with a one-inch exercise step and gradually work up to a two-inch step.

Try the treadmill. If you find that walking outside irritates your knees, try walking on a treadmill instead, says Gerald Eisenberg, M.D., director of the arthritis treatment program at Lutheran General Hospital in Park Ridge, Illinois. Some people find that it's easier on their knees, he says.

Cycle your knees. Using an exercise bike for your aerobic workout will also strengthen knee-supporting muscles. Just make sure the seat is adjusted to the correct height as shown.

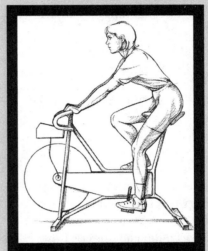

Correct position on exercise bike. The extended leg is still slightly bent.

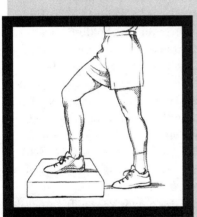

Correct position. When using a stepper, be sure to keep your back leg near the step, with your torso straight.

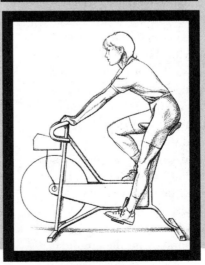

Incorrect position. The left knee is "locked"— and could be strained and injured.

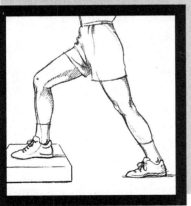

Incorrect position. Avoid stepping too far back—or leaning forward too much—when you're using a stepper. This puts strain on your knees.

the wider Q angle, says Daniel O'Neill, M.D., medical director of the St. Johns Sports Medicine Center in Nassau, Texas. It can also be caused by underdevelopment in the vastus medialis, the strip of muscle that runs along your inner thigh. The vastus medialis is constantly playing tug-of-war with muscles on the outer part of your thigh. When the inside muscle is too weak, it begins to lose this tug-of-war, and the muscle on the outer thigh yanks the patella offtrack. That can cause pain under the kneecap along its inner edge.

This problem is often seen in women who are just starting exercise programs, according to Gerald Eisenberg, M.D., director of the arthritis treatment program at Lutheran General Hospital in Park Ridge, Illinois. "Either aerobics or jogging or even vigorous walking—or other types of activities—may lead to kneecap irritation."

Easing the Knees

You don't have to buckle under to kneecap pain. To ease misery—or prevent it in the first place—here's what experts recommend.

Go gradual. "Start out on an exercise program in a graduated fashion," says Dr. Eisenberg.

Dr. O'Neill adds another guideline: Increase the intensity or duration of your exercise by no more than 10 percent each week. So if you are jogging 30 minutes one week, don't suddenly try to run an hour the next week. Instead, increase your time to about 33 minutes the second week, 36 or 37 minutes the third week, and so on. These increases sound small, but that's the point. By adding just a little bit, your knees have a chance to adjust comfortably.

Chain your feet. Exercises where your feet stay in constant contact with the ground or floor are called closed-chain exercises. They're great for building up the muscles around your knees, according to Jeff Coilek, P.T., athletic trainer in the sports medicine division at the Cleveland Clinic in Ohio. Some exercise equipment is built expressly for closed-chain exercises, including stair-climbers, slide boards, stationary bikes and exercise steps. To strengthen your quadriceps, try to use this equipment whenever possible, he says.

Do the mini-bend. One closed-chain exercise that you can do without equipment is a mini-bend, which stimulates the quadriceps muscle and helps strengthen the inner thigh muscle, says Coilek.

Stand with your feet hip-width apart. Tighten your buttocks. Keeping your feet flat on the floor, bend your knees just a little bit—to about a 30-degree angle—holding on to a table or chair for balance. Do three sets of 30 mini-bends, pausing for a few seconds between each set.

Take a stork stance. To strengthen one leg at a time, you can do the mini-bend on each leg. Standing on one leg while holding on to a table or chair for balance, do three sets of 30 repetitions. Then switch to the other leg and repeat the routine.

Strength train for better knees. If you are going to participate in a weight-bearing exercise program, it's a good idea to do a strengthening program for the quadriceps muscles too, says Dr. Eisenberg. "The stronger those muscles are, the truer the patella tends to move in the groove in the underlying femur."

Plica Pain

Though it sounds like a mineral layer under the earth's crust, synovial plica is actually a ridge of tissue that runs just underneath or along the inside border of the kneecap. It can sometimes become irritated or inflamed, according to Dr. Eisenberg. "It's a fairly common thing in joggers and skiers and other people who are fairly active."

When your knee is slightly bent, you can actually feel the plica. Run your finger along the inside border of your kneecap, and you'll touch a small cord of tissue. Dr. Eisenberg describes it as just about as big as a piece of spaghetti. It usually doesn't hurt, but if it's inflamed, it can be sore to the touch.

The solution? Just give it some rest, Dr. Eisenberg suggests. Take a break from the sport that's causing the irritation. When you start again, build up gradually to avoid another round of inflammation. If it continues in spite of the temporary rest, you might want to see your doctor for recommendations, which might include medication or physical therapies such as ultrasound.

Relieving -Itis

Kneecap pain can also be caused by inflammation of the bursa located at the knee joint. Normally, a bursa is a very efficient cushion—a fluid-filled sac that helps reduce the friction between bones and the ligaments that move across them. But if that sac becomes inflamed, you have bursitis—and it can hurt like the dickens.

Suspect bursitis if your kneecap is not only sore but also red, warm, swollen and very tender to the touch. A very common form of knee bursitis in women ages 30 to 45 is prepatellar bursitis, which causes pain on top of the kneecap, says Dr. Eisenberg. "This has in the past been known as scrub woman's knee or carpet layer's knee."

Scrubbing floors on your hands and knees

may not be your style, but knee bursitis can still sneak up on you. If you're going to be gardening or doing housework on your knees, be sure to put some kind of pad under your knees, suggests Dr. Eisenberg. You can get knee pads that fasten around your legs or a foam pad to put on the floor. They're available at many hardware stores or garden centers. Or just kneel on a pillow when you're doing housework.

Another problem is tendinitis in the knee area. You'll feel its sting when either the quadriceps tendon or the patellar tendon gets irritated or inflamed, says Dr. Eisenberg.

The best prevention is just taking it easy, especially with strenuous or unfamiliar activities. You're leaving yourself open to tendinitis if you're using too much weight when you do weight-bearing exercises or if you're exercising too vigorously to begin with, says Dr. Eisenberg. Or maybe you've taken up a brand new activity without phasing into it slowly, and you're just not used to it.

When Joints Protest Too Much

Arthritis caused by wear and tear can also affect the knee joint, although it's usually more of a problem in women over 45, says Dr. Eisenberg. Damage to structures in the knee can cause the joint to shift out of alignment, which in turn leads to degeneration of the bone. Irritation and pain are the result.

You can reduce the risk—or even prevent it—by taking a few sound steps.

Travel lightly. Even if you don't have arthritis now, you may be at risk for it later on if you're carrying extra weight, says Dr. Eisenberg. To help preserve knee health, keep your body weight under control—with low-fat eating and plenty of exercise.

Be shoe smart. Wearing well-fitting shoes

Stretches for Prevention

You can help prevent knee pain and other kinds of leg injuries if you stretch before you run or walk, says Jeff Coilek, P.T., athletic trainer in the sports medicine division at the Cleveland Clinic in Ohio. He recommends two easy stretches as shown here.

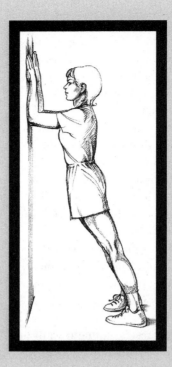

Stand facing a wall and place your elbows on the wall as shown. Keep your knees straight and your feet slightly pointed inward. Then tilt forward, moving your hips toward the wall and keeping your heels flat on the floor. You'll feel the stretch in your calves.

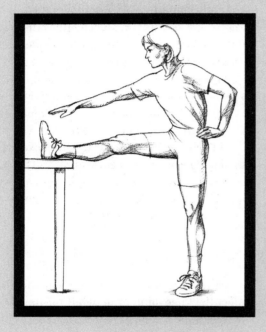

Standing on your left leg, place your right foot on a desk or table with your right knee straight. (Make sure your left knee is slightly bent—not locked.) Then reach for your toes with your right hand and hold for two to three minutes. You should feel a pull underneath your leg—but don't overextend. While the sensation should be noticeable, it should not feel painful. Switch legs and repeat.

in good condition can help keep your knees healthy. If your foot is out of alignment or improperly supported, that can translate right up to your knee and cause problems there, says Pekka Mooar, M.D., assistant professor of orthopedic surgery and chief of sports medicine at the Medical College of Pennsylvania and Hahnemann University School of Medicine in Philadelphia. Be sure to pick a shoe that is wide enough for your foot and made for the activity you're doing—a walking shoe for walking, a tennis shoe for tennis, and a running shoe for running.

Buy your shoes from somebody who understands your needs, Dr. Mooar says. If you have a friend who's into walking, ask her if she has found a shoe store with a knowledgeable staff.

Cross-train year-round. The women who think the only way to get exercise is to powerwalk or run all the time are headed for trouble, says Dr. Feagin. Cross-training—doing a variety of different types of exercises—can help prevent the wear and tear that comes from doing the same old exercise over and over. To add some variety to your exercise routine and give your joints a little relief, try step aerobics, aqua-aerobics (done in a pool) and plyometrics—exercises that involve jumping, hopping and bounding.

All Torn Up

There's a critical structure of tough tissue in your knee called the anterior cruciate ligament (ACL), and when this gets torn, it's a serious injury. This ligament plays a major role in stabilizing the knee. ACL tears are more common in high school and college athletes who play sports that require pivoting.

Women playing these kinds of sports are more likely than men to have ACL troubles. In a study conducted at Duke University, for instance, researchers found that women basketball players injured their ACLs six times more frequently than men, says Dr. Feagin. The researchers suspect that the increased injury rate to the ACL may be related to the greater Q angle and the lack of strength of women's quadriceps muscles.

For women in their thirties and forties, ACL tears are most often caused by skiing injuries. If you plan to go downhill skiing, prepare for the activity by doing quadriceps strengthening exercises for a couple of months before you go, says Dr. O'Neill. The stronger your quads are, the better they'll support your knee, and you won't fatigue as quickly, he says.

See also Joints, Muscular System, Skeletal System

Larynx and Vocal Cords

WHETHER YOUR VOICE emits the sultry growl of Lauren Bacall, the raucous whoop of Bette Midler or the babyish purr of Marilyn Monroe is mainly a matter of biology, thanks to two thin mucus membrane bands, or folds of skin, called the vocal cords.

The larynx, or voice box, attaches to both the windpipe (trachea) and the throat (pharynx). It acts as a main switching point for guiding air and food into the proper tubes. At the top of the larynx are the vocal cords. When we aren't using our voices, these reed-like sheets of tissue, no bigger than a thumbnail, are separated, forming a V-shaped opening called the glottis.

When we speak, air is forced through the cords, causing them to tighten, close and vibrate. The result: a one-of-a-kind voice that's as unique to each individual as fingerprints, says Jason Surow, M.D., otolaryngologist at Valley Hospital in Ridgewood, New Jersey, and Holy Name Hospital in Teaneck, New Jersey.

The vocal cords are like your own personal woodwind instrument, observes Dr. Surow. "The vibration of the cords is what makes the sound, but no more of a sound than the vibrating reed on a clarinet makes." When we change the shape of the throat, tongue and palate we also change the voice, creating different sounds.

In fact, these cords are so sensitive to change that your menstrual cycle could have an effect on the sound of your voice. "Some women notice a mild decrease in pitch or

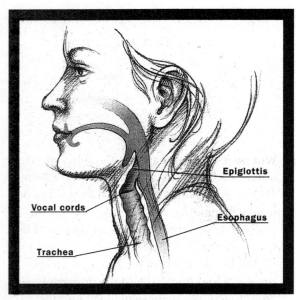

The larynx, or voice box, is the area at the top of the trachea—the passage that carries air.

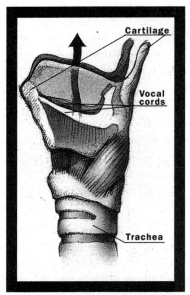

The vocal cords are stretched across the larynx, held in place by bands of cartilage.

harshness in their voices premenstrually or in the early days of their periods," explains Michael Benninger, M.D., chairman of the Department of Otolaryngology at Henry Ford Hospital in Detroit and author of *Vocal Arts Medicine*. In Europe, by contract, professional vocalists cannot sing during this time; this condition is called premenstrualis larnygopathia. Also, some women experience a postmenopausal decrease in pitch caused by a hormonal change, he adds.

Tuning Your Instrument

You do have some say in how pleasant your voice is—although the general pitch is pretty much dictated by the cords, says Dr. Surow.

A lot depends on muscles like your diaphragm and how you use those muscles, Dr. Surow notes. "Can I make you into a bass? No. Can a speech therapist change the *quality* of your voice? Yes. You could be talking

through your nose. Or maybe your nose is blocked off. Even the size of your tonsils could affect your voice."

But sometimes the instrument sounds temporarily out of tune, whether from a virus like the common cold or from overuse, like trying to shout above the din of a noisy party for a couple of hours.

The result is laryngitis, which means your cords have swollen up—leading to a lower, scratchier-than-normal voice, says Barry Baron, M.D., chairman of the Department of Otolaryngology at California Pacific Medical Center in San Francisco. "Even the slightest swelling can change the thickness of the vocal cords and your voice. The same way as when you tighten the string of a guitar in the tiniest way, it changes the sound."

Although it's impossible to dodge voice snatchers like the cold virus, there are lots of steps you can take to put the vigor back in your vibrato.

Mum's the word. Say as little as possible when your vocal cords are on strike, recommends George Simpson, M.D., professor and chairman of the Department of Otolaryngology at State University of New York at Buffalo. "In a short time your voice will return to normal, but you need to rest your voice for two or three days," he says. "Let your family know you can't talk."

Don't cheat. It's not a good idea to whisper instead of talking, says Dr. Simpson. "That bangs the vocal cords together more violently than talking."

Let the water flow. You need to knock back at least six to eight glasses of water a day to hydrate your dried-out cords, says Dr. Baron. The liquids don't touch the vocal cords, but they allow saliva to flow well, which in turn lubricates your vocal system. Better yet, squeeze some lemon juice into a glass of tea or water; it helps the glands produce thinner mucus and stirs up more saliva.

Don't smoke. Smoking is severely damaging, says Dr. Baron. "You are inhaling hot smoke directly onto the vocal cords, and it goes right on them." Over time this habit can lead to polyps—soft, fluid-filled lesions that appear on one or both cords—or even put you at high risk for cancer of the larynx.

In fact, if you're a heavy smoker, your voice is probably already taking on a husky timbre, says Dr. Surow. "Smokers get thickened, heavy vocal cords. Smoke is an irritant that causes the lining of the cords to get thicker. That heaviness causes them to vibrate at a lower frequency."

Curb throat clearing. When you clear your throat, you're grinding the vocal cords together, says Dr. Benninger. "People do it because there's an irritation, and it just causes more irritation." He advises taking a sip of water instead.

Finding Your Voice

A drill sergeant giving orders to her troops in a weak voice or a telemarketer trying to hawk magazines in an overbearing bark: Chances are, neither will be taken seriously.

There's something about the voice that tells others who you are—even more than the words you speak, says Katherine Verdolini, Ph.D., director of voice and speech at the Joint Center for Otolaryngology at Harvard Medical School. "Some people have a tiny, insecure, tight voice that sounds like they're apologizing all the time. Muscle tightening may come from fear or poor self-esteem. Freeing up your voice has a lot to do with freeing yourself."

If you think your voice sounds weak and you don't like what you hear, Dr. Verdolini's advice is to "loosen up." Try to make a naturally soft voice sound louder without changing your muscle-use patterns, and it will probably just sound strained. The same applies to big-voiced women trying to tone themselves down: Trying to force a different voice, it just sounds . . . well, forced.

"Don't squeeze your throat to get a more authoritative voice, which is usually thought of as low-pitched," says Dr. Verdolini. "The number one thing is freedom. Don't strain in any part of your body to get a free voice."

For the best possible voice, your abdomen needs to be pressed in—but not in a forced or exaggerated way—when you speak. Your throat should be open and free, and your mouth should be whatever shape gives you the most volume.

Dr. Verdolini recommends a voice coach for anyone who is truly unhappy with the way she sounds. You can call a hospital and ask for someone who specializes in voice or contact a local professional theater company and ask for its voice coach.

Don't Hoarse Around Long

If your hoarseness has lasted for more than a few weeks, you might have nodules or polyps on your vocal cords. But there is also the risk of cancer of the larynx. So you should see a doctor or throat specialist to have the condition checked out.

Nodules and polyps have many similarities. Typically harmless, they are usually the result of voice abuse, such as excessive shouting or singing without proper training.

Nodules are like calluses on the vocal cords, says Barry Baron, M.D., chairman of the Department of Otolaryngology at California Pacific Medical Center in San Francisco. "You use the vocal cords so improperly that the place where the vocal cords meet gets thicker, and nodules form."

The problem is found among those who use their voices professionally, such as actresses, singers, teachers and public speakers, according to Frederick Godley, M.D., otolaryngologist with the Harvard Community Health Plan of New England in Providence, Rhode Island.

Sometimes they'll go away on their own if you stop shouting or other bad voice habits. Nodules can usually be helped with voice therapy, in which a certified speech therapist will study your way of speaking and determine if you're abusing your voice, notes Dr. Baron. They can also be surgically removed. Surgery is usually unnecessary, however, since nodules are rarely associated with cancer, and many people don't mind having a huskier, Lauren Bacall–type voice.

Polyps—soft, fluid-filled lesions that appear on one or both cords—don't go away on their own, says Jason Surow, M.D., otolarynologist at Valley Hospital in Ridgewood, New Jersey, and Holy Name Hospital in Teaneck, New Jersey.

They can be more worrisome than nodules, because they more commonly develop into a malignancy, notes Dr. Godley.

Prolonged hoarseness could also be caused by a more serious condition such as cancer of the larynx, which is far more serious than nodules or polyps. It strikes 9,000 to 10,000 Americans a year, according to George Simpson, M.D., professor and chairman of the Department of Otolaryngology at State University of New York at Buffalo. The disease results in removal of the vocal cords in 20 to 30 percent of cases. "I'd say that 95 percent of the time, cancer of the larynx is related to smoking. Although it is prevalent in men, women are rapidly catching up, since their smoking habits match or exceed those of men."

Fortunately, if caught early, it's among the most treatable forms of cancer. If the tumor hasn't invaded the surface of the vocal cord, doctors can remove it with either laser or traditional surgery. Some small tumors can be treated with radiation therapy, according to Dr. Simpson.

Can those tomatoes. Hoarseness could be a result of stomach acid (called reflux) backing up from the esophagus and into the larynx, says Dr. Surow. Cut down on reflux causers such as tomatoes, chocolate, peppermint and caffeine and eliminate bedtime snacks.

Hydrate the air. About to hit the hay? Before you turn out the lights, turn on a humidifier, says Dr. Baron. The moisture is inhaled down onto the vocal cords.

Also, during the day, use your own personal humidifier: your nose. "The nose warms and moisturizes the air. It's a more natural way to breathe than through the mouth," notes Dr. Baron. At first you may need to train yourself to breathe through your nose instead of breathing through your mouth, but it will soon become habit.

Take a shower. One way to hydrate your sore cords is by breathing in and out while standing in a hot shower, according to Dr. Surow. In this case, breathe in through your mouth instead of your nose so the shower steam comes in direct contact with your vocal cords.

Have a piece of candy. True, a piece of hard candy or a lozenge won't cure your laryngitis, but it will stimulate your saliva glands, which help the hydration process.

Be kind to your voice. If you yell or sing loudly, you could end up injuring vocal cords from the constant abuse, says Dr. Surow.

Concentrate on good breath support, he suggests. This means breathing from the diaphragm—expanding the curved area of muscle that lies just beneath your chest but above your abdomen when you draw in breath.

"Don't breathe just from the abdomen," says Dr. Benninger. "That can cause strain, and the belly gets tired." In most cases speech therapy can correct habitual misuse of the voice.

See also Respiratory System

Lips

THE VERMILION BORDER: What's that? A border of roses around a grand British estate? Or perhaps the border of the Red Sea?

Well, hats off to good guesses, but here's a hint: Everyone has her own vermilion border. It's what doctors call the line where your skin meets your lips. Inside that red border are the lips that keep food from falling out and help form the words you live by. Of course, lips also have expression beyond words—with romantic, respectful or maternal kisses.

"The lips aren't really skin," says Diana Bihova, M.D., clinical assistant professor of dermatology at New York University Medical Center in New York City. Instead, they're more like the mucous membranes inside the mouth.

"The skin of the lips has fewer layers than the skin on the rest of the body," says Ella Toombs, M.D., a dermatologic surgeon in private practice in Washington, D.C. The thinness of the skin of the lips allows the blood vessels to be more visible, and therefore makes the lips look red.

Unlike the rest of our skin, the lips aren't protected by a densely packed layer of tissues. Because they lack this protective layer—called cornified tissue—the lips are more vulnerable to problems, notes Dr. Bihova. "They're also more prone to drying, because they have no oil glands, and they have less pigment than the skin to protect them from the sun."

Tips for Lush Lips

You probably spend a lot more time contemplating and caring for the vast canvas of

Holding the Line on Young Lips

It's spelled *rhagades*, but pronounced "raggedies." And that about describes them.

Rhagades are the first lines that develop around the mouth as we get older. Where there used to be a nice, distinct vermilion border between the lips and skin, Mother Time begins to take her toll. Hairlike creases form—at first almost unnoticeable, but gradually mussing up the clean line of our kissers.

Rhagades arrive even sooner—and show up more—if you purse your lips a lot when you frown, giggle, smoke or chew gum. Here, too, getting too much sun will cost you plenty. "Exposure to sunlight blunts the junction between the vermilion border and the skin," says Caroline Koblenzer, M.D., clinical professor of dermatology at the University of Pennsylvania in Philadelphia.

Once you start getting these lines, it's easy for lipstick to bleed into the rhagades. So what can you do?

Moisten the dry mouth zone. When you rub in face cream, you probably avoid the area right around the vermilion border because you don't want to get cream in your mouth. Makes sense—but you really *should* moisten that area, according to Dr. Koblenzer. You'll help prevent or postpone the emergence of rhagades—spelling more years of smooth-looking lipstick for you.

Use a finer liner. Lip liner can help restore definition to the vermilion border and prevent lip color from "feathering" into your skin. Apply lip liner around the edges of your lips. Then apply lipstick, blot it and apply another layer if you need to.

skin on your face than for your lips. Even if they aren't as tough as they look, lips are easy to maintain or restore to moist, rosy

health. Here's how to keep your kisser in peak condition.

Soften and screen. Arm yourself with a lip balm that contains sunscreen as well as moisturizer. The lip balm component moisturizes your lips, and the sunscreen protects them from sun damage.

"Get in the habit of wearing lip balm with sunscreen during the sunny months—from May to September—if you live in a temperate zone. During the cold months—from mid-November to mid-March," says John Romano, M.D., clinical assistant professor of dermatology at New York Hospital–Cornell University Medical Center in New York City. In winter, cold, dry air can parch your lips, and sunlight reflected off snow can burn them.

It's a good idea to apply the balm before you go outside and also to wear it overnight, Dr. Romano advises.

Don't lick. Winter is a bear on naked lips. "But most people get chapped lips mainly because they lick them. It's an unconscious habit. Every time you lick, that moisture will evaporate—and take with it some of the natural moisture in your lips. So your lips get more and more dry," says Caroline Koblenzer, M.D., clinical professor of dermatology at the University of Pennsylvania in Philadelphia.

No nibbles! If licking is a hard habit to break, so is biting your lips. That's another habit that chaps them, says Dr. Bihova.

"Even if you don't do much more than just become aware of the habit, you can apply lip balm more frequently. Then it won't be so destructive," says Dr. Koblenzer.

Grease up at bedtime. One effective way to outwit chapped lips is with a nighttime coat of full-strength petroleum jelly. Petrolatum (petroleum jelly) is the main ingredient in most lip balms. It's too goopy to wear during the day. At night, though, appearance doesn't matter—and a shellac of petroleum jelly can salve rough spots. "The petroleum jelly interferes with water loss and seals in moisture," says Dr. Bihova.

High-IQ Lipsticks

Lipstick not only looks smart, it acts smart these days. Even when shades bear names like Plum Puff or Pink Fluff, many contain ingredients that make lips healthy as well as pretty. Here's what to look for.

Go for the AHAs. Alpha hydroxy acids (AHAs) are acids made from fruit, cane sugar or milk. These acids loosen the surface layer of dry, dead skin, which then sloughs off, uncovering the soft, moist layer of skin underneath. A popular ingredient in skin creams, AHAs work on the lips as well, researchers have discovered. Look for this ingredient in lipsticks and lip balms.

"They're worth getting because they help the lips retain moisture and keep them from drying out," says Dr. Bihova.

Paint on some shine. If you like the glossy wet-lip look, you're in luck. Petrolatum is the ingredient that gives lipstick an extra-shiny finish, so you're moisturizing as well as flattering your lips with a sexy look. If you've been using a matte-coat lipstick, at least audition a shiny lipstick and see how you like it.

One caveat: Shiny lipsticks tend to bleed upwards. If that's a problem, outline your lips first with an antifeathering lip liner.

Look for long-lasting. When you read the label on a "long-lasting" lipstick, look for the most common ingredient used to make lipstick last longer: acideosine, a natural orange salt that changes to red on contact with your lips.

Even if your favorite lipstick is not long-lasting, you can still lengthen its lip life, says Dr. Bihova. Apply the first layer of lipstick, powder it lightly with your face powder, then apply a second layer. If you want to finish with a sexy touch, blot it slightly and apply a shiny wet-look lipstick to the center of your lips.

Another Sore Point

Call them cold sores, fever blisters or outbreaks of the herpes simplex Type I virus. Same thing, same story: a tingling somewhere on your lip, then a group of tiny blisters in an inflamed blotch of red. After a few days the blisters burst; then they dry out, crust over, heal and disappear in a week to ten days.

The virus that does all this damage is normally inactive—hanging around our nerve endings until we get run-down or stressed out. When our guard is down, the dormant virus strikes.

About one-third of all Americans get cold sores from time to time. They are the most common problem that the lips have.

Here are a few things that you can do to settle the score with cold sores.

Block that ray. Sunlight is the most preventable of the triggers that can set off a cold sore. To disarm the light, just use a sunblock, suggest Dr. Bihova. "But make sure that it's a sunblock and not just a sunscreen. Sometimes companies use the words interchangeably. Look for zinc oxide or titanium dioxide in the ingredients."

Don't touch. Cold sores are infectious when they blister, and you can infect both others and yourself. Be especially careful not to touch a blister and then touch your eyes, since that could infect your eyes with herpes, which sometimes leads to an open sore on the cornea. As a policy, avoid touching a cold sore with your fingers. If you do touch it for some reason, says Dr. Bihova, you should wash your hands immediately afterward.

Stay with your stick. Because the herpes virus is so easily transferred, be sure that you never borrow someone else's lipstick, says Dr. Bihova. For the same reason, you should never lend your lipstick to anyone else.

Don't pooh-pooh a white patch. Cold sores look ugly, but they soon go away. If you do happen to notice a dry, white patch that never becomes a wet, white blister, though— and if it doesn't go away after two weeks— see your doctor immediately. There's a chance that this could be a sign of lip cancer.

"Lip cancer usually begins as a scaling patch anywhere on the lower lip," says Dr. Koblenzer. "In the early stages it's just slightly whiter. So if you do see some white amongst the nice rosy red of your lips, you should call your physician."

See also Mouth

Liver

MEASURED BY BULK ALONE, the liver is the big kid on the block. It is both the largest internal organ and the largest gland in the body, weighing in at a whopping 2.5 to 3.3 pounds.

And the liver is not just big. It has clout. This glandular organ performs over 500 functions.

The Ruddy Ringmaster

The liver is a soft, reddish-brown organ that is roughly cone-shaped and sits just below the diaphragm in the upper right side of the abdominal cavity.

It's like a mainframe computer, doing a lot of things at once. But its principal job is to detoxify the blood, says Jorge Herrera, M.D., associate professor of medicine at the University of South Alabama College of Medicine in Mobile. All of the blood in the body filters through the liver, which removes any substances that shouldn't accumulate in the bloodstream. Restructuring these substances to make new water-soluble chemicals, the liver then sends them on their way in the bile, the yellowish fluid that empties into the lower intestine to help with digestion.

There are two major threats to the liver: hepatitis and heavy drinking. Both can wreak havoc and lead to cirrhosis, a disease where liver cells die from long-term inflammation and scar tissue takes their place. This scarring interferes with the normal blood flow through the liver and disrupts the organ's ability to filter toxins. Advanced cirrhosis can lead to

The ABCs of Hepatitis

If a friend or relative gets hepatitis, you should talk to your doctor as soon as possible to find out if you need to be tested. Here's what doctors know about the ways that different kinds of hepatitis can be transmitted.

Hepatitis A is transmitted most often through person-to-person contact and contaminated food and water.

Hepatitis B is a blood-borne virus that can be transmitted sexually or by sharing contaminated needles, razors or toothbrushes. People in the health care field are at risk of catching it. The disease can also be transmitted from an infected mother to her newborn.

Hepatitis C can be transmitted by people who share needles for intravenous drug use. It can also be transmitted by sexual contact—though that happens far less frequently. Also, some blood used for transfusions prior to 1990 was found to be contaminated. And those in the health care field can pick it up at work.

Hepatitis D only infects people in the presence of Hepatitis B.

Hepatitis E is rare in the United States, but it's a potential risk in some other countries.

Ph.D., chief of epidemiology in the hepatitis branch of the Centers for Disease Control and Prevention in Atlanta. So be sure that you and your family members wash your hands after every visit to the bathroom and before meals.

Vie for the vaccine. The vaccine for hepatitis A is now available, says Dr. Alter. If you are planning on traveling overseas where hepatitis risk is higher, consider getting the shot, she says. Plan ahead, because you'll need two doses, the first of which must be taken at least four weeks before you leave the United States. There is also a vaccine for hepatitis B, she says, so ask your doctor about that, too.

Go for gamma globulin. If you've been exposed to someone with hepatitis A, go to your doctor for a gamma globulin shot, says Dr. Alter. By taking it within 14 days of being exposed to hepatitis A, you can significantly reduce your risk of getting the disease.

Fool around safely. Both hepatitis B and hepatitis C can be transmitted sexually, says Dr. Alter. So if you're not sure of your partner's history, or if you have multiple sex partners, be sure to practice safe sex and use a condom.

See also Digestive System

impaired mental ability, coma and death.

It's pretty obvious how you can avoid cirrhosis caused by drinking. Dodging infectious hepatitis (which comes in several strains), however, is a less sure game. Here's what experts suggest.

Lather up. Hepatitis A, the most common type, can be transferred through contaminated food and water, says Miriam Alter,

Lungs

AS A KID YOU PROBABLY TRIED holding your breath to see how long you could go without exhaling. Maybe you were throwing a temper tantrum and wanted to give Mom and Dad a good scare. Or you were just trying to show your friends that you had the toughest lungs on the block. Your face probably started turning purple, and your lungs were probably about to explode before you finally gave up and breathed in a bountiful blast of fresh air.

Just in time, too, since your survival depends on lung inflation. These two football-size organs are made of elastic tissue filled with interlacing networks of tubes and sacs carrying air and with blood vessels carrying blood. They're the body's inhalers, filters and vacuum cleaners. The lungs supply oxygen to the body, dispose of carbon dioxide in the blood, filter and store blood and defend against invading agents of infection.

Air Travel

Unless you're winded by exercise, breathing is something most of us don't think about. Believe it or not, you take 20,000 breaths a day—that's more than seven million breaths per year! But it's all highly automated—unless you happen to be in a who-can-hold-their-breath-longer contest.

What comes automatically is actually a complex process that starts when you take in air through your nose or mouth. The air travels through your trachea, or windpipe, which divides at mid-chest into two ducts, called bronchi, that carry air to your lungs.

It's like a tree, with the windpipe being the trunk, leading to ever-tinier roots. At the end of each of these "roots" are the little sacs called alveoli. There are some 300 million alveoli, tiny air sacs where gases such as oxygen and carbon dioxide diffuse into or out of the blood.

Diaphragm Work

Some ways of breathing are better than others. And most of us are on the wrong track when it comes to the simple procedure of inhaling and exhaling.

Actually, most of us breathed better when we came into the world than we do now. As a baby, you automatically used your diaphragm, which is the largest and most efficient breathing muscle. Located beneath your lungs and forming a dome on top of your intestinal cavity, your diaphragm muscle flattens out into a saucer shape when you breathe in. That muscle action creates a vacuum inside your chest area, and air rushes into your lungs to fill the vacuum.

But when we get older, easy breathing tends to go out the window—replaced by short, shallow puffs that are activated by tensed-up chest muscles rather than the leisure-loving diaphragm. Most of us take shallow breaths between 10 and 16 times per minute, and none of those little, tense puffs really fills the lungs to capacity. With slower, relaxed, diaphragmatic breathing you can fill your lungs about 8 to 10 times per minute—with breaths that fill all the far-flung sacs of your alveoli.

Sucking It In

Deep breathing is an important technique for reducing stress, so it can become a tool to help you reduce the health problems often associated with stress—from cancer to heart disease. And the stronger your lungs, the more you increase your endurance, whether for doing aerobics, climbing stairs or swimming laps.

Here's what experts recommend to help you improve your relaxed breathing and expand your capacity.

Press your stomach. To expand your lung capacity, practice abdominal breathing, which forces you to use your diaphragm instead of your smaller, weaker chest muscles. Here's how it's done, as described in *Take a Deep Breath* by James E. Loehr, Ed.D., and Jeffrey Migdow, M.D., yoga teacher and director of the Kripalu Yoga Teacher Training Program at Kripalu Center for Yoga and Health in Lenox, Massachusetts.

- First, lie on your back and place one hand on your stomach.
- Breathe in, pushing your stomach against your hand.
- Breathe out, lowering your stomach down toward the floor as far as possible.

Ideally, you should begin by practicing this breathing for a couple of minutes each hour with a longer session in the morning and at night, notes Dr. Migdow. "If you can do that consistently for six to eight weeks, more and more during the day you'll start breathing that way automatically," Dr. Migdow says.

Hang your arms. If you spend a lot of time sitting, your muscles are likely to get stiff, and that makes breathing more difficult. To help yourself relax, do the following quick relaxation exercise while seated: As you inhale, clench your fists, shrug your shoulders, and then tighten your arms. As you exhale, let your shoulders fall. Now open your hands and let your arms hang straight down.

You can do a similar exercise with your legs and feet—first tightening them as you inhale and then relaxing them as you exhale. By the time you're finished your whole body will be more relaxed (especially your upper body), and you'll be able to breathe without tensing your chest and upper-body muscles.

Hang a thread. If you automatically sit or stand with hunched shoulders, you're keeping a lid on the best kind of breathing. When your shoulders are pulled forward, you constrict your breathing muscles. To stop the strain, try this exercise from *Miracle Healing from China . . . Qigong* by Charles T. McGee and Effie Poy Yew Chow, R.N., Ph.D., president of the East West Academy of the Healing Arts/Qigong Institute in San Francisco. While standing or sitting, visualize a straight thread extending from the ground, up your spine and to the top of your head. As you imagine the thread pulling you up, allow it to stretch your spine.

Have a roll. While standing erect, roll your shoulders back and down—away from your neck. That will make your shoulder blades drop down and allow your muscles to relax, according to Dr. Chow.

When Breathing Isn't Easy

Even if your breathing technique isn't quite up to snuff, be grateful that you're not one of those fashion victims of the nineteenth century. Back then, a woman's waist was often squished into a tightly laced corset. A 15- to 18-inch waist was the norm. Unfortunately, so was fainting—a result of the lungs being severely restricted.

While we no longer have corsets holding us back (and in), there's a breathtaking array of substances out there that can also shorten your breath. Pollen, dust, viruses, bacteria, animal dander, tobacco smoke, radon, indoor and outdoor air pollution—any of these alien agents known as allergens can find their way into your lungs.

Some people can shrug off such irritants, but for the 12.4 million Americans with asthma, they're a daily curse. Asthma results from hyperactive bronchial tubes, which can be sent into spasms by outside substances. Allergens are a big factor with children who have asthma, triggering 90 percent of their asthma attacks. But asthma-prone adults are susceptible to allergens, too, since half of adult asthma cases are allergy-related.

Other factors that can trigger an asthma attack include cold air and exercise, says Diana DeCosimo, M.D., director of the Division of General Medicine and Geriatrics in the Department of Medicine at the New Jersey Medical School and medical director of the Women's Wellness Center in Newark.

As anyone with asthma knows, having an attack can be terrifying. When muscles in the walls of the bronchial tubes go into spasms, the air passages narrow, which constricts the free flow of air. To force air through the narrow passage, someone who is having an asthma attack needs to breathe faster and harder—literally panting. The result is wheezing, coughing and breathlessness.

What's Attacking You?

How do you know if your wheezing is the allergic kind? "If you have attacks around dogs or cats, or just in the fall or spring, that strongly suggests allergies," says Garrison Ayars, M.D., allergist and clinical associate professor at the University of Washington in Seattle. You'll need to visit an allergist for tests to see if there's a substance you can avoid or eliminate. But your attacks might also be caused by nonallergen irritants, such as strong colognes, perfumes, newsprint or any strong odors, notes Dr. Ayars.

What makes one person more susceptible than another to asthma is a mystery, although it's largely inherited, says Leonard Bielory, M.D., director of the Division of Allergy and Immunology and director of the Asthma and Allergy Center at the New Jersey Medical School.

If you have one parent with asthma or allergies, you have a 30 percent chance of having the same. If both of your parents have asthma, your chances jump to 60 percent, says Dr. Bielory.

In any case, the best way to control this chronic condition is with inhaled medication such as bronchodilators and corticosteroids that reduce inflammation. Both need a doctor's prescription. "It's a reversible disease. If you think you may have asthma because of symptoms of wheezing, tightness in the chest or shortness of breath with exertion, it is always best to see your doctor rather than depending on over-the-counter medications," says Gary N. Gross, M.D., clinical professor of internal medicine at Southwestern Medical School in Dallas, Texas. "With the right medications from your doctor, you can do whatever you want," he says. "Frequent use of over-the-counter asthma sprays may be dangerous and certainly are not the best treatment."

The Best Defense

Asthma is a lifelong challenge for some people. But along with taking prescribed medications there are many other things you can do to help yourself breathe easier. Here's some advice from top doctors.

Ditch your triggers. The best way to ease your breathing is to avoid allergens, notes Dr.

Wheezing on the Run

Although exercise is recommended for many people who have asthma, some people find that they start to wheeze when they're active. For people who get exercise-induced asthma (EIA), here's what doctors recommend.

Ease into it. Warm-ups are very important, according to Phillip Corsello, M.D., staff physician at the National Jewish Center of Immunology and Respiratory Medicine in Denver. "About ten minutes of walking at a gradual pace or other gentle aerobic exercise may help prevent or reduce the severity of EIA," he says. "Also, don't exercise in cold or polluted air."

Spray before you play. If you use an inhaler before you exercise, it might help prevent an attack. "It's good to use your inhaler about five to ten minutes before you start," says Garrison Ayars, M.D., allergist and clinical associate professor at the University of Washington in Seattle. "With exercise-induced asthma, if you premedicate, you'll do fine."

Shape up. With regular aerobic exercise, you may find that you have asthma less often. "If you get into better aerobic condition, you'll eventually have less of a problem with exercise-induced asthma," says Dr. Ayars.

DeCosimo. "If you're allergic to the cat, get rid of the cat," she says. The dust mite, which feeds on shed skin cells, is another top allergen. Because these critters thrive in humidity, keep your home as dry as possible. Also, wash bedsheets in the hottest water possible to help kill the dust mites. And since all rugs and carpets are favorite mite hangouts, go for the spare look in your home—with bare floors.

Dust off for prevention. Apart from dust mites, dust itself is another big culprit. It paralyzes the clearance mechanism in the lungs, says Robert Sandhaus, M.D., director of clinical development at Cortech, a biotech firm in Denver.

Since vacuuming kicks up a dust storm in your house, you might consider a special filtered vacuum cleaner—such as the kind made by Miele Vacuum—if you have a major reaction to dust. Call Miele at 1-800-694-4868 to be connected with your local dealer. If there isn't one nearby, you'll be connected with someone at the national mail-order headquarters.

Another way to beat the dust enemy is with high-efficiency particulate absorption bags. These bags have microscopic holes that don't allow dust particles to escape, says Dr. Sandhaus. Each vacuum cleaner manufacturer makes its own version of these. But some bags can only be used with specially designed vacuum cleaners, so there may be some expense in getting the whole system.

Do brew. Because caffeine helps dilate the bronchial passages, strong black coffee can have a beneficial effect. "It releases bronchial spasms," notes Dr. Bielory. "But it's no substitute for medication."

Air out your office. With an ever-increasing number of offices being filled with recycled air, you should be aware of workplace pollution, says Dr. Sandhaus.

Because you can't open windows in most offices, chemicals from cleaning products stay in the air. "If it's a chemical that causes an odor, talk to your building manager about adding fresh air to the ventilation system. If you only have breathing problems when you're at work, you might even have to request a different office—or even consider changing jobs," he notes.

Work it out. Aerobic exercise improves asthma by opening up your airways and working out your diaphragm and chest wall muscles, which open your lungs, says Dr. Gross. He recommends a 30-minute walk or stationary bike ride three to five times a week. Don't be afraid that asthma equals inactivity. Remember, more than 10 percent of America's 1984 Olympic athletes had asthma!

Know how to inhale. Using an inhaler takes appropriate aim and timing, notes Dr. Ayars. Just before spraying you should blow out all your air. Then start to take a deep breath, and while you're breathing in deeply, activate the inhaler. Continue to breathe in deeply and slowly until your lungs are full, says Dr. Ayars. Hold your breath as long as you can so the drug can reach all the nooks and crannies of your lungs, he says.

You can also use spacers, which are three- to five-inch tubes or chambers that you put between the inhaler and your mouth. Because the spray first goes into the chamber, less spray jets onto and sticks to the back of your throat, he explains. Check with your doctor or allergist about using spacers.

Don't smoke. Smoking is bad because it irritates the airways, and people with asthma

Get Your Skin Pricked

If you're wondering whether you have asthma, allergies or a little bit of both, the best way to find out is with skin prick tests, says Garrison Ayars, M.D., allergist and clinical associate professor at the University of Washington in Seattle. Various allergens are pricked into the skin, and if a hive develops, you're allergic to that substance.

The doctor may also test your lung function with a machine called a spirometer that measures the total amount of air you breathe and how fast.

are more sensitive to irritants anyway, says Dr. Gross. "The combination of asthma and smoke makes your breathing function worsen more quickly," says Dr. Gross. "So instead of a mild course of the problem, you'll have long-term breathing problems."

Peek at your peak. To get a handle on your breathing status, use a peak flow meter, which is a thermometer-like instrument that you breathe into to measure your breathing, says Dr. Bielory. "It measures the amount of air flowing out of your lungs," he notes. "It's portable and inexpensive. Many people use them when they get up and when they go to bed. It helps you coordinate treatment so you don't end up in the emergency room."

Getting the Better of Bronchitis

If it were physically possible to cough up a lung, it would probably happen during a bout of bronchitis.

This inflammation of the airways connecting the trachea to the lungs is to coughing what chicken pox is to spots. And unfortunately, all that hacking produces loads of green or yellow phlegm. Not a real pleasant way to spend three or four days.

The usual form is called acute bronchitis, which develops suddenly and often clears up in a few days. It's usually a complication of a viral infection.

If you have a bronchitis cough that doesn't clear up after a week, you should see your doctor. "If it's not going away, it may be a bacterial infection, in which case you'll need antibiotics," says Dr. Sandhaus.

But if you battle bronchitis at the onset, it might clear up. Here's how to hold your own.

Relieve the pain. One of the things that'll make you feel better is ibuprofen, which helps ease general malaise, says Dr. De-Cosimo.

Quiet your (A.M.) cough. Use over-the-counter cough medications, which are as effective as prescription medicine, says Dr. Sandhaus. But only take the medication at night, he adds. That's because a productive cough is actually good, since you're bringing up some of that germ-laden phlegm every time you cough. "If someone has a productive cough, it's the body's way of getting rid of infectious agents; you don't want to suppress that entirely," says Dr. Sandhaus.

Dr. Sandhaus recommends cough medicine such as Robitussin DM, with a secretion-loosening ingredient such as dextromethorphan or guaifenesin.

Get steamed. Using a cool-mist vaporizer helps moisten the already too-dry air irritating your airways, says Dr. Sandhaus. But if you are prone to asthma, the cold mist can irritate your lungs and spur an attack, Dr.

Flu or Bronchitis—What's the Difference?

Bronchitis is commonly caused by a virus, and so is the flu. So how do you find out which culprit has you bedridden—hacking, sniffling and exhausted?

If you've been bitten by the flu bug, you'll have fever and muscle aches along with the coughing, according to Diana De-Cosimo, M.D., director of the Division of General Medicine and Geriatrics in the Department of Medicine at the New Jersey Medical School and medical director of the Women's Wellness Center in Newark. Flu has become a generic term for any kind of viral infection, while bronchitis is an inflammation of your airways—it specifically refers to a lower respiratory infection.

Sandhaus notes. So here's an alternative bronchitis treatment: Go in the bathroom, turn on a hot shower, let the room fill with mist and fill your lungs with it.

Flood your phlegm. Drinking clear liquids helps make that thick mucus just a bit easier to cough up, says Dr. DeCosimo. She especially recommends hot fluids such as soup or tea.

Kick the butts. It's vital for anyone with bronchitis to avoid smoking, especially while you're still coughing, notes Dr. Sandhaus. "It prolongs the illness by irritating the airways, which induces more coughing." There could be another bonus as well: When some people lay off nicotine because of bronchitis, they end up quitting for good, Dr. Sandhaus says.

Lung Cancer

Air meets blood. Breath after breath, heartbeat by heartbeat, that's what happens all day and all night. While you're awake or sleeping, a staggering 8,000 to 9,000 liters of breathed-in air meet 8,000 to 10,000 liters of blood. All that breathing is hard, steady work.

But imagine trying to perform such vital chores for someone who smokes. The lungs have to labor for breath through ever-blackening lung tissue—the result of tar deposits nestling between the air sacs.

This carcinogenic tar can later lead to lung cancer—the leading killer cancer among women. To make matters worse, smoke particles irritate the lungs' airways—causing excess mucus production and chronic irritation that result in the labored breathing of emphysema and chronic bronchitis, also known as smoker's cough.

No doubt about it—smoking is to blame for most adult lung cancers, says Dr. De-Cosimo.

"Smoking is a really serious health problem for women," says Dr. DeCosimo. "Some 2,000 girls start smoking every day. It's so tied up with looking good and staying slim; it's very seductive."

The most deadly of smoking-related illnesses is lung cancer, which strikes more than 74,000 women and 96,000 men in a typical year. The vast majority—about 90 percent—of the cases are linked with smoking, says Peter Greenwald, M.D., director of the Division of Cancer Prevention and Control at the National Cancer Institute in Bethesda, Maryland.

Lung cancer is a killer mainly because early detection is difficult. Often the only symptom is a persistent cough, and by then it

Ditching the Butts for Good

It's been linked to heart disease; cancer of the lung, bladder, mouth, lip and throat; premature births; lower survival rates for babies and wrinkled skin—not to mention bad breath, yellow teeth and smelly clothes.

Yet despite all these bad marks against cigarettes, a startling 46 million Americans keep on smoking.

Most smokers are not hardheaded or ignorant of health facts—they're simply addicted, both physically and psychologically.

In fact, a 1988 surgeon general's report compared the mechanics of nicotine addiction with those of heroin or cocaine addiction. The conclusions: "It's often *more* difficult to withdraw from nicotine than any of the others," says Thomas Glynn, Ph.D., chief of the cancer prevention and control research branch at the National Cancer Institute in Bethesda, Maryland.

In fact, of the 15 million Americans who quit smoking each year, only 3 percent stay off cigarettes. Dr. Glynn says you should realize that you are likely to relapse while trying to quit, since most people have to make three or four attempts. Don't give up, he urges; each attempt is actually a learning experience. "You know what to do better next time. It's a six-month to two-year process."

could have spread, says Dr. Greenwald.

"The most common cancer in women is breast cancer, and the five-year survival rate is more than 50 percent," says Dr. Greenwald. "But only 15 percent of women survive that long with lung cancer."

Here are a few of Dr. Glynn's top tips.

Go cold turkey. **Cutting down doesn't seem to work. When most people get down near eight or ten cigarettes a day, they resume again.**

Prepare yourself mentally. **You should be adamant about wanting to quit and know exactly why. Some people like to write down their reasons for stopping and ask friends and family to help them. It's also good to pick a specific date—particularly a birthday or anniversary—as Quit Day.**

Ditch cig "souvenirs." **Get rid of all cigarettes, matches, lighters and ashtrays in your home and office. Also, have smoky clothes cleaned professionally or have your tobacco-assaulted teeth polished by the dentist.**

Wean yourself with the patch. **A doctor can give you a prescription for the nicotine patch, which is worn like an adhesive bandage, releasing some nicotine that your skin absorbs. The patch goes on the upper arm, upper torso or shoulder and has to be replaced about once a day or so. These devices, which you wear for 12 to 16 weeks, help release you from nicotine addiction. Nicotine gum works the same way, but unlike the patch, it has a couple of drawbacks: You have to chew about 12 pieces a day, and some people gripe about the taste.**

Even if you've never lit up, you could still be at risk. Some 3,000 people a year are estimated to die from secondhand smoke, notes Dr. Greenwald. Although critics say the danger of environmental tobacco smoke has been blown out of proportion, a 1990 study in which Dr. Greenwald took part shows otherwise.

The study compared 191 nonsmokers who developed lung cancer with 191 nonsmokers without lung cancer and looked at the frequency with which their parents smoked. Those who'd been exposed to smoke during the first two decades of life had twice the risk of developing lung cancer.

A No-Tar Life

Despite the grim findings about lung cancer, there's one thing to be said for it—this is one of the most preventable cancers. Here are a few tips to help keep this cancer out of your lungs and life.

Don't smoke, don't smoke and don't smoke. It's absolutely never too late, and if one stop-smoking effort doesn't work, just try again. Not smoking is the best insurance against lung cancer. Even if you're smoking two or three packs a day, there are many methods to help you kick the habit. (See "Ditching the Butts for Good.")

Eat your fruits and veggies. People who get very little beta-carotene in their diets have two times more lung cancer than people who get plenty of it, says Harvey Simon, M.D., associate professor of medicine at Harvard Medical School, founding member of the Harvard Cardiovascular Health Center and author of *Conquering Heart Disease.* The best sources of beta-carotene are brightly colored fruits and vegetables such as carrots and red peppers, as well as dark green, leafy vegetables. "Every little bit helps, so munch away," says Dr. Simon.

Check for radon. Test your house for radon, a colorless, odorless gas that's found in rocks and soil and is responsible for some 16,000 lung cancer deaths a year, says Dr.

Simon. You can test your house for excessive radon levels with a low-priced kit available at hardware and department stores.

Beating Obstructive Diseases

If smoking wages war on your lungs, then emphysema and chronic bronchitis are the battle scars. These diseases, which fall under the category of chronic obstructive pulmonary disease (COPD), kill 87,000 people a year.

About 6 out of every 1,000 American women can be expected to get emphysema. It develops after many years of assault on the lungs—almost always by smoking. Over the years the walls between the tiniest air sacs within the lungs break down, and those compartments become enlarged, causing the lung tissue to lose its elasticity and the lungs to become distended. After that they're unable to fill and empty normally.

Eventually, breathing gets more difficult, and the person with emphysema grows weaker—at first, she'll feel breathless and, after a while, unable to do physical activity. Although the effects of emphysema can be controlled somewhat with drugs, people who have it may end up needing oxygen, even when resting.

Chronic bronchitis—also known as smoker's cough—is almost always the forerunner or companion of emphysema. It's caused by chronic irritation from tobacco smoke, which causes periodic attacks of obstructed breathing. The lungs become inflamed and clogged with mucus.

People who have chronic bronchitis never really shake the cough. If your cough produces phlegm, and it continues to bother you every day for a couple of months, it's likely that you have chronic bronchitis. Your doctor will be able to confirm this.

Aside from quitting smoking—the very best way to avoid COPD—doctors recommend a few other ways to cope.

Work out. Although nothing can reverse damaged lung tissue, aerobic exercise helps work out respiratory muscles such as the diaphragm, which strain to work when you have COPD, says Thomas Clanton, M.D., associate professor of physiology, internal medicine and allied medical professions at Ohio State University in Columbus. Dr. Clanton recommends walking or biking 20 to 30 minutes three times a week.

Lift those arms. Because simple arm exercises such as toothbrushing and drying dishes can wind folks with COPD, exercising the arm and shoulder muscles can reduce shortness of breath, says Dr. Clanton. Take an empty liter-size plastic bottle in each hand and lift them straight out to your sides. Repeat 10 to 15 times. As you get stronger, pour a little water in the bottles. Increase the measure of water in small increments as you get stronger.

Commit to C and E. Folks with smoking-induced COPD should take vitamins C and E daily, says Dr. Sandhaus. That's because cigarette smoke contains oxidants—substances that tend to attack healthy cells—while vitamins C and E are antioxidants that help counteract these effects. The recommended minimum dose of vitamin C is 250 milligrams twice a day. For vitamin E the recommended amount is 800 units twice a day, says Dr. Sandhaus. Since vitamin C can be toxic above levels of 1,200 milligrams a day, and E can become toxic above 600 IU, the high doses of vitamins C and E should be approved by your doctor.

Pucker up. To improve your breathing, try doing it with pursed lips, suggests Thomas Petty, M.D., professor of medicine at the University of Colorado Health Sciences Center and consultant to HealthONE in Denver.

"Pursed-lip breathing causes people to breathe slower and deeper, which is more efficient for good gas transfer and relieves shortness of breath," he notes. Pucker your lips as if you're whistling, then breathe in through your nose and out your pursed lips for five to ten minutes. Repeat this breathing exercise two to four times a day. Then use the technique while exercising to fend off breathing problems.

Pneumonia

It sort of feels like the flu, what with the fever, chills and cough it produces. In fact, it often begins as the flu. But pneumonia is in a league of its own, sickness-wise.

Usually caused by bacteria, and sometimes by a virus, pneumonia differs from the common flu in that its effects on the lungs are much worse. Those who suffer from pneumonia often produce large amounts of thick, gray-green or bloody mucus when they cough. And pneumonia frequently causes chest pain.

If you suspect pneumonia, have a doctor check to see if you need antibiotics, says Bradley M. Block, M.D., a family physician in private practice in Winter Park, Florida. Because it usually takes about two weeks to recover, you'll need to be patient. Make sure to stay in bed and rest up.

Tuberculosis

Just when doctors thought they were seeing the last of this lung infection, tuberculosis (TB) made a comeback. The incidence of TB was steadily falling until the early 1980s, when AIDS, which suppresses the body's immune system, reared its ugly head. The reported cases of TB rose from 22,201 in 1985 to 26,673 in 1992—a 20.1 percent increase.

To get TB you'd have to be around other people who have it, since the bacteria are airborne—spread by coughing, sneezing or just exhaling. But only one in ten infected people will develop the disease, since the body's active immune system keeps it at bay.

"Those exposed to it can get acutely ill or only a little bit sick; then it could reactivate itself later," says Dr. DeCosimo. "Many people are walking around with it in them." Those people may never have another infection until they get older, and the body doesn't fight it off as well.

Active TB takes months of antibiotic therapy to knock out. "If you take them for a while and stop, you could develop resistance to that antibiotic," says Dr. DeCosimo.

See also Circulatory System, Respiratory System

Lymphatic System

The lymphatic system teams up with your circulatory and immune systems to help your body fight off bacteria and viruses. Lymph itself is a clear fluid that contains white blood cells. Your lymphatic system includes the thymus gland, tonsils, spleen, bone marrow, lymphatic vessels that serve as the lymph transport system and lymph nodes, which cluster along the lymphatic vessels to filter the lymph.

■ **Bone marrow**, a substance found inside most of our bones, produces red blood cells. It needs the mineral iron for red blood cell production. Because women lose iron

whenever they menstruate, 3 percent of us are tired out from iron-deficiency anemia. (To get more iron in your diet, see "Stoke up on iron" on page 30.)

■ **Lymph** is rich in lymphocytes—warrior white cells that battle bacterial and viral infection. Lymphocytes also produce memory cells, stored in the lymph nodes, that remember the body's invader and help protect against future attacks. (To learn what you can do to help strengthen your immune system, see the Nutrition chapter on page 266.)

■ **Lymphocytes** multiply and are an active part of the immune system. Sometimes the immune system falters, however, and turns against the body's own tissue, as in the autoimmune disease rheumatoid arthritis. (To relieve arthritis pain, see "Anti-arthritis Advice" on page 180.)

■ **Leukemia** is a cancer of the blood-forming organs. The bone marrow, lymph nodes and spleen go awry, producing too many abnormal white blood cells and shortchanging your system of functional, disease-fighting white blood cells. (See "What Can Go Wrong" on page 30 to find out its symptoms.)

■ The simplest of the lymphatic organs, the almond-sized **tonsils** are considered expendable. Although fewer than 10 percent of all tonsillectomies are performed on adults, you may be helped by the surgery if you get repeated infections. (See "When to Bid Tonsils Good-Bye" on page 416.)

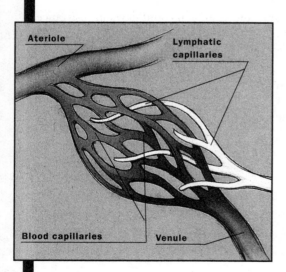

Infection-fighting white blood cells, lymphocytes, travel the lymphatic system in a stream of lymph fluid. They journey through a network of vessels, the smallest of which are the lymphatic capillaries. Here's how the tiny lymphatic capillaries are threaded among the lacework of blood capillaries.

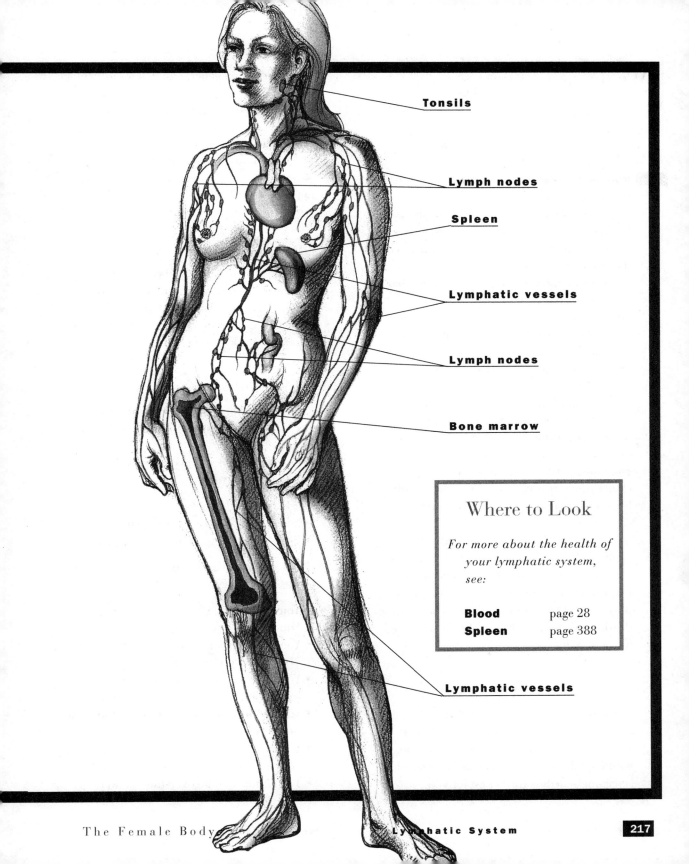

Tonsils

Lymph nodes

Spleen

Lymphatic vessels

Lymph nodes

Bone marrow

Where to Look

For more about the health of your lymphatic system, see:

Blood   page 28
Spleen   page 388

Lymphatic vessels

Medical Tests

POP QUIZ: WHAT KIND OF TEST can you *still* fail, no matter how hard you study?

Sure, calculus and organic chemistry cause brain cell blowout. But medical tests are worse. With those, late-night cramming won't do you a bit of good.

There are literally hundreds of tests that doctors can perform to help diagnose illnesses. If you've read the chapters on gynecological exams (see page 159) or pregnancy (see page 309), you've been introduced to a few of them. But these are only the tip of the medical-test iceberg.

The main function of medical tests is to save lives. So you're doing yourself a favor when you get the tests you need—on schedule. If every woman followed established guidelines for breast cancer screening, for instance, doctors estimate that some 15,000 lives would be spared each year. Similarly, screening for colon cancer could prevent many thousands of deaths annually. Even simple things such as having your blood pressure checked and your blood cholesterol levels measured and controlled regularly could help prevent up to half of the 250,000 heart attack deaths and the 100,000 stroke deaths among women each year.

Getting the Whole Story

Each woman's needs are different, based on age, genetics, medical history and lifestyle. But some basic information can help you—along with the advice of your doctor—to determine a screening schedule that's best for you.

The following general guidelines for women are approved by physicians representing the American Medical Women's Association.

Note: In addition to these, you may want testing for AIDS and other sexually transmitted diseases—recommended by many doctors. (See "Sexually Transmitted Diseases" on page 341.)

Blood Tests

Heart disease is the leading cause of death in American women, striking down half a million each year. You can detect heart disease early and take steps to reverse it if you follow the guidelines below.

Blood Pressure Test

Which is: A measurement of blood pressure done with an inflatable cuff (sphygmomanometer).

How often: Once every year if all of the following apply to you:

- You are age 19 to 40
- You have no heart disease factors
- You are not taking oral contraceptives

Twice or more every year if any of the following apply to you:

- You are over age 40
- You take oral contraceptives
- You have borderline high blood pressure (140/90 or greater)
- You have a personal or family history of high blood pressure or heart disease
- You are on blood pressure control medication
- You smoke
- You are overweight
- You regularly take over-the-counter

nonsteroidal anti-inflammatory medications (analgesics) such as aspirin or ibuprofen

- You have a physician's recommendation to take the test more than once a year

Comments: If you have healthy blood pressure, the reading should be less than 140 systolic over less than 90 diastolic. (The first number is a measure of pressure when your heart contracts; the second, when it expands.)

Blood Cholesterol Test

Which is: A small blood sample that's analyzed at the doctor's office or in a laboratory. The results tell you your total cholesterol plus HDL and LDL ratios in addition to your triglyceride level.

How often: At least once every year if:

- You are any age

Twice or more every year if any of the following apply to you:

- You have recently gained a lot of weight
- You have become sedentary
- You have become ill
- You have borderline high cholesterol (about 200 to 240 mg/dl)
- You have high cholesterol (above 240 mg/dl)
- You are on cholesterol-lowering medication
- You have diabetes or kidney disease
- You have HDL (good cholesterol) levels below 35 mg/dl
- You have had your ovaries removed
- You have recently gone through menopause
- You have heart disease or symptoms of heart disease
- You have a physician's recommendation to

have it done more often than once a year

Comments: The test should be taken after a 12-hour fast, because triglycerides are very sensitive to diet. Even children should take the test. For women, healthy readings should be in the range of 160 mg/dl for total cholesterol, with an HDL of 50 mg/dl or higher, LDL below 120 mg/dl and triglycerides below 110 mg/dl.

Exercise Stress Tests

These tests are valuable because they show how your heart performs when you're actually exercising. About 40 percent of the tests come back with a false-positive—that is, the test indicates problems when there are none. But your doctor has an arsenal of more sensitive tests that can be given for follow-up. When the finding is abnormal, your doctor might give you a stress echocardiogram—measuring with ultrasound while you exercise—or a nuclear medicine test, which involves injection of a radioactive tracing material. In fact, if you're at high risk for heart disease because of family history or a prior record of heart problems, a physician might skip the exercise stress test and go directly to the more sensitive test.

Exercise Stress Test

Which is: A test of coronary fitness. You will perform some exercise, such as walking on a treadmill or pedaling a stationary bike, while being monitored with an electrocardiogram. This test can help reveal coronary artery disease.

How often: Once for screening if:

- You have no risk factors and the test comes back negative

Repeated tests every two to five years if any of the following apply to you:

- You are over age 40
- You are over age 30 and have strong risk factors for heart disease such as high blood pressure, diabetes, obesity, smoking or family history of heart disease
- You have had your ovaries removed
- You have high cholesterol
- You have symptoms of heart disease
- You have a physician's recommendation

Comments: To prevent the onset of heart disease—particularly if you are at high risk because of your lifestyle or family history, see the exercise recommendations beginning on page 443 and nutritional guidelines beginning on page 266.

Gynecological Tests

We're all susceptible to a wide range of gynecological problems, from vaginal infections and uterine fibroids to cervical abnormalities and ovarian growths. Along with the annual pelvic exam, you should be aware of some of the other screening tests that are available to women. Here's a summary.

Pelvic Exam

Which is: Manual examination of your vaginal area to check for abnormalities of the uterus and ovaries.

How often: Once every year if:

- You are over the age of 18

Pap Test

Which is: An examination for signs of cervical cancer. The doctor takes a scraping of cells from the cervix and the cervical canal and smears it on a slide. The sample is then sent to a laboratory for analysis.

How often: Once every year if:

- You are over age 18

Comments: For greatest reliability, you need a skilled medical professional and analysis from a well-qualified laboratory. Seek a board-certified health practitioner for your test.

Transvaginal Ultrasound

Which is: A screening tool to detect changes in the lining of the uterus and ovaries that might suggest cancer. An ultrasound probe is inserted into the vagina, and the probe transmits images of the uterus and ovaries to a monitoring screen.

How often: One screening test—possibly followed by others if your physician recommends it or if any of the following apply to you:

- You are at or past menopause
- You have risk factors for endometrial cancer
- You have a strong family history or other significant risk factors for ovarian cancer

Endometrial Tissue Sample

Which is: Removal of a tiny piece of tissue from the lining of the uterus (endometrium) to check for development of cancer. To perform this test, a thin instrument is inserted through the vagina and cervical opening to remove the tissue sample from the uterus.

How often: One screening test, possibly followed by others as recommended by a doctor, if any of the following apply to you:

- You are past menopause and are considering getting—or are currently receiving—hormone replacement therapy
- You are taking tamoxifen
- You eat a very high fat diet
- You have a history of infertility
- You have a history of not ovulating
- You are very overweight
- You have a family history of endometrial cancer
- You exhibit abnormal uterine bleeding

Comments: This procedure—also called an endometrial biopsy or aspiration—can cause cramping. To avoid damage to the uterus, endometrial sampling should only be performed by an experienced physician.

Breast Examinations

More than 180,000 women are diagnosed with breast cancer every year, and as many as 46,000 die prematurely as a result of this disease. But experts from the American Medical Women's Association say that if all women followed the guidelines below, one-third of those deaths could probably be avoided.

Breast Self-Examination

Which is: Careful self-palpation (examination by touch) of each breast to check for any unusual lumps or masses.

How often: Every month, preferably the week after your period if:

- You are over age 16

Comments: Many doctors say that breast self-exam (BSE) should be a lifelong habit. To learn the skill of BSE, ask your physician for guidance or take classes at your community hospital or at a woman's health clinic.

Your local American Cancer Society office should have information. (To find out how a BSE is done, see page 58.)

Breast Examination by a Health Professional

Which is: Visual examination and careful palpation of the breasts and underarms by a qualified doctor or health professional. You should be examined both sitting up and lying down.

How often: Every two to three years if:

- You are under age 39 and have no risk factors for or symptoms of breast cancer

Once a year or more frequently at a doctor's recommendation if any of the following apply to you:

- You are over age 40
- You have lumpy breasts that are difficult to self-examine
- You do not perform monthly breast self-exams
- You have risk factors for breast cancer: a family history of the disease, no children before age 30, breast biopsies that show atypical growths or a personal history of breast cancer

Mammography

Which is: A low-dose breast x-ray. The breast is pressed firmly between two plates (uncomfortable—but necessary) for each x-ray view. Usually two or three views per breast are required for a complete screening.

How often: One baseline test, followed by additional tests every one to two years if:

- You are age 40 to 49 and don't have risk factors for or symptoms of breast cancer

Once every year or at a doctor's recommendation if either of the following applies to you:

- You are age 50 or older
- You have risk factors for breast cancer (no matter what your age)

Comments: Most doctors recommend that you schedule your mammogram the week after your menstrual period to minimize discomfort. If the doctor does find a suspicious lump, it should be biopsied for a definite diagnosis. There is a 15 percent false-negative rate for mammography: That means there's better than a one in ten chance you have no problem, even if the mammography shows a mass or lump. The biopsy is an important and necessary backup to verify the mammography.

Bone Tests

If you're an American woman, you have a one in two chance of developing fractures from osteoporosis sometime during your lifetime—most likely after menopause. Complications resulting from hip fractures account for 50,000 deaths every year. Many of these deaths may be preventable.

"There's no reason we can't prevent most hip fractures and deaths from osteoporosis if we combine early detection and treatment," says Sydney Lou Bonnick, M.D., director of osteoporosis services at the Texas Woman's University in Denton and author of *The Osteoporosis Handbook*. Many tests are available, and all the techniques are capable of detecting low bone mass and diagnosing osteoporosis, according to Sandra C. Raymond, executive director of the National Osteoporosis Foundation. But some experts believe "that for predicting fracture risk, the specific

Choosing a Doctor: Male or Female?

Does it matter whether your doctor is a man or woman? Here's what studies tell us.

A study at the University of Minnesota in Minneapolis of over 97,000 women found that female internists and family practitioners were twice as likely to give their patients Pap tests and 1½ times more likely to give mammograms than male doctors in the same fields. Less of a difference was seen between female and male gynecologists, however.

Another study conducted by researchers at Northeastern University in Boston also uncovered gender differences. When the researchers analyzed 100 routine medical visits to 50 internal medicine doctors, they found that female doctors spent more time with their patients, made more positive statements, asked more questions and smiled and nodded more. In addition, patients who saw female doctors shared more medical information with them than did patients who saw male doctors.

bone at risk for fracturing should be measured," says Raymond. That means the doctor may choose to focus on a particular area of bone, such as the hip, where fractures are likely to happen.

Many doctors recommend a bone scan before menopause. This first test provides a baseline measurement that your doctor can interpret to find out whether you should take estrogen or another medication (such as salmon calcitonin or etidronate) to prevent further bone weakening. By repeating the scan 12 to 18 months past menopause, the doctor can later determine whether you have lost too much bone. Based on the results, she may recommend that you need to begin medication or adjust your current dosage.

Not all tests are accurately interpreted, however. "It's a problem all of us recognize and are trying to improve," says Dr. Bonnick. He recommends that before having the test, you ask the technician whether she's had several years of experience with bone scans. Make sure that the physician will be reviewing the test and providing a written interpretation. Don't settle for a computer printout–based diagnosis, Dr. Bonnick cautions.

Bone Scan

Which is: Performed by machines that use low-dose radiation to measure bone mass. You sit or lie on a table with the machine positioned above or below you. The procedure is painless and, depending on the technology used, may take from 5 to 30 minutes.

How often: One baseline test just before menopause or very early in menopause with a second test 12 to 18 months after menopause.

You may need more follow-up tests, at the recommendation of your doctor, if any of the following apply to you:

- You have risk factors for osteoporosis based on your family history
- You use steroids
- You have a low-calcium diet
- You lead a sedentary lifestyle

Comments: Many different technologies are available for measuring bone density, but it's not always easy to find a facility where you can take the test. The National Osteoporosis Foundation suggests checking with a local academic health center, a major hospital or a local branch of the American Medical Association.

Tests for Colon Cancer

Colon cancer is the third leading cancer among women, after breast cancer and lung cancer—and more women than men get it every year. If you follow the screening recommendations below, you might be able to detect precancerous changes and early cancer. When it's caught early, colon cancer can usually be treated very effectively.

Digital Rectal Exam

Which is: Examination of the rectum with a gloved finger to detect abnormalities.

How often: Once every year if:

- You are age 40 or over

Fecal Occult Blood Test

Which is: A stool sample obtained at home or at the physician's office. In the lab the stool is analyzed for the presence of blood, which is a possible symptom of colorectal cancer.

How often: Once every year if:

- You are age 50 or over

Comments: This test has been criticized because of the high rate of false-positives (wrongly indicating a possibility of cancer) and false-negatives (missing cancer that's really there). A positive result might indicate ulcers, hemorrhoids or other problems—and a number of follow-up tests such as the ones below can be used to confirm the results of this test.

Sigmoidoscopy

Which is: Examination with a thin, hollow, lighted tube to look for precancerous polyps and remove them before a cancer develops.

The tube is inserted into the rectum and lower part of the colon. Flexible sigmoidoscopes are preferred, because they cause less discomfort than rigid scopes.

How often: Once every three to five years if:

- You are age 50 or over and have no colorectal cancer risk factors or symptoms

More than once every three years, at the discretion of your physician, if any of the following apply to you:

- You have a personal history of colon polyps, chronic inflammatory bowel disease or colorectal cancer
- You have a family history of these diseases—especially if your parents, siblings or children developed colon cancer before age 50
- You have symptoms of colorectal cancer, such as diarrhea, constipation or both, blood in your stools, very narrow stools, unexplained weight loss, frequent gas pains and general stomach discomfort
- You have a feeling that the bowel does not empty completely
- You have a history of breast, endometrial or ovarian cancer

Tests on the Horizon

Doctors, researchers and technicians are coming up with new medical tests so fast that it's hard to keep track of all the advances. But the general direction of the improved medical tests is toward less pain, more gain.

Among the new generation of medical tests the "ouchless" variety. Some of these are noninvasive—that is, they involve no knives, needles or tubes. Others are far less invasive or inconvenient than conventional procedures used previously. In many cases, the new procedures are faster and more accurate.

Though some of these ouchless tests are still under development, it never hurts to ask your doctor if they're available. Here's a rundown of what these procedures have to offer.

A Rodeo for Breast Checks

A technique that has been tested at Baylor University Medical Center in Dallas may help many women with suspicious breast lumps avoid the wait, worry and discomfort of breast biopsies. It involves simply placing a cone-shaped antenna over the breast for a few moments.

Rotating delivery of excitation off-resonance (RODEO) is an improved form of magnetic resonance imaging (MRI). While MRI combines magnetic fields and radio waves to produce an image of the inside of a breast, RODEO goes beyond that. It shows the contrast between normal breast tissue and cancerous tissue.

"Conventional MRI uses a contrasting agent that makes tumors appear as white," says Steven Harms, M.D., director of magnetic resonance at Baylor and co-developer of RODEO. "But since fatty tissue in the breast also shows up as white, finding a breast tumor on a standard MRI image can be like locating a snowman in a snowstorm. With RODEO a special radio field blocks out the fat, so cancerous tumors really stand out."

Speeding Up Bone Scans

Doctors can now spot bone loss indicating osteoporosis in women years earlier than they could before. The secret: dual energy x-ray absorptiometry (DEXA), the fastest and most precise radiological test developed.

DEXA uses much the same technology as

its predecessor in bone density testing, dual photon absorptiometry, or DPA. You lie on a padded table while a device resembling an x-ray machine takes a picture of your bones.

Although DEXA has been around for several years, you might have to ask your doctor to refer you to a major medical facility that provides the test.

Scoping Out Balky Bowels

Doctors at the Mayo Clinic in Rochester, Minnesota, have developed a test that can complement routine blood tests and may even eliminate the need for complex endoscopic (internal) exams in the diagnosis of irritable bowel syndrome (IBS). It's called bowel scintiscan, and it's as easy as taking an aspirin.

In IBS, problems in the stomach or small intestine can keep food from passing through the digestive system smoothly. As if that's not uncomfortable enough, the syndrome is usually diagnosed after a series of tests are negative. These include endoscopy, which involves passing a tube with a light at the end through the mouth and into the stomach and small intestine.

A separate exam with a similar tube evaluates the colon. A tiny camera passed down the tube takes pictures of what's going on inside.

Another diagnostic procedure is a bowel scintiscan—an outpatient procedure that involves swallowing a harmless radioactive capsule on an empty stomach and eating a small meal. Pictures, similar to x-rays, of the abdomen are taken immediately after the capsule and meal are swallowed and at intervals later. The pictures help a physician determine whether you have IBS or another disturbance of the contractions of the intestines.

Bowel scintiscan has several advantages over older tests, according to Michael Camilleri, M.D., professor of medicine in the Mayo Clinic's Gastroenterology Research Unit. "For a patient it's painless, and it allows us to test without inserting any tubes into the body. For the physician it provides an extended exam that effectively assesses the entire digestive tract," he says.

First offered at the Mayo Clinic, the bowel scintiscan is expected to become increasingly available at other major research and treatment centers around the country.

A Breathalyzer for Ulcers

Conventional methods for detecting duodenal ulcers may involve blood tests and endoscopic exams, which must often be conducted several weeks after treatment has started. But the latest innovation in ulcer testing not only eliminates the invasive procedures but also takes the guesswork out of diagnosis and can chart the healing process without lengthy and costly laboratory work.

The innovation is a breath test developed at Baylor College of Medicine to detect *Helicobacter pylori*, a type of bacteria that lives in the digestive tracts of duodenal ulcer patients.

To take the test, you swallow a special form of urea, a natural compound, that has been tagged with heavy, nonradioactive carbon. If *H. pylori* is present, it will feed on the urea and release the carbon. When you breathe into a test bag, the amount of heavy carbon in your breath then tells your doctor the amount of *H. pylori* you have in your digestive system.

A positive test for *H. pylori* can confirm a diagnosis of duodenal ulcer.

Bloodless Glucose Tests

Many diabetes patients must prick their fingers several times a day to get blood samples for glucose monitoring. But soon there may be a painless alternative to this sticky problem.

One kind of monitor that's being tested uses infrared light to check glucose levels in the blood. When a finger is passed through an infrared beam, circulating blood acts like a prism, dispersing the light into a spectrum. The monitor, which could be available for home use, would simply read the spectrum to determine how much glucose is present.

Spying on Heart Attack

Ultrafast computed tomography (CT) is a testing technique that targets the coronary arteries and the heart. Doctors anticipate that it may replace the conventional CT scan in heart disease screening and diagnosis.

Both ultrafast CT and conventional CT methods involve x-raying the heart and surrounding blood vessels. A CT scan takes pictures over several seconds, while ultrafast CT shoots its images within one-tenth of a second. Like a camera with a fast shutter speed, ultrafast CT freezes the motion of the beating heart and captures it in great detail.

In fact, ultrafast images are so detailed that they can allow doctors to spot minute calcium deposits in the coronary arteries—and they can intervene long before these deposits progress to full-blown heart disease. Ultrafast CT is already in use at hospitals around the country.

Testless Testing

In some cases the best replacement for tests that predict heart attack risk may be no new tests at all.

One study suggests that sometimes a program of regular physical exams, exercise stress tests and careful history taking may prove just as valuable in saving lives. The study, conducted at the Lown Cardiovascular Medical Center in Brookline, California, targeted 171 heart disease patients who had been referred for second opinions on their need for angiograms. (Angiography is a procedure used to detect blockages that involves injecting a trace substance in the arteries and then tracking its path through the blood vessels.)

Using medical histories and results of exercise tests and physical exams, the second-opinion doctors decided that 80 percent of the patients didn't need angiograms. (Only six patients were encouraged to have the procedure.)

After four years the second opinions had predicted actual outcomes very well: A majority of the patients had experienced no major problems.

No one would suggest that noninvasive, ouchless tests are the answer for every patient; many of them have yet to be perfected, and depending on your situation, more complicated conventional testing may be just what the doctor ordered. But if you think that one of these noninvasive tests may be for you, ask your doctor. Don't be surprised if the next time she tells you, "This test won't hurt a bit," it's true.

See also Blood, Breasts, Gynecological Exam, Heart, Rectum, Reproductive System, Sexually Transmitted Diseases

Menopause

JANE WAS FIT, FINE AND 42 when she went to the gynecologist for her yearly checkup. It was a medical ritual that she'd followed every year since her first pregnancy. She expected no news but the same news. All systems go.

This time, though, the gynecologist said lab tests showed that Jane was in something called perimenopause.

Jane's stomach dropped like a stone. Perimenopause—what was that? Premature menopause? She'd planned on researching menopause before it happened. And here it had snuck up on her, taking her unprepared.

Her face must have reflected her feelings, because her doctor said, "It's not the end of the world, you know."

Maybe not. But it was the beginning of a new experience for Jane—an experience that every woman will have to face.

Life after Eggs

Menopause signals that you're done with the 900,000 or so eggs that you were born with. The supply source—your ovaries—shuts down hormone production.

It doesn't happen all at once. Before fertility is officially over, the ovaries make noises about retirement and get ready to hang out the sign, "Gone fishin'." It's this stage of limbo that doctors call perimenopause.

During perimenopause a woman's supply of the hormone estrogen starts to waver. The hormone supply doesn't stop suddenly, but it declines enough to cause irregular periods. The hormone has an influence on so many of our body's functions that all sorts of changes occur when there's a shortage.

Perimenopause can last anywhere from two to ten years or so. For each woman the symptoms and signs of approaching menopause are different, and so is the time frame.

Falling levels of estrogen usually cause irregular periods, and often this is the first clue to menopause. Also, some women experience vaginal dryness and frequent urination.

About 85 percent of American women have hot flashes when they're in perimenopause. But hot flashes come in different forms. You might start sweating furiously even when the weather is cool. Or you might suddenly feel the merest flicker of heat at the back of your neck. Night sweats are another common form of hot flashes—which may in turn be responsible for some of the many other symptoms

Keep Control

If you've been using a birth control method, you need to continue to use it during perimenopause—since you're still producing some eggs and can still get pregnant. The hot flashes and funny periods of perimenopause aren't prophylactic. All it takes is one solitary egg for fertilization. That's why, to be safe, you need to practice birth control until at least a year after your very last period.

At this stage there's an added bonus in choosing the Pill as your birth control method. Because it replaces your natural hormones, the Pill helps control irregular periods. For some women it might also help control any premenstrual syndrome–like symptoms of menopause you're feeling, such as aches, irritability and food cravings.

often blamed on menopause—insomnia, fatigue, irritability, mood swings, depression and forgetfulness, says Jennifer Prouty, R.N.C., clinical faculty at Northeastern University College of Nursing in Boston and a menopause consultant.

Estrogen affects the body in other ways as well. "Everyplace you turn in a woman's body there are estrogen receptors. They're in her heart, her bones, her arteries and brain—not just in her reproductive organs and breasts," notes Bernadine Healy, M.D., a cardiologist at the Cleveland Clinic Foundation and former director of the National Institutes of Health.

But the connection to other signs generally attributed to menopause—weight gain, loss of sexual desire, joint pain, hair loss and dry skin—is much less clear. Is it menopause or just middle age or lifestyle? "We don't have enough hard data to really make those connections," says Prouty.

There's no doubt, however, that women's risk of osteoporosis and heart disease begin to soar when estrogen is depleted. Since estrogen protects your bones and is believed to also protect your heart, when it recedes, you have to consciously work to compensate for its loss—with diet, exercise and possibly hormone replacement therapy.

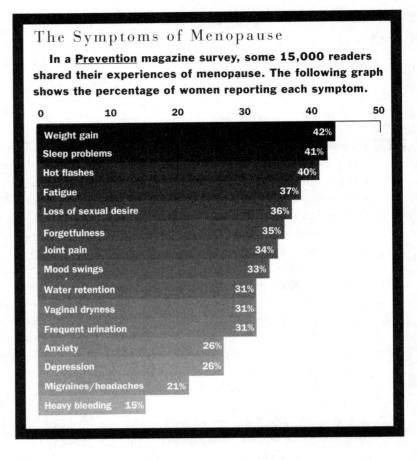

The Symptoms of Menopause

In a **Prevention** magazine survey, some 15,000 readers shared their experiences of menopause. The following graph shows the percentage of women reporting each symptom.

Symptom	Percentage
Weight gain	42%
Sleep problems	41%
Hot flashes	40%
Fatigue	37%
Loss of sexual desire	36%
Forgetfulness	35%
Joint pain	34%
Mood swings	33%
Water retention	31%
Vaginal dryness	31%
Frequent urination	31%
Anxiety	26%
Depression	26%
Migraines/headaches	21%
Heavy bleeding	15%

The Pause and After

As for menopause itself, that term just refers to the time of your final period. Of course, you don't know which is the last one. But if you go one year with no periods, you can say retrospectively that you've been through menopause.

While there's no saying exactly when it will happen, the average age is about 51. Since there's nothing special to signal your last period, you may not even know that menopause has come and gone until your box of sanitary pads starts to gather dust. By then you're in postmenopause.

But some women's bodies don't conform to general predictions. About 5 percent of all women are born with fewer eggs than the other 95 percent. These women inherit a tendency toward early menopause, shutting down egg production by age 41 or even younger.

Having your ovaries removed or destroyed by radiation or chemotherapy also produces premature menopause along with all the symptoms. Once your ovaries are gone, your estrogen drops sharply, just as if you'd gone through menopause.

If you can't remember when you had your last period, and you're not sure what stage you are in, there's a way to find out. Your doctor can give you a follicle-stimulating hormone (FSH) test. It measures how hard your pituitary gland is working to get your ovaries to function. High numbers mean that you're menopausal.

Planning Ahead

Knowing that someday your body will stop producing estrogen, you can help reduce your risks of bone loss and heart disease if you prepare for that change. "We have to prepare for what's coming—protect our bodies, preserve our health. Menopause is sobering, but it's exhilarating, too, if we plan ahead and really take charge of our health," says Anita L. Nelson, M.D., associate professor of obstetrics and gynecology at the University of California, Los Angeles, UCLA School of Medicine and director of the women's medical clinic at Harbor-UCLA Medical Center in Torrance.

The two best ways to prepare for menopause sound awfully familiar. They're the one-two combo of diet and exercise. But even if you already pay attention to both, you may need to revise them a little to get ready for the changes that menopause brings.

Bear some weight. If your diet is low in calcium and your life is low in exercise, you may actually start losing bone in your thirties. That loss accelerates as you approach menopause. But you can slow the rate of bone loss with weight-bearing exercise. "Exercise that bears the full weight of the body is what's important," says Prouty. For many women the most convenient weight-bearing exercises are walking, running or low-impact aerobic dancing. Doctors recommend that you aim for at least 20 to 30 minutes of nonstop moderate aerobic exercise three times a week.

Be upwardly mobile. While walking and running will help build the bones below your waist, you need strength training to build bone in the upper part of your body. Experts recommend resistance exercise three times a week (preferably on nonconsecutive days) using dumbbells, weight machines or exercise bands to target specific muscles or muscle groups in your body.

Attack fat. Since your risk of heart disease shoots up when your body needs estrogen, the less artery-clogging fat in your diet, the better. A diet that's low in saturated animal fat and high in fiber, fruits and vegetables is your best heart-healthy bet.

Knowing Where You Stand

Once you've started perimenopause, you need some basic information in order to plan how much or how little you need to do for a body on the brink of change. Since the risks of osteoporosis rise sharply after menopause, many doctors will recommend a test to determine the condition of your bones. A bone mineral density test will tell you if you need to take aggressive steps to ward off the bone-depleting effects of osteoporosis.

To get the test, you'll need a referral from your physician. Some doctors are reluctant to refer a woman for testing unless her family or medical history shows that she's at risk for osteoporosis. Also, insurance companies often don't cover its cost. But you really do need to know the condition of your bones as you get

Bracing for Bone Loss

A tiny old woman with a bent-over back: That's the common image of osteoporosis. But the bone-thinning disease begins much earlier, when a woman is still young and standing tall. If she's done little exercising and a lot of dieting, if she doesn't eat dairy products or calcium-rich food, if she's a small woman with northern European ancestry or if she smokes, then her bones may be too thin before she's 40.

What is it with bones and calcium? Well, bones are as busy as bees. Cells called osteoclasts dissolve old bone and carry it to the bloodstream, while cells called osteoblasts spin soft protein fibers—collagen—into honeycombs of new bone. Calcium and phosphorus crystals make those soft fibers hard—and the end product is solid bone.

Up until ages 30 to 35, osteoblasts and osteoclasts move in lockstep, so you're making new bone about as fast as the old dissolves. As the years go by, though, the destroyers gain the upper hand, with estrogen playing a role in the coup. And when estrogen plummets after menopause, the osteoclasts get the advantage. The aftermath? They can carry away up to 7 percent of our bone mass during early postmenopausal years.

Working Out Your Risk

Those most at risk of severe osteoporosis—which follows a worst-case script—are small-framed Caucasian or Asian women smokers. If you fit this description, it's especially important to take it seriously. "Osteoporosis is not only deadly, it's crippling," says Anita L. Nelson, M.D., associate professor of obstetrics and gynecology at the University of California, Los Angeles, UCLA School of Medicine and director of the women's medical clinic at Harbor-UCLA Medical Center in Torrance.

Not only will half of the women over age 50 fracture a bone because of the "silent crippler," but "by the age of 65, a woman who fractures her hip has a less than 50 percent chance of full recovery," Dr. Nelson says.

You can fight those statistics, though, and win. If you use hormone replacement therapy (HRT) during the first five post-menopausal years, you can reduce the likelihood of osteoporosis-related bone fractures by more than 50 percent.

But HRT isn't the only answer. One of the studies coming out of the National Institutes of Health's breakthrough Postmenopausal Estrogen/Progestin Interventions Trial looked at the effects of lifestyle on bone mineral density. Investigators who studied 875 women at seven clinical centers around the country found three bone-protective factors. Women with the strongest bones were those who got the most exercise, got plenty of dietary calcium and consumed small amounts of alcohol. Specifically:

- Women in the "best" group had strenuous activity at least three times a week—though mild to moderate exercise produced bone-strengthening benefits, too.
- Women in the "best" group also got at least 800 milligrams of calcium daily and drank about two glasses of wine (or

the equivalent) a week.

In the same study researchers also concluded that—other factors being equal—using estrogen produced about a 2 percent increase in bone density. (In the group they studied, the average time of estrogen use was about 3.2 years.)

Despite the lessons to be learned from this study, however, researchers caution about overindulging in wine. Two glasses is acceptable, but when people increase their consumption, the excessive alcohol begins to have a negative effect on the bone density.

Holding On to Calcium

Researchers also warn that certain kinds of foods can rob the good calcium that we eat. A diet that's heavy in animal protein and salt, for instance, will flush calcium out of your body and into your urine. The phosphorus in soda pop may do the same thing—so limit your drinking of cola, which is high in phosphorus, to one can a day.

Caffeine can interfere with calcium absorption, too, says Stephanie Beling, M.D., medical director of Canyon Ranch in the Berkshires, a health spa in Lenox, Massachusetts. But, she adds, it's okay to have one or two cups of tea or coffee every day.

Another nutrient necessary for calcium absorption is vitamin D, Dr. Beling notes. Some women get enough from the sun, but if you are unable to go outdoors, you can have vitamin D–fortified milk or cereal. And if you're taking supplements, check the label to make sure they also have vitamin D in them.

into perimenopause—so the cost is usually worth it.

The best kind of test is with a dual energy x-ray absorptiometer—better known as DEXA. To avoid the expense of a DEXA test, though, your doctor might use a cheap, new, easy urine test that measures the rate of bone loss.

Since your risks of heart disease also shoot up after menopause, it's advisable to have a lipid analysis to get the numbers on your total cholesterol—both the "good" high-density lipoproteins (HDLs) and the "bad" low-density lipoproteins (LDLs). Another number you'll need is the triglyceride figure. Triglycerides are a fat in the bloodstream that plays a part in women's heart disease.

The HDL number is an important predictor of heart disease risk in women. You want a number over 50 milligrams per deciliter (mg/dl). (Women average higher HDLs than men.) As for your LDLs, you want them below 130 mg/dl. Your triglyceride number should be below 150 mg/dl. If any of these numbers is in the danger area, or if the ratio of HDLs to LDLs isn't high enough, your doctor is likely to recommend a cholesterol-lowering diet and exercise program or even medication.

The Big Decision

If you're in your forties or even late thirties, your eye has probably been caught by the latest article on menopause and hormone replacement therapy (HRT). Every day, it seems, new research on HRT's risks and benefits hits the journals and papers.

Women on HRT take pills or use patches to replace the estrogen that's missing from their bodies. Many women don't take estrogen by itself, though, because without other hormones in the mix, it increases the risk of uterine cancer. A typical HRT regimen combines estrogen with the synthetic hormone progestin.

There's a good amount of evidence indicating that HRT stops bone loss, and it may lower the risk of heart disease by as much as 50 percent. But some other evidence shows that HRT may be associated with increased risk of breast cancer—so doctors are still weighing the risks.

As soon as you approach your perimenopause, your gynecologist will most likely raise the issue of HRT for you to consider. She may believe deeply in its benefits, because it does chill out hot flashes and may relieve other symptoms such as irritability and sleep disturbances. HRT will also improve the ratio of "good" HDL cholesterol to "bad" LDL cholesterol in your blood, and it helps put the brakes on bone loss. There are even some studies linking HRT to a lower incidence of Alzheimer's disease.

One factor to consider is how long you might be on HRT. Originally, the hormones were prescribed to quell hot flashes and other menopause symptoms. "But that's a relatively short-term consideration—five years or so," says Irma L. Mebane-Sims, Ph.D., epidemiologist and program administrator of the National Institutes of Health's ground-breaking Postmenopausal Estrogen/Progestin Interventions (PEPI) Trial.

A woman who is taking HRT for its two greatest benefits—to reduce heart disease risk and osteoporosis risk—is using it as a preventive medication for the long term. "Osteoporosis specialists give a woman at least 10 to 15 years on HRT, and then they reevaluate her. A cardiologist knows that only current users of HRT enjoy the reduction from heart attack risks," says Dr. Nelson. In other words, to get continued protection from heart disease, you need to continue HRT. As soon as

you stop HRT, you can start losing bone at a faster rate.

Despite the benefits of HRT, some doctors are reluctant to prescribe it, relying instead on exercise and diet to treat symptoms and lessen risk.

The decision to go ahead with HRT should really be based upon the profile of each individual, according to Stephanie Beling, M.D., medical director of Canyon Ranch in the Berkshires, a health spa in Lenox, Massachusetts. "If your symptoms aren't severe and you aren't at risk for osteoporosis or heart disease, then hormone replacement therapy might not be prescribed."

Other experts have come up with guidelines to help decide when they'll prescribe HRT. "If you face more than one risk for a disease that estrogen deficiency definitely causes, like heart disease and osteoporosis, then HRT unifies their treatment, so you don't have to take many different drugs," says Rena Vassilopoulou-Sellin, M.D., associate professor of endocrinology at the University of Texas M. D. Anderson Cancer Center in Houston.

A number of doctors, such as JoAnn E. Manson, M.D., associate professor of medicine at Harvard Medical School and co-director of women's health at Brigham and Women's Hospital in Boston, agree with the conclusion of a mega-study that reviewed all the data on hormone therapy since 1970: "Hormone therapy should probably be recommended for women who have had a hysterectomy and for those with coronary heart disease or at high risk for coronary heart disease. For other women the best course of action is unclear."

"A woman needs to look at her own profile of risk to make an informed decision," says Dr. Mebane-Sims. "There isn't an easy answer."

Looking at Lifestyle

Whether you choose HRT or not, doctors agree that you shouldn't neglect diet and exercise. "You shouldn't rely on pills to do things that a good lifestyle should be doing," says Dr. Vassilopoulou-Sellin. The American Medical Women's Association has declared that "for a woman entering or past the age of menopause, exercise may be the single best thing she can do for her emotional and physical health."

When *Prevention* magazine and the Center for Women's Health at Columbia Presbyterian Medical Center in New York City surveyed 15,000 *Prevention* readers, they discovered that women who exercised three times or more a week had a better experience with menopause than women who worked out less than that. They also found that eating a low-fat diet was even a bigger factor than exercise in helping women have a positive experience with menopause.

In addition to eating a low-fat diet, you can select specific foods to help compensate for an estrogen shortage. Plants have estrogens, too, called phytoestrogens, which can be quite powerful, observes Wulf Utian, M.D., Ph.D., director of the Department of Reproductive Biology at Case Western Reserve University in Cleveland.

Phytoestrogens are converted in the gut to hormonelike substances that the body can mistake for estrogen. They come in two forms—isoflavones and lignins. Isoflavones are found in soy foods, such as tofu and soy milk. Lignins show up in whole grains and flaxseed. Fruits and vegetables contain smaller amounts of lignins.

Soy is an excellent source of phytoestrogen. When researchers in Australia gave 58 women soy flour mixed into a drink, mixed into cereal or baked into a muffin, the aver-

Hormones, the Heart and Breast Cancer

A woman at risk for both heart disease and breast cancer is caught on the horns of a tricky dilemma. Hormone replacement therapy (HRT) would protect her heart, but at the same time it might increase her chances of breast cancer.

Heart disease claims many more women than breast cancer. It is the number one cause of death for women over age 65 and claims the lives of a quarter of a million women each year. Forty-six thousand women die of breast cancer each year. But many women fear breast cancer more than heart disease.

There's little evidence to support the view that HRT significantly increases the risk of breast cancer. "Most everybody in the medical community says that if there is a risk, it's so small that we're hard-pressed to find it," says Rena Vassilopoulou-Sellin, M.D., associate professor of endocrinology at the University of Texas M. D. Anderson Cancer Center in Houston. "There *is* a lot of compelling evidence that HRT cuts heart disease risk."

Other evidence of oral estrogen's heart benefits also keeps mounting. Estrogen lowers "bad" LDL cholesterol and raises "good" HDL cholesterol. It lowers a clotting factor in the blood that can cause strokes. It relaxes the blood vessels and keeps them flexible.

age number of hot flashes fell by 40 percent.

Since soybeans are such a good source, you'll probably get enough from just three to four ounces a day of tofu—which is made from soybean curd. (For some tasty ideas on how to include more soy foods in your diet, see "So Many Soy Sources" on page 281.)

Fine-Tuning Your HRT

Let's suppose that you have done a personal risk assessment and concluded that, yes, you want hormone replacement therapy (HRT). That's just the beginning. Finding the right dosage, the right form of hormones and the right schedule could take as long as menopause itself.

Oral hormones have their own side effects—and, actually, they're often similar to menopause symptoms. If you've had a hysterectomy, adjustment to HRT will be easier, because you can just take estrogen rather than estrogen plus progestin. (Since you don't have a uterus to protect from cancer, you don't need the protective effect of the progestin hormone.)

Increased estrogen can cause headaches, especially if you get migraines. Also, if you have a uterus, estrogen can activate fibroids again—benign tumors that grow on the uterine wall and sometimes cause heavy bleeding. Estrogen can also aggravate fibrocystic breast disease.

Progestin, a synthetic form of the hormone progesterone, is more problematic. While estrogen thickens the uterine wall, progestin tells it to slough off. While that protects the uterus, it also produces a period—and if you're done with menopause, that's surely unwelcome news.

If the bleeding is heavy, your doctor will probably put you on a lighter dose or a different schedule. Eventually, you will probably stop bleeding. There is no guarantee, however. Some women continue to have bleeding to the age of 60 and beyond.

Some of progestin's other side effects include bloating, food cravings, breast pain or tenderness, headaches and depression or anxiety. But sometimes these side effects go away when progestin is taken continuously in a smaller daily dose.

Cooling the Hot Flashes

One of the benefits of HRT is that it eliminates hot flashes. But even if you're not on HRT, there are a number of specific techniques you can use to help control the hot flashes that are so uncomfortable for women in perimenopause. Here's what Diana Dell, M.D., assistant professor of obstetrics and gynecology at Duke University Medical Center in Durham, North Carolina, recommends.

Breathe deeply. Hot flashes can hit unexpectedly whether you're lying in bed about to doze off or on the brink of a very important meeting with a very big client. What to do? When that telltale flush starts to prickle your skin and heat up your neck, deep breathing just might do the trick.

Expel as much breath as you can, then fill your lungs again by expanding your diaphragm—the area between your rib cage and abdomen. Release that breath fully. Repeat with a steady rhythm, and you may be able to squelch a hot flash before the sweating begins.

Douse that sizzle. Avoid sizzling foods—whether their heat comes from high temperature or red-hot chili peppers. These foods are notorious hot-flash provocateurs. They can jack up your body temperature and send a rush of heat through your face and chest.

Check your drinks. Alcohol and caffeine can make you flush. Watch your reaction to coffee, tea and colas—and give them up if they lead to hot flashes. Remember: Chocolate also has caffeine, so you may want to forfeit that, too.

Hydro Power

Some women report a lack of sexual desire that comes with menopause—which may be partly caused by vaginal discomfort. Loss of

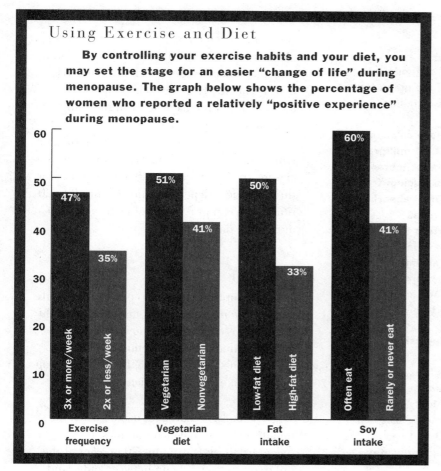

Using Exercise and Diet

By controlling your exercise habits and your diet, you may set the stage for an easier "change of life" during menopause. The graph below shows the percentage of women who reported a relatively "positive experience" during menopause.

Exercise frequency		Vegetarian diet		Fat intake		Soy intake	
3x or more/week	2x or less/week	Vegetarian	Nonvegetarian	Low-fat diet	High-fat diet	Often eat	Rarely or never eat
47%	35%	51%	41%	50%	33%	60%	41%

estrogen has a general drying effect on tissues and organs in the body, particularly in the pelvic region. If your vagina is dry, sexual activity may be uncomfortable.

Bummer, you say? Not for long. Simple solutions exist. Here's what experts recommend.

Make it moister. "There are a variety of lubricants and moisturizers on the market now," says Prouty. K-Y jelly is the classic. It has been joined by moisturizers such as Replens and Astroglide. "They have chemicals in them that create a little bit of penetration into the vaginal walls, so they're longer lasting."

Some women like evening primrose or vitamin E oils—and saliva works, too, adds Prouty. But avoid perfumed oils and petroleum jelly that may contain irritating substances.

Do a dab of estrogen. A topical estrogen cream, available by prescription, thickens the tissues around the vagina. But talk to your doctor in detail before using it long term: Since estrogen is very efficiently absorbed by the body, using it for a long time can have side effects, according to Dr. Dell.

Go orgasmic. Regular orgasms—either with a partner or through masturbation—help maintain healthy tissues, according to Prouty.

Controlling Factors

After menopause, tissues in the pelvic area get thinner and weaker, which can cause an increase of urinary tract and vaginal infections in some women. Lacking estrogen, muscles in the pelvis also start to slacken. When the bladder loses the support of surrounding tissues, you'll probably find that you need to urinate more often. And a sudden laugh or cough may produce the unsettling sensation that you're wetting yourself.

To help prevent urinary tract and vaginal infections, Dr. Dell advises wearing cotton underpants, even under pantyhose. Avoid underwear that's made of nylon, rayon and other synthetic fibers. Those fabrics trap moisture, air and bacteria—three ingredients that help increase the opportunities for infection.

If you're having problems with frequent urination or stress incontinence (meaning that

The Menopause Diet

With just a little tweaking, a good diet can easily turn into a menopause menu that counters some of the effects of falling estrogen.

For starters, you'll need more calcium—1,500 milligrams daily (or 1,000 milligrams if you're on hormone replacement therapy). Ideally, you should get all this calcium from food, because the mineral is best absorbed when it comes from food sources.

Calcium isn't the only nutrient that you need at menopause. Here are some other foods that Diana Dell, M.D., assistant professor of obstetrics and gynecology at Duke University Medical Center in Durham, North Carolina, recommends to help you through this time.

- Eight glasses of water a day can help keep that pelvic area moist.
- Foods with fatty acids, such as sunflower seeds, salmon, soybeans and leafy green vegetables moisturize the body, too.
- Potassium salt (such as Morton salt substitute) instead of table salt can reduce menopausal bloating and water retention.
- Foods with beta-carotene and vitamins C and E—the antioxidants—have been found to help reduce the risk of heart disease.
- Onions and garlic lower cholesterol.
- Foods with fiber, such as whole-wheat breads and fruits and vegetables, also help lower cholesterol and may be useful in colon cancer prevention.
- Chamomile and ginger are herbs that soothe symptoms. Both make good tea.

you sometimes urinate involuntarily), you can train your muscles to have greater control. Doing Kegel exercises will strengthen the muscles and tissues of your urinary tract and your vagina. The next time you urinate, stop the flow, then release it again. This stop-and-start movement of the muscles in the pelvic floor is called a Kegel exercise. That's the movement to practice when you're tuning those muscles up for action.

You can do the exercise sitting, standing or lying down, says Dr. Dell. Tighten your muscles for six to ten seconds; then relax them for three seconds. Repeat the movement 10 to 20 times. You can practice as often as you wish during the day.

Shaping Up

One symptom that was reported frequently in *Prevention*'s menopause survey was weight gain. But research hasn't shown that weight gain is a direct result of menopause. True, metabolism slows as we age. But much of that sloth has to do with the sedentary lifestyles we develop.

More likely, weight gain occurs when hot tomatoes turn into couch potatoes. In fact, "a sedentary lifestyle explains 70 percent of the difference in weight gain between older and younger people," says William J. Evans, Ph.D., director of the Noll Physiological Research Center at Pennsylvania State University in University Park.

The same kinds of exercise that help your heart and bones will also lead the fight against excess pounds. Fitness walking is probably your most effective fat burner, while strength training will turn up your metabolism so that you burn more calories even at rest. Eating more fruits, grains and vegetables and less meat, sweets and chips will help you shed pounds, too.

See also Endocrine System, Fertility, Menstrual Cycle, Nutrition, Toning Your Body

Menstrual Cycle

EVER WATCH A MAN who's obviously been sent to the store to buy tampons?

First, he does a flyby mission down the feminine products aisle to scan the shelf. Then, he makes another pass without stopping to double-check location. Finally, he swings by a third time—very casually, mind you—and taps the box off the shelf and into the cart, barely allowing himself to touch it. When the box lands, he's off down aisle 6 and 7 for enough items to cover the feminine hygiene product. What's he afraid of—getting caught, maybe?

The Embarrassment in Blood

Unfortunately, men aren't the only ones who get embarrassed by tampons and menstrual blood. As all women are aware, menstruation is a natural sign of good health. Yet many women feel they must hide the evidence.

Think about it. We don't walk down the hall at work toting tampons. If we have an "accident," and blood is visible on our pants or skirts, we run home to change or cover the evidence with sweaters tied around our waists. We avoid changing tampons in front of our partners. We hide tampons out of sight in the bathroom cabinet.

So even though periods come and go regularly, and even though we're living in the enlightened 1990s, women tend to feel that menstruation is something to be hidden, covered up, made invisible.

The cover-up is nothing new, of course. Reviewing menstrual taboos in 64 societies, one researcher found that nearly one-third of the groups forbid menstruating women from preparing food for men. Many of those groups isolated women in special shelters. Among Native Americans of North America, for instance, women were hidden away in special menstrual huts when they had their periods. Even the language that's been used to refer to menstruation has often been negative. Menstrual periods have been referred to as "the curse," "that time of the month," "the nuisance" and even "the plague."

The Female 400

On the average, we start menstruating at the age of 12 and continue having periods until we reach menopause at about the age of 51. We may have a few interruptions—caused by pregnancy or taking the Pill, for instance—but the average woman will have about 400 periods during her lifetime. That's a lot of tampons—probably about 6,000, in fact.

Though women often think that a menstrual period is the same as the menstrual cycle, it's not, points out Ellen S. Mitchell, Ph.D., associate professor at the University of Washington School of Nursing and a nationally certified nurse practitioner in Seattle. The term *menstrual period*, or *period*, refers to the days that a woman bleeds. A period lasts about five days, but that's only an average. About half of us bleed for three to four days, while 35 percent of women bleed for five to six days.

The term *menstrual cycle*, on the other hand, refers to the span of time from the start of one period to the start of the next. The length of the menstrual cycle can range from 21 days to 35 days, with 29 days as the average. During the menstrual cycle, we go through a series of hormonal changes, with

Going Full Cycle

Your period may be what you notice most about your menstrual cycle. But a bevy of other changes occur throughout the average cycle of 28 days. Here's a rundown of the events during that average cycle.

Using the start of your period as day one of the menstrual cycle, you can expect bleeding from that day through day five (approximately). The uterus is shedding its lining, and that process produces menstrual blood.

While bleeding continues the ovaries go through other changes. A number of follicles, or eggs, inside the ovary start to mature. Their growth is influenced by a hormone released by the pituitary gland. During this time the reproductive hormones estrogen and progesterone are at low ebb.

By day 5, one follicle has outgrown the rest and is outperforming the other follicles. It becomes the dominant egg in the ovary, and as it churns out increasing amounts of estrogen, it raises the levels of that hormone in your body. From day 6 through day 14 this follicle continues to develop and release estrogen. Under estrogen's influence, the lining of your uterus starts to grow and rebuild.

Ovulation comes next. But before that, estrogen levels drop slightly, while levels of the sex hormone androgen rise. If you find that you have increased sexual desire around mid-cycle, this is probably the reason.

Somewhere around day 14, enough estrogen has been released by the follicle to trigger a surge of luteinizing hormone, or LH, from the pituitary gland. The surge of this hormone triggers ovulation, which occurs between 34 and 36 hours after the LH surge begins and 10 to 12 hours after it peaks. (Menstruation will begin 13 to 15 days after the LH peak.)

After ovulation, the follicle transforms into something called the corpus luteum, which produces the hormones estrogen, progesterone and androgens. The increased levels of progesterone trigger changes in both the cervical mucus and the lining of the uterus. It may also be responsible for some of the mood changes that many of us experience in the second half of the cycle.

If the egg, or follicle, does not get fertilized by a sperm, the corpus luteum starts to degenerate, which causes the estrogen and progesterone levels to decline. The withdrawal of hormonal support causes the uterine lining to shed. A woman on a 28-day cycle will resume menstrual bleeding on the 29th day, when the cycle starts all over again. That 29th day becomes day 1 of the next menstrual cycle.

related changes in the ovaries and the lining of the uterus.

Knowing Your Pattern

Experts say that it's important to know what a normal menstrual cycle is for you. That will help you detect any unusual changes. Here are some ways to keep track.

Buy a date book. "Keeping a menstrual cycle calendar is an incredibly valuable thing," says Dr. Mitchell. Get a little calendar that fits in your purse that's easy to look at and can help you really see patterns, she suggests. In addition to recording when your period starts, how long it lasts and how heavy or light the flow is, track how your body feels throughout the month.

Count it right. When keeping count of your menstrual cycles, be sure to count properly. Start counting on the first day of your period and continue counting up until the day when your next period starts, says Dr. Mitchell. "A lot of women will count through their periods as part of their cycle," she says. If you do that, it looks as if your cycle is longer than it actually is. In other words, if you have a 29-day cycle, day 1 is the first day of your period and day 29 is the day before your next period starts.

Accept yourself. Once you detect your average cycle length, accept that it's normal for you. Some women think there's something wrong if they are not having cycles that are 28 days long, says Dr. Mitchell. "Menstrual cycles are not all 28 days long, as many women believe. It can be very normal between 21 and 35 days," she says.

Play detective. "If you notice there are some differences in your cycle length or in your flow, keep track of them with that calendar for a few months," says Dr. Mitchell. "Then go and talk with your health care provider about it, and take your calendar with you," she says. Your doctor or nurse practitioner can then look to see if you have a very irregular pattern of bleeding that could be a sign of a more serious problem, she says.

It's important to remember that a change doesn't always indicate a problem, says Mary Beth Hasselquist, M.D., staff obstetrician/gynecologist at Group Health Cooperative of Puget Sound, Washington, and clinical instructor in the Department of Obstetrics and

Asthma Attack? Maybe It's That Time of the Month

Okay, so you know that in the days just prior to your period, you can expect to feel bloated, crampy and grouchy. But did you also know that the hormonal changes preceding your period can influence your body in a number of other ways?

There's not enough research to tell us why. From the stories that their patients tell them and a few preliminary studies, here's what doctors have observed.

- Hormonal changes during the menstrual cycle may affect your allergies.
- If you have asthma, the days near the start of your period may be the time when you are most susceptible to severe asthma attacks.
- Some women find that they may get cold sores just before menstruation begins.
- If you have eczema, you may notice your skin condition gets worse just prior to your period.
- Gum disease, or gingivitis, tends to be worse during menstruation.
- Some women experience insomnia once a month—and it occurs just prior to their periods.
- Other women find that their voices are pitched lower—or get hoarse as if they had mild laryngitis—one to two days just prior to their periods.

Also, some women with health conditions find that their symptoms appear cyclically. A woman who has lupus, for instance, might find that her joint pain and facial rash are worse in the two weeks just before her period.

Gynecology at the University of Washington School of Medicine in Seattle. Sometimes bleeding is well within normal, and women get alarmed anyway, she says.

Premenstrual Symptoms

Women have a broad range of physical changes around the time of their periods. These are what doctors call premenstrual symptoms—but having them doesn't necessarily mean you have premenstrual syndrome, or PMS.

Some 100 symptoms caused by the menstrual cycle have been reported by women, including pain and cramping, bloating, headache, backache, food cravings, breast tenderness and mood changes. About 95 percent of reproductive-age women will experience one or more of these symptoms just prior to their periods, notes Diana Taylor, R.N., Ph.D., associate professor and director of the Women's Health Program in the Department of Family Health Care Nursing at the University of California, San Francisco.

One symptom that many women get is premenstrual headache, says Joanne Piscitelli, M.D., assistant clinical professor and the division chief of general obstetrics and gynecology at Duke University Medical Center in Durham, North Carolina. "My feeling is that it is related to the drop in estrogen and progesterone that occurs the day prior to the onset of the period." Certainly, if you're prone to migraines, you'll tend to get them more often right around the time of your period, so there seems to be some hormonal trigger, she says. Some doctors have noted that premenstrual headaches seem to become more common as a woman gets older.

Other common premenstrual symptoms range from mood changes to breast tenderness,

The PMS Diet

While **PMS** has become a common buzzword, premenstrual syndrome itself is not as common as you may think. Ninety percent of women experience one or more physical or psychological changes before their periods, but only **9 percent** meet the criteria for PMS itself.

So . . . what's up? Do you have premenstrual syndrome, premenstrual symptoms, both or neither?

If you have PMS, experts say, your premenstrual symptoms will recur in two out of three menstrual cycles—and they'll be followed by a symptom-free time before your next period. PMS symptoms will cease abruptly with the beginning of your menstrual cycle. With PMS the symptoms are so severe that they interfere with your relationships—or with some aspect of your work or lifestyle.

That's just a thumbnail description of what happens with PMS. Before undergoing treatment for it, you should be sure to get an accurate diagnosis, experts say.

After that there are a number of methods you can try to alleviate symptoms. The methods include diet, exercise, stress reduction and time management as well as behavioral and cognitive training, says **Diana Taylor, R.N., Ph.D.,** associate professor and director of the Women's Health Program in the Department of Family Health Care Nursing at the University of California, San Francisco.

Dietary changes are only part of the equation, but they can help some women. Experts commonly recommend that you keep your salt and sugar intake low if you have PMS. Here are some other dietary factors that may come into play.

Complex carbohydrates. Eating a diet high in complex carbohydrates—including dietary fiber—may help alleviate PMS symptoms, says Ellen S. Mitchell, Ph.D., associate professor at the University of Washington School of Nursing and a nationally certified nurse practitioner in Seattle. Researchers believe that there is a relationship between complex carbohydrates and the production of the brain chemical serotonin, which controls mood, appetite and sleep. Getting adequate, consistent amounts of carbohydrates into your system can help maintain serotonin levels and fend off mood swings, cravings and sleep disturbances.

Good sources of complex carbohydrates and fiber include bran, wheat, oats and other grains and grain products. You'll also get plenty of complex carbohydrates from legumes such as peas and beans and from corn and potatoes.

Caffeine. Researchers theorize that part of the nervous system is super-aroused—particularly in the second half of the cycle—in women with PMS, according to Dr. Mitchell. Since caffeine is a stimulant that directly affects the nervous system, women with PMS should keep their caffeine intake down, she says. This means cutting back on caffeinated coffee, soda and tea and also limiting the amount of chocolate you eat.

Vitamin B_6. "There's some data, although it's sketchy, that increasing your B_6 intake to about 50 milligrams a day is helpful," says Dr. Mitchell. Just how much B_6 helps alleviate PMS symptoms is controversial—and some researchers don't think that it helps—but if you stay at 50 milligrams a day, taking B_6 won't hurt, says Dr. Mitchell. (This is still very high, since the Daily Value for B_6 is just 2 milligrams.) While you may get some B_6 in your diet, you'll probably have to take a supplement to make sure you get 50 milligrams. Do not take more than this amount, however, because B_6 is toxic in high amounts.

Calcium. "There's some data that suggests that at least 1,000 milligrams of calcium is helpful in terms of PMS symptoms," says Dr. Mitchell. In particular, calcium may help alleviate the anxiety symptoms, she says.

Each eight-ounce serving of milk contains about 300 milligrams of calcium, and so does a one-cup serving of yogurt. You might choose skim milk and low-fat yogurt to limit your fat intake. With three or four daily servings of these low-fat dairy products, you'll get about 1,000 milligrams of calcium even if you don't take supplements.

Zinc and magnesium. Some research indicates that women who get PMS have less zinc and magnesium in their diets than other women. Researchers suspect that these minerals may influence the brain's production of chemicals that influence mood.

Based on the research so far, doctors aren't ready to recommend zinc and magnesium supplements—but there's no harm in reaching for zinc-rich foods such as ready-to-eat cereals, lean meats, seeds and cooked oysters. Good sources of magnesium include dark green, leafy vegetables, legumes such as cooked, dried peas and beans and whole grains.

bloating and backache. According to a national survey of 968 women conducted at the University of Arkansas in Fayetteville, 90 percent experienced premenstrual mood changes and 89 percent had bloating at some time. The same study showed that 88 percent had breast tenderness, and three-quarters of the group experienced premenstrual backache.

In the study of premenstrual symptoms that was done at the University of Arkansas, women who exercised reported less discomfort than women who were inactive. "We feel that moderate exercise, whether it's walking or running or biking, helps," says Inza Fort, Ed.D., professor of kinesiology, in the Department of Health Science, kinesiology, recreation and dance at the University of Arkansas and one of the researchers involved in the study.

To help relieve premenstrual symptoms, you should aim to get 20 minutes of exercise at least three to four times a week, Dr. Fort recommends. The most effective kind is aerobic exercise that raises your pulse and makes you sweat a little—but at a pace that's moderate enough to allow you to carry on a conversation.

For premenstrual bloating doctors recommend a number of foods to help control it. Asparagus, apple cider vinegar and herbal teas are natural diuretics that may help decrease bloating, says Dr. Taylor. If bloating is a recurrent problem, try to incorporate these natural diuretics into your diet.

Menstrual Symptoms

Apart from premenstrual problems—or in addition to them—many women get other symptoms when menstruation starts. Cramping is among the most common, says Dr. Piscitelli. Approximately 50 percent of women get menstrual cramping, and 5 to 10

percent get incapacitating pain.

Pain and cramping originate from the uterus. The pain is caused by special chemicals called prostaglandins that get released by cells in the uterine lining when it starts to shed. When you feel a menstrual cramp, it's actually a contraction of the uterus.

In most women cramps are normal, but in some they are a sign of more serious problems in the abdomen, genital tract or uterus. So if you have pain and cramping when you normally wouldn't, or if it's prolonged and severe, visit your doctor, says Dr. Piscitelli.

Even if you've come to expect cramps, there are ways to fend them off. Here's what doctors recommend.

Look over the counter. Using over-the-counter medications such as ibuprofen can help reduce cramping pain. Ibuprofen is an antiprostaglandin, so it counteracts the chemicals that cause cramps, says Dr. Mitchell.

When should you start taking it? Generally, as soon as the cramping starts, says Dr. Piscitelli. Women who experience nausea, diarrhea and vomiting with their periods may want to take ibuprofen a day or two before they expect their period to start, she says. That way they can get the medicine in their systems before they start feeling nauseous. Ibuprofen can also be effective for relieving backache and headache. Don't go overboard, though: Frequent, regular use of ibuprofen can sometimes lead to stomach trouble, so take it with food or an antacid, doctors say.

Pack up the pain. Some women find that it helps to apply heat to the area where they feel crampy and achy, says Dr. Mitchell. When you're sitting or lying down, cradle a hot pack in the area that hurts.

Let hormones do the trick. Oral contraceptives tend to make cramps less significant, says Dr. Piscitelli. The Pill prevents ovulation and reduces the thickness of the lining of the uterus, so fewer cramp-inducing prostaglandins are produced. The Pill may also help relieve menstrual-related headaches and help relieve pain and cramping caused by endometriosis and fibroids—two conditions that make menstruation particularly painful for some women.

Say yeah to yoga. In addition to aerobic exercise, yoga may help relieve menstrual symptoms, says Dr. Taylor. The "child"

pose—shown in the illustration below—may be particularly helpful.

Try a walk. While helping ease premenstrual problems, regular exercise may also help fend off menstrual symptoms. "Exercise increases the level of endorphins—your body's natural painkillers—and that may have an effect on menstrual cramp pain, but we don't know for sure," says Christine Wells, Ph.D., professor of exercise science and physical education at Arizona State University in Tempe and author of *Women, Sport and Performance*.

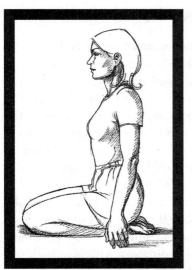

At the start of the yoga "child" pose, kneel with your arms at your sides. Sit back on your heels.

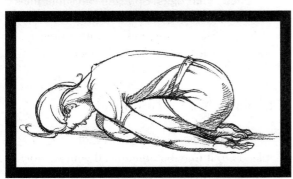

Bend over as shown. Inhale deeply through your nose, exhale through your nose, then pause a second or two before you inhale again. Hold the pose as long as you're comfortable—up to several minutes.

When Your Cycle Changes

Maybe you find you are bleeding more, less, at the wrong time or not at all. Should you be concerned?

Well, sometimes yes and sometimes no, doctors say. Spotting between periods is not a common problem, but it certainly isn't unheard of, says Dr. Hasselquist. Whether you need to be concerned about spotting depends on when in your cycle you experience it, she says.

If spotting occurs in the middle of your cycle—that's about 14 days before your next period —there's a good chance that it's caused by ovulation. In other words, it's not usually a cause for concern, says Dr. Hasselquist. During ovulation, estrogen levels drop, and that's often enough to trigger some bleeding.

Contact your doctor if the spotting does not occur around mid-cycle, Dr. Hasselquist recommends. Erratic spotting between periods could be a warning of some problem, especially if you're over 40 years old, agrees Dr. Piscitelli. Since intermittent spotting can signal a precancerous condition of the uterus, it's important for your doctor to check it out right away.

Are Your Times A-Changing?

If you're in your thirties, and your periods are different now from what they used to be, don't be alarmed. "Somewhere between the mid-thirties and the early forties there is often a very subtle change in the menstrual period or in the cycle length," says Ellen S. Mitchell, Ph.D., associate professor at the University of Washington School of Nursing and a nationally certified nurse practitioner in Seattle. "It may start getting a little lighter, maybe a day or two or three shorter. The cycles are still regular, but shorter. Many times these changes are so subtle that women don't realize it."

When the changes are so slight, it's usually not a sign that anything is wrong, according to Dr. Mitchell. "They're just part of the normal evolution of a woman's reproductive life," she says.

Near the ages of 45 to 47, you may notice that your menstrual cycles are becoming more irregular—some months your cycles may be shorter and other months they may be longer. Or you may actually skip some periods. This is the beginning of the menopausal transition. This transition period may last an average of four to six years. The irregularity will increase as a woman gets closer to menopause. Normal menopause (menopause means one year or more with no period) occurs any time from age 40 onward, even though the average age is 51. Remember, a woman can still get pregnant up until the time when she's had no period for at least one year.

But even the age range doesn't apply to all women. "You can't take a woman's age and say that something is going to happen then. The reproductive life cycle doesn't necessarily go by age," says Dr. Mitchell.

In these situations the doctor will probably want your menstrual history before deciding whether or not you need a biopsy, says Dr. Hasselquist. Here are some prudent steps that doctors recommend you take from the start of spotting.

Mark it on your calendar. If you experience some spotting, mark the day on your menstrual calendar and wait for your next period. Once your period comes, count backward to the day that you had spotting. If spotting fell on or around day 14, then it's probably mid-cycle bleeding, and you don't have much to worry about, says Dr. Hasselquist.

Consider your contraception choice. If you are on the Pill, you might have some bleeding at times other than when you have your period, according to Dr. Hasselquist. Women who get quarterly Depo-Provera birth control shots might have spotting during the first year that they're getting these hormone injections. The Norplant device—which can stay implanted under the skin for up to five years—can cause irregular spotting the whole time it's in place. If you use any of these methods, be sure to inform your doctor about any spotting and discuss it with her.

Check your eggs. Spotting can sometimes be a sign that you are pregnant, says Dr. Hasselquist. She recommends getting a pregnancy test to find out if that's the cause.

When It's Much Too Much

If you've been having heavy, prolonged bleeding, it may be time to call your doctor.

What's the measure of heavy bleeding? If you find that you soak through a full-size pad or a super tampon in just an hour, and that happens two hours in a row, that's considered heavy bleeding, says Dr. Hasselquist.

Tampon Check

Most baby boomers remember the toxic shock scare of the early 1980s. There were TV reports about women becoming incredibly ill during their periods, lots of warnings about high-absorbency tampons and news of women dying. Later, the controversy died down—which may have left you wondering whether this was just the passing of another media event.

During the ensuing years, manufacturers have changed both the fiber content and absorbency levels of tampons. Today, an estimated 1 in 100,000 women gets menstruation-related toxic shock each year. The symptoms include high fever, nausea and a sunburnlike rash mainly on the torso accompanied by low blood pressure—and if you have these symptoms, you should call your doctor. Because it's so uncommon, your chances of having toxic shock are extremely low. You can lower your risk even more if you follow this advice from doctors.

Select the right tampons. "Women who want to decrease the risk of toxic shock can use the lowest absorbency compatible with their needs," says Anne Schuchat, M.D., medical epidemiologist in the Division of Bacterial and Mycotic Diseases at the Centers for Disease Control and Prevention in Atlanta. When your flow is light, go with a lower-absorbency tampon, usually labeled "regular," and when your flow is heavy, try a "super." If your period varies, carry a variety of tampons with you so you have a choice.

Follow the instructions. Read the package insert, says Dr. Schuchat. It's important to follow the recommended time-use guidelines for your particular brand and absorbency. In general, it's recommended that you change your tampon every 4 to 8 hours. Tampons have changed over the years, so if you haven't read an insert in ages, take a look.

Go alternative. "Women who want to reduce their risk even further can alternate tampon use with pads," says Dr. Schuchat. It's best to use a pad instead of a tampon during your light days, suggests Ellen S. Mitchell, Ph.D., associate professor at the University of Washington School of Nursing and a nationally certified nurse practitioner in Seattle.

Prevent an encore. If you've had toxic shock during your period before, the CDC recommends that you avoid tampon use in the future, says Dr. Schuchat. "There is a risk of recurrence."

One possibility is that the heavy bleeding is caused by fibroids, growths that can form inside the uterus. There is nothing that you can do to prevent fibroids—and whether your doctor recommends surgery depends on their size, which she'll find out during a pelvic exam.

The abnormal bleeding caused by fibroids, however, can sometimes be managed in other ways. According to Dr. Hasselquist, birth control pills can decrease the amount of menstrual flow. And an injection of Depo-Provera, the birth control shot, will stop menstruation, says Dr. Hasselquist. If those approaches don't work, and the fibroids are large enough to require surgery, your doctor might recommend either a hysterectomy or a procedure called myomectomy. (A myomectomy is recommended for someone who wants to preserve her fertility, or does not want a hysterectomy.) But not all fibroids need to be removed. Small ones can often be left in.

Heavy bleeding could signal other changes that are likely to need a doctor's attention. Sometimes women get heavier periods because they're not ovulating, says Dr. Piscitelli. A number of things can interfere with ovulation, including polycystic ovarian syndrome, a condition where multiple cysts form inside an ovary. Also, certain medical conditions, such as thyroid disease or pituitary tumors, can interfere with ovulation.

When Your Period Goes AWOL

Prolonged periods of not bleeding—missing a period for several months in a row, or amenorrhea—are also reason for concern, says Dr. Piscitelli. If there's a chance that you're pregnant, of course, this is the first thing to check out. If not, and if you've missed your period for several months, you might want to explore other causes of amenorrhea.

Doctors have found a wide range of conditions that can cause amenorrhea. If it goes on for six months, you should see your doctor, says Dr. Hasselquist.

If your amenorrhea is related to other conditions, such as an endocrine disorder or anorexia, your cycle may return to normal as soon as the condition is taken care of.

See also Birth Control, Gynecological Exam, Ovaries, Reproductive System, Uterus

Moles

THE FACE OF SUPERMODEL-turned-MTV commentator Cindy Crawford has been seen by millions. But how many people mention that she has a protruding pigment cell over her upper lip?

Translated into nonmedical language, that's a mole.

Only 1 in 100 people is actually born with one. For the rest of us, these round, deeply pigmented growths crop up gradually and imperceptibly over the course of a lifetime—usually in our twenties and thirties. As with freckles and age spots, the main cause is exposure to sunlight, says Darrell Rigel, M.D., clinical associate professor of dermatology at New York University School of Medicine in New York City.

Usually, in order to develop a mole, "you have to be exposed to the sun and be sensitive to it," Dr. Rigel notes. "You'll see that the inside of your arm doesn't have many moles, but the outside does."

Keeping a Mole Watch

While sunlight is one cause of moles, it isn't the only one. You can develop moles anywhere on your body, including sun-protected areas such as the buttocks and breasts.

If your family tends to develop these atypical moles, which usually appear at puberty, you have to keep an eye on them, according to Ronald Scott, M.D., radiation oncologist and cancer specialist at the South Coast Tumor Institute in San Diego. That's because some of these moles have the potential for developing into skin cancer—both the benign kind or more serious ones, known as malignant melanoma.

"If your mother or father had this type of mole and developed a melanoma, your risk for this disease is almost 100 percent," says Dr. Scott.

Early detection that a mole is changing can reduce your risk of having skin cancer spread to other parts of your body. When melanoma gets larger than the size of a dime, it has more than a 50 percent chance of spreading. So it's vital to know what to look for and to catch it early, according to Dr. Rigel. It's also important to see a dermatologist as soon as possible if you notice any of the signs of potential problems.

In addition, doctors recommend that you and a dermatologist take a long, hard look at your body at regular intervals. It's the best way to get the lowdown on what your moles (as well as freckles and skin spots) look like. It's also the only way of knowing for sure when something isn't quite right.

If you're in a high-risk group, such as being a fair-skinned blond, or if you have a family history of skin cancer, you should examine yourself once a month. Stand nude before a full-length mirror and use a handheld mirror to inspect your back area, suggests Dr. Rigel.

Keep a close eye on any moles you already have so you'll know when something changes, Dr. Rigel cautions. "If it's growing, bleeding, crusting or changing, something is wrong."

He also suggests having a doctor give you an annual once-over. "On your birthday, have your birthday suit examined."

See also Skin

Learn Your A's, Bs, Cs and Ds

Taking a long, hard look at yourself every now and then has nothing to do with vanity. It's the best way to get the lowdown on what your moles, freckles or skin spots look like. If you see specific changes in moles, it could be an early signal that you should be on the lookout for melanoma, the malignant type of skin cancer.

To help you remember what to look for when you monitor your moles, doctors recommend that you use the ABCD system.

Below is a visual guide to help you identify these changes. If you notice any of the variations shown here, you should see your doctor as soon as possible. It could be a sign of potential melanoma.

A is for asymmetry. Normal moles are symmetrical—able to be split evenly down the middle—but a melanoma is oddly shaped, with halves that do not match.

B is for the border of the mole, which should be smooth and regular, rather than blurred and irregular.

C is for color. Normal moles should have uniform coloring, but a melanoma might contain a variety of colors, including red, black, brown, tan and white.

D is for the diameter of the mole, which should be no bigger than a pencil eraser.

Mouth

"LET HIM KISS ME with the kisses of his mouth; for thy love is better than wine. . . ."

"Breath like an angel's whisper. . . ."

"Open thou my lips, and my mouth shall show forth thy praise. . . ."

From Solomon to Shakespeare, poets have a way with words. Not facts.

"The mouth is actually one of the dirtiest parts of the body," says Richard H. Price, D.M.D., clinical instructor of dentistry at Boston University Henry Goldman School of Dentistry. "That's why a human bite is so serious."

So here's the real dirt on mouths: More than three dozen different species of bacteria call our mouths home. While some are good, many aren't.

The good bacteria suppress nasty fungi that also live in the mouth—such as *Candida albicans*, a common fungus that can produce yellowish sores in the mouth (it's called oral thrush). If you're taking antibiotics that suppress the good bacteria with the bad, you're much more likely to get oral thrush.

On the other hand, the bad bacteria in your mouth are definitely bad. If your immune system lets down its guard, you never know what bacteria might make a grand entrance through your mouth and begin to do their dirty work.

Since doctors are well-informed about all that bacterial activity, it's a bit surprising that they still don't know the culprit that causes the mouth's most common malady—the canker sore.

Don't Be Sore

Canker sores are simply open sores that you can get anywhere inside your mouth: on your tongue, inside your lips or on the mucous lining of your cheek. They're often a girl thing. We get them when we're teenagers and young adults and right before our periods. "Twenty percent of the population gets canker sores," says Kenneth Burrell, D.D.S., senior director of the council on scientific affairs of the American Dental Association. "And most of them are women."

As for the medical name, it's a phonic delight—aphthous ulcers. Bite your tongue, and you'll probably get an aphthous ulcer where you bit it. Apart from that, hormones, stress and nutritional deficiencies (of folic acid, iron and the B vitamins) are all thought to play a role in creating canker sores.

Let the Doc Look

Here's a conundrum. The mouth sore that hurts is usually harmless. It's the one that doesn't hurt that needs attention.

Irritating as a canker sore can be, it really isn't harmful, and it goes away in a matter of days. The sore to watch out for is a bump or an ulcer that may look like a canker sore, but it doesn't hurt and it never heals. It could be a sign of oral cancer.

You should be particularly alert to mouth bumps or ulcers if you smoke, since smoking changes the cells in the mouth. More than 19 out of every 20 people who have oral cancer are also smokers—even chewing tobacco can hurt.

A rule of thumb is that if you have any kind of sore in your mouth that doesn't heal within two weeks, see your dentist.

Halitosis: A Whiff of Trouble

Standing in a crowded bus or crammed inside a theater lobby, you may suddenly catch a whiff of pungent breath. Unfortunately, noxious fumes sometimes carry a deeper meaning to dentists.

"The smell of bad breath can sometimes tell me the amount of gum disease a person has. I want to tell her, 'Quick, go see a dentist,' " says Ray C. Williams, D.M.D., professor and chairman of the Department of Periodontics at the University of North Carolina School of Dentistry at Chapel Hill.

Or it could mean other things. Sour stomach, sinusitis and respiratory infections can also cause bad breath. So can tasty members of the allium family—garlic and onions are notorious. And so are some spice mixtures such as Indian curries.

If you're worried about the smell of your breath, here are some ways to sweeten it.

- **Rinse your mouth after eating.** Since halitosis is often caused by bacteria and food debris in your mouth, a good swish, gargle and spit get rid of the bad-breath ingredients. Better yet, follow up by brushing your teeth.
- **Chew parsley.** Like garlic and onion, parsley flavors your breath—but parsley just happens to smell good.
- **Suck on sugarless peppermint candy.** Not only does peppermint have an agreeable fragrance, the sucking action stimulates saliva, our natural mouthwashing detergent.
- **Chew sugarless cinnamon, spearmint or peppermint gum.** Like the peppermint candy, it smells good and stimulates mouth-cleaning saliva.

Here are some ways to soothe the sores.

Try a mouth bandage. A canker sore usually gets worse, because your teeth keep scraping against it. But you can give it a chance to heal if you use Orabase, says Dr. Burrell. You can buy a tube of it at most pharmacies. The ingredients make a paste that stays put in your mouth like a bandage for several hours.

Rinse with magnesia. Liquid antacids can also soothe a canker sore. Doctors recommend that you swish a tablespoon or so of Mylanta or milk of magnesia around the site of an ulcer to coat the sore and relieve its irritation.

Stir up something new. Some dentists recommend concocting a soothing mixture from half a tablespoon of liquid Benadryl—an antihistamine—and an equal amount of Kaopectate—an antidiarrhea medicine. Swish it around the sore and spit it out. "The Be-

nadryl numbs the sore, and the Kaopectate cools it and coats it. It's a very soothing concoction," says Ray C. Williams, D.M.D., professor and chairman of the Department of Periodontics at the University of North Carolina School of Dentistry at Chapel Hill.

Choose the "benz" family. Pharmacy shelves hold a number of canker sore medications. The ones to look for, says Dr. Burrell, are topical tinctures and salves that contain benzoin or benzocaine (such as Orajel). "Tincture of benzoin provides a protective layer, and benzocaine is an anesthetic."

Take your E's. Some women find relief using vitamin E as an oral salve. Just open up a vitamin E capsule and squeeze some of the contents onto your canker sore. Gently rub the gel into the sore.

See also Gums, Lips, Teeth, Tongue

Muscular System

More than 600 skeletal muscles move your skeleton and organs, heat up your body and keep you upright. A muscle is made up of bundles of fibers cinched together by connective tissue. Muscles need to move; they weaken and shrivel when they can't. When you move, muscles contract around your joints, resulting in activity of those joints, such as bending an elbow.

■ The two lats, short for **latissimus dorsi**, are your back's biggest muscles. A spasm in either one can lay you out like a log on your bed. (To find out how muscle spasms happen, and how to prevent them, see "Back-ercise" on page 13.)

■ Women's **necks** are smaller and more vulnerable than men's necks. That's one reason why 70 percent of all whiplash cases occur among women. Whiplash happens when the neck is violently thrust backward and then forward, straining or spraining muscles and ligaments in the neck. (To treat it or to help prevent it, see "Whipping Whiplash" on page 256.)

■ The **pectoral muscles** lie under a woman's breasts. Firming up those muscles can give sagging breasts a nice boost—a natural breast lift. (For two exercises that tone up the pectoral muscles, see "Chest" on page 456.)

■ The **quadriceps** are the muscles that take more verbal abuse than any other part of the body. That's because they form a good portion of the universally unloved

Where to Look	
For more about easing your muscles and keeping them well-toned, see:	
Ankles	page 3
Back	page 9
Elbows	page 92
Knees	page 192
Neck	page 252
Shoulders	page 348
Toning Your Body	page 439

thigh. (To firm up flabby quads, see the two exercises under "Thighs" on page 461.)

■ Tense **muscles in the head and neck** are responsible for tension-type headaches—the most common kind. They feel like a tight band around your head. (To relieve them, try the acupressure exercise under "Putting the Pressure On" on page 293.)

■ The **vastus medialis** is a strip of muscle along your inner thigh. If it's underdeveloped, it can cause knee pain when you first start an exercise program. (To prevent knee pain or to quell it, see "Easing the Knees" on page 194.)

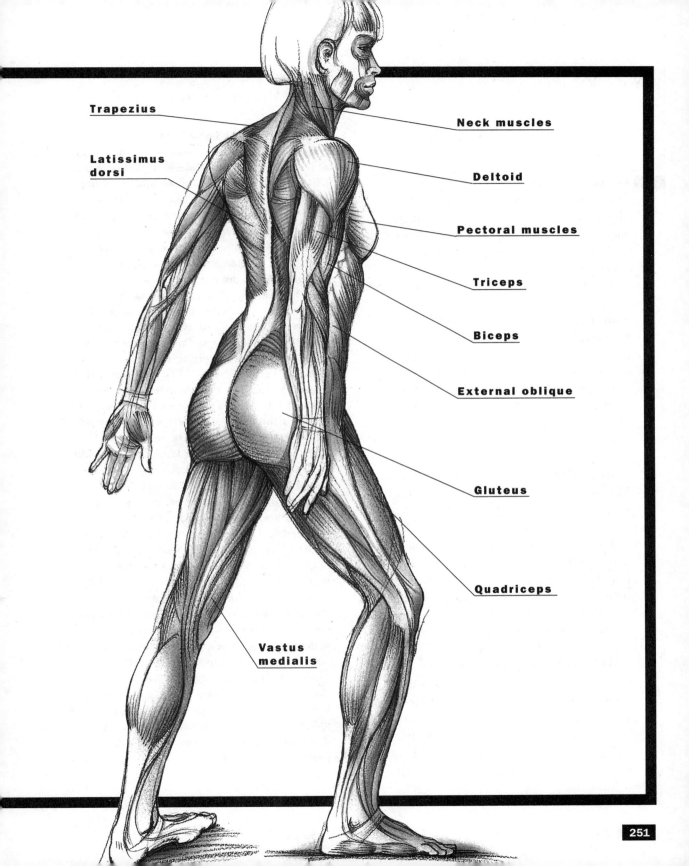

Trapezius

Latissimus
dorsi

Neck muscles

Deltoid

Pectoral muscles

Triceps

Biceps

External oblique

Gluteus

Quadriceps

Vastus
medialis

251

Neck

IN ANCIENT TIMES, people thought the soul lived in the base of the neck. They wore amulets there to ward off evil. Over the years, the amulets turned into necklaces. They lost their soul connection; they turned into the jewelry industry.

Yet the base of the neck is an apt place for the soul. Isn't that where we get choked up with emotion? And a beautiful sunset or a touching look can take our breath away.

Even today, the neck can still use some celestial protection. Consider the burden it carries—a whole head, weighted with brain matter, eyeballs and other odds and ends. "It's like a 14-pound bowling ball on a thin pole," says Annie Pivarski, orthopedic physician's assistant and ergonomics and injury prevention program supervisor at St. Francis Memorial Hospital in San Francisco. "It's subject to the forces of gravity, and it's a difficult area to keep stable."

Besides holding up your head, the neck has a lot of other important assignments. The muscles in your neck help you move your mouth and jaw. It is also a conduit for essential organs and vessels, including the vocal cords, the larynx and the major blood vessels that lead to the brain.

The slender column of the neck is the most vulnerable part of your spine, says Louis Sportelli, D.C., director of public affairs for the American Chiropractic Association and a chiropractor in Palmerton, Pennsylvania. "The neck is just seven small cervical bones— vertebrae—supported only by muscles and ligaments."

Beauty Mistreatment?

The doctor was baffled. Michael Weintraub, M.D., clinical professor of neurology at New York Medical College in Valhalla, had seen five women who all showed symptoms of stroke—and all from an unknown cause. All reported severe dizziness, numbness in the face and a sense of imbalance. Then he found out what they had in common. Each woman said the symptoms first occurred in the beauty parlor, when she bent her head backward over a sink.

Since he first published his findings, Dr. Weintraub has learned of about 75 more cases—all in beauty parlors and hair salons when women were getting shampoos.

When you bend your head backward, that angle compresses certain arteries in the back of the neck. That slows the passage of blood to the brain. The symptoms described by Dr. Weintraub's patients could pass quickly, but if they last a long time, it could mean that the decreased blood flow (ischemia) is severe enough to potentially cause a mild stroke (infarction), he says.

Beauty parlor shampoos aren't the only triggers. Other activities that put the neck in that extreme position, such as painting a ceiling, could produce the same effect, Dr. Weintraub says.

Are you at risk for beauty parlor stroke? You might be if you are developing hardening of the arteries (atherosclerosis) or arthritis in your neck or if you were born with an underdeveloped (hypoplastic) artery. So if you know you have any of these conditions, avoid bending your neck back beyond a 15-degree angle, says Dr. Weintraub. He recommends bending your head forward over the sink when you're getting shampooed.

Like the rest of the spine, the neck has spinal disks nestled in the facet joints between each cervical bone. "Those joints are designed to move," says Scott Haldeman, M.D., D.C., Ph.D., associate clinical professor of neurology at the University of California, Irvine, and adjunct professor at Los Angeles Chiropractic College in Whittier. "The joints get nutrition through movement. The cartilage in the joints doesn't have a blood supply of its own, but the ligaments and the bone have a blood supply bringing nutrients to the joints. The flow of nutrients increases when the joints move."

Basic Neck Rules

We sometimes move our necks all wrong. And when we're deep in concentration, we don't move them at all. That's often how we end up getting a pain in the neck.

"Don't let an episode of neck pain alarm you," says Jeffrey Susman, M.D., member of the U.S. Public Health Service Agency for Health Care Policy and Research and vice-chairman of family medicine at the University of Nebraska College of Medicine in Omaha. "The good news is that 90 percent of the time, you'll be well again within a month. Neck pain does tend to recur, but it's not disabling; it almost always resolves spontaneously. And it's not something that needs extended treatment or evaluation."

Here are two things that you can try to avoid that first episode—or to prevent a recurrence.

Don't stick your neck out. You stick your neck out hundreds of times a day, says Wayne Rath, P.T., co-director of Summit Physical Therapy in Syracuse, New York. "You get up in the morning, and you poke your head up out of bed. You brush your teeth, and you poke your head forward over the sink. When you eat, you poke your head forward, too."

Then, if you sit at a desk or work over a table, you round your shoulders and tilt your head and neck forward again. That angle plays havoc with the ligaments in the back of your neck and upper back, as they strain to hold their unnatural position. No wonder your neck protests—with stiffness, pain or a crick.

Some New Nods for a Nimbler Neck

You're being cruel to your neck if you hold it in one position too long or keep it under strain. Try this exercise recommended by Annie Pivarski, orthopedic physician's assistant and ergonomics and injury prevention program supervisor at St. Francis Memorial Hospital in San Francisco. She suggests that you do it to keep your neck limber—and at the end of every day to relieve stress.

1. Use a mirror and look straight ahead, with your ears aligned over your shoulders.

2. Slowly drop your head toward your chest and hold for 30 seconds. Then return your head to starting position.

3. Slowly rotate your head to the left as far as you comfortably can, and hold it there for 30 seconds. Return to the starting position.

4. Rotate your head to the right side and hold for 30 seconds. Return to the starting position.

5. Slowly drop your left ear toward your left shoulder; hold for 30 seconds. Return to the starting position.

6. Drop your right ear to your right shoulder, hold for 30 seconds and return to the starting position.

To prevent that protest, remember that the neck is least stressed when you have your ears aligned over your shoulders, not in front of them. Whenever possible, try to keep your head lined up in that position to avoid neck ache, suggests Rath.

Move it. You're caught up in a movie, a Scrabble game, a book. You don't move a muscle. But not moving is a bad move, too. In addition to slouching and sticking our necks out, "holding a static position is one of the worst crimes that women commit against their necks," says Pivarski.

When you don't move your neck, the ligaments tighten and your neck stiffens up, says Dr. Haldeman. The lubrication to the joints of your neck begins to decrease. Parched, the tissue fibers stick together and move only grudgingly. So whatever you're doing, take a break now and then to mobilize your neck and get the fluids flowing again.

Kicking the Cricks from Desk Work

Most of the desk work we do is a period of purgatory for our necks. In fact, people who spend their days behind a desk lose about 30 percent of their neck strength, according to research findings of Wayne Westcott, Ph.D., national strength training consultant for the YMCA.

All neck experts recommend a regular neck break for people who work at their desks all day. "It's important. Take a five-second break, sit up straight and go through two or three flexibility motions," says Philip Paul Tygiel, P.T., owner of Tygiel Physical Therapy in Tucson, Arizona.

In addition, here are some other ways to make your desk work more neck-friendly.

Prop your papers. While some head movement is desirable, you don't want to pivot

Are You Rubbernecking at Work?

It is said that every parent favors one child over the rest. But why do you favor one eyeball over the other?

Turns out, most of us have left-eye or right-eye dominance, according to Emil Pascarelli, M.D., professor of clinical medicine at Columbia Presbyterian Medical Center in New York City. Unless you recognize which eye is dominant, you could be causing neck or shoulder pain without even knowing it.

If you are right-eye dominant, you should avoid reading from pages placed on the left side of a computer terminal, says Dr. Pascarelli. You'll be constantly over-twisting as you try to bring that page into view. It's the over-twisting of your neck that can lead to shoulder pain as well as neck pain, he says.

To find out whether you are right- or left-eye dominant, try a simple test described by Dr. Pascarelli. Holding both arms straight in front of you, press the index fingers and thumbs of each hand together to form a small, square hole. Bend your arms and "pull" the hole towards your eyes, while gazing at a single object. Whatever eye your hands go towards naturally is your dominant eye.

If you do this test and find that you're right-eye dominant, you may be able to reduce shoulder and neck pain by placing your reading material to the right side of your computer, says Dr. Pascarelli. If you're left-eye dominant, place the material to the left. That way your dominant eye is closest to the material and neck twisting is reduced to a minimum.

your head and rotate your neck all day long. You can buy devices that clip onto your computer to hold your documents at eye level so you don't have to tilt your neck. Or use a slant board, which raises the papers so you don't have to tilt your head as much.

Pivarski thinks that the best technique is to position your documents between the keyboard and the computer monitor. "Then you can just glance up at the screen, instead of rotating your head to one side all day."

Eyeball the computer. While some experts believe that looking down may be easy on your eyes, others think it's easier to look straight ahead because you maintain the alignment of your neck. The idea is to keep the head in a relaxed, neutral position, according to Dr. Susman.

Stretch the other way. If you do turn your head to one side frequently—to sip a drink, look out the window or grab the phone—make sure you also turn your head in the opposite direction from time to time, says Pivarski. If you have a water bottle on your right, for instance, swap it to the other side of the computer for half the day. Or, if you just automatically turn to the right a lot, take a break, turn your head to the left and hold for 30 seconds.

Pillow Talk

Since most of us sleep on pillows, we need to entrust our necks to reliable ones. Some pillows are neck nightmares. Sleeping with no pillow is reasonable if you're sleeping on your back, according to John E. Dunn, M.D., clinical professor of orthopedic surgery at the University of Washington School of Medicine in Seattle.

The best sleeping position mirrors—horizontally—the best standing position. When you lie down tonight, notice whether each ear is directly lined up with each shoulder. That's the way it should be. It's important that your head is aligned with your shoulders and body, whether you're lying on your side or on your back, says Dr. Dunn.

Try sleeping on your back with a pillow beneath your knees. That's the most comfortable position, says Edward Hanley, M.D., chairman of the orthopaedics department at Carolinas Medical Center in Charlotte, North Carolina. "If you can, look at yourself lying down. Your body should make a straight line down the mattress. Just make sure that your pillow doesn't cock your head up, the way some large, foam-filled pillows do."

Here are some other ideas to make your neck more comfortable all night long.

Coddle your head. Pillows made especially for neck comfort and support come in a number of variations. Some full-size pillows have separate sections to support both the head and the neck. Others have elevated neck-roll sections or indentations for the neck.

Audition a neck pillow. For easy neck rest when you're sitting in a car or plane, check out the curve-shaped pillows that hold your neck in place. With one of those, even if you doze off while you're traveling, your head won't fall over to one side.

Where to shop? Many catalog companies that specialize in bedding (such as the Company Store) offer neck pillows. They're also available in medical supply stores or from sources such as Backsaver that specialize in back devices. Or you can make your own by rolling up a towel in cylinder shape. Experiment with different sizes and thicknesses until you find the most comfortable and supportive size.

Getting Stiff-Armed by Stiffness

Every once in a while, out of the blue, you wake up with a stiff neck. It's like a fly in the house. How did it get in? What's it doing here?

If you like quick, sure answers, better not hold your breath. Doctors aren't sure what a stiff neck is, much less what causes one.

"The traditional orthopedic thinking is that stiff necks happen when muscles spasm so hard that they tear some of the fibers. But to be honest, I'm not really sure about that," says Dr. Dunn.

Experts have made some good guesses, however. They suspect that bad posture (especially at a desk), an awkward sleeping position and stress are possible causes.

Whatever is prompting your stiffness, here's what doctors recommend for relief.

Wait it out. "It won't last long," says Dr. Dunn. "If the pain is killing you, take aspirin or acetaminophen to break the pain spasm cycle." Just follow the directions on the label.

Wash that crick right out of your neck. A long, hot shower may provide a balm of relief, as long as the pain is not acute. Just stand under the shower head and let it rain warmth on your neck, suggests Pivarski. "It relaxes the muscles in the neck."

Or go cold. "There's a lot of controversy about whether to use ice or heat for neck pain," says Dr. Hanley. If the pain gets worse, you might try an ice pack or an ice bag wrapped in a towel. "In general, acute pain responds better to ice."

Wrap a bag of ice or an ice pack in a towel and press it to the sore area of your neck for about ten minutes. Take 20-minute breaks between treatments, so your skin doesn't get numb from the cold, adds Dr. Hanley.

Whipping Whiplash

Jokers call it "litigation neurosis," but whiplash is no joke if you have it. If you get rear-ended in a car accident, there's a good chance that you'll end up with the tender, swollen neck and the pain that come with whiplash. It happens when the violent motion of a collision throws the neck forward and backward, usually straining or spraining the muscles and ligaments in the neck area.

But you can give yourself whiplash, too—and sometimes it doesn't take much. Trying to look cool, for instance: "When young boys started wearing their hair long, they'd flip their heads to get the hair out of their eyes and strain the neck muscles and ligaments similar to a 'whiplash,'" recalls Dr. Sportelli.

Marilyn Kassirer, M.D., assistant clinical professor of neurology at Boston University School of Medicine identified "head bangers' whiplash," caused by eighth-grade dancers jerking their heads to and fro at a dance marathon. Most of the teenage whiplash cases—nine out of ten—were girls, and Dr. Kassirer thinks that is because they had longer hair to whip.

Fortunately, "about 80 percent of mild whiplash pain resolves itself in 1 to 12 weeks," says Dr. Sportelli.

Women wind up with more whiplash than men, though, says Randolph W. Evans, M.D., clinical associate professor of neurology at the University of Texas Medical School at Houston. "The ratio is about 70 percent to 30 percent. The reason might be that women have narrower necks than men." A smaller neck means less muscle mass—so there's simply less support for all the weight of the head.

If your doctor says that you have whiplash, she might prescribe anti-inflammatory medication, limited use of a neck collar and neck exercises to build up strength and flexibility.

Of course, it's best if you never get whiplash. One way to avoid it is to properly adjust the headrest in your car.

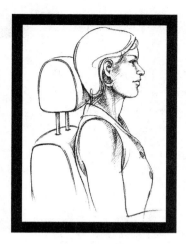

To avoid the risk of whiplash, raise the head-rest to the position shown—so it meets the back curve of your skull.

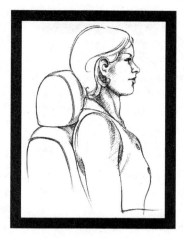

In this position the head-rest is too low and won't prevent your head from snapping backward in a collision.

A headrest isn't something to rest your head against when you're stopped at a red light, Dr. Evans points out. Its original name was "head restraint," and that's exactly what it's meant to do—restrain your head in case of an accident. A properly adjusted head restraint can reduce the incidence of neck pain by 24 percent, according to Dr. Evans. "But 75 percent of all head restraints are left unadjusted, in the down position. And they don't protect a person of average height."

To position the restraint correctly, raise it so the back curve of your skull is against the head cushion. If the cushion is pressing against the upper part of your skull, the restraint is too high, and if it's poised at the nape of your neck, it's too low. Just remember to readjust it when you're a passenger, too, suggests Dr. Evans.

Better Luck with Neck Time

You can tell a woman's age by her neck, says Seth Matarasso, M.D., assistant professor of dermatology at the University of California, San Francisco, School of Medicine. "The fat below the skin on your neck atrophies as you age. That skin gets paper-thin and starts to wrinkle. Sun exposure causes fine lines, too." His advice is to be just as diligent about applying sunscreen on your neck as you are about spreading it on your face or shoulders.

Another way to keep your neck looking younger is to use an exfoliant cream or lotion, such as the prescription drug tretinoin (Retin-A) as a "facial peel." Any products that contain glycolic acid, such as Avon's Anew creams, will "peel" the top thin layer of dead skin cells from the surface of your neck, which minimizes fine lines and makes age blotches or freckles less prominent. "There is some evidence that exfoliants thicken the skin, too," says Dr. Matarasso.

See also Muscular System, Nervous System, Skeletal System

Nervous System

The brain, the spinal cord and the nerves and fibers that extend from the spinal cord to the muscles and internal organs make up the nervous system. All our thoughts, sensations and actions are orchestrated by this system.

■ The **sciatic nerve** is the longest nerve in your body—and sciatica is the popular name given to any disorder that causes pain from that nerve. (To find out how to treat sciatica, and other back pain, see "Sciatica—Pulp Friction" on page 386.)

■ A **pinched nerve** in the back can happen when one of the spongy disks that cushions each part of the backbone bulges or bursts. The swollen or exploded matter can then press against one of the 31 pairs of nerves that spread from the spinal cord. (To keep your spinal disks healthy, read "Dodging Disk Damage" on page 382.)

■ The vulnerable neck is just seven small bones, a few little muscles and ligaments and eight pairs of **cervical nerves** that shout "ouch!" all too often. (To banish the common pain in the neck, see "Basic Neck Rules" on page 253.)

■ If you have a sore neck and shoulders plus weakness in your upper arms and back, you might have **thoracic outlet syndrome**. Women with long, graceful necks develop it the most often. (See "Where Pain and Posture Mix" on page 351.)

■ While you can't make new brain cells, the ones that you have can grow bigger with exercise. And exercise makes brain cells grow not only in the motor areas but also in other areas of the **cerebral cortex**

Where to Look

To find out how to keep your brain sharp and senses alert—and how to keep pain to a minimum—see:

Back	page 9
Brain	page 44
Ears	page 84
Eyes	page 108
Neck	page 252
Pain Relief	page 290
Ribs	page 326
Skin	page 360
Spine	page 379
Tongue	page 411

and in the temporal lobes, where thinking, learning and memory take place. (See "Pumping Up the Power" on page 49.)

■ Scientists have found that many of our memories are stored in the **temporal lobes**, and memory experts have developed techniques to help you pack in even more. (See "Remember the Alamo [and Everything Else]" on page 50.)

■ The ancient seat of emotion and behavior is the **limbic system**. This is the brain area where researchers have discovered important differences between men's and women's brains. Because of the difference in the limbic system, women tend to verbalize, while men are more prone to act. (See "More between the Sexes" on page 49.)

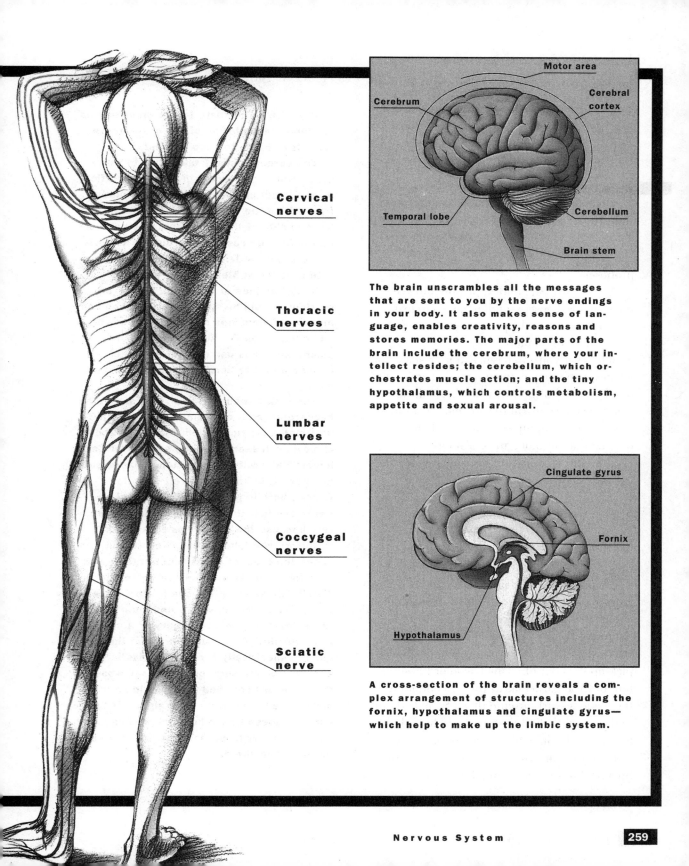

Cervical nerves

Thoracic nerves

Lumbar nerves

Coccygeal nerves

Sciatic nerve

Motor area

Cerebrum

Cerebral cortex

Temporal lobe

Cerebellum

Brain stem

The brain unscrambles all the messages that are sent to you by the nerve endings in your body. It also makes sense of language, enables creativity, reasons and stores memories. The major parts of the brain include the cerebrum, where your intellect resides; the cerebellum, which orchestrates muscle action; and the tiny hypothalamus, which controls metabolism, appetite and sexual arousal.

Cingulate gyrus

Fornix

Hypothalamus

A cross-section of the brain reveals a complex arrangement of structures including the fornix, hypothalamus and cingulate gyrus—which help to make up the limbic system.

Nose

WHAT DO BARBRA STREISAND, Steffi Graf and Anjelica Huston have in common? Besides the fact that they're all powerful and successful women, they share a facial characteristic that's not the vogue: a sizable proboscis.

While Barb, Stef and Anjie opted to keep their outsized noses—and managed to look quite attractive in the process—many women decide that less is more.

Whatever your preference in nose sizes—or whatever the shape of your own—there's a lot to admire about the way it works. This intake chamber has to warm the air that comes in, filter it and pump up the humidity before passing that air along to your lungs.

In addition to heating, moistening and vacuuming, your nose is a notoriously keen-scented sniffer—able to detect a man wearing Aramis, a well-spiced soup or the "change me" signals from a baby's diapers. Those are just a few of the 4,000 or so distinctive odors that your alert schnozz can detect.

The nasal hound dogs that track down fragrance are two smell receptor sites, each about the size of a nickel, stuck way up near the top of the nasal cavity. The scent perception is done by millions of nerve fibers, which pick up the odor of frying bacon or the subtle hint of fresh gardenias as the air containing these odors swirls around them. Signals shout to the sprightly limbic system and hypothalamus in the brain, which quickly sort things out to make sure you don't eat gardenias for breakfast or put bacon in a fresh bouquet.

Is a New Nose Good News?

If you're a candidate for a rhinoplasty operation—resculpturing of the nose—there are a few things to keep in mind.

The surgery usually takes two to three hours and is performed in a doctor's office or at a hospital. Most incisions are made from within the nose, and the bones on the top and side of the nose are broken and adjusted in most cases, according to Victoria Vitale-Lewis, M.D., a plastic surgeon in private practice in Melbourne, Florida.

To get an idea of what your nose's proportions should be, the plastic surgeon can measure dimensions of your forehead, nose and chin, notes Dr. Vitale-Lewis. Some plastic surgeons use computers to get an idea of what the finished product will look like.

The result should fit your face and ethnic background and, most important, look natural, notes Darrick Antell, M.D., assistant clinical professor of plastic surgery at Columbia University and attending plastic surgeon at St. Luke's Roosevelt Hospital Center, both in New York City. "Most patients say that their friends couldn't even tell, because the result was so natural."

Before you take the leap you should check the credentials of your surgeon with your local county medical society, notes Dr. Antell. "Make sure that she is a board-certified plastic surgeon with a minimum of three years of general surgery or a similar prerequisite." Also make sure that the surgeon is specifically certified in plastic surgery. "Some surgeons don't say what they're board certified in—it could be in podiatry," he notes. A warning signal: If the surgeon doesn't have hospital privileges for plastic surgery, it probably means that she's not board certified.

Appearances, Appearances

Too often, though, we're too busy critiquing the nose's exterior to pause and praise its inside work. In fact, when it comes to major reconstruction, many women like to do a major number on their noses. Rhinoplasty, commonly referred to as a nose job, is the fifth most popular plastic surgery performed on 30- to 50-year-old women in the United States.

Many people who want nose jobs have a bump on the nasal bridge that you can see from the side, notes Victoria Vitale-Lewis, M.D., a plastic surgeon in private practice in Melbourne, Florida. Rather than give women tiny pixie noses the way surgeons did in the 1950s, the trend is to go for the natural look. "In the past, a lot of times, doctors used to oversculpt the nose. Now we only take down some of the hump until it's straight and put the tip out a little bit," she notes. "It's not scooped out or phony-looking."

No One Knows the Trouble It Sees

The poor nose. It's blown, rubbed, subjected to smoke, air pollution and dry air and picked and scratched almost on a daily basis.

The problem with your proboscis is often with the mucous membrane that lines the interior of the nose and is covered with minute hairlike projections called cilia. Blood vessels in the nasal cavity are the space heaters that warm the air to about 95°F. For the cleaning work, you have mucous membranes, which secrete about a quart of gooey mucus every day, plus millions of cilia. Cilia are relentless mucus movers, thrashing away at all that goop at the rate of 12 to 15 beats per second as they move it along toward the throat. Like a miniature wet-dry vacuum, the moving mucus flushes away dust and debris and is swallowed, so it steers clear of your pollution-sensitive lungs.

"The lining of the nose is quite thin. In cases where the air is dry or the lining becomes irritated, it may be the source of bleeding," notes Anthony J. Yonkers, M.D., professor and chairman of the Department of Otolaryngology–Head and Neck Surgery at the University of Nebraska Medical Center in Omaha. "The result can be a wide range of troubles ranging from crusting to recurrent bouts of bleeding."

Although most nosebleeds tend to be spotters rather than frightening gushers, they can still be annoying. Here are a few tips to stop them before they start.

Humidify. Using a hot-air humidifier in the bedroom helps keep the nasal tissues moist, notes Alexander C. Chester, M.D., clinical professor of medicine at Georgetown University Medical Center in Washington, D.C. "Many of the new office buildings have no humidifiers at all, so you could bring a humidifier to work as well."

Pass the jelly. Wiping a thin layer of petroleum jelly just inside the nose is another good membrane moistener, notes Dr. Chester. Another solution is a bacteria-killing ointment such as mupirocin (Bactroban). It's only available through prescription.

Measure your pressure. If you get chronic nosebleeds, it is important to have your blood pressure checked, says Dr. Yonkers, "Nosebleeds may be an indicator of high blood pressure."

Pinch an inch. If bleeding does occur, despite preventive measures, Dr. Yonkers recommends holding your head level while pinching your nose closed with the thumb

Sniff Power

The nose knows disrespect. Few people doubt the importance of the sense of hearing or sight, and even taste and touch are considered vital to quality of life. But smell? Well—so what if you can't smell a rose or a cake baking in the oven, right?

That's what Immanuel Kant thought, anyway. In the hierarchy of the senses, the idealist German philosopher rated smell last. Unlike sight, hearing and touch, which really tell it like it is, said Kant, the sense of smell is purely subjective.

Smell has to do with more than superficial things such as perfume and potpourri. It's a powerful link with our emotions and memories, says Alan Hirsch, M.D., psychiatrist, neurologist and neurological director of the Smell and Taste Treatment and Research Foundation in Chicago. "The quickest and surest way to produce an emotional response is with smell."

What's in a Sniffer?

We actually have two olfactory (smell) systems. One is connected to the conscious part of the brain. The second goes to the limbic system of the brain, which is directly connected to our emotions and to the unconscious.

To understand smell, you have to know the nose. Its most vital function is to perform warm-up for the respiratory system. As you breathe, your nose raises the temperature of the air to 95°F and filters dust and debris through its mucus.

Two postage stamp–size smell receptor sites are located at the top of the upper chamber of the nasal cavities, packed with five million yellowish hairlike fibers. When you smell, air swirls over these nerve fibers and is registered in the limbic system and the hypothalamus of the brain.

It's this direct connection with the limbic system, or the emotional part of the brain, that causes scent to stir up visceral reactions in people, notes Dr. Hirsch. After all, who can catch a whiff of floor wax and chalk dust without thinking of grade school? And doesn't the smell of a certain aftershave bring back memories?

Such responses are especially strong in women, whose sense of smell is more discerning than that of men. If you have a normal female nose—and are free of the sniffles—you can detect about 4,000 different odors on a good day.

In a survey he did of 989 people from 45 states and 39 countries, Dr. Hirsch discovered that nostalgic odors vary depending on a number of factors. Among the variables were gender, birthplace and year of birth.

Men, he found, tended to remember the smell of meat barbecuing, while women recalled the smell of baked bread. People born before 1930 remembered more natural smells, such as pine, roses, manure and hay, while those born between 1930 and 1980 recalled more artificial smells, such as Play-Doh, crayons and Windex.

Besides the link with our emotions, the sense of smell has practical applications. Try eating an apple with your nose pinched shut. For all you know, you could be eating an onion. Smell is responsible for 90 percent of our sense of taste, notes Dr. Hirsch.

And don't forget being able to sniff out spoiled milk or leaking gas or even the odor of a baby's soiled diapers.

More to It Than Meets the Nose

An innate preference for certain smells is an instinct that kicks in at birth. In a research study of 30 infants, 22 chose an unwashed nipple over a washed one while breastfeeding. Researchers concluded that the babies were responding to attractive odors produced by glands in the unwashed breast.

That blind date you found very attractive but nonetheless weren't attracted to? Blame your crass indifference on pheromones, those subtle scents we emit that attract or repel humans of the opposite sex. "It could go back to what was imprinted in your emotional brain while you breastfed," says Robert Francoeur, Ph.D., professor of human sexuality at Fairleigh Dickinson University in Madison, New Jersey, and co-author of The Scent of Eros. "You could react to a similar smell later in life."

In fact, many doctors also link what could arguably be called the most important application of all—sexual attraction—to the sense of smell. It's a fact of life in animal circles. Male moths, for instance, can be driven to distraction by the sex attractant chemical that's produced by a female from two miles away.

and forefinger of one hand. With your other hand, hold a towel or handkerchief under your nostrils to stop the dripping. If bleeding persists after 10 to 15 minutes, seek a doctor's help, he says. If all else fails, doctors can pack your nose with gauze or with water-filled balloons that help stop the bleeding. But don't try to do this yourself, doctors caution.

Grab a towel and cubes. A towel soaked in cold water or an ice bag pressed to the back of the neck can ease the bleed as well, notes Dr. Yonkers.

A Swollen Lining

Another troublemaker is the nasal polyp, a benign growth in the mucous membrane of the nose that can lead to sinusitis and nasal obstruction, notes David Zwillenberg, M.D., otolaryngologist at Thomas Jefferson University Hospital in Philadelphia.

"It's an inflammatory reaction. The lining of the nose gets so swollen from irritation that it herniates downward. I've seen them so big that they hang down from the back of the throat," he says.

About half of all polyps develop as the result of an allergy, so managing sniffles and congestion is a key to treatment, notes Dr. Zwillenberg.

Another polyp aggravator is aspirin, notes Dr. Chester. "Some people with polyps are highly sensitive to aspirin as well as certain dyes and foods such as apples, melons and citrus fruit. They should be aware of it and use Tylenol."

Often, polyps can be treated with a nasal steroid that's injected in the area where the polyps are growing. They can also be removed surgically, but about 50 percent of the time, they'll grow back.

Common-Scents Advice
for Improving Your Life

To think that all this time you've been wasting your time dabbing Chanel No. 5 behind your ears and wrists! All you really had to do was dig into a slice of pumpkin pie and rub it in.

That's right—the way to a man's heart really is through his stomach. That's just one of the fragrant tidbits that Alan Hirsch, M.D., psychiatrist, neurologist and neurological director of the Smell and Taste Treatment and Research Foundation in Chicago, has uncovered during his study of scents.

On the other hand, scents are so powerful, there may be times when you don't want to use them, notes Dr. Hirsch.

If you have a job interview or want to impress a male boss, it's better to wear no scent at all, he says. "Otherwise, they could interpret it as your trying to manipulate them."

Here are some other details on the ways that scent can affect the course of relationships . . . and other things.

Love life. Measuring penile blood flow of men wearing masks scented with various odors, Dr. Hirsch discovered that pumpkin pie mixed with lavender was tops—causing a 40 percent increase in blood flow.

Doughnuts and black licorice were also turn-ons—causing a 32 percent increase, with the combination of doughnuts and pumpkin pie stirring up a 20 percent increase. On the other hand, floral perfume only speeded things up a measly 3½ percent.

Why does food work such magic? It's probably because such odors elicit vivid, fond memories of the past, notes Dr. Hirsch. It might also have to do with the fact that, throughout history, people congregated at the sites of food kills, which is where they had the best chance of meeting a mate and procreating. (Which doesn't explain the pumpkin pie phenomenon—unless our ancestors did a lot of their necking on Thanksgiving.)

Learning. A mixed floral scent doubles the rate of learning, notes Dr. Hirsch, so if you have a job where you're constantly having to take in new information, try wearing a mixed floral perfume.

Room size. If you have a small office or apartment and want people to perceive it as larger, try a green apple scent or a cucumber scent. For some reason, one or the other of these scents makes rooms seem larger.

On the other hand, barbecue-smoke scent makes a room seem smaller.

Relaxation. Lavender increases alpha waves in the back of the brain and helps relieve stress. On the flip side, jasmine stirs up beta waves in the front of the brain and makes you more alert and awake.

Weight loss. Can scents make you eat less? Dr. Hirsch says maybe. For six months 3,193 people were given blasts of green apple, banana or peppermint spray whenever they were hungry. For people who inhaled between 18 and 285 sniffs a day, the average weight loss was five pounds a month. One reason it works is

A Whiff of That
Special Someone

The same type of chemical that drives a male moth mad with longing could also have the desired effect on the male of your choice. A lot of it is in the pheromones, scientists say.

A pheromone is a hormone-derived aromatic messenger that subconsciously influences the sexual development and behavior of a species of animal. It's also a big player on the sexual stage.

In the brain, pheromones influence the production of gonadotropin-releasing hormone (GnRH), which is responsible for starting the cycle of sex hormones that originate in the pituitary gland and filter down to the adrenal glands, ovaries and testes.

Although we can't smell them, pheromones have a subconscious influence over us, notes Robert Francoeur, Ph.D., professor of human sexuality at Fairleigh Dickinson University in Madison,

New Jersey, and co-author of *The Scent of Eros*.

An example of their effect? Well, consider how women living in the same dorm room begin to have synchronized menstrual cycles, notes Dr. Francoeur. "They're constantly smelling the pheromones of the other women, and the woman with the dominant scent becomes the point of synchronization for all the other women."

What effect does smell have on the love act itself? Dr. Hirsch says that it rates right up there with the water bed and candles. "During sexual excitement, the nose gets engorged and one starts to breathe through the mouth. This means that you have a better ability to detect odors at that time."

Another scent-sational fact: Some 90 percent of people who lost their sense of smell through head injury reported some sexual dysfunction, says Dr. Hirsch.

that the brain interprets the amount you've smelled as the amount you've eaten, Dr. Hirsch notes.

Exercise. Whiffing the scents of strawberries and buttered popcorn increases the number of calories you burn in a three-minute period, notes Dr. Hirsch. "It could

be that they distract you or reduce your level of fatigue. In theory, you could put a bowl of strawberries or buttered popcorn near your treadmill."

Sleeplessness. Lavender increases alpha waves, which make people more relaxed and help them fall asleep quicker.

A Bad Curve?

Another nose plugger is the deviated septum. The septum is the partition separating the two nasal cavities from each other, and you have the condition known as deviated septum when that partition is bent or twisted.

The most common problem resulting from deviated septum is an inability to breathe well through the nose, which can cause problems with snoring and dry mouth, notes Randy Oppenheimer, M.D., clinical instructor of otolaryngology at the University of California, San Diego. How easy is a diagnosis? "We just look up with a nasal speculum, and we can tell in one second. It's a very common problem. A lot of people have deviated septums and don't even know it."

To straighten a deviated septum, doctors remove or restructure the pieces of cartilage and bone that are causing blockage. It's a simple hour-long procedure done on an outpatient basis, notes Dr. Oppenheimer.

See also Respiratory System

Nutrition

RIGHT NOW, OVER 50 TRILLION tiny cells—collectively known as you—are humming away to keep you alive. All they ask? A little exercise, water—and food!

Give them junk food, and they're resourceful enough to keep you going—for a while. But give them healthy fare and your payoff is terrific. You feel and look your best. Your energy brims. Plus, you help keep at bay problems such as heart disease, cancer, osteoporosis, diabetes and overweight—major conditions that can impair or end a woman's life.

If you think healthy eating takes too much time or requires strategizing or giving up favorite foods, relax. Down-to-earth advice from experts—designed for women who live in the real world—makes healthy eating hassle-free. Read on and see for yourself.

Getting with the Good-Health Program

What's a great first step to the healthiest diet? Striking a smart balance among carbohydrates, protein and fat, says Doris Derelian, R.D., Ph.D., president of the American Dietetic Association. All these major food ingredients provide us with calories for energy. But studies around the world show that diets low in fat but high in carbohydrates are linked to the lowest rates of heart disease. These diets are also associated with people who have the lowest rates of some cancers.

That's why experts take a hard look at the overly abundant amount of fat that most women get in their diets. When you look at the statistics, you have to ask yourself: Why are we raising our risks by eating more fat than is good for us?

One way to measure fat is by asking how many of our total calories come from calories of fat. Studies show that Americans get about 34 percent of their calories from fat. That means many of us are getting more than one-third of our total calories from the fat in foods such as salad dressings, hamburgers, potato chips, french fries and high-fat desserts and snacks.

That would be fine if it were healthy to live on a diet that's one-third fat. But health is not being dealt a strong hand when fat intake is that high. Instead, this is the kind of fat intake that puts us at high risk for heart disease, certain kinds of cancer and other problems. What we should be getting, says Holly McCord, R.D., nutrition editor for *Prevention* magazine in Emmaus, Pennsylvania, is a maximum of 25 percent of total calories from fat.

Equally important, women need to boost carbohydrates (from vegetables, fruit and whole grains, not from sugar or white flour) to 55 percent of calories—or even more, says McCord. That leaves protein providing 15 to 20 percent of calories.

Trouble is, no woman sits down to a hearty meal of percents. The female body needs food. So how do you translate all those numbers into menus without resorting to a computer? You use the easy-to-follow *Prevention* 3-2-1 Plan.

Three Times a Day, Get with the Plan

Here's how the 3-2-1 Plan works. Simply think of your day in 3 segments—breakfast and morning, lunch and afternoon and dinner and evening. Then, sometime during each segment, make sure you get your "3-2-1." That means, try to eat three servings of a starchy vegetable such as potatoes or legumes (beans, dried peas or lentils) or a food made from grain (preferably a whole grain). Also have two servings of fruit or nonstarchy vegetables and one serving of either low-fat meat, fish, poultry or beans or a low-fat or nonfat dairy food. (To learn what constitutes a serving, see "3-2-1 Servings" on page 268.) Throughout your day, make sure that you use low-fat or fat-free condiments.

You don't have to eat all your 3-2-1 servings at one meal. Here's an example of how one lunch/afternoon segment might go. Say you had a turkey sandwich with tomato slices on whole-wheat bread for lunch—that's two grains (two slices of bread), one vegetable (two big tomato slices) and one meat (sliced turkey). Later, you could have a handful of whole-wheat pretzels and an apple for a mid-afternoon snack—that's one more grain and one fruit Thus your total for this segment of the day is three grains, one vegetable plus one fruit and one meat. You've hit your 3-2-1 goal!

Here's why the 3-2-1 Plan puts you ahead of the nutrition game.

- It automatically steers you to the right ratio of carbohydrates, protein and fat as the day progresses—provided you choose low-fat meats, dairy products and condiments.
- It makes it easy for you to keep a mental note of your "score" as the day goes along by dividing your eating into three "3-2-1" segments.
- It apportions your food intake evenly throughout the day, which helps keep your energy level brimming and your appetite under control.

- It ensures that you get a minimum total of six servings of nutrient-rich fruits and vegetables and nine servings of grains (preferably whole grains) or legumes every day. If you're still hungry, make extra fruits and veggies your first choice for snacks, suggests McCord.

Vitamins and Minerals Women Need Most

To keep you ticking, your food must deliver much more than calories. Your body requires precious substances called vitamins and minerals—essential players in the countless chemical reactions that make life possi-

3-2-1 Servings

Prevention magazine's 3-2-1 Plan makes it easy to ensure that your daily diet includes the right proportions of carbohydrates, protein and fat. During each segment of the day—morning, afternoon and evening—be sure to have three servings from the first group, two from the next two groups and one from the last two groups. The following lists show what counts as one serving in the 3-2-1 Plan.

3 Servings

Grain/Legume/Starchy Vegetable Group

- **1 slice bread**
- **½ hamburger bun, bagel or English muffin**
- **1 ounce ready-to-eat cereal**
- **½ cup cooked rice, pasta or noodles**
- **½ cup cooked cereal**
- **1 ounce pretzels (a small handful)**
- **1 small baked potato**
- **½ cup cooked beans, lentils or split peas**

2 Servings

Fruit Group

- **1 medium fruit (apple, banana, orange)**
- **½ cup berries or cut-up fruit**
- **½ cup cooked or canned fruit**
- **¾ cup fruit juice**

Nonstarchy Vegetable Group

- **1 cup raw leafy vegetables (lettuce, spinach)**
- **½ cup cooked vegetables**
- **½ cup chopped raw vegetables**
- **¾ cup vegetable juice**

1 Serving

Dairy Group

- **1 cup skim or 1 percent low-fat milk**
- **1 cup low-fat or nonfat yogurt**
- **2 slices low-fat or fat-free cheese (about 1½ ounces total)**

Meat/Poultry/Fish/Eggs

- **2 to 3 ounces cooked extra-lean beef, fish or skinless poultry (about the size of a deck of cards)**
- **½ cup cholesterol-free egg substitute**
- **1 cup cooked dried beans**

ble. Some minerals such as calcium are needed for body-building material, too.

The 3-2-1 Plan helps you meet crucial vitamin and mineral needs. But study after study shows that even careful eaters may come up short on certain micronutrients—nutrients that are important to your health even though they're found in extremely minute amounts in food. Women are especially at risk of getting less of these micronutrients than they need, says Margo Woods, D.Sc., who teaches nutrition at Tufts University School of Medicine in Boston.

We have this shortage partly because our food intake is small—often 1,800 or fewer calories per day. Yet studies have found that even registered dietitians find it tough to design low-fat diets that meet all of an adult woman's vitamin and mineral requirements without exceeding 2,200 calories—more than most women need.

Another problem is that some women have become super-conscientious about cutting out fat—but they've totally forgotten about choosing the rest of their foods wisely. "Women have to remember that their diets are about more than just fat," says Dr. Derelian.

So here's the bottom line: It's crucial for females to choose foods dense with vitamins and minerals. "I know it's easy to come home after a stressful day and say, 'I need to take care of myself with a brownie.' But what you really could do to take care of yourself is eat a banana and drink a glass of milk. Try to satisfy your emotional hunger, knowing that you've treated your body with respect and love," says Dr. Woods.

You might need to go the extra mile to get some of the vitamins and minerals that women need, but it's worth it. These important nutrients include calcium combined with

Calcium Champs

To get hearty doses of calcium, you need to choose foods that are champs in providing this crucial mineral. Experts recommend that premenopausal women have 1,000 milligrams per day—entirely from food sources, if possible.

The following foods have 300 milligrams of calcium (30 percent of the Daily Value) per serving or more. You'll want to aim for three servings a day to get all the calcium you need. Here are some of your top choices.
- **1 serving instant breakfast drink made with nonfat milk**
- **1 cup nonfat or low-fat yogurt**
- **1 cup nonfat or 1 percent low-fat milk**
- **1 cup buttermilk**
- **1 cup nonfat lactose-reduced milk**
- **2 one-ounce slices fat-free or low-fat cheese**
- **1 cup calcium-fortified orange juice**
- **2 slices light calcium-enriched bread**
- **1 cup calcium-fortified soy or rice beverage**
- **1 cup pudding made from mix**

enough vitamin D, folic acid and the antioxidant vitamins: vitamin A (as beta-carotene), vitamin C and vitamin E. There are a few others as well—vitamin B_6, zinc and iron—that are only found in certain foods. But you need them all, according to Dr. Woods.

Should You Double Your Calcium?

Researchers say that half of all women over age 50 will suffer from osteoporosis—gradual bone loss that proceeds so stealthily that it's been called the silent crippler. People with osteoporosis lose so much bone mass and, as a result, calcium (a vital component of our skeletons), that their bones break with just a slight bump. How can you prevent this? One important way is by getting enough calcium before menopause begins. Experts believe this helps keep bones in the strongest state to withstand the rapid bone loss of menopause.

Yet most women get only half the 1,000 milligrams of calcium a day before age 50 recommended by the National Institutes of Health. Admittedly, consuming that much calcium takes planning. The best strategy? Eat three servings a day of foods high in calcium, suggests McCord.

If—in spite of good intentions—you don't get three Calcium Champs daily, make up any shortfall with a calcium supplement, suggests Robert Heaney, M.D., professor of medicine at Creighton University School of Medicine in Omaha, Nebraska. Many women take 500 milligrams a day.

Calcium needs an assistant to make sure that you absorb as much as your bones need: That's why you also require 400 international units (IUs) of vitamin D per day. Once again, studies show that many women probably aren't getting enough.

Actually, your body can make its own vitamin D if enough sunlight strikes your skin. But if you're putting on sunscreen to prevent skin damage (which is certainly advisable), you're also blocking the sun power that helps your body make this "sunshine vitamin." So—are we getting enough sunshine to keep us from being D-ficient? For some women, busy schedules and SPF 15 sunscreens may make it iffy.

Here's another problem with vitamin D: It's not widely distributed in food. Some of the best sources include an eight-ounce glass

More Boost for Your Bones

If you can't get all the calcium you need from food, it helps to have some supplement savvy. Here are tips from Robert Heaney, M.D., professor of medicine at Creighton University School of Medicine in Omaha, Nebraska, to help you get the most boost for your bones.

- To know how much calcium you're getting, check the label for the amount of calcium per tablet.
- Take your calcium supplement at bedtime. Experts say this may help protect bones from calcium loss while you sleep.
- If you take more than 500 milligrams in a supplement, divide your dose for best absorption. For instance, take a 500-milligram tablet in the morning and another 500 milligrams at night.
- Which supplement should you choose? Calcium carbonate is best absorbed with food. Calcium citrate can be taken on an empty stomach.
- Avoid bonemeal, dolomite and any calcium carbonate supplements labeled "oyster shell" or "natural." They often cost more than other supplements, but they aren't any better.
- Don't take supplements with more than 2,000 milligrams in a day unless your doctor prescribes it.
- If you have kidney stones, or if you've had them in the past, you should check with your doctor before taking any amount of calcium in a supplement.

of milk, which is fortified with 100 IU of vitamin D, and some breakfast cereals, which are also are D-fortified (check the label for the amount). For insurance, Dr. Heaney says a multi-supplement with 100 percent of the Daily Value (DV) for vitamin D isn't a bad idea. (Regular intakes should not exceed 600 IUs per day, however.)

Don't Forget Folate

Here's a common micronutrient shortfall that all women of childbearing age should want to reverse, says Dr. Woods. American women are getting only half the 400 micrograms of folic acid—the supplement form of folate—now recommended by the U.S. Public Health Service to prevent serious brain and spinal cord defects in newborn babies. If you try to make up the shortfall after you're pregnant, it may be too late. The defects that are related to lack of this B vitamin occur in the first two weeks of pregnancy, before a woman may realize she has conceived.

Pregnancy aside, doctors say that folate may have some protective benefits for your own health. Researchers have found that women who lack folate in their diets may increase their risks of heart disease and colon and cervical cancer.

Where should the extra folate come from? Food is always the best source of any nutrient, including folate, says McCord. Foods with 100 micrograms or more of folate include eight ounces of orange juice from frozen concentrate, one serving of certain fortified breakfast cereals (check labels to find out if cereals are fortified), one cup of raw spinach and a half-cup of cooked asparagus.

Many health authorities agree that it may be difficult for women to get enough of this superstar vitamin in their daily diets. So you might need a daily supplement to provide the sensible backup insurance you need. Walter Willet, M.D., Ph.D., chairman of the Department of Nutrition at Harvard Medical School, recommends a multi supplement with 400 micrograms of folic acid, which is 100 percent of the DV. On the label, folic acid is sometimes also identified as folate or folacin.

Be Pro-Antioxidant

Antioxidant vitamins have been on the health scene for decades, but lately, they seem to have exciting new careers. The stars of the show are vitamin A, which comes from beta-carotene in food sources, vitamin C and vitamin E.

Nutrition science has known for years that each of these vitamins plays a crucial role in the body. Yet even though we know a lot about them, more is being discovered all the time. Vitamin A is vital for eyesight and keeping the skin healthy, while vitamin C helps keep blood vessels and immune systems strong. As for vitamin E, nutritionists have always called it an antioxidant, but they know that this vitamin is critically important.

What's the big deal? Simply this: Antioxidants have the power to neutralize fast-moving, submicroscopic particles called free radicals. Like manic roadrunners looking for trouble, free radicals zip through living cells, accelerating a chain reaction that puts cell deterioration into fast forward.

Free radicals are produced continuously in our bodies by perfectly natural internal processes. Their numbers are multiplied drastically by outside forces such as air pollution, cigarette smoke and sunlight.

Once formed, free radicals are highly unstable, reacting with healthy body tissue and causing cell damage as they speed up the chemical process called oxidation. It's now known that this damage may lead to serious illness such as cancer and the clogged arteries of heart disease. At the same time, oxidation may also speed up the aging process.

Unless, that is, the antioxidants come to our rescue by reacting with free radicals before they can react with us. If we have enough beta-carotene, vitamin C and vitamin E inside our bodies, free radicals can be quenched before they wreak too much oxidative havoc.

Studies show that people whose diets are rich in foods that contain antioxidant vitamins often have lower rates of heart disease, lung and colon cancers, cataracts and stroke. Among the richest sources of these vitamins are fruits and vegetables. In fact, the antioxidant-rich foods are so protective that the National Cancer Institute recommends you try to eat at least one food that's high in beta-carotene and one food high in vitamin C every day.

Mega sources of beta-carotene (which our bodies turn into vitamin A) are carrots, pumpkin, sweet potatoes, spinach, collard greens, winter squash and cantaloupe. The DV for vitamin A is 5,000 IUs, and to get that much, you need to consume three milligrams of beta-carotene. It's possible (though not proven) that supplements of beta-carotene at higher levels may be beneficial, and researchers are testing amounts up to 50 milligrams. But experts don't know the full effect of beta-carotene at that level.

They do know, however, that taking excessive amounts of preformed vitamin A at 15,000 IUs can be toxic. Women who are pregnant or trying to conceive should be especially careful about taking vitamin A. One study showed that consuming more than 10,000 IUs of vitamin A a day can cause a variety of birth defects including cleft lip,

cleft palate, hydrocephalus and heart defects. Consuming large amounts of beta-carotene does not seem to have the same effect.

Superstar food sources of vitamin C include oranges, orange juice, grapefruit and

A Nutritional Safety Net

You missed lunch because your meeting ran long. Or you ate a pint of frozen chocolate yogurt in place of dinner last night. Or—simply because you're a woman—your appropriate calorie intake may be too low to supply you with the vitamins and minerals you need.

What's the best solution when you have a shortfall in your diet? First, eat the most nutrient-dense foods you can. They'll deliver a potent mixture of protective compounds, many of which you can't get anywhere else. Second, you can turn to supplements for an extra helping of nutrients.

"Especially for women, a balanced multivitamin-mineral supplement makes sense," says Walter Willett, M.D., Ph.D., chairman of the Department of Nutrition at Harvard Medical School. "Don't substitute it for a healthy diet. Think of it as a small insurance policy against nutritional gaps that are beyond your control."

What kind of supplement should you choose? Look for one with close to 100 percent of the Daily Value for most vitamins and minerals. Just remember: No single-dose multi will have 100 percent of the DV for calcium. Such a pill would be far too big to swallow. So even if you're taking a multi, make sure you're getting enough calcium from food or take a separate calcium supplement.

grapefruit juice. Other sources are red bell peppers, kiwifruit, strawberries, broccoli, brussels sprouts and cantaloupe.

For vitamin C the DV is 60 milligrams. There's some evidence that taking in higher levels of vitamin C may confer protection against heart disease, some cancers and secondhand cigarette smoke. Supplements of vitamin C up to 500 milligrams a day appear to be safe, says Dr. Willet.

As for the third antioxidant, vitamin E, it's hard to get enough of it in a healthy, low-fat diet. That's because vitamin E is mainly found in high-fat nuts and vegetable oils. As a result, some health experts think it makes sense to take vitamin E supplements—and they often recommend levels above the DV of 30 IUs.

Two large studies have linked taking vitamin E supplements of 100 IUs or more to a 40 percent reduced risk of heart disease. Supplements up to 400 IUs a day appear to be safe, according to Dr. Willet. But if you're taking blood-thinning medicine, you should first check with your doctor before taking a vitamin E supplement.

Mining More Micros

A number of vitamins and minerals are major-league players in our bodies even though they come in micro quantities in our food. Among the core group of micronutrients that women often need more of are vitamin B_6, zinc and iron, says Dr. Woods.

Vitamin B_6 has a number of important tasks. It helps the body transform food into energy and ensures healthy function of nerve tissue. Studies suggest that B_6 also helps strengthen our immune systems.

Most women do not get the two milligrams recommended as the DV. But there are many everyday foods that will boost your B_6 supply, including potatoes, bananas, avocados, chicken, turkey, Atlantic salmon, brown rice and watermelon.

Zinc is necessary for proper wound healing and a strong immune system. But studies show that, next to calcium, zinc is the mineral most often lacking in women's diets.

Aim for the DV of 15 milligrams, experts say. Oysters are a super source, and some other kinds of seafood are also top zinc foods—including lobster and crab. Or try to eat more lima beans, lentils and split peas, with occasional servings of lean beef, which is also an excellent source of zinc.

When it comes to iron, we've seen recommendations change with the times. In the past, women were taught that they routinely needed supplements of iron—the mineral that helps our blood carry oxygen throughout the body. Today, we know that most women do get enough iron in their diets. But important exceptions may be women who have heavy periods or female athletes who train rigorously. If you fall into either of these categories, you may need to take a supplement. Just be careful not to exceed the DV of 18 milligrams unless a blood test shows that you are clinically iron-deficient.

Good iron sources include lean beef, cooked dried beans, lima beans and prune juice.

Low-Fat Foods for a Happier Heart

Not so long ago, many of us thought a broken heart could only mean one thing—love troubles. Now we know better. Serious heart trouble of the physical kind is all too common among women. In fact, heart disease is the number one cause of death for women, just as it is for men. Here's how you can fight back.

A Guide to Multi Supplements

Scan any supplement-laden shelf in the drugstore, and you'll be dazzled by the variety of choices you have in multi supplements. The labels tell you what vitamins and minerals are in them.

But what else do you need to know to make a choice? How should you store them? What are the best ways to take them? Here are some guidelines from Richard J. Wood, Ph.D., laboratory chief in the mineral bioavailability lab at the Jean Mayer USDA Human Nutrition Research Center on Aging in Boston.

Daily Value (DV). This term—used on the label to tell you the contents—replaces the old term, USRDA (Recommended Daily Allowance). Daily Value and USRDA amounts are identical.

Timed-release multis. They're supposed to sustain steady blood levels of nutrients. The problem is that they may release nutrients past the point in the digestive tract where you can absorb them.

Expiration date. You can find this date on the label, though sometimes it's so obscure you may need the pharmacist's help to locate it. When you're deciding how much to buy, figure out how many supplements you'll take before that date. For optimum potency, you should take them all before expiration.

Ability to dissolve. Look for multis that display the letters "USP," a promise to dissolve 75 percent after one hour in body fluids. (USP stands for U.S. Pharmacopeia, a nongovernmental group that sets standards for supplements.)

Natural versus synthetic. Experts agree there's no important difference. If iron is a concern, look for it as ferrous sulfate or ferrous fumarate. The chemical form of other nutrients in multis doesn't make a significant difference, most experts agree.

When to take. For maximum absorption, take your multi with a low-fiber meal, not on an empty stomach. Also, make sure your meal isn't totally fat-free. The fat-soluble vitamins in multis (for example, beta-carotene/vitamin A) need an estimated three to five grams of fat to stay inside you. That's the equivalent of about a teaspoon of olive oil or margarine.

Storage. To keep multis potent, avoid storing them in hot or humid places such as the bathroom, a sunny windowsill, the ledge over the sink or anywhere near the stove. Once a bottle is opened, don't refrigerate it; this could result in condensation inside the bottle. Many experts suggest that you store supplements in the same cupboard where you keep spices.

The cotton. Toss it—it's only there to prevent damage during shipping.

Though women are usually through menopause before heart disease is diagnosed, it develops over a lifetime, according to Dr. Derelian. "So it's never too early to adopt heart-healthy habits to protect yourself." Along with exercise, the top strategy she recommends for safeguarding your heart is a diet that's low in fat—especially saturated fat.

Younger women do benefit from this heart-smart lifestyle. In one study, women in their forties had lower total and LDL (the bad kind) cholesterol levels following the adoption of a low-fat diet with exercise. Not only that, each of the women lost an average of ten pounds in six months.

Gram for gram, fat has more than twice as many calories as protein or carbohydrate. (Be careful, though, not to binge on low-fat foods, or you may wind up eating even more calories than you saved by cutting out fat in the first place, says McCord. Adios, weight loss.)

Another potential gain from going low-fat? Cancer experts point to studies showing that countries such as China and Japan with diets lowest in fat—and especially low in saturated fat—have the lowest rates of breast cancer. Countries with higher fat diets have more breast cancer.

Though the link between fat and breast cancer is not certain, Dr. Woods says there is strong evidence suggesting that you can help protect yourself against breast cancer if your diet has less than 20 percent of calories from fat. Also linked to low-fat diets: lower rates of cancer of the colon, cancer of the endometrium (the lining of the uterus) and ovarian cancer.

Fat-Slashing Strategies

It's true that low-fat diets used to be spartan affairs—lots of lettuce, cottage cheese and skim milk. Plus, you needed a shelf of reference books to help you research the fat grams in food. But a low-fat diet is easy today, thanks to terrific new products at the supermarket and easy-to-read new food labels on almost everything. Here are some tips from McCord and other experts to help you make fat-reducing choices.

Know your fat budget. Each day, make sure your calories from total fat don't exceed 25 percent of all your calories. (Some experts, such as Dr. Woods, say it's even better if you can keep your diet under 20 percent calories from fat.) Also, your calories from saturated fat should not exceed 7 percent of all your calories. Using "Fat Budget Finder" on page 277, first find your own calorie level—and then the maximum grams of fat and saturated fat you should be getting each day. Just remember that having some fat in your diet is

Top Five Fat Trip-Ups

You may be surprised at the top five sources of fat in women's diets. You'd guess that chocolate is number one? Not even close. In fact, chocolate is not to be found among the top five.

Starting with the worst offenders, here are the leading fat contributors along with smart substitutions to help slash fat from your meals.

Instead of . . .	Fat (g.)	Substitute . . .	Fat (g.)
2 Tbsp. French dressing	20	2 Tbsp. fat-free French dressing	0
2 slices American cheese	10	2 slices fat-free American cheese	0
1 Tbsp. soft margarine	11	1 Tbsp. fat-free soft margarine	0
3 oz. 90% lean ground beef	11	3 oz. ground skinless turkey breast	1
2 slices bologna	16	2 slices fat-free bologna	0

How Many Calories Do You Need?

If you're at a healthy weight level—or if you know what your ideal weight should be—you can easily calculate how many calories you need in your diet every day to achieve or maintain that weight. But one factor that you have to consider is your average daily activity level. If you are more active, naturally, you'll burn more calories, so you need more in your diet. Here are the three steps that will help you come up with your daily calorie needs.

1. Find your activity level.

<u>Sedentary.</u> Your job or lifestyle involves light walking at most. You exercise only occasionally.

<u>Active.</u> Your job requires more than light walking (such as full-time housecleaning). Or you get 30 to 60 minutes of aerobic exercise three times every week.

<u>Very active.</u> You exercise for at least 60 minutes four or more times a week.

2. Find the activity factor that corresponds to your activity level.

Sedentary	12
Active	15
Very active	18

3. Determine your calorie needs by taking your activity factor from step 2 and multiplying it by your weight in pounds (activity factor × weight in pounds = calorie needs). If you're overweight, use a healthy weight for this step.

Here's an example. Suppose you are an active woman—which means that your activity factor is 15—and your healthy weight is 134 pounds. In order to calculate what your calorie needs are, you should multiply 15 by 134, which gives you 2,010 calories. So 2,010 calories is your ideal daily intake.

In other words, as long as you stay at your current activity level, you'll want to get about 2,000 calories per day. For best health, those calories should come from a variety of food sources, including vegetables, fruits, grains, low-fat or nonfat dairy products and limited quantities of meat, fish and poultry.

Remember, though, that if your activity level changes, you'll have to recalculate your daily calorie needs, again using the formula in step 3.

---

essential to good health.

Frequent the food label. Once you know your fat budget, check the labels of all the foods you eat in one day. That way, you can keep a running tab of grams of fat and saturated fat, making sure you don't exceed your fat budget. You'll soon know the high- and low-fat foods by heart, and you'll soon have a good sense of whether a particular high-fat food is worth all the other foods you give up to fit it in your diet.

Learn label lingo. Terms you can rely on are *fat-free* and *low-fat*. Fat-free means one-half gram of fat or less per serving, while low-fat means three grams or less per serving. Beware the terms *reduced-fat* and *light*: They can be deceiving, because these terms are used only in comparison with a higher-fat food. ("Reduced-fat" on a bag of chips, for instance, simply means that particular brand of chips has 25 percent less fat than a regular chip—even though the percentage of fat is still astronomically high.)

Do the produce promenade. Fruits and vegetables (except for avocados) are a sure bet for ultra low fat fare. When you're in the fresh produce section of your supermarket, you're in the best location for easy, no-label food shopping.

Shop for substitutes. Many low-fat substitutes for high-fat foods are available. Your supermarket probably has low-fat or fat-free salad dressings, mayonnaise, margarine, cheese, cream cheese, sour cream, cottage cheese, milk, yogurt, evaporated milk, frozen yogurt, ice cream, hot dogs, sausage, cold cuts, puddings, crackers, chips, cookies and frozen entrées. Check the labels before you buy and compare the low-fat to the regular products. You'll be amazed at how far many of these products have come.

Slice it low-fat. To cut the fat that still haunts many main meals, it might be necessary to make meat a lesser part of your diet. For instance, you can serve meat as a side dish instead of a main dish. Or be a part-time vegetarian. When you're looking for a boost of protein, go the low-fat route by choosing fish or shellfish, chicken or turkey breast without skin, pork tenderloin or cuts of beef labeled "extra lean."

Take out the trans. Another type of fat that may promote heart disease is trans-fatty acid, or trans fat. You won't be able to find the grams of trans fat by reading food labels, because the government doesn't require food producers to include that information. But even without label reading, you can avoid most trans fat by steering clear of commercial french fries or any food that lists

Fat Budget Finder

Here's a quick way to calculate how many grams of fat and saturated fat you should allow in your daily fat budget. First of all, you'll need to know your daily calorie level. (See "How Many Calories Do You Need?" on page 276.) Then find the maximum grams of total fat and saturated fat that correspond to your daily calorie level. During the day, keep track of how many grams of fat you have in each meal and snack. If you make sure the total fat and saturated fat don't exceed the number of grams shown here, you'll always stay within your fat budget.

Calories	Total Fat (g.)	Saturated Fat (g.)
1,200	33	9
1,400	38	10
1,600	44	12
1,800	50	14
2,000	55	15
2,200	61	17
2,500	69	19

How to Favor Fiber

Eating plenty of fruits and vegetables delivers a huge health bonus: bountiful fiber. You get especially high doses from legumes such as cooked dried beans, peas or lentils or from a high-bran breakfast cereal. And you're boosting your diet with fiber whenever you have whole grains—any food made from a grain that hasn't had the outer bran layer removed, such as whole-wheat bread, brown rice and oatmeal. But if your diet is typical of most women, you're eating only half as much fiber as you should.

What's so fabulous about fiber? Aside from the fact that it helps fill us up and makes weight management a much more pleasant affair? Aside from the fact that it gets you going and keeps constipation and diverticulosis on the run? If that's not enough, how about the way fiber seems to protect against heart disease and cancer?

Many population studies have linked diets high in fiber with lower rates of colon cancer, the third most common cancer in women. Fiber may even help block breast cancer, several studies have found. In one study in Australia, women who ate about 30 grams of fiber a day had half the risk of breast cancer as women who ate about 15 grams a day.

As for heart disease, it is a well-established fact that adding soluble fiber to the diet lowers high cholesterol levels in many people. (Soluble fiber, which is especially high in sources such as beans and oats, is the kind that dissolves in water to form a gel.)

Scientists aren't sure yet just how fiber protects us. Probably, it works in several ways. By speeding the passage of waste through the intestines, fiber gives cancer-causing substances in food and digestive juices less time to promote colon cancer. Diets high in wheat fiber appear to lower blood levels of estrogen, a factor that may protect against breast cancer.

Soluble fiber appears to bind up cholesterol and carry it out of the body. Also, soluble fiber may be transformed by helpful bacteria in the digestive tract into substances that inhibit high cholesterol. Finally, eating a high-fiber diet means eating whole grains, veggies, fruits and beans, all of which are top sources of other protective wonder-ingredients.

Daily Tactics

The bottom line? We need 20 to 35 grams of fiber a day, experts say—and from a variety of high-fiber *foods*, not supplements.

To track your own fiber intake, consult package labels for grams of dietary fiber in each serving of food you eat during the day. For fresh fruits and vegetables, which usually aren't labeled, you can estimate an average of two grams per serving.

Or, just by following these easy guidelines from Holly McCord, R.D., nutrition editor for Prevention magazine in Emmaus, Pennsylvania, you'll make your high-fiber quota without counting.

Start the day with cereal. Having a high-fiber cereal at breakfast may be the single biggest step you can take to reach your fiber goal, says McCord. Look for a cereal with seven grams of fiber or more per serving.

Hunt for whole wheat. Shop for whole-wheat bread, rolls, English muffins, pretzels, crackers, cookies, pasta and couscous in natural food stores and some supermarkets. To make sure a product is 100 percent whole wheat, don't judge by the name. Look for the words "whole wheat" or "whole-wheat flour" in the ingredient list on the label, suggests McCord.

The benefit? Whole-wheat foods should average about two grams of fiber per serving. But if the ingredient list names "wheat flour" or "enriched wheat flour" instead of "whole-wheat flour," the product was made from refined flour and will average only zero to one gram of fiber per serving (unless it's fiber-fortified). Over the course of a day, this difference adds up.

Have beans every day. Or peas, or lentils. You can count legumes as a filling five grams of fiber per half-cup—and much of this is soluble fiber, the heart-healthy kind that's hardest to get. If a serving of beans a day sounds like a lot, remember how many of our favorite foods are bean dishes: baked beans, bean soup, pea soup, lentil soup, chili, three-bean salad, minestrone and burritos. McCord suggests adding cooked beans to beef up vegetable soups and tossed salads.

Get a minimum of six fruits and veggies a day. For each serving you can count an average two grams of fiber, making a total of 12 grams toward your daily total.

Eat the skins. That includes baked potatoes, sweet potatoes, peaches and apples. Otherwise, you'll miss lots of the fiber. (Be sure to wash them well first.)

Snack on cereal. If you miss having cereal for breakfast, why not make a high-fiber cereal into a healthy, filling snack? Or even a light lunch or dinner, with milk and fruit?

partially hydrogenated oil among its first three ingredients. This includes stick margarine and many frozen foods and baked goods.

Be stingy with oil. Low-fat cooking methods include grilling, broiling, poaching, steaming, microwaving and roasting. Sautéing is often listed as a low-fat way to cook, too. But you're just asking for fat if you sauté your food in a pan swimming with oil.

If a recipe calls for sautéing, use no-stick pans with no-stick spray. (The spray is oil, all right, but you use a lot less of it because you're just misting the pan a bit.) Many people don't realize you can "liquid sauté" just as effectively by having a layer of water, broth or fruit juice instead of oil in the bottom of the pan. If you do use oil, McCord recommends that you sauté with flavored oils so you get more flavor while using less. If you use butter, be sure to use it very sparingly, since it's loaded with saturated fat.

Streamline your baking recipes. If you have a cake or muffin recipe that calls for oil, butter or other high-fat shortening, use a low-fat or nonfat substitute that will give you a new taste sensation as well as a lower-fat dessert. Instead of the shortening called for in the recipe, try apple sauce, mashed bananas, prune baby food or canned cooked pumpkin. Start by switching half the shortening to a low-fat substitute. You'll find that some recipes work well with even more of the nonfat substitute, so keep on experimenting. To make sure the baking goodies don't stick to the pan, all you need is a light coating of no-stick spray.

Chill out. Do you have a favorite homemade soup or stew? There's a way you can get out most of the fat before you serve it. Let the soup or stew cool in the refrigerator so that the fat can rise to the top. Once the layer of fat has congealed, just lift it off.

Get inspired. Keep an eye out for lean but luscious recipes in low-fat cookbooks and magazines.

Veggies, Fruit and Fiber— A Woman's Best Friends

If there's one single piece of nutrition advice every researcher and physician agrees with, it's this: The more vegetables and fruits you eat, the healthier you will be. That's based on study after study showing that something in fruits and vegetables appears to protect us against all sorts of disease.

One analysis of over 200 studies concluded that people who eat five or more servings of produce a day have less than half the overall cancer risk of people who eat only one serving of produce a day. Five daily servings is the minimum amount recommended by the National Cancer Institute. By following the *Prevention* 3-2-1 Plan, however, you'll actually top that goal by getting a minimum of six servings of fruits and vegetables a day.

Keep in mind that when it comes to fruits and vegetables, more is better. In addition to the studies that show reduced cancer risk, other research has linked diets that are high in fruits and vegetables with less risk of heart disease, stroke, eye diseases and rheumatoid arthritis.

What's the magic ingredient in produce that confers all this protection? Most researchers believe there's no single component working alone. At this point scientists theorize that the "magic" comes from some combination of the thousands of compounds in any given plant. Some are vitamins. Some are types of fiber. Others are newly researched compounds with names that only chemists could love, like

Our Bosom Buddies

Some preliminary evidence suggests that the cruciferous vegetable clan—broccoli and its cousins—may be one of women's best weapons against breast cancer. This potent veggie family boasts two compounds—sulforaphane and indole-3 carbinol—that may work to fight breast cancer. Small wonder the National Cancer Institute recommends we eat several servings of these good guys a week.

Besides broccoli, go for cabbage, cauliflower, brussels sprouts, bok choy, kale, mustard greens, collard greens and turnip greens—all members of this cancer-fighting family. There are many ways you can work them into your diet. Here are some ideas from Holly McCord, R.D., nutrition editor for **Prevention** magazine in Emmaus, Pennsylvania.

- Steam petite broccoli florets to top your homemade or carry-out pizza. The florets come frozen and bagged, ready to cook and pop on your pizza.
- Sauté julienned broccoli stems—available as "broccoslaw" in the produce department—in stir-fries.
- If your restaurant entrée is garnished with a dark green, curly edged veggie, eat it! It's probably kale, one of the most nutritious crucifers of all.
- Brush broccoli spears with olive oil and grill. You won't believe how delicious they taste.
- With bags of shredded cabbage and red cabbage, it just takes a moment to make instant coleslaw. (Use low-fat or nonfat mayonnaise in the dressing.)
- Make plain steamed cauliflower yummier with a dab of low-fat margarine and a sprinkle of nutmeg.

flavonoids and isothiocyanates. Without doubt, there are many more "magic ingredients" yet to be discovered.

So here's the point. You can't get these thousands of protective compounds—known and unknown—by swallowing a vitamin pill. You have to eat more fruits and vegetables. If you're like the average woman, though, you're only eating three to four servings a day rather than the five servings recommended by the National Cancer Institute or the six servings (minimum) in the *Prevention* 3-2-1 Plan.

Produce Results: Tactics for More Servings

If you think it's too hard to make room for more fruits and veggies in your life, just take a look at these easy-as-pie tips from McCord and Jerianne Heimendinger, Ph.D., research scientist and acting director of the Lifestyles Research Center at AMC Cancer Research Center in Denver and former director of the National Cancer Institute's Five a Day for Better Health program.

Get a jump start with breakfast. In one fell swoop, breakfast can easily supply two fruit servings: Just have a glass of orange juice to start, then slice up a banana on your cereal. If you miss breakfast, you may have some catching up to do to get five or more servings into your day, Dr. Heimendinger points out. But it's still not that difficult—just have a pear for a mid-morning snack and a glass of juice with your salad at lunch. Then try broccoli, beets and potatoes for dinner. You did it!

Plan your snack back-ups. Plan ahead so you have a fruit or veggie snack with you whenever you're away from home. Pop a bag

(continued on page 284)

So Many Soy Sources

Getting more soy in your diet could turn out to be one way to lower your risk of breast cancer. In countries such as Japan and China, where soybean foods are part of the everyday diet, women have much lower rates of breast cancer than in the United States. Scientists think that may be caused in part by compounds in soy called isoflavones that help curb the effect of estrogen in promoting breast tumors.

How do you get more soy in your diet? One excellent source is tofu, because it's such a concentrated source of soybean curd. Some experts estimate that the amount of soy in a half-cup of tofu per day could be effective.

Apart from that, here are some other easy ideas from Holly McCord, R.D., nutrition editor for Prevention magazine in Emmaus, Pennsylvania.

- Use soy milk on your cereal. Make sure that you shop for a brand that is 1 percent low-fat or nonfat. To get as much calcium as there is in regular milk, get calcium-fortified soy milk.
- Enjoy a cup of flavored soy yogurt.
- Make cream soups with soy milk.
- Blend a frosty. Mix 3 cups vanilla soy milk with 1 diced, ripe banana and 1 cup fresh or frozen strawberries. (If you use frozen strawberries, thaw them before blending.) Blend until smooth.
- Make oatmeal cereal using soy milk instead of water.
- Whip up blueberry fluff. Combine 2½ cups frozen blueberries with 10 ounces silken tofu and 2 tablespoons sugar. Blend until smooth. Pour in dessert dishes. Chill.
- Prepare instant pudding with soy milk or from special new mixes designed to blend with silken tofu.

It's no secret that slimming down successfully can be a real challenge, and many of us need all the help we can get. So we turned to top obesity expert Wayne Callaway, M.D., associate clinical professor of medicine at the George Washington University School of Medicine and Health Sciences in Washington, D.C., for additional tips that will give you the upper hand on weight control. Here are his suggestions.

Get moving. The first secret to controlling weight is being more active. With regular exercise—and that doesn't mean super-exertion—we can burn the calories we consume instead of storing them as fat.

When it comes to blocking our exercise path, many of our conveniences are also our biggest barriers. "Thanks to cars, elevators, escalators, automatic garage-door openers, remote control televisions, portable telephones, riding mowers, you name it—we're engineering movement right out of our lives," observes Dr. Callaway. "The result is an activity deficiency. To slim down and stay slim, getting more exercise should be your number one lifelong priority."

Trim your diet in mini-steps. Make any diet changes only one or two at a time— enough to save about 125 calories a day. For example, that could mean switching from mayonnaise to mustard on your sandwich at lunch. The next day, use 1 percent low-fat milk instead of half-and-half in your coffee. When those changes have become habits, add another small change or two.

With this method, you aren't trying to change an entire lifetime of eating habits all at once, so you won't be setting yourself up for relapse and binge. And, by the way, losing one-quarter pound a week means that you'd lose about 12 pounds in one year!

By taking small steps, you have a much greater chance of acquiring new habits that will sustain weight loss. "To lose 10 to 12 pounds a year and keep it off, you can't do it with a gimmick. You have to do it slowly on a day-to-day basis," he says.

Shed your scales. "I think we should burn scales," says Dr. Callaway. "They give a very superficial measurement that doesn't tell you anything about muscle mass or fluid retention." Getting on a scale that says you haven't lost any weight after you've been faithful to your eating plan can be discouraging enough to make you give up. A better gauge is to look at how your clothes fit.

Don't have a fat-free free-for-all. Remember that fat-free foods are not invitations to binge. "This is a critical point," says Dr. Callaway. "Many women have cut way back on fat but overcompensated with low-fat or fat-free carbohydrate foods."

Fat-free potato chips, cookies and frozen yogurt—even pasta and pretzels—do have calories, and if you eat too much, you'll gain weight. Even with fat-free food, you can't repeal the law of calorie reality: 3,500 excess calories equals one pound of extra weight.

Make breakfast and lunch your mainstays. Skipping these meals sets you up for overeating later in the day. "When you undereat, the next meal will make you more hungry," observes Dr. Callaway. "If you do pig out at night, don't get up the next day and skip breakfast and lunch to try and make up for it. The more you cut

The Sneaky Way to Lose Weight

What a difference you can make by modifying old favorites instead of giving them up. Little by little, these changes do add up to a slimmer you.

To prove you can eat traditional favorites while you're shedding calories from your diet and trimming fat from your body, Holly McCord, R.D., nutrition editor for <u>Prevention</u> magazine in Emmaus, Pennsylvania, calculated how much you'll save by making a few easy switches. In fact, you'll avoid 1,745 calories (enough to lose half a pound) with the following tips.

- Instead of having a strawberry milkshake made with ice cream and whole milk, blend four frozen strawberries, one cup skim milk and two packets artificial sweetener. Turn the blender on high for about two minutes, until the strawberries are completely blended. Savings: 180 calories.
- Instead of cooking one regular hot dog, treat yourself to a low-fat frank. Savings: 100 calories.
- Instead of one slice of pound cake, enjoy a slice of fat-free loaf cake. Savings: 90 calories.
- Instead of spreading half a bagel with regular cream cheese, use fat-free cream cheese. Savings: 75 calories.
- Instead of preparing a helping of tuna salad with a quarter-cup regular mayonnaise, make tuna salad with a quarter-cup nonfat mayonnaise. Savings: 360 calories.
- Instead of a salad with four tablespoons regular French dressing, use four tablespoons fat-free French dressing. Savings: 280 calories.
- Instead of a ham sandwich made with two slices of regular American cheese, use two slices of fat-free American cheese. Savings: 80 calories.
- At the fast-food counter, instead of ordering a quarter-pound burger, order a regular hamburger with ketchup, mustard and a pickle. Savings: 150 calories.
- Instead of having one cup of premium chocolate ice cream, dip up nonfat chocolate frozen yogurt. Savings: 380 calories.
- Instead of a three-ounce chicken-breast half with skin, savor the same chicken minus the skin. Savings: 50 calories.

back, the more you're going to pig out."

Pace yourself for success. "Here's another critical factor," says Dr. Callaway. "When I see a woman who has a lot going on—a divorce, a job change, a sick child—I say, 'Look, if you really want to begin right now, let's start with something really simple. Just do one thing positive every day—it may be to eat breakfast or take a ten-minute walk.' " Then there's the satisfaction of knowing that at least you got that done.

"That may be all that you can do for the time being," he adds. But that's fine. "Don't beat up on yourself for not being able to do it all." Begin your weight-loss campaign only when you have some extra emotional energy to spend.

of mini carrots into your briefcase. Grab an apple to munch on during the drive home from work.

Have some "see food" in your fridge. You're more likely to snack on fruits and vegetables if you keep them visible in your refrigerator, not hidden away in crisper drawers to be forgotten, says Dr. Heimendinger. Put cantaloupe cubes or celery sticks in clear glass containers at the front of the top shelf.

Get fixin's. In delis and fast-food restaurants, always request extra lettuce and tomatoes on your sandwich.

Give orders. In restaurants, order a cooked vegetable as a side dish or even as an appetizer. Too often restaurant entrées include only a token bit of vegetable.

Drink a serving. A glass of tomato juice or vegetable juice cocktail counts as a vegetable serving. Keep some cold in the refrigerator—and make vegetable juice your appetizer selection when you eat out.

Go ahead and save time. Take advantage of time-saving precut produce at the supermarket, such as broccoli florets, carrot coins, watermelon cubes, pineapple spears and salad greens. Other super time savers are frozen bags of veggies, which are often packaged in delicious combos. (Frozen veggies, by the way, may have higher vitamin levels than fresh produce—unless it's just-picked fresh.)

Bake some sweet potatoes. Once baked, sweet potatoes make delicious, quick snacks. You can keep them in the refrigerator to eat out-of-hand like a piece of fruit.

Double your measure. Instead of taking one serving of a vegetable at a time, take two—a cup of carrots instead of a half-cup. It really isn't that much.

Be berry creative. Don't forget about fruit for a wonderful dessert. Layer berries or peaches with low-fat or nonfat yogurt or frozen yogurt for a healthy parfait.

Lighten Up Your Life

Weight statistics for American women make for some pretty heavy reading. In the mid-1980s one out of four women was more than 20 percent over her recommended weight. Ten years later, that number had risen to one out of three. Even young women in the age range of 20 to 30 years old are ten pounds heavier than the average weight of 20- to 30-year-old women in the 1980s.

Why the startling increase? We're eating as much—or more—as we always have, but we're moving less, obesity experts agree.

To be honest, this flab-i-demic is costing women dearly. We pay emotionally as well as physically. Studies show that we don't like ourselves as much, because we don't like the way our bodies look (even though some of the fashion industry standards may be unrealistic). But it's our health that really takes a beating. By weighing too much we put ourselves at higher risk for heart disease and endometrial cancer, diabetes, high blood pressure—even gallstones and arthritis. Many of these conditions ultimately can rob us of independence or even life itself.

So staying slim isn't just a matter of fashion. Keeping a healthy, stable weight turns out to be one of a woman's smartest strategies for long-term well-being, says Dr. Derelian.

How do you find your healthiest weight?

The easy guideline suggested by Dr. Derelian is to allow 100 pounds for the first 5 feet of your height, then add 5 pounds for every inch over 5 feet. Once you have this figure, add 10 percent to find your upper range and subtract 10 percent to find your lower range. For example, a woman who is 5 feet 4 inches tall should weigh approximately 120 pounds, plus or minus 12 pounds. That makes her healthy weight range 108 to 132 pounds. If you are under five feet tall, Dr. Derelian suggests finding your healthy weight by starting with 100 pounds and adding 10 pounds for every 10 years of age after age 30. For example a 70-year-old woman who is 4 feet 8 inches tall should weigh approximately 140 pounds.

Suppose today that your mirror or your doctor says it's time to shed some pounds. Guess what? If you remember the advice you've just been reading about the best diet to avoid heart disease and cancer, you already have a lifelong prescription for slimming down and staying there. The key points are:

- Follow the *Prevention* 3-2-1 Plan.
- Stick with low-fat foods.
- Load up on vegetables and fruits.
- Eat plenty of whole grains and beans for fiber.

If you do those things, chances are excellent that you'll naturally lose some excess weight, says McCord. (If you want to count calories as well, see "How Many Calories Do You Need?" on page 276 to estimate how many calories you'll need to maintain a healthy weight. Then, by reading food labels you can keep track of your daily calorie intake.)

Just remember that maintaining a healthy weight is only half the story when it comes to reaping the greatest health benefits. Experts agree that maintaining a high level of fitness is equally important. "Some thin people are very unfit," says Dr. Derelian, "and they, too, are at risk for degenerative disease." (Dr. Derelian advocates getting a half-hour of moderate to strenuous aerobic exercise three to four times a week for fitness. But remember to always check with your doctor before starting any fitness program.)

Ovaries

FUNNY, WHEN A WOMAN pulls a gutsy move, her chutzpah usually gets attributed to parts of the male anatomy. Rarely, if ever, do you hear, "Boy, she's got ovaries."

For whatever reason, the ovaries—the female reproductive glands—have never made it into the popular vernacular as a power symbol the way their male counterparts have.

Yet there they are. These two small structures, situated on either side of a woman's uterus, influence practically every aspect of a woman's health.

The ovaries churn out hormones that are instrumental in regulating the menstrual cycle. One of those hormones, estrogen, plays a key role in maintaining the health of a woman's skin, heart, breasts and bones. It also helps regulate her metabolism and body temperature.

Then there's the miraculous process of ovulation. The release of an egg for fertilization is a central ovarian function and key to a woman's fertility.

And to think that all that clout springs from two glands about the size and shape of almonds.

Powerful, but Susceptible

Yet, with all their powerful attributes, the ovaries are susceptible to dysfunction and disease. Most ovarian problems are not preventable, but by understanding what can go wrong, you'll be better able to recognize problems early and seek the care you need.

The prime task of the ovaries—ovulation—

Look for the Signs

You may know women who say they know when they're ovulating. Is this really possible?

Well, yes, there are some ways to tell, doctors say. Aside from estimating when we ovulate—it usually occurs somewhere between 12 and 16 days after the first day of your last period—there are body signals you can look for.

The first is a phenomenon doctors call mittelschmerz, which loosely translated means "middle pain." The term refers to the twinge or cramp in the lower abdomen or back that some women feel when an egg is released from the ovary.

Second, changes in the quality of your cervical mucus—which is produced by the cells that line the cervical canal—can also indicate if you're ovulating. Around the time of ovulation, your cervical mucus tends to become more watery and profuse.

A more definite way to tell if you're ovulating—it's the method used by couples who are having trouble conceiving—is to measure your basal body temperature, or BBT. Over the course of your cycle, your body temperature changes. Prior to ovulation, it's lower. (For most people it's about 98.6°F, but not exactly—so you need to find out your own basal rate.)

Around the time of ovulation, the BBT rises. If your body temperature has remained elevated at least four-tenths of a degree Fahrenheit for up to three days, that indicates that ovulation has occurred. (If your temperature continues to be elevated for more than two weeks, it could be an indication of pregnancy.)

Urine tests (similar in design to pregnancy tests) that can help you predict ovulation are available at local drugstores.

involves an intricate interplay between hormones. The big players in this hormone interaction are the estrogen released by the ovaries and other hormones released by the brain and the pituitary, a small, pea-size gland located at the base of the brain that regulates the activity of other endocrine glands (the endocrine system) throughout the body.

Located inside each ovary are hundreds of thousands of follicles—tiny clusters of cells that function as storehouses for immature eggs. There are about 1 million follicles present in the ovaries at birth, but their number declines with age, until there are less than half—about 400,000—by the time a woman starts menstruating. For an egg to mature inside a follicle and be released from the ovary, it needs stimulation from certain hormones.

It's kind of a tag-team process, where one hormone triggers the release of other hormones, and they in turn promote the growth and release of an egg. The first hormone, a gonadotropin-releasing hormone, is released by the brain, travels down to the ovaries and tickles the pituitary gland located at the base of the brain. The pituitary then releases two more hormones, which go to work on the ovary and its follicles.

When a follicle is stimulated by a gonadotropin-releasing hormone, the cells surrounding the egg begin to grow and release estrogen. This works to start building the lining of the uterus so that it can be ready for implantation if the egg is fertilized.

The entire follicle fills with fluid and swells to reach the surface of the ovary. When it gets a surge of the hormone called the luteinizing hormone, the follicle releases the egg. Once the egg is released from the ovary, the remnants of the follicle become the corpus luteum, which releases the female sex hormone progesterone. This further prepares the uterine lining for the possible reception of an egg.

While many women will always have healthy ovaries, sometimes things can go awry. Among the problems women may encounter are unusual cyst formation, polycystic ovaries, ovarian failure, benign ovarian tumors, obstruction by endometriosis (a disease of the uterine lining), inflammation and cancer.

When a Cyst Is the Matter

Ovarian cysts are fluid-filled sacs that form inside the ovary. Not all ovarian cysts are problematic, says Daniel Cramer, M.D., Sc.D., associate professor of obstetrics and gynecology at Brigham and Women's Hospital in Boston.

A cyst, called a follicular cyst, generally forms every month during a normal cycle. After ovulation this cyst is converted into a corpus luteum cyst. If no pregnancy occurs, the corpus luteum cyst disappears.

But if an egg is not released and stays inside the ovary and continues to enlarge, that may become a problem. A doctor is likely to advise you to have the cyst removed if it grows to be larger than ten centimeters (about four inches) or if it turns into a complex cyst, which is a fluid-filled sac with growths inside.

Your doctor can usually feel an oversized cyst during a pelvic exam and tell just how big it is by doing an ultrasound exam. The ultrasound will also reveal whether or not the cyst is a complex one, because the test allows your doctor to see its contents.

Some women suffer from polycystic ovarian syndrome, a condition in which follicles do not get released from the ovaries and multiple cysts form instead. The syndrome can cause irregular menstrual periods, excessive hair growth and infertility.

The heart of the problem is hormone imbalance. While the follicles produce sufficient estrogen, they do not produce enough of the second kind of hormone that's needed to complete the egg release and fertilization process—progesterone.

Progesterone is key in helping the uterine lining shed, so without enough of it, the lining may stay in place and a woman may skip her period for several months at time. When the uterine lining (endometrium) doesn't shed, a woman's risk of endometrial cancer increases. In addition to not producing enough progesterone women with polycystic ovarian syndrome produce excessive amounts of the male hormone testosterone, and this can lead to excessive hair growth on the face and chest.

Other problems can also interfere with ovulation, including defects in the ovary itself, diseases that compromise the immune system and exposure to radiation or chemotherapy. Not ovulating is one of several problems that can result in infertility.

Beyond the category of ovarian cysts are benign ovarian tumors, says Dr. Cramer. The most common form of benign tumors are called dermoid tumors, which arise from the growth cells in the ovary. There's also a collection of tumors that arise from the epithelium, another layer of cells in the ovary.

Endometriosis and Inflammation

Endometriosis—a disease in which the endometrial lining of the uterus grows outside the uterus where it doesn't belong—can also interfere with ovulation. Sometimes endometriosis implants adhere to the ovaries. While the disease starts off as small spots of tissue, it can grow into large clumps. If it covers the surface of the ovary through which an egg is to be released, then ovulation can be blocked, says Edmond Confino, M.D., associate professor and director of the In Vitro Fertilization Program at Northwestern University in Evanston, Illinois. It can also spread and attach to other organs such as the fallopian tubes or bowels.

The ovaries are also susceptible to a condition called oophoritis, which is basically swelling and inflammation of the ovary itself. Pelvic inflammatory disease, an infection of the upper reproductive tract, can cause it, as can the mumps virus.

The Silent Cancer

Finally, the ovaries are susceptible to cancer. Researchers don't know exactly what causes ovarian cancer, but they theorize that there may be some link between incessant ovulation and ovarian cancer. That is, women who ovulate repeatedly year after year without a break—that is, they haven't gotten pregnant or haven't been on the Pill—appear to be at increased risk.

One possible explanation is that because ovulation causes a cycle of rapid growth of the ovarian cells immediately followed by cell division, the cells of the ovary may be most vulnerable during ovulation. Therefore, incessant ovulation increases the opportunities for mutation to occur, says Susan Harlap, M.D., chief of the epidemiology service at Memorial Sloan Kettering Cancer Center in New York City. The more often ovulation occurs, then, the more susceptible a woman may be.

Another factor that can contribute to ovarian cancer is having a family history of the disease.

The frustrating thing about ovarian cancer is that the disease is virtually a silent one— that is, women don't feel any pain from it. In fact, with ovarian cancer there are usually no

Ovarian Cancer: Know the Risks

Generally speaking, a 35-year-old woman with no family history of cancer has about a 2 percent chance of developing ovarian cancer sometime during the course of her life. There are some things that can increase that risk.

Family history. If you have a mother or sister with ovarian cancer, statistics show that your risk for the disease over the course of your lifetime jumps to about 5 percent, experts say. Your risks are even greater if both your mother and a sister have it, or if two or more sisters have the disease. If your family profile resembles this, it is absolutely imperative for you to receive genetic counseling and advice, because there are steps that you can take to lower your risk, says Susan Harlap, M.D., chief of the epidemiology service at Memorial Sloan Kettering Cancer Center in New York City.

No children. Not having had kids increases your risk for ovarian cancer. "Women who have had children are at reduced risk," says Dr. Harlap. "Having the first child reduces their risk by 17 percent. Every subsequent child causes another 13 percent reduction." Women who breastfeed reduce their risk even more.

Age. The incidence of ovarian cancer increases with age, says Dr. Harlap. So if you are 30 or 40 years old, your risk for the disease is greater than it was when you were in your twenties. If you have a family history of ovarian cancer and are considered to be at increased risk, you may want to participate in studies about screening and treatment for ovarian cancer, says Dr. Harlap. To find out about ongoing studies in your area, contact the closest major cancer center.

signs until very late in the disease. The symptoms that do finally appear include abdominal discomfort and swelling.

Mind Ovary Matters

There's no self-exam that can help you detect ovarian cancer, but here are some general guidelines, recommended by experts, to help you protect your ovaries.

Consider the Pill. The Pill is the most beneficial thing we know of in terms of preventing ovarian cancer, says Dr. Harlap. "The longer a woman has used the Pill, the greater the protection," she says.

Most studies indicate that at least four years of Pill use is required before it reduces your risk for ovarian cancer. According to other studies, however, some protection has been seen with even shorter periods of use. In addition, the Pill can help prevent ovarian cysts and benign growths, says Dr. Harlap.

While use of the Pill is beneficial for ovarian cancer protection, "women need to be aware that there are some risks associated with it," says Mary Daley, M.D., director of the Margaret Dyson Family Risk Assessment Program at Fox Chase Cancer Center in Philadelphia. If you are particularly prone to blood clots, for example, the Pill may not be for you. Ask your doctor if you have any risk factors that preclude you from taking the Pill, she says.

Have an annual exam. During an annual pelvic exam, your doctor can palpate your ovaries by pressing up from your vagina and down on your abdomen. The size of your ovaries and any pain you feel when she does this exam can help detect ovarian cysts, benign ovarian tumors or enlargement of the ovaries from cancer. So schedule a pelvic exam annually, experts say.

Ban the butts and munch the crunchies. Chances are that the causes of ovarian cancer aren't very different from the causes of other cancers, says Dr. Harlap. So follow the general cancer prevention practices. Get regular exercise, quit smoking and follow a healthful diet that includes five to eight portions of fruits and vegetables every day.

Don't powder up. One theory about ovarian cancer is that certain substances may trigger cell mutation. Doctors suspect that talcum powder may be one culprit. So avoid the use of talcum powder in the genital area, says Dr. Cramer.

Interview Grandma. It's important for women to be aware of their family history, not only of ovarian cancer but of breast cancer, says Dr. Daley. "The two are related."

You can start the process of learning your history by asking family members if anyone has ever had ovarian cancer, Dr. Daley says. It is particularly important to do this on your paternal side as well as on your maternal side, as you would still have a high risk of ovarian cancer if your father's mother or grandmother had the disease.

Get guidance. If a woman finds she has a family history of cancer, the next step is to confirm the diagnosis of the relative by obtaining her medical records. This can be a complicated process right from the start, since often the relative is deceased and the medical records are stored at the hospital. Try requesting the records on your own, but if you have a hard time tracking them down, you may want to enlist professional guidance from a major cancer center, says Dr. Daley.

Cancer centers often have counselors who are familiar with hospital systems and know some of the ins and outs of finding records.

Hire an interpreter. Once you have the records, you have to make sense of them—so you may want to see a genetic counselor. Some cancer centers, such as Memorial Sloan Kettering in New York City, have genetic counselors available who can read the records, help interpret your family history of cancer, assess your own personal risk and determine a prevention plan for you, says Dr. Harlap.

The cancer center you contact may have a genetic counselor on staff who can help you, but be sure to ask the cost. If you're not near a cancer center, call the teaching hospital nearest you or a branch of the American Cancer Society.

Ask for authorities. The gurus of cancer detection are those who study it all the time. If you or your doctor suspects ovarian cancer, go to a gynecologic oncologist for your treatment, experts say. While gynecologists are trained to diagnose cancers, gynecologic oncologists have several years of additional training on how to treat the disease. For help in finding one, contact the closest major cancer center, recommends William Hoskins, M.D., chief of gynecology service at the Memorial Sloan Kettering Cancer Center in New York City. Or call the Society of Gynecologic Oncologists in Chicago at 1-800-444-4441. The Society will provide a list of gynecologic oncologists in your geographic area through either voicemail or fax.

See also Birth Control, Endocrine System, Fertility, Gynecological Exam, Hormones, Menstrual Cycle, Reproductive System

Pain Relief

"RUB IT," MAMA SAYS when her bambino falls down and goes bump. It's a common mom command. Like "Stand up straight" or "Eat your veggies," it's one of those mom-isms that has turned out to be medically correct.

The father of medicine would have made a good mother, too. "The physician must be experienced in many things but most assuredly in rubbing," said Hippocrates, "for rubbing can bind a joint that is too loose and loosen a joint that is too rigid."

The way rubbing works actually tells us a lot about the way pain—and pain relief—travel through our bodies, according to Margaret A. Caudill, M.D., Ph.D., co-director of the Arnold Pain Center at Deaconess Hospital in Boston, assistant clinical professor of medicine at Harvard Medical School and author of *Managing Pain before It Manages You*.

Say you bark your shin on a low coffee table. Three different kinds of fibers—all serving various functions—immediately come into play.

First, pain receptors on your skin yelp the news to sensory nerves rich in A-delta fibers that pick up the message. The yelp speeds along the nerve highway at the equivalent of 40 miles per hour and swerves into your spinal cord, which rockets the pain message to other nerves or to your brain.

Right after that sharp flash, you feel another kind of pain—a low, aching, dull throb. That little number is made up of a power brigade of signals that tread along the nerve highway of C fibers at a more placid three miles per hour.

But suppose you rub your shin as soon as you hit it. The rub sets off touch fibers—the A-betas. "Those fibers race at 200 miles an hour to the spinal cord and, theoretically, compete with the pain message," says Dr. Caudill. You'll know those touch fibers won the race when the rub soothes away the pain.

The Chemistry of Pain

But pain is useful, too. Pain warns you to take your hand off the stove burner, to take care of your back or to find out why your head aches. Often what makes you hurt also starts to cure you. Those pain messages provoke production of a chemical that sounds like an old sitcom—bradykinin.

This powerful chemical unleashes a torrent of inflammatory chemicals, such as histamines and prostaglandins. They heal but they also hurt.

Once you've been warned, and pain has your attention, your body's phenomenal pharmacy starts to kick in. Scientists have discovered that every one of us can make at least eight natural morphinelike opiates, all stronger than the opium from any poppy plant in China. In fact, narcotics such as

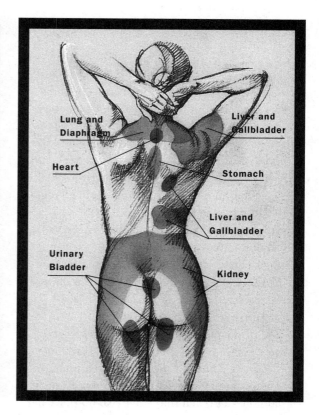

You can feel some kinds of "referred pain" in surface areas of your body that are far away from the organ that's actually hurting. The illustration above shows where referred pain can be felt on the front of your body.

Some skin regions on the back of your body also get referred pain from internal organs, as shown above. If these areas hurt frequently, be sure to alert your doctor.

morphine and codeine work by mimicking our inborn opiate action.

Endorphin is one brain chemical in our home-brewed batch—it's responsible for the famed runner's high. Enkephalin is another. "Actually, we found the morphine receptors in the body before we found the opiates. We wondered why in the world they were there, until we found endorphin," says Dr. Caudill.

Endorphin and its sisters start to loosen the pinch of pain. Another brain chemical, serotonin, dubbed the "feel-good" chemical, starts tamping down the pain, too. Normally, that's the typical tale of pain. As we get better, the pain diminishes.

When Pain Keeps Preying

Sometimes, though, pain settles in and gets stuck on the replay button. That's the case with more than 45 million Americans who suffer from chronic headaches and another 22 million who have recurring back or neck pain—our most common problems.

"What happens with chronic pain is that the pain mechanism itself goes awry. The symptom itself becomes the disease," says Dr. Caudill. Often chronic pain has no clear-cut cause or source. But researchers are discovering the mechanics of chronic pain: an injured pain nerve that gets stuck on go, "like a broken thermostat," she says.

Chronic pain can bring in its wake even more symptoms—exhaustion and sore muscles (if they haven't shown up already) and even insomnia and depression. Luckily, most pain doesn't reach that stage. No matter what kind of pain plagues you, there are remedies that you can try at home. (See your doctor if they don't provide relief.)

Rub-A-Dub-Dub

Massage may be the most ancient and natural pain reliever of them all. Even in 2598 B.C., massage was known—and mentioned in a Chinese tome, *The Yellow Emperor's Classic of Internal Medicine*. Temple carvings in India show the great Buddha himself in a state of bliss as he gets a massage.

"Everybody is capable of doing massage on herself or others," says Joan Johnson, author of *The Healing Art of Sports Massage* and director of Sports Massage of the Rockies in Boulder, Colorado. Here are a few of her self-massage pain-relief techniques.

Play lower-back tennis. To loosen a stiff back, lie on the floor with your knees bent, your feet apart and your hands on your chest. Then position a tennis ball directly under the area you want to massage. Rest as much of your body weight on the ball as you can without feeling uncomfortable. Roll your back in a small circle around the tennis ball, then reposition the ball on other areas of your back for more self-massage. Massage each spot for a minute or two—but let your body be your guide.

Be nice to your neck. To massage a stiff neck, stand up straight and reach your right hand over your right shoulder and around to the back of your neck as shown on the opposite page (top left). Press four fingers firmly into the area of your neck directly below your skull, about an inch from the big knob that you can feel on your backbone. The points you want to massage, midway between the bottom of your skull and the top of your shoulder blade, are part of the trapezius muscle.

Hold your fingers at the starting point for a few seconds, then slowly tilt your head away from your hand while you drag your fingers down closer to your shoulder. Repeat on your

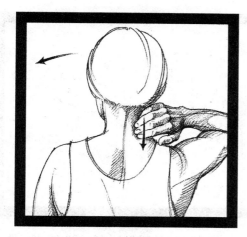

For a great neck massage, press and drag your fingers in the area shown while tilting your head away.

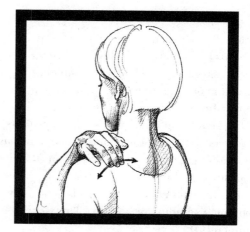

To massage the tension out of taut shoulder muscles, rock your fingers back and forth as indicated by the arrow.

left side using your left hand. Do this massage for several minutes, alternating sides.

Rock your shoulders. Sometimes your shoulders are so tense, you can almost feel the weight of the world pressing on them. To banish that burden, stand up straight, reach your right arm across your chest and press the fingertips of your right hand into the muscle at the top of your left shoulder as shown (top right). Rock your fingertips backward and forward to massage the muscle. Then repeat using the left fingertips on your right shoulder. Continue to massage for several minutes.

Putting the Pressure On

Western medicine is slowly accepting the hallowed pain-relief methods of the Chinese: acupuncture and its do-at-home variation, acupressure. Both forms rely on stimulating any of the body's 361 acupoints, which lie along 14 lines of energy that the Chinese call meridians. In Eastern therapy, pressure at any of these points restores the proper circulation of the body energy called qi (pro-

nounced chee), says Patrick J. LaRiccia, M.D., director of the acupuncture pain clinic at the Hospital of the University of Pennsylvania in Philadelphia.

"The Western theory is that acupressure releases endorphins, the body's own painkillers," says Dr. LaRiccia. Researchers have found that many acupoints correspond to neuron motor points, where large nerves meet muscle or bone. And meridians may be what scientists now call nerve pathways. In any case, numerous studies have found the venerable practice helps 56 to 85 percent of people with chronic pain.

Here are some ways to find relief.

Heal your head. Next time you have a headache, use this acupressure technique from David Nickel, O.M.D., doctor of oriental medicine, licensed acupuncturist and author of *Acupressure for Athletes*. Sit down and loosely cup your hands over your ears and the sides of your head. Position your thumbs at the base of your skull, about 1½ inches from the center of the back of your head.

Using your thumbs, apply pressure slowly,

gradually increasing force. "Press for five seconds and gradually release for five seconds," says Dr. Nickel. "Exhale forcefully through your mouth as you press, and inhale gently through your nose as you release. If you notice significant relief, that's all you need to do. If you want to induce more relaxation or if you didn't get quick results, keep your thumbs in position and repeat the routine.

Harass heel pain. If your heels ache after too much standing or walking, Dr. Nickel recommends this exercise.

Sit down on a rug or mat with your legs comfortably open and move the foot that hurts close to your body—but not uncomfortably so. Grasp that foot with both hands.

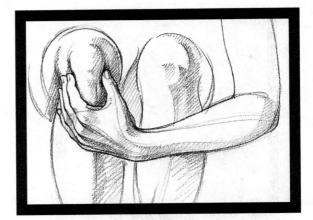

Pinch the area around your kneecap as shown to help relieve the pain of knee injury.

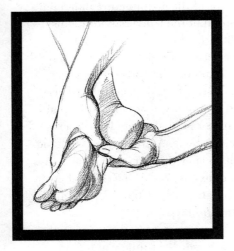

Relieve heel pain by pressing as shown on the acupressure point on the sole of your foot.

Your fingers should be on the top of your foot and your two thumbs on the bottom—over the end of the heel bone that's closest to the center of your foot. Position one thumb over the other for more pressure, then press for five seconds and release for five seconds. Continue for up to a minute, using Dr. Nickel's breathing technique at the same time—exhaling through your mouth as you press, inhaling through your nose as you release.

Rework runner's knee. If you've injured your knee while running or jumping, here's an exercise from Dr. Nickel to press away the pain.

Sit down on a chair with your legs bent at the knees. If your right knee hurts, use your left hand to pinch your knee with your thumb and forefinger at the base of your kneecap as shown above.

Your thumb and finger should be about 2½ inches apart. Using Dr. Nickel's breathing technique—exhaling through the mouth, inhaling through the nose—alternately apply and release pressure for five seconds each, for up to a minute.

Ice your ivories. The acupoint on your hand for tooth pain is in the "web" of skin between your thumb and index finger. With your right thumb, feel along the web of your left hand until you're pressing an area near the bone, as shown on the opposite page (top). That's the point the Chinese call Ho-ku. At that point, press the area for five-second intervals, again using Dr. Nickel's breathing technique. Press that area with an ice cube that's wrapped in a napkin or paper towel, as shown on the opposite page (bottom).

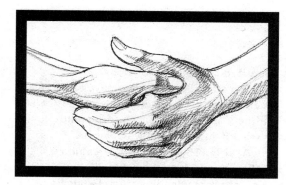

The acupressure point called Ho-ku is located on the "web" of your hand.

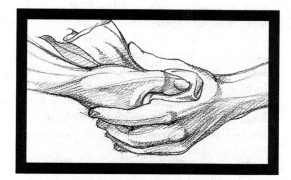

To relieve toothache pain, press the Ho-ku point with a wrapped-up ice cube.

Folding and Holding

If you bruise a bone or twist a joint, the muscles around the injury tense up like full-backs guarding the painful spot. Those hunched-up muscles fire off pain messages, too.

But there is a way to calm down those muscles. "Essentially, you first relax the muscle, pamper it, let the muscle rest and then ask it to gently stretch," says Dale L. Anderson, M.D., biomechanical medicine physician on the complementary (alternative) medicine committee of Park Nicollet Clinic in Minneapolis and author of *Muscle Pain Relief in 90 Seconds.* "What you're really doing is co-operating with Mother Nature and unleashing the 'physician within.' "

Here's the technique.

1. Find the tender spot. For most aches and pains, you can usually find a small area of the body that feels very tender. "That's the epicenter of the pain—the zinger," says Dr. Anderson.

To find the zinger, press into and around the general area that hurts until you touch the point that hurts most. Then "fold" your body as comfortably as you can around the spot in the direction of the pain. That shortens and relaxes the muscle as much as possible. The muscle will start to feel comfortable and the pain will start to leave.

2. Hold the position for 90 seconds. Ninety seconds is the minimum, not the maximum, Dr. Anderson says. You will probably want to continue the hold because your muscle will feel like melting butter. In the fold position, the body is treating itself.

3. Return to normal slowly. In the folded position your muscle forgets its pain, says Dr. Anderson. So awaken it very slowly and gently as you unfold it. "You don't want to excite that waking muscle into spasm again."

Learning to Relax

If you have chronic pain, your lifestyle may be contributing to your suffering. Relaxation and sleep could be the keys to relief.

"Many women who suffer from some kind of chronic pain just push through daily living until the pain tips them over the edge," says Dr. Caudill. "But there are basic, common-sense things to do—relaxation techniques, taking time for bubble baths, maintaining friendships and keeping up your social network." In order to find the time to do that, "it's very important for women to pace themselves and delegate activities to decrease stress and pain," she says.

(continued on page 298)

The Painkillers

Stretching, acupressure, massage and positive attitudes are among the best natural pain soothers. But sometimes the natural remedies don't help.

Enter medication.

Of course, many pain-soothing medicines have been around for a long time, and many have their origin in natural substances. Hippocrates, the father of modern medicine, advised ancient Greeks to chew on willow bark whenever they hurt or felt feverish. It turns out that white willow bark was full of salicylic acid—unrefined aspirin. Even the powerful prescription drug morphine is derived from a flower—the poppy.

The Master Medicines

There are an abundance of choices among prescription and over-the-counter drugs. Here's what some of them can do for you.

<u>Acetaminophen.</u> Like aspirin, acetaminophen is an analgesic—that is, a painkiller. Unlike aspirin, it's not an anti-inflammatory. Acetaminophen products such as Tylenol work by blocking pain messages to the brain.

They're a good aspirin substitute for people who have tricky stomachs, according to Tim Covington, Pharm.D., Bruno professor of Pharmacology at Samford University in Birmingham, Alabama.

<u>Antidepressants.</u> Tricyclic antidepressants (such as Elavil) work by affecting brain chemicals that control the perception of pain, says Richard M. Linchitz, M.D., medical director of the Pain Alleviation Center in New York City. Doctors often prescribe them for headaches, arthritis pain and neuropathy, a type of nerve pain that is often caused by diabetes.

The tricyclics may take days or weeks to become effective. Also, they can cause side effects such as dizziness, dry mouth, increased appetite and weight gain.

<u>Aspirin.</u> This century-old wonder drug relieves pain by quickly blocking production of prostaglandins, the chemicals in your body that contribute to pain and inflammation. It can relieve the inflammatory pain of joint injuries or arthritis flare-ups as well as headache.

The drawback is that aspirin can upset your stomach, and long-term use can cause internal bleeding. If your stomach is sensitive, use buffered aspirin—but be aware that it takes longer to work, because it slips through the stomach and isn't absorbed until it reaches the intestine, says Dr. Covington.

<u>Ibuprofen.</u> With product names like Advil and Nuprin, ibuprofen is an anti-inflammatory—and the pill of choice for menstrual cramps and toothaches.

Like aspirin, ibuprofen can cause bleeding problems. "However, the side effects of aspirin can last for 10 to 14 days, while the bleeding problems caused by ibuprofen are much more short-lived," says Peter Staats, M.D., assistant in the Division of Pain Medicine, Department of Anesthesiology and Critical Care Medicine at Johns Hopkins University School of Medicine in Baltimore.

If you take ibuprofen regularly, it can upset your stomach as aspirin does. Take it with meals, suggests Dr. Staats.

<u>Narcotics.</u> Also called opiates, the two common narcotics are codeine and morphine, which are strictly available as prescription drugs. They block pain signals, too, but they're much more powerful than

acetaminophen. For severe pain, doctors may combine these with other analgesics such as acetaminophen. Narcotics can be addictive. They can also cause drowsiness, dizziness and nausea.

Main Meds for Most Maladies

With aspirin, acetaminophen and ibuprofen, you have three inexpensive nonprescription pain relievers for almost every occasion. Which is best for each kind of pain? Here's an overview.

Headaches. For everyday tension-type headaches, each of the three drugstore pain relievers can do the job, says Frederick Freitag, D.O., member of the board of the National Headache Foundation.

Minor aches and fever. All three relievers work, but you might want to consider acetaminophen, because it's easier on your stomach lining than the others.

Toothaches. Ibuprofen is your best bet. It outperformed aspirin and acetaminophen in one study.

Sore muscles. Ibuprofen and aspirin have the edge. They are anti-inflammatory agents that help reduce swelling of sore or bruised muscles. Ibuprofen is less irritating than aspirin to most people's stomachs.

Sprains and tendinitis. Again, aspirin and ibuprofen get the nod, because they help reduce swelling.

Menstrual cramps. Ibuprofen is the drug of choice. For best results, start taking ibuprofen three days before you start your period.

Cautions

Any drug that's used for chronic pain can have a potential "tolerance" effect, says Margaret A. Caudill, M.D., Ph.D., co-director of the Arnold Pain Center at Deaconess Hospital in Boston, assistant clinical professor of medicine at Harvard Medical School and author of Managing Pain before It Manages You. "Taking daily painkillers can really cause you problems," she says. "The body has a way of building up tolerance to any drug used to kill pain. Your body may need more and more medication to relieve pain—and it can produce side effects."

To prevent a rebound problem, take pain medication no more than three days a week, suggests Alan Rapoport, M.D., co-director of the New England Center for Headache in Stamford, Connecticut, assistant clinical professor of neurology at Yale University School of Medicine and co-author of Headache Relief for Women.

This is particularly important for women, who might react more strongly than men to standard doses of many medications. The standard doses are usually based on studies done on men, who are generally larger and heavier than most women.

Women have drug side effects about twice as often as men do, doctors say. And women tend to absorb and use more of the medication in an average drug dose. Women also eliminate drugs from their systems more slowly than men do.

Sleep problems can make pain problems worse, adds Dr. Caudill. She recommends a period of unwinding before you go to bed. "Write in a diary or do breathing exercises."

One method to help release tension is the relaxation response described by Dr. Caudill's colleague, Herbert Benson, M.D., at Harvard Medical School in the early 1970s. Here's how to do it: Sit or lie down in a comfortable position, relax all your muscles and breathe slowly and deeply. Focus on a phrase or a word and repeat it in your mind each time you exhale. If your mind wanders, gently guide it back to your word.

Don't pay attention to thoughts that intrude; just let them passively float through your mind. Practice the relaxation response for 20 minutes once a day or for 10 minutes twice a day, advises Dr. Caudill.

If there are some days when you don't have ten consecutive minutes to yourself, here's a quick relaxer from Dr. Caudill: Take a moment to tense all your muscles at once, then take a deep breath and slowly breathe out, letting all the tension go.

Tools of the Trade

Gimmicks and gadgets galore promise to vanquish your pain. Some of them only cause more pain—in your purse. Here are two tools that really work, experts say.

Say ahhh with a Thera Cane. The Thera Cane is a hook-shaped plastic rod with small bumps at both ends. Along its length are four smooth-tipped pressure applicators, or pitons. By pressing the pitons against different areas of your body, you can deep-massage muscles that are difficult to reach, including the ones in your back. Simply press the piton into the muscle and slowly rock it back and forth across the tender spot. The tool comes

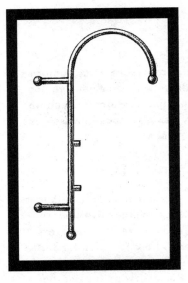

Made of hard plastic, the Thera Cane has a number of bumps, knobs and handles—so you can apply "deep pressure massage" to different areas of your body.

with directions and a video. To find out where you can buy one, you can contact the Thera Cane Company by calling 1-800-947-1470.

Get some feedback. With biofeedback techniques, you can actually learn how to control and diminish pain by altering your

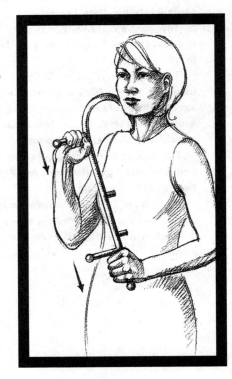

To get pain relief in the back and shoulder, hold the Thera Cane as shown, applying pressure as shown to "deep massage" the shoulder muscle. Instructions with the Thera Cane describe other positions and pressure points for pain relief.

Take Flight from Plane Pain

If airplane ear pain puts you off flying, or makes every flight extremely uncomfortable, here's a way to tame the problem.

Thirty minutes before your flight leaves, take a decongestant that contains pseudoephedrine. In a study of 190 fliers with recurrent ear pain, only 32 percent of the people who received pseudoephedrine before takeoff had ear pain, compared with 62 percent in the placebo group. This research confirms anecdotal reports of the effectiveness of this pain prevention strategy. Decongestants dilate the eustachian tubes and make it easier to clear the ears of the pressure built up inside. The medicine also helps decrease secretions that might block the tubes, says study co-author Jeffrey Jones, M.D., director of the Department of Emergency Medicine at Butterworth Hospital in Grand Rapids, Michigan.

But researchers warn against this decongestant if you have thyroid disease, heart disease, high blood pressure or diabetes. In these cases Dr. Jones recommends other ear-clearing techniques, such as chewing gum or yawning.

body's response to pain signals.

Here's how it works. A trained biofeedback therapist hooks you up to sensors connected to a biofeedback machine. The machine can measure muscle tension, temperature, breathing patterns, heart rate or blood flow. If you have back pain or a headache, the biofeedback machine registers it and immediately feeds you audible or visual signals—in the form of beeps or flashing lights.

Over a period of two to six months, the therapist trains you how to use your body to regulate and control the lights and sounds—and hence your pain. By achieving pain-free state feels like. Eventually, you can reproduce that state yourself and graduate from the machine.

Pain-Free Food

For people who get headaches there are specific foods that can cause pain. Migraine triggers such as red wine and chocolate are infamous. But studies show that some foods do the opposite—and actually increase your pain tolerance, says Dr. Caudill. Here's how to sort through the good and the bad.

Talk turkey. Foods such as turkey and milk that contain the essential amino acid tryptophan are terrific. Tryptophan is a precursor to the pain-squashing brain chemical serotonin. It has been used to treat premenstrual problems, depression and drug and alcohol cravings.

A diet rich in tryptophan, high in complex carbohydrates and low in proteins may increase pain tolerance, says Dr. Caudill. She recommends tryptophan titans such as turkey and other lean meats, fish and low-fat or nonfat milk. But the secret to good health and pain relief is simple, general nutrition. "You should always eat a balanced diet and never skip meals," she advises.

Abort alcohol. Many of Dr. Caudill's chronic pain patients have found that alcohol makes their problems worse. If you get frequent headaches or muscle pain, try eliminating alcohol and see if you feel better.

If alcohol seems to trigger headaches at some times and not at others, try limiting your cocktails to one glass of dry white wine

(continued on page 302)

Your Guide to Pain-Free Dentistry

If you ever saw the dental-torture scene in the movie Marathon Man, you'll never forget it. Laurence Olivier bends over Dustin Hoffman with a drill—and an agenda: As soon as Hoffman spills the beans, Olivier will stop the drill. It's a classic fear-monger's moment.

For most women it doesn't take a movie to inspire dental terror. Many of us will do almost anything to avoid going to a dentist. Chances are, no matter how minor the procedure, we're probably going to feel a little pain.

Well, you can't stop it all. But some strategies can help you avoid feeling like a marathon woman in the hot seat.

Talking about your specific concerns is the first step toward heading off dental discomfort. "A straightforward statement to the dentist early on can make a difference," says Raymond Dionne, D.D.S., Ph.D., clinical researcher at the National Institute of Dental Research at the National Institutes of Health in Bethesda, Maryland.

"Let the dentist know that you're concerned about discomfort and that you'd like her to do everything possible to make the procedure less painful for you," Dr. Dionne adds.

Here are other things you can do to help make your time in the chair more comfortable:

Tell all. You can help the dentist—and help develop a rapport—if you say what you're most concerned about.

"Tell the dentist what it is about the treatment that may bother you—even something as simple as sitting too long in the same position," says Herman Segal, D.D.S., director of courses in behavioral management of pain and anxiety in the Department of Oral Medicine at the University of Pennsylvania School of Dental Medicine in Philadelphia. "That can help your dentist figure out the barriers to treatment and how to defuse the problem."

Numb out. Ask your dentist to numb the area before injecting an anesthetic, suggests Stuart Fountain, D.D.S., president of the American Association of Endodontists. If she applies an anesthetic spray or ointment to your gums first and waits a few minutes while the area numbs before inserting the needle, the procedure may be much more tolerable.

Note: This technique isn't routine—so be sure to ask for it before your dentist gets to work.

Slow the action. Slow-motion injections are less painful than quick ones, so ask your dentist for the slow treatment. "When the injection is hurried, there's a sudden pressure buildup within the tissues," says Dr. Fountain. Injecting the needle slowly takes away the pressure and makes the injection much more comfortable."

Ask for ice. The dentist can place ice on your tooth to test if it's thoroughly anesthetized before beginning treatment. "If you don't feel the cold, you won't feel what the dentist does to the tooth," Dr. Fountain says. "If you flunk the ice test, ask for more local anesthetic."

Don't grimace and bear it. If you feel

any pain at all during the procedure, there's a chance you didn't get enough anesthetic to begin with, or it's starting to wear off.

"It's good to talk about this before the procedure begins," says Dr. Segal. If you prearrange a signal, the dentist will know you're feeling pain. For instance, you might tell the dentist that you'll raise your hand if you begin to feel pain.

Tote a Walkman. "A lot of people have a problem with the noise of the drill," Dr. Fountain says. "So more and more people are bringing in headphones and a portable radio or tape deck with their favorite music to block out the noise and help them relax."

Go digital. Before you have root canal work, your dentist might check the response of the tooth's tissue to determine whether the procedure is necessary. Using an electric tester with digital controls, your dentist can measure how much sensation you experience in the sensitive area.

Try conscious sedation. You can get an intravenous sedative that lets you stay awake, even though your body's relaxed and you're not fully aware of the procedure.

Conscious sedation is nearly as effective as general anesthesia, without as high a risk of slowed breathing, according to a study headed up by Dr. Dionne. "If you're going to have a very unpleasant procedure like impacted wisdom tooth removal, or if you're very phobic, it's a good alternative," he says.

Take the local. It's not often that your procedure requires a general anesthetic, but when it does, you can ask for a local anesthetic, too. That may reduce the amount of pain you feel after procedures that can require general anesthesia, such as wisdom tooth removal. "Pain signals still get through under general anesthesia, even though you don't feel them because you're asleep," Dr. Dionne says.

Prep to stop pain. Take a nonsteroidal anti-inflammatory drug (NSAID), such as ibuprofen, before or just after the procedure to reduce postoperative pain. "Tooth pain is related to pressure from inflammation that makes fluid accumulate around the tooth," Dr. Fountain says. NSAIDs can lessen the accumulation.

Follow your dentist's advice about how much ibuprofen you should take and how often.

"As little as 400 milligrams of ibuprofen before the procedure has a dramatic effect on suppressing the amount of pain people have in the post-op period," Dr. Dionne says.

Ask your dentist about laughing gas. If you're really nervous, nitrous oxide (called laughing gas because it can relax you to the point that you giggle at just about anything) is a mild form of general anesthetic that you inhale.

Nitrous oxide isn't potent enough to put you out, but it can help take the edge off. Its effects disappear within a few minutes after you stop breathing it. Not everyone can take laughing gas, but your dentist can help you decide whether it might help with the pain.

at a time, suggests Alan Rapoport, M.D., co-director of the New England Center for Headache in Stamford, Connecticut, assistant clinical professor of neurology at Yale University School of Medicine and co-author of *Headache Relief for Women*.

In general, the lighter the color of alcohol, the lighter the pain reaction. Even if you just have one glass of wine, drink several glasses of water before you go to bed and more water when you get up to rehydrate, suggests Dr. Rapoport.

When the Head Aches

The ancient gods punished offenders for their sins by giving them headaches, our early sisters thought. Later on, Egyptians wrapped their aching heads in their best linen to relieve pain. On top of the wrapped heads, they placed clay crocodiles, with some wheat in the crocs' mouths from the gods' sacred storeroom.

Modern versions of the cloth and croc still exist. Some women remember their grandmothers tying a rag around a throbbing head. Folks in Latin America sometimes use a live toad on the head instead of a clay crocodile.

Whether divine, demonic or just plain human, headaches are as common as sin. About 90 percent of all the people in the world have had a tension-type headache, says Dr. Rapoport.

Tension-type, migraine and cluster headaches make up 90 percent of all the headaches that people have. The allergy or sinus kind is much more rare. Also rare are the headaches caused by strokes, tumors or infections.

The term *tension-type* refers to tense muscles in the head and neck, but it might just as well mean tension from stress—a common headache trigger. Once you're in its grip, those

Head Off Stress

Though no one asks for headaches, we may be heading for them if we let stress get out of hand, says Joseph Primavera III, Ph.D., co-director of the Comprehensive Headache Center at Germantown Hospital and Medical Center in Philadelphia. "If you're under stress and out of shape, at some point your body is going to speak loudly to you. If you're genetically inclined, headache may be the voice that comes in loud and clear."

Unfortunately, as they sense a headache coming on, many people try to get as much done as they can before it gets worse. "That's like stepping on the gas in your car when the gas tank is on empty," says Alvin Lake, Ph.D., division director of psychology and associate program director of the head-pain treatment unit at Michigan Head Pain and Neurological Institute in Ann Arbor.

Instead, try some quick de-stressors that Dr. Primavera recommends.

tense muscles make a tension-type headache feel like a tight band around your head.

Migraine headaches usually start on one side of the head—above the eye, for instance. Once you have a migraine, you might be acutely sensitive to the slightest sound or light. Some women also experience nausea and vomiting.

Some of those who get migraines—migraineurs, doctors call them—get a warning in the form of auras, which are flickering points of light and jagged lines that distort vision.

Migraine headaches are vascular headaches, meaning that they involve your blood vessels. First, those blood vessels con-

- **While you're stopped at a traffic light, drop your shoulders, lift your breastbone and breathe deeply. Also, set your rearview mirror in a position that will force you to sit up straighter.**
- **At the office, pause in your work about once an hour. Close your eyes for one minute and take some deep breaths.**
- **Take a stretch break in the morning and again in the afternoon.**

At the first sign of a headache, stop what you're doing for just a few minutes, breathe deeply and relax with one of the following:

- **Close your eyes and give your face, scalp and neck a mini-massage.**
- **Think of a favorite place: a quiet, grassy patch of woods or a warm, sunny beach.**
- **Sit or lie down comfortably—then progressively relax your muscles, starting from your toes and working your way up to the top of your head.**

strict, which can set off the auras and also make you super-sensitive to sound and light. Then the blood vessels dilate, producing pain.

The tendency to get migraines is inherited, so if you get them, it's likely that someone in your family gets them, too. For some women the trigger that sets off the headache can be biological, such as hormonal swings in the menstrual cycle. Other possible triggers include your environment, stress or alcohol. Also, there are people who get migraines in response to drops in barometric pressure.

Migraine and tension-type headaches can be hard to tell apart, and some experts believe the two types are part of a continuum, with no clear boundary between them, says Dr. Caudill.

A cluster headache feels like a sharp, piercing, throbbing, burning pain that bores into one side of your head or around or behind your eyes. Cluster headaches are uncommon in women, though.

What Triggers the Assault?

Among the three major triggers of migraines in women are the menstrual cycle, food and stress. In the food category, certain ingredients are more likely than others to be linked with migraine attacks. Alcohol is the biggest bully, but many people are sensitive to caffeine or products containing aspartame (such as NutraSweet) or monosodium glutamate, or MSG.

Other possible triggers are foods that contain tyramine, such as aged cheeses, fresh bread, pickled or fermented foods, liver, red wine, yogurt, figs and bananas. Or you might have to watch out for foods that contain nitrites, a chemical that preserves processed meats, such as bologna, salami, pepperoni, bacon, ham and hot dogs. Other foods that some people have to avoid include nuts, peanut butter, onions, sour cream and avocados.

See also Nervous System

Pancreas

IF THE PANCREAS WERE NOMINATED for an Emmy, most likely it would be in the category of best supporting gland. It's often considered a behind-the-scenes player—not one of those star organs like the heart that captures the limelight of publicity.

Yet the role it plays is crucial.

The golden-colored gland is only about seven to eight inches long and three to four inches wide. It sits just behind the stomach, and the broadest end, the "head," is connected to the small intestine. The tail—the narrower part that's down at the lower end of the gland—is located near the spleen. Between the head and the tail is what's called the body of the pancreas—the main part of the gland. All in all, a drawing of a pancreas kind of resembles an oversize tongue.

Cell Director

Even though it seems like a small bit player in the body, the pancreas deserves our applause, because it contains special cells called beta cells that, in small clusters, are known as the islets of Langerhans. These beta cells secrete the hormone insulin. Insulin basically acts as stage director when it comes to our energy metabolism. It's essential to our body's ability to utilize food.

After we eat, a complex process takes place in which food gets broken down into a form of sugar—called glucose, or blood sugar—and also into fat. In the muscle cells that take in the glucose, it's converted to yet another chemical form called glycogen. The muscles then store the glycogen for use as an energy source. Fat cells take in the fat.

Throughout these processes, insulin plays the role of director. Insulin tells the fat cells to take in the fat and store it, and the muscle cells to take in the sugar.

Without insulin, or without enough of it, the body gets into serious trouble. The sugar in the bloodstream can't get transported into our muscle cells. So even though that blood sugar is available, it has nowhere to go, says Lawrence Hunsicker, M.D., professor of internal medicine at the University of Iowa College of Medicine in Iowa City. The same goes for the fat. Sugar and fat show up outside a muscle or fat cell, but they might as well be underage teenagers at a well-policed nightclub. Without their IDs—in the form of insulin—sugar can't get in, and the fat can get a table but can't get served.

When Insulin Poops Out

Diabetes is a disease where insulin either doesn't show up or is unable to do its job—depending on what kind of diabetes it is. One type of diabetes is insulin-dependent (called Type I): that's when the pancreas stops making insulin because those special islets of Langerhans cell clusters have been destroyed. This type of diabetes usually develops before a person is 20 years old.

With the second type of diabetes, non-insulin-dependent (called Type II) diabetes, the pancreas usually makes some insulin, but either there is not enough of it produced, or the fat and muscle cells in the body become resistant to it and keep it from doing its job. Type II diabetes generally develops in adulthood and often arises around the age of 40.

When Babies Grab Glucose

The hormonal changes that take place during pregnancy sometimes trigger diabetes in women who have never had it before. The condition, known as gestational diabetes, presents a risk both to the fetus and to the mother, says Yvonne S. Thornton, M.D., visiting associate physician at Rockefeller University Hospital in New York City and director of the perinatal diagnostic testing center at Morristown Memorial Hospital in New Jersey.

If you're pregnant, there's about a 3 to 5 percent chance that you'll develop gestational diabetes, according to Dr. Thornton. The risk is higher for Mexican-American and Native American women than it is for other women. While you can't prevent gestational diabetes, regular blood tests can lead to early detection, which is important for your health and the future health of your child.

How does it happen?

Normally, insulin helps escort glucose from the bloodstream into the cells that store it, so insulin is leaving the blood at the same time as the blood sugar. But when gestational diabetes develops, the placenta battles the pancreas for insulin needed for a growing baby and wins the war. With the pancreas exhausted and un-able to keep up with the increasing demands for insulin, diabetes develops.

The risk to the fetus is that it is likely to be a large baby that requires cesarean section or suffers birth trauma, she says. A large child also runs the risk of obesity in childhood and all the risks for chronic disease that come with obesity. As far as the mother is concerned, there's about a 30 to 50 percent chance that she will develop Type II (non-insulin-dependent) diabetes within the first five years after she has delivered the baby.

Unfortunately, there's not a whole lot that women who are pregnant can do to prevent gestational diabetes, says Dr. Thornton. Because undetected diabetes can lead to unexplained stillborns, it is essential to get screened with a blood sugar test between the 24th and 28th weeks of pregnancy. That test will tell your doctors if your blood sugar is high and enable them to make dietary recommendations to address the problem.

For women who develop gestational diabetes during pregnancy and want to prevent progressing on to Type II diabetes after pregnancy, the best thing to do is make sure to return to an ideal body weight, says Dr. Thornton.

An estimated 13 million people in the United States have diabetes, and about 90 percent of them have Type II diabetes.

Type II diabetes can be dangerous, because you end up with excess sugar in the bloodstream, either because you don't have sufficient insulin or because your cells are resistant to it. High sugar levels are responsible for damage to the kidneys, eyes and other organs, says Dr. Hunsicker. And since fat isn't being properly slurped up by your cells, fat levels in the bloodstream can build up and contribute to the development of atherosclerosis, or hardening of the arteries. That's one reason why heart disease is frequently a major complication of diabetes.

Finding Out Where You Stand

Researchers hope that before long, they'll develop a way to help prevent Type I diabetes—because once the beta cells in the islets of Langherans are destroyed, they're gone for good. For the much more common Type II diabetes, however, experts already know steps that you can take to lower your chances of developing the disease.

The first thing to do is assess your risk of getting Type II diabetes. Here's what doctors recommend.

Take a hint from your folks. Having a family history of Type II diabetes places you at increased risk for the disease, says John Bantle, M.D., of the Division of Diabetes, Endocrinology and Metabolism at the University of Minnesota in Minneapolis. "If you have a parent with diabetes, your risk goes up." Chances are about one in three that you'll develop the disease if one parent had it. If both did, your chances are about 50/50. Anyone with a family history of the disease needs to be extra vigilant about taking preventive measures.

Watch for clues. An estimated half of those who have Type II diabetes don't know it. Often that is because there aren't any symptoms. But sometimes there are symptoms; you just need to know how to recognize them so that you can get help early. The three classic signs of diabetes are unusual thirst, frequent urination and unexplained weight loss, says Dr. Bantle. So if you experience these symptoms, be sure to tell your doctor.

Get screened. Since you can also have diabetes even if you don't have symptoms, find out for sure by asking your doctor to check how your pancreas is performing. This can be done with a blood sugar test. This test measures the amount of glucose in your blood to

determine whether you might have the disease. If you have diabetes in your family, it's important to have your blood sugar checked once a year, says Dr. Hunsicker.

Watch that waist-to-hip ratio. There is evidence to suggest that the waist-to-hip ratio and, particularly, the waist circumference are important in determining whether you're likely to get Type II diabetes, says Gregory

---

Snack for Stability

If we were all smart, we'd eat like cows. That's because grazing may be a major key to keeping insulin levels stable.

One study illustrating the glories of grazing had 12 people with Type II (non-insulin-dependent) diabetes eating either two large or six small meals over an eight-hour period on two different occasions. When they ate the two big meals, their insulin levels rose much higher than when they ate the six meals over the eight-hour period. The two large meals also induced a yo-yo effect, with an 84 percent difference between the lowest and highest levels of glucose.

"This attitude of 'Suzy, don't snack' is dead wrong for us today," says Aaron Vinik, M.D., Ph.D., director of the Diabetes Research Institute in Norfolk, Virginia. "Research suggests that you get much healthier blood sugar and insulin levels from multiple feedings—having three small meals and three snacks throughout the day."

Between a small breakfast and light lunch add fruit or a nonfat yogurt snack. Between lunch and a light dinner add another snack—a bowl of rice or some vegetable sticks. Then round out the evening with a postdinner snack—nonfat frozen yogurt or a small bowl of nonfat cereal with skim milk.

Dwyer, Ph.D., exercise physiology professor at Ball State University in Muncie, Indiana.

Women who carry their weight around their waists are a prime target for the disease, he says. To determine your waist-to-hip ratio, take the measurement of your waist and divide it by the measurement of your hips. If the result is 0.86 or higher, then you are at high risk, says Dr. Dwyer. For example, if your waist is 28 inches and your hips measure 34 inches, your waist-to-hip ratio is 0.82, so you're on the safe side. If you let your waist size swell to 30 inches, however, the ratio becomes 0.88—which may be asking for diabetes trouble. Time for a weight-loss plan.

Playing the Prevention Game

Researchers have a good idea of the dietary and exercise factors that put you at greater risk of Type II diabetes. Based on those studies, doctors recommend a number of important lifestyle habits that will help you fend off the disease.

Watch the weight gain. When it comes to preventing diabetes, the best strategy is to maintain an ideal body weight, says Dr. Bantle. Data suggest that if you are modestly overweight—that is, you need to lose about 10 pounds—losing those pounds won't make a dramatic difference. But if you're supposed to weigh about 125 pounds, and you're actually closer to 150, it's time to reduce. In general, anything greater than 120 percent of your ideal body weight puts you at increased risk, according to Dr. Bantle. Dropping some pounds is one thing that is clearly beneficial in preventing diabetes, he says. But you want to do it with steady weight loss, not by going on a crash diet—unless it's a diet your physician recommends and monitors for you.

Well, are you in that risk area of being overweight? Instead of just looking at what you weigh now, ask yourself how much weight you have gained since you were in your twenties, suggests Lesley Fels Tinker, M.D., nutrition scientist working on the Women's Health Initiative for the Clinical Coordinating Center at the Fred Hutchinson Cancer Research Center in Seattle. With some exceptions that's the age when most of us hover near our ideal weight.

If you are overweight, consider increasing your physical activity and decreasing your food intake, suggests Dr. Tinker.

Make a motion. Research shows that if you're more active, over the course of your lifetime, you'll have a much lower risk for diabetes than your couch-potato neighbor, ac-

Stroll for Control

If you have diabetes and you're a walker, you're a step ahead in combating the effects of your condition. "Exercise helps improve blood sugar control by making the muscles more sensitive to insulin," says Neil F. Gordon, M.D., Ph.D., director of preventive cardiology at the Dallas Heart Group and Institute of Exercise and Environmental Medicine at Presbyterian Hospital and author of <u>Diabetes: Your Complete Exercise Guide</u>. "But even if the blood sugar level is not affected, we know that exercise reduces the risk of coronary heart disease, which is what most people with diabetes eventually die of."

People with Type II (non-insulin-dependent) diabetes who aren't taking any medications can feel safe developing a walking program after a complete physical to rule out any heart or neurological problems, says Dr. Gordon.

cording to Dr. Dwyer. A study of nearly 6,000 male alumni of the University of Pennsylvania in Philadelphia conducted by the University of California School of Public Health at Berkeley strongly suggests that physical activity may help prevent Type II diabetes. Two additional studies conducted at Harvard University—one of men and the other of more than 87,000 women—also suggest the protective effect of walking, running, bicycling and other steadily maintained activities. While there are no specific guidelines for how many hours of exercise you need to get each week to prevent the disease, says Dr. Dwyer, the message is that the more active you are, the better.

When Enzymes Run Rampant

While the islets of Langerhans are known for insulin production, the pancreas also produces other important chemicals—specifically, the digestive enzymes that we need to digest our food. But sometimes the pancreas gets an inflammation—for reasons unknown—that disrupts the release of digestive enzymes, says Joseph Lyon, M.D., professor in the Department of Family and Preventive Medicine at the University of Utah School of Medicine in Salt Lake City.

Because those digestive enzymes are powerful—after all, they're the chemical crunchers that break down food in your intestines—they can create a bad scene if they get misdirected. This happens when you have pancreatitis. Normally, your pancreas releases enzymes in an inactive state into the upper portion of the small intestine, and it is there where they become activated and go to work on food. When pancreatitis develops, however, the enzymes spill into the abdomen instead, says Dr. Lyon. The enzymes basically start attacking your internal digestive organs.

The problem is that nobody knows what causes pancreatitis. It's been associated with gallstones. There is some evidence that high levels of alcohol intake can trigger it. "But there is nothing really in the way of a prevention strategy for pancreatitis," says Dr. Lyon. "You just hope that you don't get it."

When it strikes, pancreatitis causes severe abdominal pain and vomiting. The pain is intense, and you'll know that you need medical help, says Dr. Lyon. Once it is diagnosed, there are a number of effective treatments.

When Cancer Strikes

Television celebs Michael Landon and Donna Reed got it. So did Jimmy Carter's brother, Billy. So pancreatic cancer has made the headlines now and then.

While pancreatic cancer isn't as prevalent as lung cancer or skin cancer, it's more likely to be fatal than many kinds of cancer that are more common. Even though it's the ninth most common malignancy in the United States, it's the fourth most common cause of cancer death.

Doctors have found a consistent link between smoking and pancreatic cancer. Since this cancer is so dangerous and smoking is clearly a risk factor, it just makes sense to give up the habit, says Dr. Lyon.

In addition to the smoking risk, some doctors say, there's a link between a high-fat diet and pancreatic cancer. The connection is less clear, says Dr. Lyon. But because a low-fat diet helps ward off many other health problems as well, sticking to a low-fat diet certainly couldn't hurt, he observes.

See also Digestive System, Endocrine System

Pelvis

Pregnancy

WHEN ELVIS "THE PELVIS" PRESLEY first displayed his pelvic gyrations to the public, what did everybody think of?

Sex.

And when Michael Jackson or Madonna starts swiveling and thrusting, what can't you help thinking about?

Sex.

But the pelvis itself—a ring of bones in the lower trunk—is really designed to bear your weight and protect your internal organs. In women the pelvis is uniquely designed for childbirth. So much for pelvic erotica.

The pelvis, or pelvic girdle, as it is officially called in medical lingo, is located between your belly button and your crotch. When you place your hands on your hips, you are actually resting them on top of your pelvis. The true hip—the hip joint, that is—is located lower down and further inward.

In women the pelvis tends to be wider, lighter, shallower and rounder than it is in men. The center opening is larger and rounder so that the head and body of a fetus can fit through at birth. Also, the joint where the two sides meet is less rigid in women, so that the pelvis can expand during childbirth.

The pelvis is a tough bone, but it can get fractured. In older women, fractures are most often related to osteoporosis. Automobile accidents are another common cause, says Ira H. Kirschenbaum, M.D., arthritis and joint replacement surgeon at Westchester Bone and Joint Associates in White Plains, New York.

See also Skeletal System

THERE'S NO MISTAKING the telltale signs of baby fever.

If it's your first, you may have found yourself gravitating toward piles of Oshkosh B'-Gosh overalls instead of Levi's 501 jeans. Or maybe you catch yourself looking at infants when you're in the supermarket.

If this is your second or third pregnancy, the telltale signs probably take the form of practical planning. Maybe you're talking to your husband about the best times to get pregnant or when you'll move your toddler into her "big girl" bed to free up the crib. Or you're telling your friends, "We're thinking about having another one."

Preparing for Pregnancy

Whether you're aiming to get pregnant next year or in the next few months, you should be getting ready now. This means eating right, getting plenty of exercise and maintaining a healthy weight, says Kathleen Kuhlman, M.D., maternal fetal medicine specialist at Thomas Jefferson University in Philadelphia. "There is just really no substitute for being healthy going into the pregnancy."

This is particularly true for women over age 30. When you're past the nearly foolproof bloom of youth, family-inherited medical problems such as diabetes and high blood pressure may develop. If that happens, your pregnancy can get much more difficult.

While most women see their doctors after they get pregnant, it's best to get a checkup ahead of time in order to spot any underlying, potentially complicating conditions, such as high blood pressure, says Dr. Kuhlman. Here's what your doctor may recommend.

Take a history lesson. A woman should know as much as she can about her genetic background, says Dr. Kuhlman. If someone in your family has cystic fibrosis or mental retardation, it's important to let your doctor know. She may advise you to undergo genetic counseling to determine what the various risks are. In some rare cases your best bet may be *not* to get pregnant—but this is something you'll want to take up with an expert.

Aim for your ideal. Ask your doctor what your healthy weight should be, then do your best to reach that target before getting pregnant. Women who are underweight have a higher chance of having a preterm delivery or giving birth to a smaller baby, says Dr. Kuhlman.

Overweight women tend to have larger babies, "which are more likely to cause problems with delivery or cesarean section," says Jennifer Niebyl, M.D., professor and head of obstetrics and gynecology at the University of Iowa Hospital and Clinics in Iowa City.

There are also other risks associated with being overweight during pregnancy. That extra weight can put you at higher risk for diabetes, high blood pressure and back pain.

Slim slow and steady. While being overweight during pregnancy can cause problems, you don't want to crash diet and try to lose weight all at once. A weight-loss program should never be started during pregnancy, says Dr. Kuhlman. If you are overweight and not yet pregnant, talk to your doctor about starting a sensible weight-loss plan.

Don't forget the folic acid. One of the most important things a woman can do to protect her baby is take extra folic acid, according to Dr. Kuhlman. This vitamin has been shown to significantly reduce the risk of having a baby with a neural tube defect, such as spina bifida, which is a defect in the spinal column.

It doesn't take much folic acid to help prevent this condition, which can leave a child

---

Hints for Maturer Moms

Although most women over age 35 go through normal pregnancies without any complications, they still need to be more wary than their younger counterparts. This is because they're more likely to develop conditions such as Type II (non-insulin-dependent) diabetes or high blood pressure—conditions that could have a significant effect on the pregnancy. They also have a higher risk of miscarriage, blood clots in the legs and bleeding during pregnancy.

"Anybody in her mid-thirties or beyond who is even contemplating getting pregnant ought to have a very thorough evaluation," says Lawrence Devoe, M.D., professor of obstetrics and gynecology and director of maternal fetal medicine at the Medical College of Georgia in Augusta.

Although we don't normally think of women in their thirties as being at risk for high blood pressure, this problem occurs in almost one out of every ten pregnancies, according to Dr. Devoe. High blood pressure doesn't cause visible symptoms for years or even decades—but because it can lead to heart attack and other problems, it's critical to catch it early.

Women over 35 are also at a higher-than-average risk for gestational diabetes, a form of diabetes that only occurs during pregnancy. By age 35 the risks begin to rise for birth defects like Down's syndrome.

To Test or Not to Test

Many prenatal tests are available, but which ones you choose to have will depend on you and your doctor. Although your doctor can advise you, the ultimate decision is really yours. So here are some of the tests your doctor might recommend.

Ultrasound. By beaming ultrasound waves into the woman's body, an image of the fetus is generated on a screen. This can help tell you how the fetus is positioned in the womb, whether it's growing and developing normally and if there's more than one fetus.

Alpha-fetoprotein (AFP) screening. By testing your blood between the 13th and 18th weeks of pregnancy for a substance produced by the baby's liver, doctors can detect potential birth defects, such as neural tube defect and Down's syndrome. If abnormalities are found with an AFP test, further tests—such as a repeat AFP or ultrasound—may be done. Fortunately, 95 percent of women who receive an abnormal AFP test result give birth to babies without a neural tube defect.

Triple testing. This test, which includes AFP and can be administered at the same stage of pregnancy, screens for neural tube defect, just as AFP can. It also screens for Down's syndrome—and it can improve the detection rate for Down's syndrome threefold.

Amniocentesis. Most often used for women who are age 35 or older or who are experiencing a high-risk pregnancy, amniocentesis is usually performed during the 16th week. The doctor can insert a needle into the uterus and withdraw amniotic fluid, which can then be tested for genetic birth defects, such as chromosome abnormalities. Though the test is quite safe, it does slightly increase the risk of miscarriage.

Chorionic villi sampling (CVS). Also used to detect possible birth defects, CVS is generally performed between the 10th and 12th weeks. The doctor takes a small sample of the placental tissue, called chorionic villi, which can be tested for genetic defects. The risk of miscarriage from CVS is a bit higher than with amniocentesis, but the test can be performed as many as six weeks earlier.

Fetal monitoring. This is used to check the heart health of the fetus in some high-risk pregnancies. A "nonstress" test is performed by monitoring fetal heart rate and fluctuations in fetal activity. The "contraction stress" test also measures the heart rate—but it's during uterine contractions that have been induced.

seriously handicapped. To be on the safe side, doctors recommend getting 0.4 milligram a day, either as a supplement (the folic acid form) or in foods that are high in folate, the the natural form of folic acid. Foods high in folate include lentils, lima beans, spinach and wheat germ.

Begin taking folic acid before you get pregnant, says Dr. Kuhlman. The neural tube begins to form around the time a pregnant woman misses her period, and it's closed at 28 days after conception. So if you wait until you're already pregnant before taking folic acid, that may be too late to get the extra protection.

Ask about medicines. While some medications are perfectly safe for a pregnant woman, others are not. The risk varies with timing:

Often the greatest danger is during the first six weeks—a time when many women don't even know that they're pregnant. If you are planning on getting pregnant soon, says Dr. Kuhlman, ask your doctor ahead of time what medications you can take and which you should steer clear of.

Iron out anemia. If you already have iron-deficiency anemia when you get pregnant, you may have an increased risk for preterm delivery. Unless you do something to compensate for the lack of iron and other dietary inadequacies, you might have a low-birth-weight baby, according to Theresa Scholl, Ph.D., professor of obstetrics and gynecology at the University of Medicine and Dentistry of New Jersey Robert Wood Johnson Medical School in Piscataway.

Doctors recommend that you have a blood test to find out if you're iron deficient before you're pregnant. "It's really hard to catch up if you're anemic when you start pregnancy," says Dr. Niebyl. If your iron is at low ebb, your doctor will probably recommend taking supplements.

Toss the cigs and spare the child. Women should aim to begin pregnancy in a state of the best possible health, says Lawrence Devoe, M.D., professor of obstetrics and gynecology and director of maternal fetal medicine at the Medical College of Georgia in Augusta. It's especially important to stop smoking before you get pregnant, since cigarettes are associated with so many health problems, ranging from high blood pressure to lung cancer.

Look at your bloodline. If you're Jewish, you should be tested to find out if you have the gene causing Tay-Sachs disease, says Dr. Kuhlman. This is an inherited condition that can cause mental retardation, paralysis and early death. You don't have to be 100 percent Jewish to be at risk, she adds.

Tay-Sachs disease is only inherited if both the father and the mother carry the affected gene. If you're a carrier, your husband should be tested, too—and if it turns out that he isn't a carrier, you can rest assured that your baby won't be at risk.

Surprise, Surprise

While many woman plan their pregnancies months or even years ahead, more than half the time the stork pays a surprise visit. Women often assume it's something that only happens to teens, but it's not, says Anita L. Nelson, M.D., associate professor of obstetrics and gynecology at the University of California, Los Angeles, UCLA School of Medicine and director of the women's medical clinic at Harbor-UCLA Medical Center in Torrance. Two-thirds of unintended pregnancies happen in women over 20.

Accidental pregnancies may occur when birth control methods fail or, more commonly, when a couple neglects to use any contraception, says Paul Blumenthal, M.D., assistant professor of obstetrics and gynecology at Johns Hopkins University Medical Center in Baltimore. Some women assume that they are less likely to get pregnant as they approach their forties, so they may be more casual about using contraceptives.

If you want a planned rather than an unplanned pregnancy, it's important to continue using your birth control method until you're ready for a child, stresses Dr. Blumenthal. Though a child may be welcome, an unintended pregnancy can be stressful for anyone.

Until you reach menopause, you need to assume that you can still get pregnant, advises Kimberly Yonkers, M.D., assistant professor of psychiatry and gynecology at the

University of Texas Southwestern Medical Center in Dallas.

Weighting Around

Once you get pregnant, your body will undergo tremendous changes, some almost immediately. No one enjoys the morning sickness, back pain, fatigue and emotional ups and downs, but for many women those discomforts are offset by the thoughts and expectations associated with having a healthy baby.

"Women sort of feel like their bodies have taken over and are totally out of control," says Christine Olson, Ph.D., professor of nutrition in the Division of Nutritional Sciences at Cornell University in Ithaca, New York.

Contributing to the out-of-control feeling during pregnancy is weight gain. A woman generally puts on 15 to 35 pounds in nine months. How much of this extra weight is "ideal" depends on how much you weighed before you got pregnant.

"The more underweight you are, the more you have to gain during a pregnancy," says Dr. Kuhlman. "The more overweight you are, the less you need to gain."

A woman who was below her ideal body weight before she got pregnant is usually advised to gain 25 to 40 pounds. If you're right at your ideal weight when pregnancy begins, plan on gaining 25 to 30 pounds, doctors advise. An overweight woman should have a gain of somewhere between 15 and 25 pounds.

Where's all that weight going? Well, if you gain 30 pounds, about 11 pounds goes to the baby, while 6 pounds ends up in your own womb, breasts, buttocks and thighs. Another 7 pounds or so is blood and fluid, and the rest is the amniotic fluid and placenta.

While every woman gains weight during pregnancy, the pounds pile on at different rates. "Some women who are really bothered by nausea will probably lose several pounds in the first trimester," explains Dr. Olson. "That is perfectly within the range of 'normal' and not something that should cause panic."

In the second and third trimesters, however, the pounds steadily accumulate. A woman typically gains between half a pound and a pound per week. "So it's pretty rapid

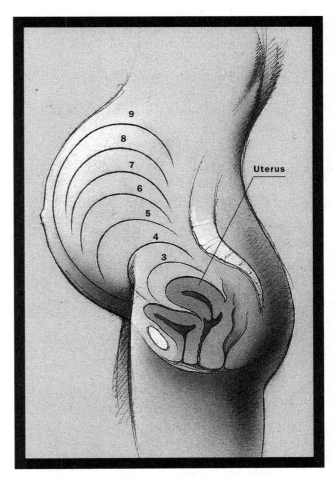

How a child grows. Here's the development of the womb during a normal pregnancy—showing the position of the uterus from the third to ninth month.

during the second and third trimesters," Dr. Olson says.

Keeping Up with Change

To help you keep track of the changes in your body—and evaluate whether your pregnancy is on course—here are some methods that doctors recommend.

Query your doc. If your doctor forgets to bring up the issue of weight, don't hesitate to ask her, says Dr. Olson. She can help you calculate how much you're likely to gain—and understand your goals during the coming months.

Keep a chart. During each checkup—and before you leave the doctor's office—ask for a copy of the weight-gain table that's included in your medical chart, suggests Dr. Olson. That way you can also chart the changes yourself, weighing yourself daily or weekly so you and the doctor have a continuous profile.

Don't fear the future. Although weight gain during pregnancy is a good thing, many women worry that they won't ever get back to their prepregnancy weight after childbirth. In most cases this isn't a problem: Women can usually get back to their prepregnancy weight within six months to a year after giving birth, says Dr. Olson.

Intestinal Blues

We have all heard stories of pregnant women who endure horrible nausea—who feel so ill during the first three months of pregnancy that the very thought of food is almost more than they can bear. Less dramatic, but certainly more common, are those who never get terribly sick, but have stomach upset that just doesn't go away—especially during the first three months of the pregnancy.

Hepatitis and Pregnancy

While many prenatal tests are optional and not always necessary, all pregnant women should be tested for hepatitis B, says Miriam Alter, Ph.D., chief of epidemiology in the hepatitis branch of the Centers for Disease Control and Prevention in Atlanta.

A woman infected with hepatitis B will likely pass the disease on to her infant. Once that occurs, the infant has a 90 percent chance of staying infected and a 25 percent chance of dying from liver disease.

Caught early, however, hepatitis B is easy to stop. Once a pregnant woman tests positive, her baby will be treated at birth with hepatitis B immune globulin—a fast-acting serum that immediately reinforces the immune system—as well as hepatitis B vaccine. The infant also receives two additional inoculations of the vaccine. The first is given after one month and the second at six months. In 95 percent of cases, this prevents the infant from contracting the disease, says Dr. Alter.

Despite the term *morning sickness*, pregnant women may have to fight this inner battle at any time of the day and night. True, it's often worst when the stomach is empty—that's why morning can be such a difficult time for many pregnant women.

There are some techniques to help keep your stomach calm. Here's what experts recommend.

Don't fast. "Keep some food in your stomach at all times," advises Dr. Niebyl. "Having crackers in the morning or cheese or protein snacks at night can help." To prevent nausea, it's generally best to eat small meals frequently rather than have a few large meals with long intervals between.

Quell queasiness with complex carbs. For some women spicy foods such as sausage pizza trigger morning sickness. For others, heavy, fatty foods such as doughnuts may cause problems, says Dr. Niebyl. As a rule, it's best to eat mainly rice, grains and complex carbohydrates—foods that are readily digested and that are easy on the stomach.

Treat yourself gingerly. Ginger has been shown to help ease morning sickness, says Dr. Niebyl. You can buy ginger tea in health food stores. Or try ginger ale or a snack of low-fat ginger cookies.

Take a B₆ balm. Studies have shown that taking vitamin B_6 can help relieve nausea, says Dr. Niebyl. She recommends taking 25 milligrams of the vitamin three times a day. "It's very cheap and very safe, and it works in a significant proportion of patients." Just be sure to check with your doctor first, since this amount of B_6 is far above the Daily Value of 2 milligrams.

The Span of Expansion

Throughout the nine months of pregnancy, your breasts will enlarge—in some cases to twice their prepregnancy size. Your nipples will also get larger, as well as darker.

Even before then—in fact, from the very beginning of pregnancy—your breasts may begin to feel sore and tender. Indeed, nipple tenderness, erectness or sensitivity might be your first, early indicator that you're pregnant.

Apart from breast changes, you'll find that your skin undergoes many changes as well. Itching is common. Stretch marks may appear on your belly as well as on your breasts. Or you might observe temporary changes in the color of your skin—a dark line running down the center of your stomach, for exam-ple. Some women get a brownish "stain," called chlorasma, across their faces when they're pregnant. (These changes in skin color generally go away during pregnancy or after childbirth.)

While all these changes are going on, you need some strategies to deal with the vagaries of your new body. Here are some ways to get relief.

Move up a cup. Good support is critical for relieving breast pain. As your breasts enlarge during pregnancy, you'll want to move up to a larger bra size as well, suggests Dr. Kuhlman. Experts recommend cotton bras with wide shoulder straps and deep bands under the cups to provide extra comfort and support.

Make peace with new marks. You can't prevent stretch marks, and there's no way to eliminate them once they occur, says Dr. Niebyl. And they're unpredictable. "Some women carry twins and don't get a single stretch mark, while another woman might carry a small baby and get many of them. You just have to wait and see."

Warming Up to the Idea

Having a baby is one of life's truly uplifting moments. The months leading up to it, however, can be emotionally turbulent.

"The first and third trimesters tend to be times when women are more anxious and perhaps a little bit more sad than usual," says Katherine L. Wisner, M.D., director of Women's Services in the Mood Disorders Program at Case Western Reserve University in Cleveland. What's more, many women don't sleep well during much of pregnancy, which can exacerbate feelings of sadness and fatigue.

During the first trimester—particularly if it's your first pregnancy—don't be surprised if

When Pregnancy Feels Off-Key

If you thought pregnancy was bliss, it could be a shock if you find yourself feeling far from cheery. In fact some women feel downright, well, down.

Can pregnancy cause depression?

A full-blown depression has a wide variety of symptoms, ranging from poor sleeping habits to weight loss, feelings of helplessness, inability to concentrate and other characteristics. In the past doctors and researchers viewed pregnancy as a time when women were relatively protected from the onset of new episodes of depression, says Kimberly Yonkers, M.D., assistant professor of psychiatry and gynecology at the University of Texas Southwestern Medical Center in Dallas. But studies suggest that pregnancy may not really be protective.

How can you know if you are depressed?

The first thing to look for is what doctors call functional impairment. That is, if your low mood and lack of interest and motivation affect your ability to do your chores or enjoy your daily life, that's a marker for depression, says Dr. Yonkers. "Just as major depression can occur at any other time of a person's life, it certainly can occur during pregnancy." Some women have their first episode of depression during pregnancy. Others, who have experienced depression before, may be faced with a repeat performance when they're pregnant.

Research suggests that 5 to 10 percent of women can experience significant levels of depression during the course of pregnancy, says Katherine L. Wisner, M.D., director of Women's Services in the Mood Disorders Program at Case Western Reserve University in Cleveland.

If you think you may be depressed, experts recommend that you talk to your doctor. "If a woman has prolonged sadness for longer than two weeks, or mood swings or loss of interest in life events that persists for more than two weeks, then she ought to seek care from her physician," says Sharon Dobie, M.D., assistant professor in the Department of Family Medicine at the University of Washington in Seattle.

Depression during or after pregnancy can be treated in a number of different ways, including therapy and medication, says Dr. Wisner.

you worry about the whole prospect of motherhood. Your concerns may range from how you'll manage financially to how you'll cope with changes in your lifestyle. Many women worry about the changes their bodies are going through, as well as the possibility of miscarriage.

This phase usually doesn't last, and with the second trimester often comes a time of relative peace and comfort, says Dr. Wisner. This is the time when women are excited, because they begin to feel the baby move and aren't yet burdened by the physical heaviness of the pregnancy, she adds.

By the third trimester, women are usually less worried about their future as moms and more anxious about what labor will be like, says Dr. Wisner.

As your pregnancy progresses it's important to keep your feelings in perspective. Here are some ways to do that.

Get ready for the roller coaster. One thing is certain: You will have emotional ups and downs, says Dr. Wisner. Some days you may cry a lot, or be angry or simply not want to get out of bed. Remind yourself that this is normal, that you're not alone—and that the feelings will pass, says Dr. Wisner.

Reach out to others. Being with other pregnant women during your pregnancy—and with new moms after your baby is born—is a great way to deal with the challenges. You'll discover which problems are universal, and which seem to be yours alone. "Using other women for support is very, very important," says Dr. Wisner.

Find experts you can trust. It's not always easy finding a doctor you feel comfortable with and can talk to, but this is perhaps the best way to allay anxiety and help keep your worries in check, says Dr. Wisner. Make sure you have a doctor who will answer all your questions and will take your calls when you don't feel right about something that's happening.

Feeding Your Growing Family

Women have always joked about their appetites during pregnancy. Although some women feel so queasy that they never want to eat, others have appetites that they never dreamed were possible. Then there are those cravings that some women get—for chocolate, for example, or "comfort" foods such as meat loaf or mashed potatoes.

"Cravings are natural during pregnancy, as long as they don't get out of hand," says Dr. Kuhlman. Eating too much of one food or craving nonfoods such as dirt or cornstarch is a signal to consult with your doctor, she says.

Since you're eating for two, experts generally recommend getting an additional 300 calories a day over your usual intake. This goal doesn't take exercise into account, however. If you're walking or working out several times a week, you may need to eat even more.

Here are the basics of keeping your body well-stocked for your baby—and for you.

Find the farm food. Soda and candy are out. Fruits, vegetables and low-fat dairy products are in. According to Dr. Olson, it's important to eat several servings a day of vegetables, fruits, whole grains and dairy foods, such as low-fat or skim milk and cheeses.

Even if you're in an office all day and the only "pantry" is the vending machine down the hall, try to make smart choices, advises Dr. Olson. Pick juice or milk instead of soda, for example. Instead of a candy bar, have the peanuts or have crackers with peanut butter. Better yet, start the habit of bringing fresh vegetables or fruit to the office.

Crank up on calcium. The same stuff that keeps your bones strong is also crucial for the growing fetus, says Dr. Scholl. So it's important to get more of this mineral than you ordinarily would.

Experts recommend that pregnant women get 1,200 milligrams of calcium a day. An eight-ounce glass of milk or an eight-ounce serving of yogurt contains about 300 milligrams. If you aren't getting enough calcium in your diet, your doctor may recommend taking a supplement. A possible bonus is that calcium supplements may help reduce the risk of pregnancy-related high blood pressure and preterm delivery, says Dr. Scholl.

Pregnancy in Motion

As the months go by and your body gets progressively heavier, the very idea of exercise may seem laughable. But for many women—particularly those who normally enjoy walking, biking or other forms of exercise—going an entire nine months without a workout can feel like cruel punishment.

"Pregnancy should not be a state of confinement," says Raul Artal, M.D., professor and chairman of the Department of Obstetrics and Gynecology at State University of New York at Syracuse Health Science Center and College of Medicine and author of *Pregnancy and Exercise*. If you enjoy exercise and want to continue your workouts, there's generally no reason not to—assuming, of course, that your overall health remains good.

Some women, however, develop pregnancy-related conditions that make it unwise to exercise. If you have high blood pressure, your doctor may advise you not to exercise until you've come to term. Exercise may also be out of the question if you've had preterm labor during this pregnancy or a previous one—or if you've had persistent bleeding during the second or third trimester. Doctors will usually advise against strenuous exercise if there's any retardation in the growth of the fetus, signs or risk of premature labor or any potential complications related to the condition of the cervix.

Even if your doctor says that it's fine to exercise, it's important to remember that your body has been undergoing a host of changes that may make it necessary to tailor your workouts. Here are some of the subtle and not-so-subtle changes that could affect your workout or your daily walk.

Cardiovascular changes. Pregnancy causes the heart to pump more blood even at rest, which means you may get tired more easily.

Larger uterus and breasts. Your center of gravity shifts, so it's easier to lose your balance.

Changes in breathing. Your body needs more oxygen to function even when you're resting. This means less oxygen is available during aerobic exercise.

Higher metabolism. Your body has to work more vigorously during pregnancy, so it's not that surprising that it produces more heat. Even light exercise may elevate your body temperature to an uncomfortable level.

Working Out New Workouts

With a consistent but somewhat modified exercise schedule, you have a good chance of staying fit right through your pregnancy. Keeping in mind any cautions from your doctor—as well as the body changes that could affect your usual workout—here are some exercise guidelines tailored for the pregnant you.

Do what you've done before. If you've been active prior to your pregnancy, there's no reason to stop, says Dr. Artal. If you didn't exercise before, however, pregnancy isn't the time to take up vigorous sports. You can always do that later, after the baby is born.

Watch your back. Since pressure from the fetus can interfere with circulation, it's best to avoid exercises that require you to lie on your back, according to Dr. Artal. When you lie on your back, the additional weight of the fetus puts pressure on a vein that returns blood to the heart.

Keep it moderate. Remember, the oxygen in your body is less available to your muscles, because it is needed by the growing fetus—so don't overdo it. Don't push yourself to the point of exhaustion, says Dr. Artal. As soon as you start feeling tired, take a break. You can always start up again once you're rested.

Stay cool. Because your body temperature is already elevated during pregnancy, you want to avoid raising it too much more during exercise, cautions Dr. Artal. You can keep the temperature lower if you wear loose-fitting clothing. Also, don't exercise in extremely hot weather and always drink plenty of water to keep yourself hydrated.

Honor gravity. Remember, some exercises

Moms, Backs and Babies

Your first bout with back pain may come with your first pregnancy. "Half of all pregnancies result in back pain," says John J. Triano, D.C., staff chiropractor at the Texas Back Institute in Plano.

There's a good reason why so many moms end up with back trouble. As your body prepares for birth, the hormone relaxin loosens the ligaments that control the joints in your pelvis. Your belly expands, stretches the abdominal muscles and exaggerates the normal curve in the small of your back. It's a condition called swayback, or lordosis, which means the curve is unnaturally large. Swayback hurts your posture, and it can stretch and weaken your muscles if they aren't exercised.

You can outwit expectant-mom back pain, though. Here are the best ways to do it.

Keep on truckin'. "Try to maintain an active lifestyle," says Jeffrey Susman, M.D., member of the U.S. Public Health Service Agency for Health Care Policy and Research and director of primary care and vice-chairman of family medicine at the University of Nebraska College of Medicine in Omaha. "It's best to be fit before you go into pregnancy, and maintaining that level of fitness is probably the best treatment for back problems then."

So if you're used to a vigorous walk, ride or swim, keep it up. "Especially if your legs swell near term, and if walking is irritating, swimming could work for you," says William Case, P.T., president of Case Physical Therapy in Houston.

Be sure to discuss any new exercise regimen with your doctor, recommends Case, especially if you haven't been active.

Belt back pain. If your back does bother you in spite of your best efforts, try a back support belt for pregnant women, suggests Alan Bensman, M.D., medical director of Glenwood Rehabilitation Center in Minneapolis. "It has an expandable pouch in the front and a back support with stays." An inexpensive support belt from a maternity shop may be all you need, he says. If your pain persists or gets worse, he recommends a visit to your doctor, who may recommend a sturdier prescription version available from medical supply stores.

Sleep easy. In the ninth month of pregnancy, you're sure to have restless nights. Beached upon a percale shore, you can't seem to get comfortable no matter how you lie.

Here's a position to try, suggested by Mary Pullig Schatz, M.D., author of Back Care Basics: Place a firm pillow under your head and (optionally) a rolled towel under your neck as shown in the illustration below. Pregnant women are generally advised to lie on their left side to assure good circulation, according to Debra R. Judelson, M.D., a cardiologist in Beverly Hills, California, and president of the American Medical Women's Association.

Place a folded blanket underneath your belly and another folded blanket under your top knee. Your bottom knee should be bent slightly. Your top knee and calf should rest on the blanket. Arrange your arms as comfortably as you can.

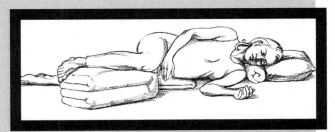

Ideal sleeping position: With pillows and blankets arranged as shown, your body is supported all around and the pressure is off your back.

will be more challenging, because your center of gravity has shifted. Choose exercises where balance isn't so critical, such as walking, swimming or riding a stationary bike rather than playing tennis or racquetball, recommends Dr. Artal.

Heft the light weights. "It's good to do toning exercises and to get involved in some degree of weight lifting," says Dr. Artal. But limit the load to small weights—under five pounds is his recommendation.

"Heavier weights may have a negative impact on pregnancy and may have an effect on the blood circulation," Dr. Artel explains.

Keeping the Spark Alive

Can you have sex while you are pregnant? Will you want to?

"Some women have less sexual desire, some women have more. It's not really predictable," says Sharon Dobie, M.D., assistant professor in the Department of Family Medicine at the University of Washington in Seattle.

As long as you don't have physical problems, there is no reason not to have sex, according to Dr. Dobie.

But you may be advised by your doctor to avoid intercourse or orgasm if you've had premature contractions or a condition called placenta previa, in which the placenta drops over the opening to the cervix.

Finding a comfortable position can be a challenge. Some couples find that a side-by-side position works best, says Dr. Dobie. Another possibility is sitting astride your partner during intercourse. The so-called missionary position, for obvious reasons, is often uncomfortable.

See also Childbirth, Reproductive System

Rectum

Sure, it's a dirty job, but some body part has to do it. The chore in question belongs to the rectum—a short, muscular tube at the bottom of the large intestine that gathers feces and stores them. To finish its task, the rectum passes things along to the anus. You know the rest of the story.

But there's often an unhappy ending to this short saga. As many as half the people in the United States suffer from piles, or hemorrhoids. "Hemorrhoids are quite common, especially in women who've had multiple pregnancies and deliveries," says Bruce Wolf, M.D., chairman of the public relations committee for the American Society of Colon and Rectal Surgeons.

We all have small veins in the anal area, called the hemorrhoidal plexus. When these veins become abnormally swollen, they cause symptoms such as pain and bleeding.

Some hemorrhoids are external. They can be felt with a finger—and resemble soft swellings around the anal opening.

Internal hemorrhoids, however, if they are small, cannot be felt or seen without instruments, because they are hidden inside the anal canal.

Many people assume that any anal or rectal malady indicates hemorrhoids. But such assumptions can be dangerous. Pain, bleeding and other symptoms may indicate other disorders. It would be wise to get checked by a proctologist or gastroenterologist who can diagnose your problem accurately, says Sidney Wanderman, M.D., co-author of the book *Hemorrhoids*.

Sitting Easier

Although hemorrhoids can itch and burn when they're at their worst, helping ease the discomfort is not too difficult, says Dr. Wanderman.

Get into a soothing sitz-uation. Take a 15-minute sitz bath several times a day, after bowel movements if possible. Just fill the tub with a few inches of hot—but not burning hot—water. Ease in and take a rest. The hot water reduces swelling and eases spasms of anal sphincter muscles. Do not add anything to the bath water, such as bubble bath, Epsom salts, bath oil or soap. These extras can irritate swollen hemorrhoids, says Dr. Wanderman.

Ease onto your knees. The position may not be graceful, but doctors say it helps temporarily relieve the pull of gravity on hemorrhoidal veins. Kneel on the floor, bend forward and rest your left shoulder and the left side of your face on the floor, with your buttocks lifted in the air. Breathe slowly and deeply. Staying in this position for even a few minutes is beneficial. If you can keep the pose for a half-hour or so—while reading or watching television—that's even better, says Dr. Wanderman.

Wipe with care. Wiping too hard with toilet paper can irritate hemorrhoids and cause bleeding. Doctors suggest you try using moistened cotton balls. Or rinse with water after a bowel movement and pat dry. Tucks anal pads are also useful.

Soften things up. When a hard, dry stool passes from the body, it may irritate hemorrhoids and cause bleeding. A stool softener (not a laxative) softens the stool by making it absorb more liquid. The stool then becomes easier to pass and creates less friction on hemorrhoids.

Ensure a smooth passage. The basic ingredient in any hemorrhoid medication is a lubricant that lessens friction and irritation. Modern hemorrhoid remedies contain cod-liver oil, vegetable oil, cocoa butter, lanolin, glycerin, petrolatum and, most peculiarly, shark-liver oil. Plain petroleum jelly inserted into the anal canal with a finger is just as effective as any of these, according to doctors. It's also cheaper. Be sure to wash your hands thoroughly afterward.

Piles Prevention

Just because so many women have them doesn't mean you need to join the group. Here are the top tactics for preventing hemorrhoids that doctors recommend, says Dr. Wanderman.

Bulk up your diet. Add bulk and roughage to your diet by eating raw vegetables and fruits, bran and other whole grains. Bran is especially useful, because it absorbs many times its weight in water, making stools softer and easier to pass.

Refined, processed foods with little fiber content and meats and animal fats do not provide the bulk and roughage that the intestines need to form an easily passed stool, says Dr. Wanderman.

Don't allow drought. People on weight-loss diets that call for eight glasses of water a day have often been surprised by the resulting improvement in bowel movements. The water helps soften the stool so it's not as much of a strain to pass, notes Dr. Wanderman.

See also Digestive System

Reproductive System

Without the reproductive system, the history of the human race would be Adam, Eve, The End. But thanks to the fallopian tubes, ovaries, uterus, cervix and vagina, history has been made and the human race continues. Each month in almost every woman of childbearing age, an ovary releases an egg, which moves through a fallopian tube to the uterus. If the egg is fertilized, it burrows into the lining of the uterus, grows into a fetus and comes out the cervix and vagina a full-fledged human being.

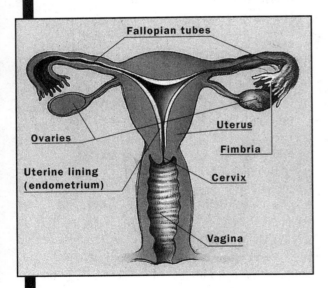

Painful, useful and pleasurable, the uterus gives us cramps, childbirth and orgasms. It can transfigure itself from a muscle-walled one-inch cavity to a womb big enough to hold a six- to ten-pound baby. But its removal is the second most performed surgery in the United States. (See "Hysterectomy—And Other Options" on page 424.)

Where to Look

To keep your reproductive system in good order—whether or not childbearing is still in the picture—see:

Birth Control	page 19
Childbirth	page 68
Fallopian Tubes	page 118
Fertility	page 141
Gynecological Exam	page 159
Hormones	page 182
Medical Tests	page 218
Menopause	page 227
Menstrual Cycle	page 237
Ovaries	page 285
Pregnancy	page 309
Sex	page 330
Sexually Transmitted Diseases	page 341
Uterus	page 421
Vagina	page 427

■ Half of all women of childbearing age get menstrual cramps, caused by contractions of the **uterus**—that incredible expansive organ of muscular tissue. (To learn how to relieve monthly cramps, see "Menstrual Symptoms" on page 242.)

■ Yeast infections are a common form of an inflammation of the **vagina** called vaginitis. They itch like mad and produce redness, odor and a discharge. (For tips on how to control yeast, see "From Yeast to Rest" on page 428.)

■ The **endometrium** is the lining of the uterus. But sometimes endometrial tissue grows where it shouldn't—on the fallopian tubes or the ovaries, for instance—and blocks conception. It's a common cause of

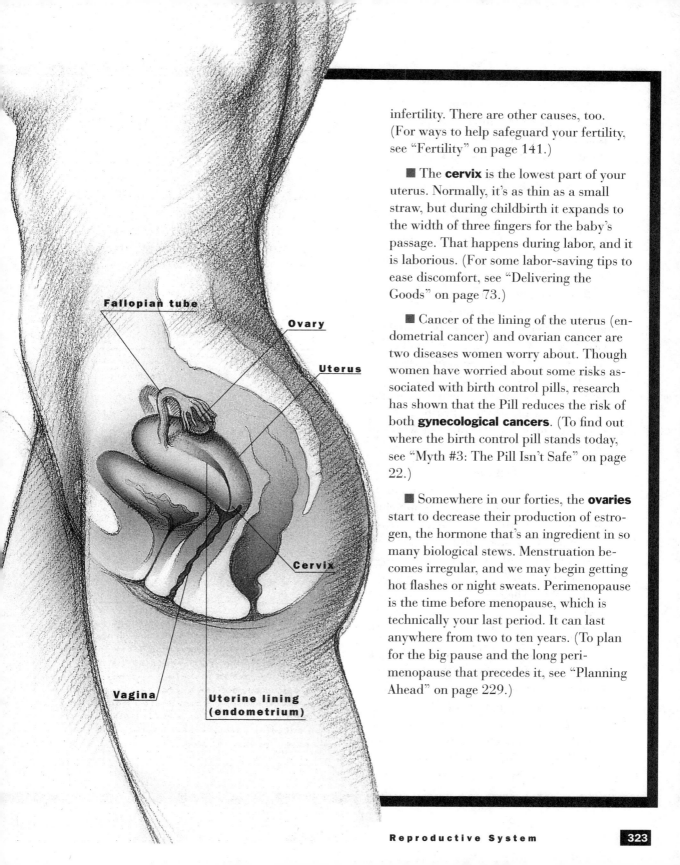

Fallopian tube

Ovary

Uterus

Cervix

Vagina

Uterine lining (endometrium)

infertility. There are other causes, too. (For ways to help safeguard your fertility, see "Fertility" on page 141.)

■ The **cervix** is the lowest part of your uterus. Normally, it's as thin as a small straw, but during childbirth it expands to the width of three fingers for the baby's passage. That happens during labor, and it is laborious. (For some labor-saving tips to ease discomfort, see "Delivering the Goods" on page 73.)

■ Cancer of the lining of the uterus (endometrial cancer) and ovarian cancer are two diseases women worry about. Though women have worried about some risks associated with birth control pills, research has shown that the Pill reduces the risk of both **gynecological cancers**. (To find out where the birth control pill stands today, see "Myth #3: The Pill Isn't Safe" on page 22.)

■ Somewhere in our forties, the **ovaries** start to decrease their production of estrogen, the hormone that's an ingredient in so many biological stews. Menstruation becomes irregular, and we may begin getting hot flashes or night sweats. Perimenopause is the time before menopause, which is technically your last period. It can last anywhere from two to ten years. (To plan for the big pause and the long perimenopause that precedes it, see "Planning Ahead" on page 229.)

Respiratory System

The respiratory system gives us the breath of life. Air—and the oxygen in it—is as vital as food and its nutrients. With the nose, throat, sinuses, larynx, vocal cords, trachea (windpipe), bronchial tubes, lungs and diaphragm, we have a complex ventilation system that enables us to inhale oxygen molecules and send them to each cell in our body. As we exhale we expel some of the body's metabolic trash—carbon dioxide.

■ The **diaphragm** is the main breathing muscle. When you breathe from your diaphragm, you expand your abdominal cavity instead of the chest area, pulling air to the deepest parts of the lungs. Deep breathing is also a major stress-reducing technique. Most of us, though, take inefficient shallow breaths. (To brush up on your breathing, see "Diaphragm Work" on page 206.)

■ The **bronchial tubes** are the two big bronchi that split off from the windpipe (the trachea) and the secondary bronchi that branch out from them. Hyperactive bronchial tubes—too sensitive to pollen, dust, animal dander, cold air or exercise—can provoke asthma attacks. (To handle asthma, see "The Best Defense" on page 208.)

■ The airways of each lung look like a sideway tree of many branches. The trunk of the tree is the big bronchus, the larger branches are the secondary and tertiary bronchi and the smaller branches are called bronchioles. Bronchitis is an inflammation of the bronchial airways (the trunk and large branches), usually caused by complications from a viral infection. (To find out how to battle bronchitis, see "Getting the Better of Bronchitis" on page 210.)

■ Your voice box—the **larynx**—sits at the top of your windpipe (the trachea). And your vocal cords—two thin bands—stretch across the top of your voice box. Sometimes overuse or the common cold makes these cords swell—a condition called laryngitis. (When that happens, see the tips under "Tuning Your Instrument" on page 198 for relief.)

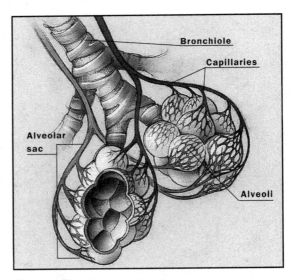

The air you breathe comes in through your mouth, goes down your throat and drops into your windpipe. Then it wends its way through the bronchial airways to reach 300 million tiny air sacs called alveoli. Tiny blood vessels called capillaries exchange gases with the alveoli through a thin shared membrane. Oxygen passes from the alveoli to the blood, and outgoing carbon dioxide moves into the lungs where it's exhaled.

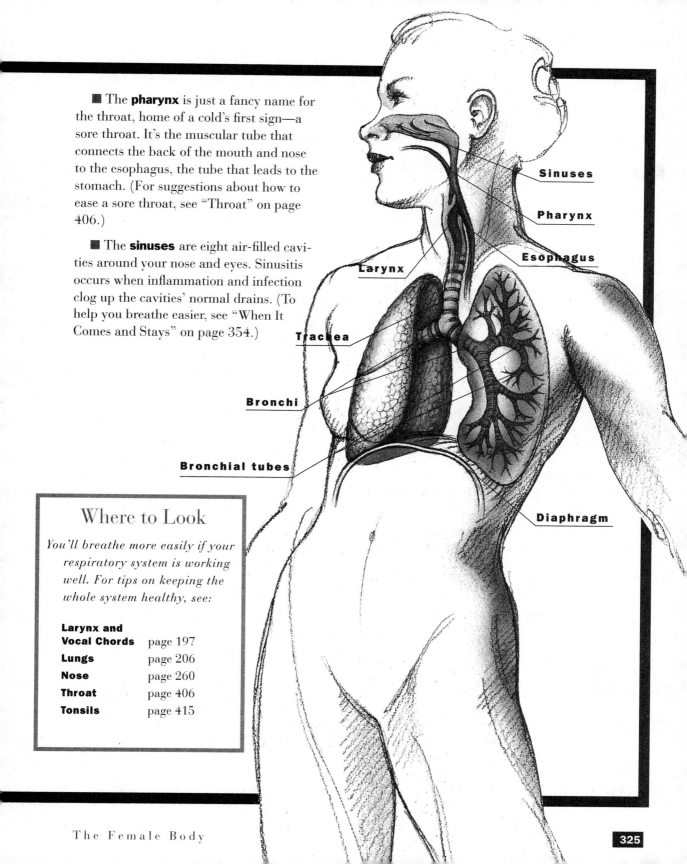

The **pharynx** is just a fancy name for the throat, home of a cold's first sign—a sore throat. It's the muscular tube that connects the back of the mouth and nose to the esophagus, the tube that leads to the stomach. (For suggestions about how to ease a sore throat, see "Throat" on page 406.)

The **sinuses** are eight air-filled cavities around your nose and eyes. Sinusitis occurs when inflammation and infection clog up the cavities' normal drains. (To help you breathe easier, see "When It Comes and Stays" on page 354.)

Sinuses

Pharynx

Esophagus

Larynx

Trachea

Bronchi

Bronchial tubes

Diaphragm

Where to Look

You'll breathe more easily if your respiratory system is working well. For tips on keeping the whole system healthy, see:

Larynx and Vocal Chords   page 197
Lungs   page 206
Nose   page 260
Throat   page 406
Tonsils   page 415

Ribs

IF YOU DON'T HAVE A DEGREE in anthropology, you might fall for it yourself.

At an historical museum a guide pointed out to Susan Larson—who has a Ph.D. in anthropology—that you can tell a female skeleton from a male one because it has an extra rib. But because Dr. Larson knows her bones—she's assistant professor of anatomy at the State University of New York at Stony Brook—she knew that it wasn't true.

"Men and women have the same number of ribs," says Dr. Larson. The idea that women have an extra one is a myth, one that most likely originated with the biblical story of God taking a rib from Adam to create Eve. So if the Creator gets blamed for rib robbery, it's a bad rap: The thievery never happened.

Your ribs—12 pairs of them—are flat, curved bones that branch off from your spinal column. Seven pairs curve around in front and attach to the sternum, or breastbone. The three lower pairs—referred to by doctors as "false ribs"—curve around front, curve upward and attach to the rib above. The last two pairs don't attach to anything—thus the name "floating ribs."

All together, the ribs form a cage that protects the heart, lungs and other organs. Thin sheets of muscle located between the ribs allow the cage to expand and relax as the lungs inflate and deflate during breathing.

If you fracture one of those protective bones, you'll know right away that something is wrong. "When you do break a rib, it is extremely painful," says Bruce Janiak, M.D., director of the Emergency Center at the Toledo Hospital in Ohio. Rib fractures usually result from a fall or a blow. If one area is painful to touch, a doctor will be able to confirm whether or not one or more ribs are broken, sometimes without an x-ray. "It is frequently unnecessary to x-ray for a broken rib. The physician should make the appropriate judgment," he says.

If you've only broken one rib, there isn't much that the doctor can do to help you. Ice packs and anti-inflammatory medications will usually relieve the pain, says Dr. Janiak, and your doctor will advise you about rest and movement. But if your ribs have moved out of alignment—what's called a fragmented fracture—your doctor might have to perform surgery to wire the ribs in position.

Sometimes the rib cartilage—the rubbery tissue that connects the rib to the breastbone—can become inflamed, says Dr. Janiak. Because the cartilage contains nerves, inflammation can cause rib pain and tenderness.

Researchers aren't exactly sure what causes the inflammation, but it may be from a virus or physical stress to the ribs. If you can't tell whether it's rib pain or chest pain, talk to your doctor, who can prescribe medication to reduce inflammation, says Dr. Janiak.

Sometimes arm and shoulder pain is indirectly a rib problem. Some people are born with a pair of "extra" ribs just above the uppermost rib. The result is a condition known as thoracic outlet syndrome. Along with the arm and shoulder pain, it may cause pins-and-needles sensations in the fingers and weakness in your hand grip. Thoracic outlet syndrome can often be treated with exercises. In some rare cases a doctor might prescribe special devices that limit elevation of the arms, says Dr. Janiak. If necessary, surgery can be performed.

See also Nervous System, Skeletal System

Salivary Glands

IF ANYBODY EVER WRITES A SONG about the salivary glands and saliva, they should borrow a phrase from Joni Mitchell. Her 1960s lyrics—"Don't it always seem to go, that you don't know what you've got till it's gone"— seem to say it all.

For saliva is something we take for granted until we don't have it, says Leo Streebny, D.D.S., Ph.D., professor in the Department of Oral Biology and Pathology at the State University of New York at Stony Brook. "Only when we don't have it do we realize how important it is." This special chemical solution is vital in protecting our teeth, fighting off mouth infections and enabling us to speak, swallow, taste and even kiss. "Saliva is an incredible solution," he says.

Wetting Your Whistle

Saliva is churned out by the three major salivary glands plus hundreds of smaller ones throughout the mouth, says Dr. Streebny. These are located on the side of the face, underneath the lower jaw and under the tongue, he says. They normally produce as much as 1 to 1½ quarts of saliva a day.

But if the salivary glands don't produce their saliva quota, a condition known as dry mouth—or xerostomia—can develop. And dryness isn't the worst of it. If you have xerostomia, you're more prone to mouth infections, you may have trouble tasting and swallowing your food and you may even have difficulties talking clearly. The problem affects women more than men by a ratio of about nine to one.

The principal cause of dry mouth is medications, says Dr. Streebny. "There are more than 450 medications that have the capacity to cause it."

But dry mouth can sometimes be caused by Sjögren's syndrome, an autoimmune disease that affects as many as four million people—90 percent of them women over age 50. The disease creates a sort of global drying of the body. You'll not only have dry mouth but also dry eyes, skin, lips, throat and vaginal tissue, says Dr. Streebny.

Dry mouth can also be caused by dehydration. Menopause may also have something to do with it. Whatever the cause, though, here's what you can do about dry mouth.

Go for the chewables. Eat foods that require vigorous chewing, suggests Dr. Streebny. Foods such as celery, bagels and carrots help stimulate saliva flow.

Gum it up. Chewing gum is a wonderful way to stimulate saliva flow, says Dr. Streebny. Just make sure that it's sugar-free.

Get your daily ounces. Dry mouth could be nothing more than dehydration, according to Dr. Streebny. Keep a water bottle filled and drink eight ounces every hour or so.

Go on a reconnaissance mission. If you get dry mouth and it's temporary—lasting only two to three days—you probably don't have too much to worry about, says Dr. Streebny. If it's continuous, however, he recommends that you see your doctor.

Give it a squirt. Dry mouth sufferers can get relief with a saliva stimulant called Pro-Flow. Dr. Streebny recommends spraying it in your mouth as often as necessary. A salivary stimulant—pilocarpine—is also being tested. In addition to helping with dry mouth, this drug may lessen some of the dryness symptoms elsewhere in the body.

See also Mouth

Scalp

To womenfolk in the Wild West, getting scalped was a whole lot worse than just a bad hair day.

While scalpings have gone out with the flintlock, the irony is that we're still losing a sizable portion of our tightly stretched top-knots, flake by flake, every day.

The scalp is a tough sheet of skin richly mined with blood vessels. Normally, hair grows profusely from follicles located all over the top of it, but under that tangled forest a layer of skin is constantly shedding. As with other parts of our outer covering, dry cells are constantly getting sloughed off and tumbling through hair shafts like dust through a cornfield.

Two kinds of common skin problems can accelerate that shedding process. One is an inflammation that affects the scalp and other areas of the body called seborrheic dermatitis. It's better known as problem dandruff—which is different from regular dandruff.

"True dandruff is common and harmless," notes Jerome Shupack, M.D., professor of clinical dermatology at New York University Medical Center in New York City. Seborrheic dermatitis, on the other hand, is a real problem that won't go away without special treatment.

Psoriasis is the other dead-skin problem that can make your scalp flake. If you have psoriasis, it's even more likely than seborrheic dermatitis to show up on other parts of your body—often in the form of red, itchy or scaly patches.

"Psoriasis makes a thicker type of crust

Let Your Fingers Do the Pressing

A gentle massage that stimulates your scalp can help prevent dandruff—plus it could have side benefits of relieving headache and helping you relax. Here's one scalp massage routine recommended by Edith Malin, shiatsu practitioner and teacher at the International School of Shiatsu in Doylestown, Pennsylvania.

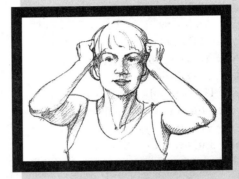

1. With the fingertips of both hands, tap your head at random all around about 30 times. Then repeat with lightly clenched fists, tapping your scalp with the flat area of your fingers (between your first and second knuckles) and the heel of your hand.

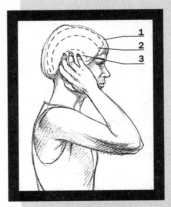

2. With the fingertips of both hands, make circles on your scalp. First, move down the center line of your scalp from your forehead to your neck (see line 1 in the illustration). Use a circling motion to slide your scalp around. After you have covered your center line, repeat the movement in two lines on the side of your head (see lines 2 and 3).

Then repeat this massage, this time moving your fingers in a pressing motion along the same three lines. Be sure to cover your center line (1) and your two side lines (2 and 3).

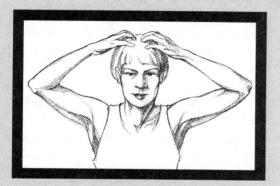

3. With the four fingertips of both hands, press your scalp three or four times as you move from front to back along the center line. Then, starting at your temples, repeat the pressing, working toward the back of your head.

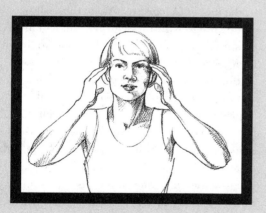

4. Center your thumbs about three inches apart where the base of your skull meets your neck. Press for 30 to 60 seconds.

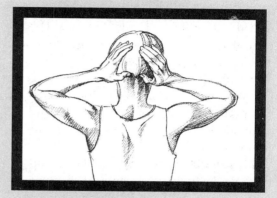

5. Hold your forehead with your left hand while firmly cupping the base of your skull just above your neck with your right hand. Hold for 30 to 60 seconds. "Think 'lift,' instead of actually lifting," suggests Malin. "By just visualizing the gesture, you will give a subtle, rather than an overt, lift to your head."

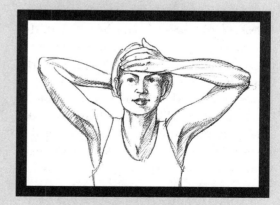

Finally, place your hands on your head just above your ears and apply steady, gentle pressure for another 30 to 60 seconds.

than seborrheic dermatitis," says Dr. Shu-pack. "If you try to scrape it off, it bleeds."

You'll probably want to have a doctor check out psoriasis if you suspect you have it. But dandruff and mild seborrheic dermatitis don't necessarily require any special medical attention. Both can be "beautifully con-trolled," according to Diana Bihova, M.D., clinical assistant professor of dermatology at New York University Medical Center in New York City. Here's how.

Lather up. Any shampoo will wash away dead skin cells, says Dr. Shupack. "If you shampoo every day, you'll mechanically re-move the scales."

Do something special. If regular shampoos don't do the trick, use a dandruff shampoo twice a week—and regular shampoo the other days—to control normal scaling, suggests Dr. Shupack.

But dandruff shampoos may be harsh and can damage hair—especially fine hair—and they can discolor blond, white or gray hair, Dr. Bihova cautions. Use a hair conditioner to prevent any dryness or damage.

Rotate shampoos. Even when a dandruff shampoo clears up flaking without a hitch, you'll probably find that the flakes will start falling again after a few months. Switch shampoos about three times a year, Dr. Bi-hova suggests. "Each kind of shampoo works differently. You have to find the right one that works for you at any particular time through a process of trial and error."

See also Hair

Sex

FROM GLANCING AT TELEVISION, the movies or advertising, you'd think the average woman was a walking hurricane of run-amok hor-mones, dying for a Fabio look-alike to ravish her at the drop of a loin cloth.

Look at the come-hither, close-to-nude babes in the high-gloss ads for amazing fra-grances and stupendous styles.

So what if you have naked people advertis-ing clothing?

Sex—especially sexy women—sells.

Temptresses fill both the small and large screen, from the man-eating executive Amanda Woodward on television's *Melrose Place* to the same type of man-eater (with ad-ditional cleavage in the form of Demi Moore) in the movie *Disclosure*. While these shows come and go with the seasons, you can always be sure that new starlets will appear to flaunt their attributes.

But the blame for our obsession with sex can't fall entirely on the media. After all, the appeal of the sex act is very real—even though for women, it has more to do with our deep-seated desire for connection than with outright lust, notes Barbara Levinson, R.N., Ph.D., licensed marriage and family therapist and owner of the Center for Healthy Sexuality in Houston.

"It's about the urge to procreate and to couple. We are a coupling society. The urge to be with other people is in our collective unconscious," says Dr. Levinson. "It's a way we've learned to love and be intimate. It gives a connection with a partner and also with oneself."

Who's Doing What to Whom and How Often?

The only thing more fascinating than our own sex lives is other people's sex lives. But sometimes what you think others are up to is twice as interesting as what's really going on.

In the book Sex in America, based on a 120-page survey of 3,159 people, researchers found exactly that.

Rather than a nation of bed hoppers, we're by and large monogamous. The majority of women—75 percent—have only had one sex partner in the previous 12 months. It's about the same for men. According to the survey, 67 percent of men reported having only one sex partner in the previous year. Also, more than 80 percent of married women and between 65 and 85 percent of married men report being faithful.

The notion that single people are living it up, engaging in sex with a different partner every week while married people's love lives stagnate, is also false. According to the study, the average married woman has sex seven times a month, as opposed to single women, who average five times a month.

Despite the idea that hot sex involves the unusual or kinky, the study shows that 78 percent of women and 83 percent of men find vaginal intercourse the most appealing sex act. Their second-favorite activity is watching a partner undress, followed by receiving oral sex. Such exotic fare as group sex was rated not at all appealing by 78 percent of women and 33 percent of men.

Well-Connected?

Bonding with a soul mate is fine and dandy, but pleasure is definitely nothing to sneeze at. And when we start to ask for details, women are much more likely than men to report a problem coming to climax. In fact, although 65 percent of men report always reaching orgasm during lovemaking, only 15 percent of women report the same thing.

Not surprisingly, many of us are still hampered sexually by the age-old attitude that nice girls don't, notes Gina Ogden, Ph.D., licensed marriage and family therapist in Cambridge, Massachusetts, and author of *Women Who Love Sex*. "Many women are subjected to negative messages about sex. Women who love sex are called sluts," she says. "We have earned the right to say no to sexual abuse but not the right to say yes to sexual pleasure. It's

as if the country is in a kind of cultural missionary position—with men on top."

Our attitudes toward sex—whether conscious or unconscious—are largely shaped by the families we grew up in, says Dr. Levinson. Look back at how you learned about sex. What was the sexual atmosphere in the house? Were boundaries violated? Some families overvalue sex by talking about it constantly, while others undervalue it by being completely silent. All these factors could influence how you view sex today, she says.

"Ask yourself what your value system is. Were you told that sex is dirty?" Dr. Levinson asks. "Or were your parents open about it, letting you feel good about your body and giving you the appropriate information?"

Regardless of what messages you've been hit with, you can discover a fulfilling sex life.

Reaching the Top

When it comes to climbing the heights to sexual fulfillment, you might say that women take the stairs while men take the elevator. Or, to put it in culinary terms, men are microwaves and women are Crock-Pots. We just need a lot more time to reach that ever-elusive peak.

In a way, women's sexual responses are similar to men's. Each goes through the four stages of desire—excitement, plateau, orgasm and resolution—with distinct changes in blood flow accompanying these stages.

For men the increase in blood flow leads to a prominent result: an erection. In women arousal is almost invisible. In fact, many women aren't even aware when they are aroused. One reason is because there are so many things going on in the female body during this phase that it's hard to recognize any one distinct change. But certainly, there's something going on.

The process starts when the erectile tissue within the clitoris fills with blood and the clitoris becomes hard. Both the inner and outer vaginal lips swell, and the inner lips may turn dark wine red or bright red. The vagina also gets wet—the result of a fluid that comes from the vaginal walls. The muscles that support the uterus may start to clench, causing the uterus to lift up off the vagina, and the far end of the vagina—the cul-de-sac—to be revealed.

As you get closer to orgasm, the areolae, or dark skin surrounding your nipples, become prominently swollen, which may create the visual illusion that your nipples are no longer erect. In women who have never breastfed a child, breast size might increase by 20 to 25 percent. Breathing becomes shallow and rapid.

When you finally hit orgasm, all kinds of things are going on in your body: The muscles around your uterus and cervix spasm so that your abdomen sucks in. Your blood pressure, breathing and heart rate reach a peak. You may feel a tingling sensation in some parts of your body, and a feeling of warmth moves from your genitals up to your face, chest and neck.

Finding Out What Turns You On

As we all know, the elusive "Big O" is about much more than physical responses—especially for women, says Marilyn Volker, Ed.D., a sexologist in private practice in Coral Gables, Florida.

"Orgasm is a biological, psychological, social and sexual response. Most people take it for granted, but it's very complex," says Dr. Volker. What can get in the way, she notes, are messages—good or bad.

There's pressure nowadays for women to climax—something that sometimes makes women fudge a bit. It's not difficult to fake an orgasm or two, as Meg Ryan proved in the classic moaning-and-groaning-in-the-deli scene in *When Harry Met Sally*. But don't give in to that temptation, says Dr. Volker.

"If you fake it, say to yourself, 'If he asks me afterward if I had one, will I tell the truth?' Like many people who have had to face issues about orgasm, you may find that honesty can lead to better understanding. A lot of women fake because they don't want to have the kind of intimacy that says they need more stimulation," she says. Also, pretending that you're satisfied is sending your partner the message that whatever he's been doing works for you.

Magazine articles, talks with friends and personal experience may have convinced you that most women simply don't have earth-shattering orgasms.

Steaming Up the Sheets during a Cold Snap

If the most exciting sound coming from your bedroom is your husband's snoring, it might be time to get real. Spicing up a sex life could be as simple as learning to communicate, notes Barbara Levinson, R.N., Ph.D., licensed marriage and family therapist and owner of the Center for Healthy Sexuality in Houston. "It's all about connectedness, intimacy and loving each other. Intimacy is the foundation. You can tell your partner what you want. In this sexual age of ours, wonderful sex happens in the context of an open, honest relationship."

But if you've been together long enough, even open and loving relationships could use a jump start. Here are a few of Dr. Levinson's tips for ensuring togetherness.

- **Use fantasy and playacting, dressing up and setting different scenarios.**
- **Switch positions in the middle of sex or do it in different rooms of the house.**
- **Take baths together.**
- **Put candles in the bedroom.**
- **Dedicate a whole day to lovemaking.**
- **Watch soft-core porn videos together.**

"Your sexual life is only limited by your own imagination," notes Dr. Levinson. "Women in their forties and fifties are not 'over the hill.' " She points out that women of any age can be extremely sexual—and comfortable with their own sexuality. "Sex doesn't stop after 60. It can continue as long as one has the imagination, the will and the inclination. Our worst enemies are our own limiting beliefs about ourselves," she says.

Some of the women's magazines you may have read for sexual advice stress affection rather than physical pleasure. Each in its own way may pronounce that most women care less about penis size than the color of a man's eyes.

And you may have read that most women don't (and won't ever) have vaginal orgasms during intercourse. Many articles even assure readers that an absence of orgasm during sex is okay.

"Women aren't supposed to admit that they enjoy healthy, exuberant sex," says Rene Denfeld, author of *The New Victorians*. "Even when we're talking to friends or thumbing the pages of magazines, it's supposed to be about romance, not sex."

This lack of candor contributes to a general shortage of knowledge about how our bodies are designed and how our muscles can best be strengthened to maximize sexual sensation.

Which Path to the Peak?

When it comes to achieving orgasm, there's one thing we know for sure: Everyone is unique. Although some women's strongest orgasms are torrid, ecstatic experiences, these same women say that their typical orgasms are less intense and are more sensual. On the other hand, about 12 percent of women say they have never experienced orgasm at all.

Many women—up to 70 percent—require direct clitoral stimulation to reach orgasm. But even though clitoral orgasms are most common, you can also climax from stimulation of the G-spot, the well-publicized term for an area of extreme sensitivity somewhere in the vagina. Stimulating that vaginal area can produce an intense orgasmic response in some women. Occasionally, that response is accompanied by a female ejaculation—the expulsion of a large amount of thin, clear liquid that's composed of a substance similar to semen without the sperm.

It was the famed sex researcher, the late Alfred Kinsey, D.Sc., originally a zoologist at Indiana University, who pioneered the view that the clitoris provides the only route to female orgasm.

In experiments using cotton-tipped probes to gently stroke the inner walls of the vagina, Kinsey concluded that the vagina has so few nerve endings that it's about as sensitive as a kidney. William Masters, M.D., and Virginia Johnson, then a husband-and-wife research team, supported Dr. Kinsey's premise during the 1960s when they proclaimed that a woman's sexual response resides in the clitoris alone.

"No matter how an orgasm is produced (by masturbation, oral sex, vaginal intercourse, anal intercourse or use of a dildo or vibrator), most women describe their subjective orgasmic sensations as emanating initially from a sudden burst of warmth and pleasure in the clitoris," reported Dr. Masters and Johnson and Robert Kolodny, M.D., in their book *Heterosexuality*.

Although women often report having that type of orgasm, others have the kind that arises from deep within the vagina—similar to the type described by psychologist John D. Perry, Ph.D., and his co-authors in their best-seller *The G-Spot*. Dr. Perry argued that many women have a sensitive area on the upper or front wall of their vaginas and that touching or rubbing this so-called G-spot could trigger what Sigmund Freud would have referred to as vaginal orgasms.

Sounds specific enough, but the idea of a distinct spot designated solely for sexual pleasure confused a lot of women. Most of us couldn't find it—couldn't even figure out how to search for it—and the concept of an elusive place guaranteed to produce absolute ecstasy for all those who chance upon it fell out of favor.

Good Vibrations

Twelve years after *The G-Spot* came out, Dr. Perry tried to clarify what he meant by a G-spot. It turns out that the G-spot is a little less gimmicky than it sounds. "It's really not important where or what the spot is," Dr. Perry says. "Our whole point was that the vagina is sensitive—and it is."

The resulting orgasm is different from a clitoral orgasm. Dr. Masters and Johnson describe the bodily changes that occur during clitoral orgasms as "tenting." The internal organs (such as the bladder and uterus) are pulled up toward the breasts, expanding the top of the vagina.

During a vaginal orgasm, on the other hand, the internal organs are pushed downward, contracting the upper half of the vagina. "The top of the vagina contracts and the bottom expands to create a pushing-out effect," explains Alice Ladas, Ed.D., a New York City sex therapist and a co-author of *The G-Spot*. "In fact, if you're having intercourse and you have a vaginal orgasm, the man may be forced out."

Unfortunately, the front wall of the vagina isn't the only neglected pleasure zone in our clitoris-centric climate. The cervix, that bulging plug about the size of a quarter forming the entrance to the uterus, is highly sensitive in some women. You might also be highly sensitive in the area of the cul-de-sac—the very far end of the vaginal canal that surrounds the cervix—which may be closed off, depending on your state of arousal or position.

Action to Satisfaction

Every couple is different in terms of physiology and inclination. Even minor changes in position such as bending your knees, tilting your pelvis or raising your legs can result in huge pleasure payoffs—simply by altering the angles your body creates so that your lover's penis rubs against your newly identified pleasure spots. But general guidelines for targeting your most sensitive spots do apply. Here are a few.

Find the front wall. Any movement that brings the front wall of the vagina down to meet the penis can heighten pleasure for some women. The best way to stimulate that area depends on the length of your partner's penis, your position during sex and the location of your sensitive area, says Dr. Ladas.

For some women the sensitive area is on the front wall toward the opening of the vagina. Others find that it is deep inside the vagina, toward the back.

If your partner's penis points straight out or downward when it's erect, rear entry is often ideal for front-wall stimulation. This won't work, however, if your partner's penis is short and your area of sensitivity is deep inside your vagina.

If your partner's penis is long and your sensitive area is toward the front of your vagina, then you may not want him to push deep inside you at first, says Dr. Ladas. With less penetration his penis will come in contact with that sensitive front area during arousal.

If your partner's penis points up toward his stomach when it's erect, a modified missionary position may be ideal for you. Try lying on your back with your lower back pushed down, your pelvis tilted up and your knees bent up toward your chest, so your legs can rock in sync with your pelvic movements.

"This position tends to give the woman the most stimulation in the pubococcygeal muscle area (the area around the vaginal opening), the clitoral area and the front wall, and it provides the best chance of opening up the cul-de-sac," says Barbara Keesling, Ph.D., sex therapist in Orange, California, and author of *Sexual Pleasure*. "So it's a great position all around."

Other adjustments may do the trick, too—no matter what the angle or size of your partner's penis. Try supporting the small of your back with your hands or a pillow while you have sex, says Dr. Keesling. Or ask your partner to lift you slightly as he thrusts. Also, try bringing one leg forward—almost as though you're doing a split. "This can change the shape of the vagina and create a new sensation," she says.

Survey the cervix. If the cervix is one of your hot spots, consider trying a position that allows your partner's penis to penetrate deeply. Rear entry is one way. Or, try a modified missionary position, raising your legs up over your partner's shoulders as he enters. Or, if your partner has a very short penis, you can use a penile extender, says Dr. Ladas. This little cap fits over the head of the penis to lengthen its reach. Penile extensions are available in sex shops or by mail order.

Reach the cul-de-sac. The key to stimulating this area is also depth of penetration. A rear-entry position in which the woman leans her head and breasts on the bed and loops her legs around her partner's allows especially good access to the cul-de-sac, says Dr. Keesling.

Build Some PC Power

Great sex requires more than an emotional connection. It demands real physical strength as well.

It's important to learn to identify and use the four groups of muscles—the pubococcygeal muscles, the uterine muscle, the diaphragm and the pelvic muscles—that can heighten your pleasure during sex. Building strength in those muscles will increase your newfound sexual enjoyment. A good place to begin is with the two sets of muscles that ring the vaginal opening and the set that surrounds the anus. These are collectively referred to as the PC muscles (short for pubococcygeal). Proper toning of these muscles can heighten a clitoral orgasm even though the clitoris itself is not directly attached to, but rather bounded by, those PC muscles.

"An exercised muscle receives more blood, more oxygen and more nutrients than a sedentary muscle," says James White, Ph.D., professor emeritus of exercise physiology at the University of California, San Diego. "As a result, you experience greater arousal and a heightened sensation of pleasure when you're working with exercised PC muscles."

"The case for PC workouts is even stronger if you're interested in having vaginal orgasms," says Dr. Ladas. "Research shows that the weaker your PC muscles, the less likely you are to be vaginally orgasmic."

Here's why: Vaginal orgasms depend on contractions of the PC muscles to create sensation. So the more developed your PC muscles, the more intense your orgasms. "I'm convinced that a lot of women with very weak PC muscles may have orgasms and just not feel them," says Dr. Perry. "The weakness of the muscles may render their orgasms imperceptible to them."

To identify your PC muscles, sit on the toilet with your knees apart. Urinate and then try to stop the flow. Or lie down on your back and try to contract your vagina around two fingers.

As you do so, try to distinguish between two sets of muscles—the set located at the entrance to the vagina and the other set positioned deeper inside. Ideally, you should be able to flex and release each group separately. The third set of muscles that constitute the PC group is the muscles that ring your anus. Contract and release these to identify them as well.

To do the most effective PC exercises, you should contract the vaginal muscles around resistance provided by your fingers or your partner's penis. But you can increase the muscles' strength even if you contract them without resistance. Here are the two basic exercises.

Flexes (also called Kegels). Tighten your PC muscles for one second, then relax them for one second. Repeat this exercise 10 times. As your strength improves, increase the amount of time you contract and relax. Gradually work up to ten seconds of holding and ten seconds of relaxing at a time.

Flutters. Contract and release the PC group as quickly as possible. Start by doing 10 at a time. Gradually work up to 100.

Work Out the Others

In addition to the PCs, other muscles associated with sexual pleasure can be tuned up to boost your satisfaction. Here's how.

Use your uterine muscle. Believe it or not, uterine contractions can contribute to orgasmic sensation, so building the strength of the uterine muscle can help intensify pleasure. The trouble is that the uterine muscle is tough to target. So try this, suggests Dr. Keesling: Lie on your back and raise your knees, then tighten the various muscles in your lower abdomen. If you feel air entering or exiting your vagina as you contract, you have found the uterine muscle.

Double your diaphragm power. Another key player in the vaginal orgasm is the diaphragm, a muscular parachute that arches over the liver and is called upon to push out bowel movements and bear down during childbirth. By contracting your diaphragm, you compress the space in which your internal organs reside, says Dr. White. They bunch together, pushing the front wall of your vagina downward toward your partner's penis. The result? Increased vaginal sensation.

Dr. Ladas recommends a specific exercise to target both the PCs and the diaphragm: Tighten the muscles around the rim of your vagina, then contract the muscles located deeper inside the vaginal canal. After holding for a few seconds, push out as though you're having a bowel movement. Then release all the muscle groups and relax for a few seconds. Repeat five times.

Do some pelvic workouts. The position of your pelvis, the heart-shaped bone that creates your hips, determines the angle of your vaginal canal and the positioning of your clitoris. If you strengthen and stretch the muscles in your buttocks, abdomen and lower back, you can control how your pelvis—and your pleasure zones—are positioned. In other words, you can make your physiology work for you.

First, stand in front of a mirror and put your hands on your hips, keeping your knees relaxed, not locked. Then try rotating your hips without moving your shoulders or upper body.

If you can isolate your hips and move them forward, backward, to either side and around in a circle, you can control your pelvic positioning, says Dr. Ladas. If your body moves woodenly, experts recommend the following exercises to increase your range of movement.

Pelvic rolls. Lie on your back with your knees bent. Slowly rock your pelvis up without lifting the small of your back from the floor. You should feel your gluteal (butt) mus-

cles contract and those in your lower back stretch, says Dr. Keesling. Repeat ten times.

Abdominal crunches. Lie on your back with your knees bent and your feet flat on the floor. Rest your fingertips lightly beside your ears. Contract and pull in your abdominal muscles, then curl your head and shoulders upward until your lower back is pressed into the floor. Pause for three to five seconds, then continue to contract your abdominal muscles as you gradually lower your torso to the floor. Repeat ten times.

Reverse leg lifts. Lie on your stomach and lift one leg, keeping your knee slightly bent. Hold for ten seconds and return to the starting position. Repeat ten times with each leg.

Know What You Need

Even if your PCs and other muscles are as toned as an 18-year-old's, there's more to reaching your sexual potential than physical prowess.

In fact, that gray matter between your ears is probably the single most important sexual organ in your body, notes Dr. Volker. "You could do all the exercises in the world, but if you've been raped or are the victim of incest—or if there are trust issues or a power play going on with your partner—the exercises won't do any good," she notes.

If your sex life is less than satisfying, and you know that you've been sexually abused in the past, counseling and therapy are the most logical answer.

"Making love is a learned experience," notes Dr. Levinson. "Animals do it instinctively, but humans need to be taught. I don't think anyone is destined to be a bad lover."

Whatever your thoughts and feelings about sex, it helps to know your own body and your own responses as well as possible. There are

Desire Drainers

Seeing your guy wearing droopy shorts and black socks with sandals might not set you on fire sexually, but it probably doesn't douse the flames, either. When it comes to desire, your libido is affected more by drugs, alcohol, health problems and past experiences than your mate's resemblance—or lack of resemblance—to Tom Cruise.

Although a couple of beers might help loosen you up before a sexual encounter, alcohol is, for the most part, bad news. Far from being a stimulant, it actually depresses the central nervous system, slowing your responses, dulling your sense of touch and making you sleepy. It can reduce a woman's sex drive and her ability to reach orgasm.

Sleeping pills, tranquilizers, antiseizure medications or blood pressure medication can also numb sexual desire. Disorders such as hormonal imbalances caused by an underactive thyroid or overactive segment of the pituitary gland can block your sex drive as well.

Hysterectomy, the surgical removal of the uterus and sometimes the ovaries and fallopian tubes, has also been known to affect desire, but only if the ovaries are removed. Hormone replacement therapy helps restore lubrication and reverse thinning of the vaginal walls, says Domeena Renshaw, M.D., director of the Loyola Sexual Dysfunction Clinic in Chicago and author of Seven Weeks to Better Sex. Even if your ovaries have been removed, your ability to have an orgasm will not be affected, because arousal happens in your clitoris or vagina and in your mind.

Don't discount psychological ties to lovemaking. Current sexual relationships are directly tied to past ones and the messages we got when we were in those past relationships, notes Gina Ogden, Ph.D., licensed marriage and family therapist in Cambridge, Massachusetts, and author of Women Who Love Sex.

"If a woman has experienced some kind of sexual abuse or terror or control in the past, she'll take that into the bedroom with her, even if her partner is the most gentle person in the world," Dr. Ogden notes. "She needs to work on those issues before she can fully let go into sexual pleasure. In addition, her partner needs to be part of this working out. A couple may find that with extra sensitivity they can deepen their relationship.

"However, many couples find it helpful to seek counseling for these issues," Dr. Ogden adds. She recommends that couples look for a counselor who is trained in both sex therapy and abuse counseling.

---

lots of ways to work at maximizing your sex life on your own. Here are some therapists' suggestions.

Be your own lover. Most women learn to have orgasms through self-stimulation before they can have them with a partner, notes Dr. Volker. They touch themselves and find a way to show their partner, maybe by guiding the partner's hand. "You can do it playfully or very erotically. It can be fun."

Here's a brief how-to: Begin by touching your body with your hands, exploring every part—including the most sensitive areas, such as your nipples and pubic region, says Domeena Renshaw, M.D., director of the Loyola Sexual Dysfunction Clinic in Chicago and author of *Seven Weeks to Better Sex*. Then focus on your sexual organs, exploring leisurely, moving at your own pace. Note what kind of motion and pressure your clitoris responds to most. Move your finger down to the vaginal opening and slide it in. Be sure that your genitals are lubricated. If needed, body oil (such as coconut oil), saliva or petroleum jelly works fine. (But remember: Don't use petroleum jelly or baby oil during intercourse if you are using a barrier contraceptive such as condoms or diaphragms. They break down latex rubber.) You can also stimulate your genitals by friction against clothes or an object such as a pillow or a vibrator.

Peek at your clitoris. Take a hand-held mirror, hold it down to your genitals and take note, says Dr. Levinson. "You should know what your genitals look like. It's amazing how many women are afraid to look at them. How do you expect to guide your lover to pleasure you if you don't know what you look or feel like?"

Befriend your body. Take inventory of your body—see what you like and what you don't like, think about what's a realistic standard and what's not, and think about what you can improve and can't improve, suggests Dr. Levinson. "It's hard to enjoy sex when you're busy hiding yourself under the covers. Men don't really care about your fat thighs when they're making love. Accept your body as it is. When a woman feels sexy, she acts sexy," she says.

Playing with a Partner

Just as you explore your own body, it's also important to explore different possibilities with your partner. Here's some variety that experts suggest to add spice to your sex life.

Try outercourse. Don't assume that every sexual episode has to culminate in intercourse, notes Dr. Volker. Most women can have an orgasm through manual or oral stimulation, so there are other facets to sex. "Don't use the term foreplay—it assumes intercourse always has to happen. The message is that you don't have real orgasms except through intercourse."

Pick a powerful position. When it comes to memorable intercourse, putting yourself on top could make all the difference, notes Dr. Volker. That provides maximum clitoral stimulation—something that the man-on-top, or missionary, position offers the least. Another winner is rear vaginal entry, which allows for direct stimulation of the vagina, and you or your partner stimulates the clitoris during intercourse.

Don't just go below the belt. Any part of a woman's (or man's) body is a possible erogenous zone, notes Dr. Ogden. Why not give or get a full-body massage, focusing on parts of the body that aren't genital but are still arousing, such as the insides of the thighs or the elbows or the back?

"One exercise I give couples with sexual desire problems is to have the guy make love to his wife for one hour without going above the ankles," she notes. "Either they say, 'The hell with this,' and go ahead and make love, or they come back and say that it's the most sensual experience they've ever had."

Be Lewis and Clark. To learn what both you and your lover want, try body mapping—where one partner touches the other, who then rates how it felt, notes Dr. Ogden. Do it everywhere, so you'll know whether you need to touch faster, slower, firmer or softer and where. "It's a nonjudgmental way of teaching about what kind of touch feels good where," notes Dr. Ogden. "Lots of times, you'll say, 'Don't do this, don't do that,' but

Not This Month, Dear, I'll Have a Headache

Some women can gobble five chocolate chip cookies without pausing for air. Others nibble at one for 20 minutes and still end up leaving half of it uneaten.

Different people. Different appetites. That theory also applies to sexual desire, says Arlene Goldman, Ph.D., psychologist, sex therapist and coordinator of the Jefferson Sexual Function Center in Philadelphia. "We all have different appetites for sex. Some might want sex every day; others save it for special occasions."

If you rarely crave sex anymore, and you used to want it, say, every other day, you might suffer from inhibited sexual desire. Fatigue, unexpressed anger and the routine of married life can do a number on the libido, but here are a few ways that Dr. Goldman says you can reawaken the sexual you.

Uncork your anger. "Most of us, unless we're masochists, don't want to make love with someone we're angry at," she says. You need to resolve the issue by talking about what's bothering you. Leave it out of the bedroom.

Don't imitate Ward and June. Take time with your husband as a lover, not just a husband and parent. Make time for romance. "At the beginning many of your thoughts are of your partner and wanting to hold him and be sexual, but once you're married, it's 'Who'll pick up the kids after work?' Very little time is spent on the sexual aspect," Dr. Goldman notes.

Call your partner during the day and talk in a loving way. Spend time alone together, with the kids out of the house. Talking about sex is a turn-on, so share your fantasies and desires.

Don't leave it to spontaneity. The idea that sex has to be spontaneous to be good is a myth. "In your busy life, maybe you need to plan. You might need to get up earlier in the morning before the kids get up, leave your kids at the in-laws and have a night alone together," Dr. Goldman says. One babysitting idea is to find other couples you can exchange babysitting with so you'll have that time.

Give him a hand. Sometimes sexual intercourse isn't the only option. When one partner consistently wants sex more than the other, "you feel like your partner is always pushing you to be sexual, and you lose the normal desire you had to begin with," she says.

"You could suggest masturbating him or letting him masturbate while you watch," she notes. "Sometimes women just want to be held, kissed or cuddled but are afraid that if they start something, they'll have to finish it."

mapping allows you to say what feels good."

Don't expect fireworks. You shouldn't think that every sexual encounter has to end in orgasm, says Dr. Ogden. If you feel like you're just not into it, be honest and ask if there's anything you can do for your partner's satisfaction. "Who made the rules here? The most creative lovers are the ones who can negotiate. It's like ordering an appetizer while just watching the other person eat a full platter. You can enjoy it just as much."

See also Clitoris, Reproductive System, Sexually Transmitted Diseases, Vagina

Sexually Transmitted Diseases

■ **CAN YOU IMAGINE** what it must have been like trying to buy condoms on Walton's Mountain? Must have been tough for John-Boy or Jim-Bob to spit out the big question to ole Ike Godsey: "I want to buy some ccc . . . ccc . . . cccondoms, please."

My, how times have changed.

Instead of being stashed away behind the counter, condoms now congregate in clusters of showy packaging, filling drugstore shelves of their own. Why, there are even entire stores—such as Condom Kingdom in Philadelphia—dedicated to selling them. They come in different shapes and sizes, even various colors and flavors. There's even a female condom. Wonder what Mary Ellen Walton would have made of that.

Mention condoms, and it won't be long before the terms *HIV* and *AIDS* enter the discussion. AIDS certainly brought condoms out of the closet and into the limelight. During this age of AIDS, condoms have gone from being just a means of pregnancy prevention to the prime mode—aside from abstinence—of disease prevention. And that's important, because AIDS isn't the only threat out there.

Unequal Opportunity Infections

There are more than 50 sexually transmitted diseases (STDs), including gonorrhea, trichomoniasis, bacterial vaginosis, chlamydia, hepatitis B, the herpesvirus, genital warts, HIV/AIDS, pelvic inflammatory disease (PID), syphilis, chancroid and others.

When it comes to certain STDs, women "seem to have an unfair disadvantage when compared with men" says Cheryl Walker, M.D., assistant professor of obstetrics and gynecology at the University of California, Irvine. Of the estimated 12 million people who get an STD every year, about 6 million, or 50 percent, are women. The problem with just looking at the numbers is that they don't reveal the whole story: In the case of certain STDs—namely, chlamydia and gonorrhea—women are twice as likely to get them as men are. The toll that these infections take on women's health can be far greater than it is for men. Women's fertility can be threatened, childbirth can be complicated and a newborn's health can be endangered.

Since it's essential to protect yourself, here's what experts recommend.

Be sure you're disease-free. If you've had unprotected sex with a partner who's carrying a sexually transmitted virus or bacteria, you may have already been exposed to an STD. But with some STDs, you may have the infection without any symptoms. To be on the safe side, you should ask your doctor to do a full battery of tests for STDs, says Eddie Sollie, M.D., associate clinical professor in the Department of Obstetrics and Gynecology at the University of Texas Southwestern Medical Center at Dallas and author of *Straight Talk with Your Gynecologist*. Detecting infection can enable you to get the treatment you need.

Send him to the doctor. Before sleeping with a new partner, ask him to undergo STD testing, experts recommend. It's not just a matter of trusting someone to tell the truth. A man can be infected and not know it.

Make condoms the only way. Before beginning sexual relations with a new partner,

How to Use a Condom

When asked whether most women know how to put a condom on a man, Katherine Forrest, M.D., principal research scientist at the American Institutes for Research in Palo Alto, California, will answer you plain and simply: "Nope."

"I think that most women are not learning how to do this," says Dr. Forrest. "When they do learn how to do it, it's usually by trial and error."

But using a condom properly shouldn't be left to chance. Here's what Dr. Forrest recommends.

<u>Rehearse ahead of time.</u> Before you are in a situation where a condom is needed, go get some condoms and practice, says Dr. Forrest. Practice taking the condom out of the package so that it's oriented properly, learn how to open the package without tearing it with your teeth and learn how to hold it and how to unroll it.

Need a prop? You can practice on a large carrot or banana, says Dr. Forrest.

<u>Have it ready.</u> If you are going on a date and anticipate that you might have sex, take condoms with you, says Dr. Forrest. If you are at home and anticipate an evening of lovemaking, you can get one condom ready an hour or so ahead of time and have others available. To get ready, open the condom packet, orient the condom so it will unroll easily and put it in the drawer of the bedside table. That way finding and using the condom will be easier.

<u>Check the lube tube.</u> Be sure to use only water-based sexual lubricants, such as K-Y jelly or Replens, since other kinds can deteriorate the latex. Look for the term "water-based" on the label. If the lubricant contains oil, you don't want it. Examples of substances you should <u>not</u> use are hand lotion, massage oil or petroleum

jelly, explains Dr. Forrest. Check the expiration date, which should be marked on the package. Because latex weakens with age and could break, don't trust a condom if the expiration date is long past.

<u>Keep them cool and fresh.</u> Condoms should be stored in a cool, dark place, since heat and strong light can damage them.

<u>Squeeze and roll.</u> To put a condom on properly, follow the steps shown above. Start by unrolling the condom just enough so you can press the air out of the tip between your thumb and forefinger. Set the condom on the end of your partner's erect penis and unroll it smoothly as shown above.

Once it's in place, there should be about ½ inch of empty space at the tip of the condom. After your partner ejaculates, hold the condom at the base of his penis while he withdraws from your vagina; this will prevent the condom from coming off inside of you and spilling the semen. Your partner should pull out before his penis is completely soft, says Dr. Forrest.

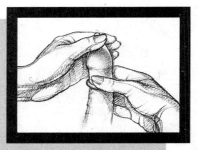

1. Start by unrolling the condom just enough so you can press the air out of the tip between your thumb and forefinger.

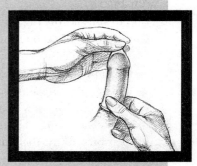

2. Unroll the condom smoothly down the shaft, from the tip all the way to the base. Try not to allow air bubbles between the condom and skin.

make up your mind that you'll only have sex if he uses condoms, says Katherine Forrest, M.D., principal research scientist at the American Institutes for Research in Palo Alto, California. Establish that understanding with him, "before you get in bed, before your clothes come off," she says. "Alternatively, now that female condoms exist, you can make that a rule that applies to you rather than to him. Condoms should be used for anal and oral sex, as well as for vaginal sex."

Bring in the reserves. While latex condoms are the best means of preventing STD infection, barrier methods such as the diaphragm and contraceptive foams, gels and creams also offer some protection, Dr. Forrest says. By covering the cervix and blocking this entryway into the uterus, the diaphragm can help prevent organisms from infecting the upper genital tract. Laboratory studies also suggest that nonoxynol 9, the spermicidal agent in some vaginal contraceptives, may protect from disease as well.

Do it with the lights on. The first time you have sex with a new partner, make love with the lights on, says Dr. Forrest. That way it's easier to see your partner's skin and penis and detect any signs of STD infection before you have intercourse, she says. Things to look for include irregularities in the skin surface, sores, bumps, discharge from the opening of the penis or any signs of irritation and inflammation.

The Big Threats

There are so many STDs that it's hard to know what to worry about most. Certainly, all STDs are of concern, but the top three threats for women today are chlamydia, the human papillomavirus (HPV) and HIV/AIDS, says Dr. Forrest.

Chlamydia

This is a type of bacteria that poses a major threat to women, because it threatens their fertility, says Dr. Forrest. The disease is extremely prevalent—an estimated half a million cases are diagnosed and reported to the Centers for Disease Control and Prevention (CDC) in Atlanta each year, says Dr. Walker. That figure might be misleading, however, because chlamydia infections are not officially reportable diseases. Some doctors estimate that the real figure is between three and ten million cases each year in the United States.

The tricky thing about chlamydia is that you can have it and not even know it, says Dr. Forrest. There are often no symptoms to help a woman detect the infection. If chlamydia goes untreated, it can travel up into the fallopian tubes, causing blockage and scarring. This upper tract infection, called pelvic inflammatory disease, or PID, is what often causes infertility. Tubal scarring from chlamydia infections can also lead to ectopic pregnancy.

Here's what you can do about chlamydia.

Take a yearly test. If you've had a new partner in the past year, or if your partner has had other partners, get checked for chlamydia once a year, says Dr. Forrest. "Get tested even if you don't have symptoms."

Don't skimp on treating it. Chlamydia can be treated with an antibiotic, but it's essential to follow the doctor's directions. Be sure to complete the full course of the antibiotic, even if you have no symptoms and are feeling fine, says Dr. Forrest.

Make your man go. If you've contracted chlamydia, be sure your partner goes to the doctor and gets tested and treated, too, says Dr. Forrest. If he's infected, treating you alone won't do much good, because he can just reinfect you.

Tests You Need to Ask For

Every year you have a Pap smear. The results come back normal, so you're free of sexually transmitted diseases, right?

Not necessarily, experts caution. The Pap smear can't detect chlamydia, gonorrhea, HIV/AIDS or syphilis, to name a few. If you want to know your status on these diseases, you need to ask for other tests. Among them:

Gonorrhea and chlamydia culture. Since the Pap test won't show whether you have chlamydia or gonorrhea, you need to ask your doctor to take a culture for these sexually transmitted diseases. This test is not automatically part of your annual gynecological exam.

HIV/AIDS test. To find out if you are infected with the HIV/AIDS virus, you need to have an HIV blood test. You can choose between anonymous and confidential HIV testing.

In anonymous testing you never give your name; instead, you are assigned a number. The advantage of this kind of testing is that no one else can find out your HIV status unless you tell them. The down-side is that you may forget the number and not be able to get your test results. Also, counseling about your risks and how to protect yourself may not be automatically provided. Be sure to request this information, says Katherine Forrest, M.D., principal research scientist at the American Institutes for Research in Palo Alto, California.

With confidential testing, the facility doing the testing knows your name but agrees to keep the results confidential. The advantage of this kind of testing is that counseling is usually automatically provided, both before testing and at the time the results are given to you. But there's a drawback that you have to consider: If the results go in your medical record, your insurance company may find out that you are infected with HIV and deny future medical coverage.

Syphilis test. Syphilis can be detected through a blood test at your doctor's office. Syphilis testing is not done routinely as part of an annual exam, though it is required in many states before you can get a marriage license.

Human Papillomavirus

More commonly known as genital warts, human papillomavirus (HPV) is another disease that should be of particular concern to women, says Dr. Forrest. That's because certain strains of the virus are associated with the development of cervical cancer.

"HPV infection is by far the most common STD in women," says King Holmes, M.D., Ph.D., director of the Center for AIDS and STDs at the University of Washington School of Medicine in Seattle. An estimated 24 mil-lion people are believed to be infected with the virus, according to officials at the CDC. Yet, "most women who have it don't know they have it," says Dr. Holmes. That's because women may be infected without developing warts. Or the warts may be located where women can't see them.

Here's what doctors recommend for HPV.

Have an exam. See your doctor yearly for a pelvic examination and Pap smear. The Pap smear can often detect the virus, and if you have the strain of HPV that causes warts, your doctor may be able to see them during a pelvic exam. The virus currently has no cure—once you're infected you have it for life—but your doctor can remove any warts and monitor you more frequently for any cervical changes. If you have the virus, some doctors advocate having a Pap smear every six months, because of the increased risk of cervical cancer associated with HPV.

Go for the greens. If you have HPV, reach for green leafy vegetables and citrus fruits and juices. Researchers at the University of Alabama at Birmingham found that women with one type of HPV were less likely to develop precancerous cervical changes if they had high levels of folate in their systems. While food sources of folate are best, such as spinach, oranges and lentils, many multivitamins also contain folate in the form of folic acid. The Daily Value is 0.4 milligram.

Human Immunodeficiency Virus (HIV)

The virus that leads to AIDS is among the top three STDs that women should be particularly concerned about. That's because of the fatal nature of the disease, says Dr. Forrest. By 1992 the disease was the fourth leading cause of death in women ages 25 to 44, with the death rates in women steadily climbing.

One possible reason for the sharp increase is that many women have assumed they were in a low-risk group. The fact is, if you have unprotected heterosexual sex with an infected partner, you run a risk of contracting the disease. More than one-third of HIV-infected women have contracted the virus through heterosexual sex.

Having a monogamous relationship with a partner who is also monogamous (and HIV-free) is one way to avoid this virus. If you're not in that kind of relationship, here are some other ways to protect yourself.

Stock up on condoms. The best means for preventing HIV infection, other than abstinence, is to use latex condoms during sex, experts say. "There is no doubt whatsoever, when used consistently and correctly, that latex condoms are highly effective in preventing the transmission of HIV," says Herbert Peterson, M.D., chief of the women's health and fertility branch at the CDC.

Get tested. HIV can be present in your

Battle of the Condoms: Male or Female?

Finally, we have a choice. In addition to male condoms, female condoms are now available in stores. Called Reality, the female condom consists of two plastic rings connected by a polyurethane sheath; one ring is inserted inside a woman's vagina where it goes around the cervix, and the other ring stays outside.

Studies show that the male and female condoms may be nearly comparable in preventing pregnancy, says Katherine Forrest, M.D., principal research scientist at the American Institutes for Research in Palo Alto, California. But not enough research has been done on the female condom to know whether it protects against sexually transmitted diseases as effectively as the male version, she says. Preliminary study suggests that the female condom should help decrease risk, experts say.

The female condom may be more protective against STDs that are spread by skin-to-skin contact, says Dr. Forrest. That's because the end of the female condom that stays outside of the vagina can prevent the skin around the opening of your vagina from coming in contact with your partner's penis.

---

system for years before you show any symptoms, doctors say. The sooner that you get treated for the infection, the better. So if you've had unprotected sex with a partner whose sexual history you're not sure of, go for an AIDS test.

Know your partner. "That means more than just knowing he's a nice guy and seems clean and honest," says Dr. Forrest. It means knowing about all the people he has had sex with in the past—which is extremely difficult. But anything that you can find out about his sexual history can help you know him better and help you make your decision about whether or not you want to have sex with him. Questions to ask him about himself should include: Has he ever had an STD, has he always used condoms and has he been checked for HIV and other STDs recently?

See also Reproductive System, Sex

Shins

SPRINT TO CATCH A TRAIN. Leap to the deck of a boat. Powerwalk through the park. None of these steps are drastic—but all of them put pressure on the second-biggest bone in the body.

The tibia, the kick plate that fronts the lower leg, is almost always called by its nickname—the shinbone.

Most of us don't pay much attention to the shin until we happen to whack it against something. Despite its easy bruise-ability, the shin wasn't intended to play the role of bumper car.

"The function of the tibia is really propulsion," says Gary M. Gordon, D.P.M., director of the running and walking clinic at the Joseph Torg Center for Sports Medicine at Hahnemann University Hospital in Philadelphia. The tibia absorbs all the weight of the body from the thighbone, passing the burden on to the ankle and, finally, the foot.

Splints Prevention

As weight-bearing responsibility is passed down the line, some of the tension is picked up by the bridges of muscles, tendons and ligaments that connect the shinbone to other parts of the leg and foot. Sometimes, when the shin just won't take it anymore, we wind up with a condition called shinsplints.

"*Shinsplints* is a catch-all term for pain in the front of the lower leg," says William Case, P.T., physical therapist and president of Case Physical Therapy in Houston. The term covers most causes of shin pain: an inflamed tendon, an inflamed muscle or a stress fracture.

Most often shinsplints mean a case of tendinitis, an inflammation of the tough fibers that connect the muscles in the lower leg to the shinbone. The inflammation occurs because we've overused the tendons in the shin. That could happen if we run too many miles, for instance, or if we wear worn-out athletic shoes. Here's how you can avoid getting shinsplints in the first place—or slow the pain before it gets worse.

Wear a springy shoe. "The main thing that prevents painful shins is shoes that are in tip-top shape," says Dr. Gordon. "When your shoes lose their shock-absorbing power, your muscles, tendons and bones absorb that shock. You want your shoes to take the pounding away from your body."

If you run more than 25 miles a week or take three or more aerobics classes each week, Dr. Gordon recommends replacing your shoes every two to three months. A more moderate exerciser can get four to six months out of a pair. If your shins start hurting during a workout, Case says one reason may be that you need a new pair of athletic shoes.

Change your routines. Sometimes our aching shins remind us that we need to change more than just our worn-out pair of sneaks. If twinges of shin pain are sneaking up on you, Case strongly recommends taking a second look at your exercise routine. Pounding the pavement six days in a row or sweating through the highest level of your workout tape day after day can beat up more than just your footwear.

If your shins protest during or after your workout, chances are you're overdoing it. Try switching your workouts to alternate days of the week, lowering your overall workout time, or toning down the volume of your exercise routines, suggests Case.

Always warm up. Tendons need warm-ups even more than muscles. Before you go out for a run or any kind of workout, Case recommends that you do at least five to ten minutes of warming up and stretching to prevent tendinitis. Walking and riding a stationary bike are two good ways to warm up your shins.

Helping the Pain Wane

Sore shins can sneak up on the avid athletes among us. They also come to almost any dress shoe–shod woman who walks around the mean streets of the big metropolis all day. Here's how to soothe them.

Do the Dixie. Fill a half-dozen or so Dixie cups or Styrofoam cups with water and keep them in your freezer for bad shin days. When pain hits, grab one of those chilled Dixies as soon as possible. Peel off the cup's rim and rub the ice up and down your shin for five to ten minutes to numb the ache and control the inflammation. As the ice melts, peel away more of the rim.

Call for help. If your shin pain doesn't feel better after six or eight weeks, cease and desist the activity that could be causing the pain. The reason: You may have a stress fracture of the tibia, not tendinitis. See your doctor, who will probably schedule an x-ray or bone scan to diagnose a fracture.

See also Skeletal System

Shoulders

IF YOU THINK WOMEN JUST CAN'T throw a ball, take a look at Birmingham, Alabama, native Lee Anne Ketcham.

Ketcham was the starting pitcher for the Colorado Silver Bullets, the first postwar all-female pro baseball team to be recognized by the National Association of Professional Baseball Leagues. She was also the first female pitcher to play for the Maui Sting Rays, an all-men's professional team in Hawaii.

Her fastball has been clocked at 80 miles per hour, which would qualify it for a speeding ticket in almost every state in the union.

When anyone's shoulder is pushed to the limits like that, it needs tender loving care. To perform the way she does, Ketcham spends one-third of her weight-lifting time strengthening a series of muscles that surround the shoulder joint. That's important for keeping her shoulder not only strong but stable as well.

Inside Your Shoulder

The shoulder and arm that can help catapult a ball at 80 miles per hour obviously has excellent working parts designed for efficiency and power. The central pivot of this mechanism is a ball-and-socket joint in which the ball-shaped head of the upper arm bone, or humerus, fits into a cuplike socket called the glenoid cavity. The shoulder joint is like a golf ball sitting on a golf tee. The socket part of the joint is very shallow, which means that the ball-shaped head of the humerus can rotate freely in the cavity, and the shoulder can move through a large range of motion.

Because the cavity of the socket is shallow and the "ball" part of the shoulder joint has plenty of mobility, that ball would slip right out if it weren't strapped in by ligaments and tendons. If your shoulder starts to hurt, maybe it's because these structures are getting a heavy-duty workout. Even if you're not hurling a hardball at the speed of a Porsche in the passing lane, you can still mess up the muscle tendons around that joint—especially the group of four muscles that doctors call the rotator cuff.

The Cuff Link

The most common shoulder problem among women ages 30 to 45 is rotator cuff tendinitis, also called impingement syndrome, according to James Kramer, M.D., assistant clinical instructor in the family practice residency program at the Moses H. Cone Memorial Hospital in Greensboro, North Carolina. This injury occurs when one of the tendons of the rotator cuff gets pinched between two bony parts of the shoulder. "As the arm bone swings out to the side and up above, the head of the humerus rides up and, essentially, pinches the tendon on the bony covering above it," says Dr. Kramer. Activities that can bring on rotator cuff tendinitis involve a lot of overhead motion—such as pitching, swimming, playing tennis or reaching overhead when you're on the job. You're especially vulnerable if you repeat the same motion over and over again for six weeks or more.

How do you know you have it? This type of tendinitis usually begins with a deep aching in the shoulder, and there may also be pain on the upper outside portion of the shoulder, says Dr. Kramer. You might not feel the pain while your arms are down, but as soon as you reach overhead, you get a sharp

Building Your Cuff

With some therapeutic shoulder range-of-motion exercises, you can help relieve the pain of rotator cuff injury. These exercises both increase flexibility and strengthen the muscles around the shoulder, which can help prevent future injury, according to James Kramer, M.D., assistant clinical instructor in the family practice residency program at the Moses H. Cone Memorial Hospital in Greensboro, North Carolina.

Figures 1 through 4 show some exercises that can be done with a two- to three-foot strip of surgical tubing or exercise elastic that's wrapped around a doorknob. Just be sure to consult with your doctor before doing these exercises—and stop if you begin to feel shoulder pain. After completing these exercises, do the stretches shown below.

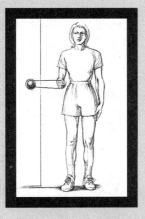

1. Hold one end of the elastic in your fist, with the other end around a door handle as shown.

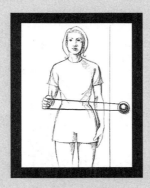

3. Change position so you can hold the elastic as shown above, stretched across the front of your body.

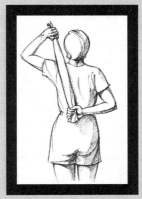

To stretch after exercising, hold a towel as shown and pull on each end slowly two or three times.

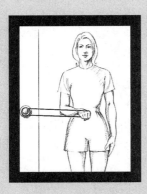

2. Rotate your hand so the thumb points down and inward.

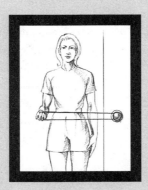

4. Rotate your hand outward, so the thumb points up.

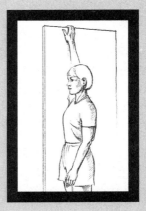

A second stretch: Reach to the top of the doorjamb and hold, then relax. Repeat two or three times.

When Things Get Out of Joint

Dislocating a shoulder is an unforget-table experience. You start to take a tum-ble, reach out your hand and, suddenly, something pops out of place. This is what happens when the ball-shaped head of the humerus completely slips out of the socket.

There is also a minor-league form of dis-location called subluxation: That's when the ball slips out of the socket for an instant, then slides back in.

Both injuries can be painful in a big way—but they're not the same as separat-ing your shoulder, according to James Kramer, M.D., assistant clinical instructor in the family practice residency program at the Moses H. Cone Memorial Hospital in Greensboro, North Carolina. That happens higher up, on top of the shoulder, where the collarbone is attached to part of the scapula with a ligament. When you land so hard that the ligament gets torn, you have a separated shoulder.

Whether or not you know the differences between these injuries, you should see your doctor to find out if you need x-rays and treatment.

Heed your body's hints. When you're doing an unfamiliar activity like apple pick-ing or painting a ceiling, you may find that your shoulders start to ache. "Don't push through that," says Dr. Kramer. "If you really notice your shoulders starting to ache, slow down or stop what you are doing at that par-ticular time."

Apply for relief. If you feel shoulder pain from doing overhead activities, applying ice should help. Use a bag of ice cubes, a bag of frozen dried beans or an ice pack wrapped in a towel to protect your skin from direct contact. Hold it to your shoulder for 10 to 20 minutes, suggests Dr. Kramer. You can repeat as often as you like, but allow some time for your skin to warm up between each application.

Put out the fire. Take an anti-inflamma-tory such as ibuprofen to reduce inflamma-tion and alleviate the pain, says Dr. Kramer.

When Pain Leaves You Frozen Stiff

When it's uncomfortable to move, natu-rally, you try to do the opposite. "The more it hurts to move your shoulder, the more you tend to keep it still," says Dr. Kramer. But that could lead to other problems. One possible consequence is something doctors call adhe-sive capsulitis, also known as frozen shoulder.

You have frozen shoulder when the capsule around the joint starts to stiffen. Some people also develop adhesions in the frozen shoulder, which is what happens when pieces of body tissue form in the wrong places and cling like duct tape to the moving parts.

Even if you're feeling some pain in the shoulder area because of adhesions, experts recommend that you perform range-of-motion exercises to keep the joint limber and supple.

If you try a number of shoulder exercises and find that you can't reach or stretch as far

complaint from your shoulder. You may also feel pain while you're sleeping at night.

If you can't get the upper hand on your overhead activities, here are some actions doctors recommend to end the pain or guard against it.

Get within reach. If you can identify what activities you do that require repetitive over-head motions and cut them out of your daily routine, that's the first thing to do, says Dr. Kramer. If you have to pull files from a high shelf, for example, use a step stool so the shelf is within easy reach.

as you used to, it's a sign that you've lost some range of motion in that shoulder. You should see a doctor, since the loss may be caused by adhesions.

Where Pain and Posture Mix

Some women feel shoulder and neck pain combined with a feeling of weakness in their upper arms and backs. They may also have numbness and tingling all the way down their arms into their hands. If you have some of these symptoms, you should probably see your doctor to find out whether you have thoracic outlet syndrome.

This syndrome is more common in women than men—and you're more likely to get it if you have a long, swanlike neck and droopy shoulders or postural problems, says Dr. Pascarelli. Also, if some of your neck muscles are tight with tension, that could be a trigger for the condition, according to Dr. Pascarelli. And it often goes unrecognized. The symptoms are caused by traction or compression of nerves around the neck or compression of blood vessels.

Here are some ways to decompress if you have the syndrome.

Be straight with yourself. Avoid slumping at your chair, says Dr. Pascarelli. Thoracic outlet syndrome often develops in secretaries who are sitting at their computer keyboards with their shoulders hunched and necks jutting forward. Maintain good posture, and you're less likely to have the problem.

Ride erect. When you're in the car, sit up

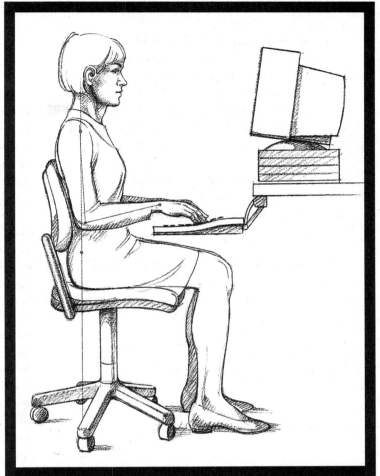

In a no-strain work position, your chair should be adjusted so you can sit upright with your shoulders back, feet flat on the floor and elbows bent at a 90-degree angle.

straight and keep your hands in a light grip at the 10 o'clock and 2 o'clock positions on the steering wheel. If you have a height-adjustable steering wheel, put it in the lowest position when you're driving. Elevate the driver's seat if you can—or get a seat pad to raise yourself so your hands can rest comfortably on the wheel while you're driving. "If the steering wheel is too high, that's going to throw a tremendous amount of tension on your neck and shoulders," says Dr. Pascarelli.

Compute at ease. If the desk holding the computer is too high, that means you'll be looking up at the screen—which could put unwanted compression on the nerves that aggravate thoracic outlet syndrome. Check to make sure your desk and chair are the right height for you, suggests Dr. Pascarelli. Then adjust the height of your chair so that you can sit comfortably with your neck and back in alignment when you're working. The center of the screen should be about six inches below eye level.

See also Joints, Muscular System, Skeletal System

Sinuses

IF YOUR BODY'S BREATHING SYSTEM were a theater ensemble, the Tony Awards should go to your sinuses. They're the supporting cast—without which you'd be gasping for air. Every minute of every day, they're delivering a command performance.

Though these eight air-filled cavities—located behind and around the nose and eyes—may be a long way from the lungs, they're actually their best guardians. They perform like filters, protecting the lungs from invading viruses, allergens, dust, dirt, or any airborne particles. They also moisten dry air that could irritate the lungs as well as cool very hot air and warm extremely cold air that could shock the lungs.

Other special duties: They give the voice resonance, and—because they're actually cavities carved out of solid bone—they make the skull lighter than it would be otherwise. All those caves in your skull make it easier for you to hold up your head.

They're also mini mucus manufacturers. The membrane-lined cavities of the respiratory system create between a pint and a quart of mucus a day. This sticky secretion traps particles that enter the nasal passage, while the cilia—microscopic hairlike filaments—sweep those particles toward the back of the nose.

Stuffed to the Gills

When you consider the array of maladies that can clog your sinuses, it's amazing that they are ever clear at all. Who among us hasn't suffered the stopped-up discomfort of a cold or the wheezing, sneezing and dripping of an allergy?

When it comes to head-throbbing aches, the top affliction is sinusitis—a disruption of normal sinus drainage that results in facial pain, greenish nasal and postnasal discharge, extreme fatigue and head congestion. Thanks to this annoying infection and inflammation, the sinuses rival the lower back for causing the most pain and discomfort of any body part.

In fact, nearly 40 million Americans suffer chronic sinus problems, with sinusitis being the number one chronic condition of women ages 30 to 45 and the second-highest chronic condition for women over 45. Even if it isn't an ongoing problem, many women are likely to be struck sometime by the severe form of the infection known as acute sinusitis, which can last from ten days to several months.

Millions of cases of sinusitis are caused when colds, bronchitis, asthma, allergies, the flu or airborne irritants cause the drainage openings of the sinuses to swell or get blocked. Fluid accumulates and microorganisms infect the sinuses. About 80 percent of cases are caused by bacteria, and viruses cause 20 percent.

Another culprit is the climate. Damp weather usually aggravates sinusitis. When the barometric pressure drops—which generally happens before a rainstorm—anyone who has a history of sinusitis problems is likely to have a flare-up.

When you have a common cold, sinusitis problems may start when your breathing is obstructed, causing the nasal mucous membrane to become inflamed and swollen. The cold virus inactivates the cilia of the nasal membrane, causing the mucus in the nose and sinuses to stagnate rather than flow.

The ostia, which are drainage ducts the size of pencil lead, connect the sinuses to the

Where They Are

If you've ever had a sinus headache, you probably have a good idea of where your mucus-producing sinuses are located. The frontal sinuses are above your eyes and nose and behind your forehead. You also have maxillaries, which are pyramid-shaped sinuses, located inside each cheekbone. The ethmoids are multicompartmental sinuses lying behind the maxillaries and between the bony orbits of your eyes.

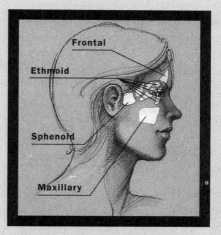

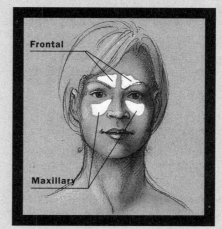

Sinuses of the nasal passage: side view (top) and front view (bottom)

nasal passages. When these tiny ducts are clogged with mucus and can no longer drain properly, the sinuses become a breeding ground for bacteria.

The mucous membrane and its cilia are left damaged and weakened following a bout of sinusitis. Sometimes—especially in polluted or dry air—the membrane never completely recovers, leaving it much more susceptible to future infections.

When It Comes and Stays

Chronic sinusitis is when you have either ongoing sinusitis that lasts longer than three months or at least three or more sinus infections in a six-month period, says Robert Ivker, D.O., clinical instructor in the Departments of Otolaryngology and Family Medicine at the University of Colorado School of Medicine in Denver and author of *Sinus Survival*.

The number of people with chronic sinusitis is climbing—partly because of the increasing number of pollutants in both the indoor and outdoor air, says Dr. Ivker. "The nose and sinuses are our bodies' primary air filters, and the air we filter is getting dirtier and more toxic. Try rubbing sandpaper over the back of your hand 23,000 times a day. Can you imagine the quality of that skin? The same things happen to the membranes of the nose and sinuses."

Although a bout of sinusitis can be a roadblock to comfortable living, there are many ways for you to pull the plug on congestion and breathe easier. Here are some hints from doctors.

Get all steamed up. Steam is just what the doctor ordered to loosen up a mucus-packed nose and help drain the sinuses, says Anthony J. Yonkers, M.D., professor and chairman of the Department of Otolaryngology–Head and Neck Surgery at the University of Nebraska Medical Center in Omaha. "You should go into a steamy shower and just stay there for a while."

Bow over vapor. Another way to get steamed is by leaning over a pot of piping hot water with a towel over your head. Do it four times a day for five to ten minutes, says Alexander C. Chester, M.D., clinical professor of medicine at Georgetown University Medical Center in Washington, D.C. Adding a few drops of eucalyptus oil can pack some decongesting punch as well. The oil is available at many health food stores, but only use it as an inhalant, since eucalyptus oil is poisonous if it's ingested.

Warning: If you heat a pot of water on the stove, be careful, because a rush of rising steam can give you severe burns. Be sure to take the pot off the stove. If it's covered with a lid, lift the lid to release any built-up steam before you lean over the pot.

Ax the antihistamines. Don't use antihistamines—they thicken and dry mucus, says Dr. Ivker. "The thicker the mucus, the harder it is to drain from the sinuses."

Do decongest. Take single-action tablets that contain only decongestants, such as pseudoephedrine (Sudafed), says David Zwillenberg, M.D., otolaryngologist at Thomas Jefferson University Hospital in Philadelphia. Decongestants constrict the blood vessels, put air through the nose and alleviate pressure.

Don't overdo. Using a decongestant nasal spray for more than three days can make you stuffier than you were before, says Dr. Yonkers. "Any long-term use of decongestant sprays causes a chemical rebound problem with the lining of the nose. This means that your nose becomes congested again, making you want to use the spray again and again, until you are caught up in a long cycle."

Take a hike. Getting at least 20 minutes of aerobic exercise three times a week could help you breathe easier, notes Dr. Yonkers. "One of the problems with sinusitis is that you have decreased oxygen levels in the tissue. This helps certain bacteria grow better. By increasing the metabolic rate, you might change that."

Salt your schnozz. To help flush the sinuses, Dr. Ivker recommends irrigating them with saltwater. Mix one-third teaspoon of noniodized table salt with one cup of lukewarm water and a pinch of baking soda. Bottled water without chlorine is preferred, says Dr. Ivker. Stir well, until the salt and baking soda are completely dissolved, and pour the solution into a shot glass. Tilt your head back slightly and to the left. Then, slowly pour half of the water into your right nostril. The water will flow out of your left nostril or down the back of your throat if your left nostril is clogged. Spit out the water if it goes down your throat. Repeat this procedure on the left side. You can also try a commercial saltwater mist spray like Ocean or Ayr for a similar effect.

Stop smoking. Cigarette smoke contains irritants that damage the nasal lining, says Dr. Yonkers. "If you smoke at home, the smoke sits around your house, and you rebreathe it. If you must smoke, do it outside and keep your home air sacred. The same goes for the car."

Pop out of bed. Getting too much shut-eye can exacerbate congestion, says Dr. Chester. The lying-down position increases nasal congestion, because drainage is slowed. Propping your head up with several pillows or raising the head of your bed may help.

Don't make a spectacle of your sinuses. Eyeglasses sometimes pinch the nasal bridge and aggravate nasal congestion, says Dr. Chester. Try contact lenses or looser-fitting glasses.

Call for reinforcements. If all else fails, your doctor can help cut a sinus infection short with antibiotics. For acute sinus infections, first-line therapy is usually prescription medicines like amoxicillin (such as Amoxil) or erythromycin (such as E-Mycin) for ten days. In chronic cases you might be given antibiotics and decongestants for at least a month. As a last resort, surgical drainage might be used to widen your sinus openings.

The Uncommonly Annoying Cold

It's bad enough that you end up looking like Rudolph the Red-Nosed Reindeer and sounding like Elmer Fudd; why does the common cold have to be so, well, common? Chances are, this year you'll be struck by cold viruses—and succumb to humanity's most prevalent sickness—at least twice and up to four times.

When a nasty virus stops you cold, try the following tips.

Wash up. Since colds are transmitted by hand-to-face contact, it's a good idea to wash your hands frequently. Try not to touch things that you know someone with a cold has touched, says Dr. Yonkers. "Everyone worries about people sneezing around them in the office, because they think that they'll breathe in germs and get infected. But if you touch the doorknob that they just touched and put your hand to your eye or nasal chamber, it's much more likely that you'll be infected."

Be extra aware in the air. One of the more common places to pick up cold viruses is in airplanes, notes Anne Simons, M.D., assistant clinical professor of family and community medicine at the University of California, San Francisco, and author of *Before You Call the*

What Makes a Cold a Cold?

Believe it or not, the runny nose, sore throat and dry cough that may accompany a cold are not caused by one of the some 200 cold viruses that are floating around out there. They're actually a reaction to the body's fight against the viruses. Once the infection starts, fluid and mucus accumulate as a result of successive waves of white blood cells flowing to the area to fight off infection.

You catch a cold by breathing in virus-containing droplets that are sneezed or coughed into the air or by rubbing your eyes or nose after touching some virus-contaminated object.

For the most part a cold lasts about five days, but when stuffy nose and congestion hang on longer than that, you may have acute sinusitis, notes Alexander C. Chester, M.D., clinical professor of medicine at Georgetown University Medical Center in Washington, D.C. The infection can spread to other mucus-lined areas, causing laryngitis, bronchitis or other infections. "The membranes of the nose are damaged by the virus, which causes a bacterial infection. You'll want to see a doctor about taking antibiotics."

Spice it up. Spicy foods make the nose run, which helps loosen mucus and moisten the lining of the nose, says Dr. Yonkers. Try eating spicy Mexican foods or a spoon of horseradish.

Drink up. Drinking at least six glasses of water a day is important, according Dr. Chester. "Anything that will keep the membranes hydrated and the mucus from drying out is a very good idea."

C's the day-saver. Vitamin C can be a sure cold fighter, notes Dr. Chester. "The theory is that it has a decongesting effect; that's why it aborts a cold." He recommends taking 2,000 milligrams a day—in doses of 500 milligrams taken four times a day. This is far above the Daily Value of 60 milligrams, so you should check with your doctor before taking higher amounts.

Get souped up. You might have thought that it was an old wives' tale, but chicken soup really does work on colds, says Dr. Zwillenberg. Having a steaming bowl of chicken soup every day cuts down on the amount of time that people show symptoms.

Allergies: Alien Invaders

If you've never so much as sniffled during hay fever season, and you've hugged many a dog or cat without sneezing, count yourself lucky. For tens of millions of Americans, allergies aren't just something to sneeze at; they're also something to cough, wheeze and be miserable over.

Allergies are tricky things. They can develop at any age. The dust on your nightstand that never bothered you before might suddenly have you sniffing and coughing.

Although allergies tend to run in families, the cause isn't clear. All doctors know is that the immune system mistakes otherwise harm-

Doctor. Because so many people are packed together in planes, and the flight attendants are handing out and collecting cups and utensils, be especially careful about hand-to-face contact when you're flying.

Don't forget that flying with a cold can cause a short-term blockage between the sinuses and the nose, notes Dr. Yonkers. If you have to fly with a cold, use nasal spray and take decongestants to shrink your nasal lining before the plane takes off.

Mucus Revelations

Trying to read your mucus isn't as interesting as reading, say, *People* magazine, but it could help you find out what's wrong with you.

With the common cold and allergies your mucus is thin, clear or white. But the nasal secretions of a sinus infection are an unmistakable thick, greenish yellow.

How do you distinguish a cold from an allergy? There's no difference in mucus color, but other symptoms can tell you. With an allergy the symptoms are likely to be sporadic rather than constant, often involving sneezing and itching. A cold, on the other hand, is more likely to be accompanied by a headache, sore throat and low-grade fever.

less things like pollens, molds, dusts and animal dander for invaders. Aggravated into reaction, the immune system then mounts different defensive reactions against them. Those reactions cause symptoms such as runny nose, watery eyes and nasal congestion.

If you're coughing and sneezing for what seems like no reason, you just might have an allergy. Your doctor can take a medical and environmental history, including information about pets, bedding, living conditions and seasonal variations in symptoms. All this information helps the doctor detect what you are allergic to.

If itchy eyes and a drippy nose are driving you to distraction, here are a few simple suggestions from doctors.

Be a dust buster. Because dust and dust mites are major allergens, it's smart to get rid of as many sources of these irritants as possible, says Dr. Chester. Use washable curtains and tight-weave rugs that don't hold dust. Also, avoid collecting knickknacks, because they can accumulate dust, and change the filters in your air conditioner and heating systems monthly. In addition to washing your sheets and pillowcases as frequently as feasible, you should wash your mattress pad, bedspreads and blankets every month.

Flush out the mold. Having a vaporizer in your bedroom is good for keeping your nasal tissues moist, but don't forget to clean it every three days to prevent the buildup of allergy-causing molds, says Dr. Zwillenberg. Rinse it with a weak bleach solution made from one teaspoon of bleach and one quart of water or use a 50-50 solution of vinegar and water.

Have a bleach party. Another way to avoid molds is by washing areas around sinks and bathtubs with bleach, says Dr. Simons. You can use straight bleach or make a diluted solution by adding some water to the bleach.

Take a non–sleeping pill. To ease nasal congestion and dripping, try a nonsedating prescription antihistamine such as terfenadine (Seldane), loratadine (Claritin) or astemizole (Hismanal), says Dr. Zwillenberg. Some of these might make you drowsy. "But they're much less sedating than regular antihistamines."

Get a dryer. If pollen is your poison, it's a good idea not to line-dry clothing, says Dr. Zwillenberg. "Clothes dried outside tend to trap pollen. It's just one more irritant to deal with."

See also Nose, Respiratory System

Skeletal System

The skeletal system includes 206 bones, the cartilage that covers the ends of the bones, the joints where bones meet and the ligaments that connect bone to bone. The skeleton supports the body and its internal organs—but the bones do more, storing calcium and producing red blood cells from the marrow.

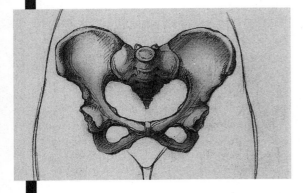

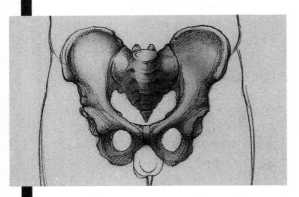

The difference between a man's pelvis and a woman's pelvis. The woman's pelvis (top) is wider and shallower than the man's (bottom). Also, the woman's bones are lighter, thinner and smoother.

■ The **back** is a complicated flexible structure—26 spool-like bones separated by cushy spinal disks and joined to muscles and ligaments. Although back pain results in more doctor visits than anything but the common cold, most back pain clears up on its own if you follow a few basic guidelines. (See "Relief Happens" on page 10.)

■ The **knee joint**, connecting the thigh- and shinbones, is the biggest and most complex joint we have. Women are more vulnerable to knee problems than men are. (To keep that joint in good shape, see "What Joint Health Hinges On" on page 189.)

■ **Rheumatoid arthritis**, a disease that causes inflammation of the joints, can affect joints throughout the body, but it generally shows up first in the small joints of the fingers, wrists, ankles and feet. (See "The Many Aches of Eves" on page 188.)

■ The thin **femoral neck bone** in the hip is the vulnerable site of many fractures caused by the bone-thinning disease osteoporosis. Since women are at far greater risk than men of getting disabling hip fractures as they age, it is important to build strong bones while you are still young. (See "Amassing More Bone" on page 179.)

■ The **joint at the base of the big toe** is home base for the bony growth of a bunion. (To relieve feet that are killing you, read "What's Good for the Sole" on page 132.)

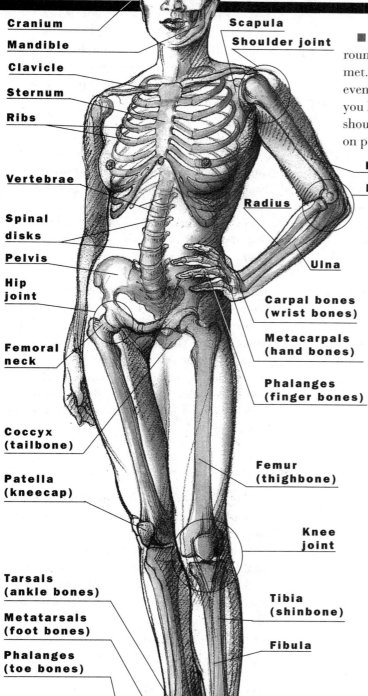

Cranium

Mandible

Clavicle

Sternum

Ribs

Vertebrae

Spinal disks

Pelvis

Hip joint

Femoral neck

Coccyx (tailbone)

Patella (kneecap)

Tarsals (ankle bones)

Metatarsals (foot bones)

Phalanges (toe bones)

Scapula

Shoulder joint

Humerus

Elbow joint

Radius

Ulna

Carpal bones (wrist bones)

Metacarpals (hand bones)

Phalanges (finger bones)

Femur (thighbone)

Knee joint

Tibia (shinbone)

Fibula

■ The eight bones of the **cranium** surround and protect your brain like a helmet. But to avoid skull fractures, you need even more protection for your head when you bicycle. (To see how a bike helmet should fit, turn to "No More Bike Bonk" on page 378.)

Where to Look

To avoid bone injury and keep your joints shipshape and your skeletal system healthy, see:

Ankles	page 3
Back	page 9
Body Type	page 38
Collarbone	page 82
Elbows	page 92
Feet	page 131
Hands	page 165
Hips	page 177
Jaw	page 185
Joints	page 187
Knees	page 192
Neck	page 252
Pelvis	page 309
Ribs	page 326
Shoulders	page 348
Skull	page 377
Spine	page 379
Tailbone	page 397
Wrists	page 436

Skin

SKIN IS THE WRAPPING that holds your body together. It keeps out harmful environmental elements such as radiation, bacteria, viruses and dangerous chemicals. Without it you would literally fall apart.

Of course, none of that covering is either permanent or wrinkle-free. Smile lines around your eyes tell the world that you've been living and laughing for a long time—certainly nothing to be ashamed of. Expression lines eventually crease your forehead, the skin between your eyes and the delicate skin around your eyes. They are the result of constantly moving your face in the same patterns over a long period of time.

But of all the potential agers facing your skin, none is a tenth as destructive as the sun. A common figure cited by several doctors is that 80 percent or more of the visible aging that occurs on the skin is a result of sun exposure—a process called photoaging.

Fry Now, Pay Later

Behind every wrinkle, every age spot, every freckle and every skin cancer there is an afternoon spent at the beach or a picnic or a simple walk in the sunshine. More accurately, a lifetime of such moments waits until your thirties and forties to show up on your face.

Unfortunately, lots of women don't realize that every unprotected minute spent in the sun as a child—and for most of us, there were thousands of them—would show up on their faces years later, says William Coleman, M.D., clinical associate professor of dermatology at Tulane University in New Orleans. People who have stayed out of the sun look a lot younger than those who haven't, he observes. "Research shows that many children, by age ten, have enough sun damage to develop severe wrinkling and skin cancer later on. It's a delayed phenomenon."

Were it not for a lifetime of sun exposure, it's possible that your skin could be relatively youthful-looking up until your seventies. That's the age when intrinsic aging of skin kicks in, and studies back this up.

For an objective test, one panel of judges viewed pictures of 41 Caucasian women who lived in Tucson, Arizona—one of the sunniest places in the United States. The women in one group had been exposed to fewer than two hours of sun a week. In the second group the women had been exposed to more than 12 hours weekly. Viewing the pictures, the judges consistently guessed that the women with the greater sun exposure were, on average, 11 years older than their actual ages. The women in the low-exposure group were thought to be only 5 years older than they were.

Rays from the Sun

How could the good old sun—that comforting, glowing orb that feels so good—turn out to be such a traitor?

When the sun is at peak power—between 10:00 A.M. and 3:00 P.M. each day—you're getting a blast of ultraviolet (UV) rays that do the dirty work. The UV rays are divided into three segments: UVA, UVB and UVC. Luckily for us, atmospheric oxygen and the ozone filter out UVC rays, which are the shortest, most powerful and most highly destructive rays, before they reach the Earth.

Of the radiation that gets to us, UVB rays are more destructive to the skin and are thought to cause most of the aging. UVA rays have a relatively low energy content, but since there are more UVAs than UVBs in sunlight, UVA damage can be significant, too.

When the sun hits the skin, ultraviolet radiation penetrates into the nucleus of each cell. That's where much of the damage is done. The nucleus stores DNA, the string of molecules that makes up the "message center," controlling the activity of each individual cell as well as the information that travels to other cells. The radiation breaks down the DNA, damaging the cells that produce collagen and elastin, proteins that make up the bulk of your skin and help keep it taut and resilient. "It's like microwaving the collagen until you end up with broken and destroyed tissue," says Melvin Elson, M.D., medical director of the Dermatology Center in Nashville and director of the Cosmeceutical Research Institute in New York City.

Thinning Skin

To see the effect of the sun, doctors have looked at what happens to the outer two layers of skin, the dermis and the epidermis.

The dermis is the thicker layer, which houses the sebaceous glands, or oil ducts, and the sweat glands. This layer is also filled with the collagen and elastin that make your skin tight but flexible. At the base of all that is the subcutaneous fat, which separates the dermis from the muscle and bone, insulating you from the cold.

That layer is topped off by the epidermis, a protective shield that is constantly reinforced as cells at its bottom divide and multiply, pushing the cells above them to the surface. When the very top cells get sloughed off, they're just dry and useless flakes—a miniature, invisible dust storm. These used-up cells

are the material that makes up your bathtub ring and some of the dust in your house.

As sunlight exposure continues, the ridges between your epidermis and dermis keep flattening out until they completely disappear. To make things worse, the thinner the skin gets, the less tissue there is to absorb the UV rays, and the more harmful even a small dose can be.

Even reflected sunlight is damaging—and the light can be reflected off everything it touches. Sand reflects 17 percent of the UV rays. Freshly fallen snow reflects more than 80 percent. This reflection can send sunlight upward to delicate areas that burn very easily, such as the top of your nose and underside of your chin.

Photoaging doesn't just show up in the form of wrinkles. Age spots, also known as solar lentigines, are brown splotches that commonly appear on the hands and face. They're a result of the skin trying to protect itself from sun overexposure by producing an overabundance of melanin—the pigmented cells in your skin that are responsible for tanning—in uneven patches. Photoaging is also the cause of 90 percent of all skin cancer.

Exposure: It All Adds Up

The reality is that you can avoid the sun. Every minute spent in it has a cumulative effect over a lifetime.

Say you spend 7 minutes walking to and from work every day. That's 14 minutes in the sun a day. Then you go out for lunch and sit for 10 minutes outside, or you spend 5 minutes outside talking to someone. It all adds up, says Michael Martin, M.D., assistant clinical professor in the Department of Epidemiology and Biostatistics at the University of California, San Francisco, and author of

It's All in the Pigment

The darker your skin, the better your built-in protection against skin cancer. The following chart summarizes findings about some specific ethnic groups. The lightly pigmented groups, such as the Irish and Scottish, are at much higher risk of getting skin cancer than the darker groups, such as the Greek or Spanish.

Highest Risk	Moderate Risk	Lowest Risk	
Scottish	Scandinavian	Polish	African
Irish	German	Italian	Spanish
English-Welsh	French	Greek	
Russian	Slavic		

How to Outsmart the Sun. "Think of it like the fading of a piece of furniture. Put it in direct light, and it happens fairly quickly, but with a little bit of exposure over a period of time, it still fades. Add up 30 two-minute exposures, and it's as damaging to your skin as a continuous full hour of sun."

How much will that affect you?

In part the answer depends on heredity. You inherit your skin type, your ability to tan and your resistance to burning—the factors that largely determine how you will wrinkle. If you're a sun-loving, fair-skinned blond with northern European ancestors, you'll probably age more quickly than an African-American.

It comes down to melanocytes, which are pigmented cells in your skin that produce color, or melanin. When the sun hits your skin, the melanocytes go to work, putting some color in your skin to protect it from harmful UV rays. The additional color helps prevent the rays from penetrating the deeper layers of skin.

One way to measure skin tolerance is by calculating the sun protection factor (SPF), the measurement used on sunscreens. The darkest African-American has a built-in SPF of 10 in her skin, which means that it takes ten times as long for her skin to burn as a Caucasian woman's.

While a lifetime of sun exposure won't age the African-American much, the blond Caucasian has practically no natural melanin. This means that the UV rays will go directly to the deep layers of skin and cause tissue damage.

Saving Face—With Prevention

As far as sun damage goes, what's done is done. But it's never too late to ward off crow's-feet and worry lines, says Michael Bilkis, M.D., assistant professor of dermatology at New York University Medical School in New York City. Here are some tactics.

Slather on sunscreen. Dermatologists sound like broken records on this point: Of everything you can do to ward off wrinkles and age spots, wearing sunscreen is the most important.

Go 15 or over. Choosing the right sunscreen can be a challenge, with SPF numbers ranging from 5 all the way up to 50. How can you determine how much protection you'll get from a sunscreen?

It all depends on your skin type. Take the number of minutes that it takes your skin to turn red and multiply it by the SPF. If you normally burn after 20 minutes in the sun, an SPF 15 will protect you for 300 minutes, or five hours.

Most doctors recommend an SPF of 15 or higher, says Jonathon Weiss, M.D., assistant clinical professor of dermatology at Emory University School of Medicine and Clinic in Atlanta. "I prefer one with a factor of 30 or higher."

Don't wait to renew. If you're wondering how often to put on more sunscreen, the answer is, the more frequently the better. Sunscreen gradually loses its protective power. If an SPF 15 sunscreen promises to block out 92 percent of UV radiation, for instance, it's only doing that at first. After a period of time (two hours or less), it may have diminished to an SPF of about 7. Every sunscreen has a half-life, when it's only half as effective, according to Dr. Weiss.

Up the ante to avoid beach burns. For folks who wear sunscreen every day and spend most of their days indoors, a nonwaterproof SPF 15 is adequate. Long days outside and on the beach, however, require heavy-duty protection of at least SPF 30, says Dr. Bilkis. If you spend a considerable part of your day under the sun, apply a nonwaterproof SPF 30, reapplying the sunscreen often as the day goes on.

"The lower number is for when you're not in the sun or sweating for a long time," he notes. "The other is for the beach. If you're outside sweating, you want something that will stay on your skin." A sunscreen that is truly waterproof—indicated by the label—should maintain its SPF after 80 minutes of water exposure.

Never trust a cloud. You need protection even on cloudy days, says Dr. Bilkis. Some of the ultraviolet rays aren't absorbed by the clouds; they come right through. And because you don't feel the heat, your body doesn't tell you when it's time to come inside. "The worst sunburn I ever saw was on a man who was out on his boat on a foggy day."

Make it a daily habit. Get used to putting on a dab of sunscreen every morning, suggests Harold Brody, M.D., clinical associate professor of dermatology at Emory University School of Medicine in Atlanta. He recommends a combination sunscreen moisturizer with an SPF of 15, applied after you've washed and dried your face in the morning—preferably, at least 30 minutes before you go outside. Just rub a pea-size drop on each cheek and another on your forehead. Then moisten your fingertips and work the sunscreen, along with the water, into your skin.

Beware: If a moisturizer simply says that it prevents aging or contains a sunscreen but doesn't list an SPF, chances are that it won't be an effective sunscreen on its own.

Have it made with shades. Wear sunglasses every time you head outside, says Dr. Weiss. They protect the eye skin to some extent and help prevent squinting, which plays a big role in expression wrinkles.

Dress for sun excess. Choose clothes that won't let those harmful rays in. Darker colors protect better than lighter ones, and tight-weave clothes are better than loose-weave clothes, notes Dr. Weiss. "A wet white T-shirt allows UVB rays to penetrate."

One good test for a protective garment: If you can see through it only by holding it very close to your eyes, it has an SPF of at least 15.

Delay that jog. Rather than worry about sweating off your sunscreen, plan outdoor exercises like biking or jogging either before or after the sun's peak burning hours of 10:00

A.M. to 3:00 P.M. Even then, you should be smeared with sunscreen, since daily application should be a regular habit.

Keep a hat on. A hat with at least a two-inch brim that goes all around the head offers good protection. "It should protect your ears and neck as well as your face," says Dr. Martin.

Screen your kids. If you have children, it's never too early to start slathering sunscreen on their exposed noses, shoulders, tummies—and don't forget the tops of their ears and feet. "You should definitely start putting sunscreen on as a child," notes Barbara Gilchrest, M.D., professor and chairman of dermatology at Boston University Medical Center. "People get most of their lifetime sun exposure when they're outside playing."

Avoid fry shops. Spending time in a tanning salon is absolutely the worst thing that you can do to your skin, says Dr. Weiss.

These places hype the fact that their light-bulbs emit relatively low-energy UVA rays rather than UVBs. UVA rays go deeper into the skin, actually penetrating to the level of some hair follicles and sweat glands. This can cause damage that could lead to cancers of the skin. Also, the tan from a tanning bed doesn't protect you from a UVB burn once you go outside.

Doing Your Part

In spite of the sun's significant influence on your skin's health, looking younger is not only about protecting your skin from UV rays. There are lots of other strategies that can stop the boots of time from marching across your face.

Stop yo-yoing. Constantly losing and gaining weight can eventually affect the elasticity of your skin, says Dr. Elson. The cells in the

subcutaneous fat layer of the skin don't multiply—they enlarge. Excess weight pushes on the skin. "After seesawing for 40 years, the skin won't snap back anymore. Maintain a normal weight."

Quit smoking. Smoking is a major cause of wrinkling, says Dr. Elson. It's damaging in two ways: Constant facial movements result in lines, and a buildup of tar narrows the blood vessels that in turn nourish the skin. The result is that the skin doesn't recover as well from injuries like sun damage.

Beware of anti-aging exercises. Exercises that promise to tone the muscles of the face are a bad idea, says Dr. Martin. "Any facial exercise has the effect that smiling does; you're creasing the skin over and over again in odd ways that you normally wouldn't use with facial expressions."

Stop smooshing your face. Sleeping on your stomach or side leads to facial creases, says Dr. Elson. One solution is to get a wrinkle pillow, available in many department stores. It holds your head in a certain position so that you can't roll back and forth.

Also, a satin pillowcase can help cut down on creasing of the skin, says Dr. Elson. Or try setting two pillows side by side and placing your head in the crevice where they meet to help force yourself to sleep on your back.

Skin Cancer: More Than a Scare

Crow's-feet and age spots might not be the cutest things in the world, but at least they don't hurt you. Another direct result of the sun isn't so benign: skin cancer. If you are white and live to age 65, your chances of getting it are about 50-50.

The incidence of skin cancer increases the closer you live to the equator. Someone in Texas, for example, would be expected to develop skin cancer about ten years earlier than someone in Minnesota.

It's the most common form of cancer in the United States; nearly 40 percent of all diagnosed cancers are skin-related. Despite the anxiety and fear it causes, however, when it is detected early and removed, skin cancer can be beaten by timely intervention.

There are three types of cancer: basal cell, squamous cell and malignant melanoma. Basal cell, which appears as a small, fleshy bump or nodule on the head, neck and hands, is the most common form of skin cancer. Left untreated, it will begin to repeatedly bleed and crust over. It rarely spreads to other parts of the body, but it can cause considerable local damage if let go. It is not life-threatening, however.

Squamous cell appears either as nodules or as red, scaly patches in the rims of the ears and on the face, lips and mouth. Unlike basal cell, it can spread, and it is estimated that more than 2,000 people a year die from it. If removal is potentially disfiguring, as when the cancer is located on the nose or under an eye, the lesion can be treated with radiation rather than cut off.

Unfortunately, basal cell and squamous cell cancers can recur. "Sun-damaged skin is sun-damaged skin," says Ronald Scott, M.D., Ph.D., radiation oncologist and cancer specialist at the South Coast Tumor Institute in San Diego. The incidence of recurrence is highest at the middle of the face—the nose is the top spot for skin cancer.

Then there is malignant melanoma—the pit bull of skin cancers—which strikes 32,000 Americans a year and kills nearly 7,000. Because it is almost always curable in its early stages, early detection is critical. Melanoma begins in or near a mole or other dark spot, so it is vital to be familiar with every mark on

Where to Look First

When you do a self-exam for changes, discolorations or new growths in your skin, some areas deserve special attention. See the illustration to identify the places where skin cancers most frequently occur on a woman's body. If some areas are hard to see when you do a self-exam, use handheld and full-length mirrors.

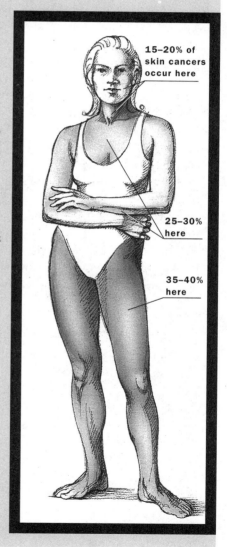

15–20% of skin cancers occur here

Thirty-five to 40 percent of skin cancers occur on the lower extremities. Other risk areas include the upper extremities and the face, neck and head.

25–30% here

35–40% here

your body and to check yourself often.

Unlike the other two types of cancer, melanoma usually appears on places that are covered by clothing, says Dr. Martin. This is because melanomas are closely linked with severe sunburns—the kind that a pale person gets when she bakes on the beach for three hours. Melanoma also hits at a younger age; 20 percent of them strike people under age 40.

Your chance of getting a melanoma has skyrocketed. Fifty years ago, a person had only a 1 in 1,500 chance of acquiring one. The lifetime risk has increased to 1 in 135.

The increase is partly a result of some changes in lifestyle that have occurred over the decades. "We can travel more easily now; we can beat up our skin in a weekend," observes Dr. Coleman. "That, and wearing less clothing and exposing more of the body, contribute to melanoma."

Should you have every lump and bump that pops up on your skin removed? "Everyone gets skin growths, and they don't all turn into cancer," says Dr. Scott. If you have a strange growth that you never noticed before, have a doctor check it out. Also, be sure to notice any moles that change shape or size.

Facing Up to Wrinkle Control

Women who worship the sun often end up regretting it—and looking for solutions. Crow's-feet, fine wrinkles and the deep folds that run from the nose to near the chin are all the most common—and easiest—to erase through modern medical intervention, says Barry Resnik, M.D., clinical instructor of dermatology at the University of Miami School of Medicine. Among the available treatments are collagen injections, chemical peels and tretinoin cream, according to Dr. Resnik. In fact, collagen injections are the

What Does Collagen Do?

If you have a collagen injection to help remove wrinkles, your doctor will inject bovine collagen—which comes from cows—into your skin in the wrinkled area. The illustrations below show a woman with nasal labial fold lines—the deep wrinkles that run from the nose to the mouth—and the results after a collagen injection treatment.

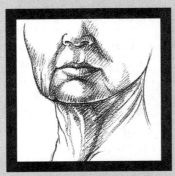

Before collagen injection.

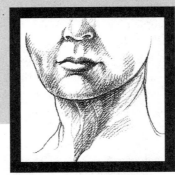

After treatment.

fourth most popular procedure for people ages 19 to 34.

With collagen injections the wrinkles are, in effect, puttied over from the inside with bovine collagen that is injected into the skin. (Collagen from cows is used, because it is most similar to that found in humans.) It lasts for anywhere from six months to a year, when the collagen is absorbed into the body. If you are allergic to bovine collagen, as 3 percent of the population is, you can ask about microlipoinjection, a nasty sounding but fairly simple procedure, which involves taking fat from the hip or abdomen and injecting it into the wrinkle.

Another procedure involves treatment with a prescription vitamin A–derivative cream called tretinoin (Retin-A), which can smooth out fine lines and even out skin tone.

Using it is extremely simple: Apply a pea-size amount to your face and the backs of your hands every night. These are the areas that are most exposed to the sun. Tretinoin penetrates the damaged skin cells and spurs them to start making collagen again, which fills in fine wrinkles. It also increases blood flow in the skin to give it a youthful, pink tone.

"It's a slow process," says Edward Jeffes, M.D., assistant chief of dermatology at the Long Beach Veterans Administration Medical Center and associate professor of dermatology at the University of California, Irvine. "It doesn't reverse severe damage, but it does erase fine lines." But be patient: It takes at least six months to see the full benefits.

Because tretinoin increases sensitivity, it means that you must always use sunscreen when you go outside. And the only way to keep reaping its benefits is to keep using it. In some people there are various unpleasant side effects, including dryness, peeling, reddening and blistering of the skin. If your reaction is severe, your doctor might advise you to use tretinoin every other day or to stop the therapy altogether for a few days.

Chemical peels are another procedure for smoothing out unwanted wrinkles. The chemicals are applied by a dermatologist, and the skin reacts to the application by sloughing off several layers of skin cells. Then new skin is regenerated, which not only looks better but also is less prone to skin cancer.

Different chemical solutions, including glycolic acid, lactic acid, trichloroacetic acid, salicylic acid and phenol, are used alone or in combination to achieve the desired effect. The strength and type of solution that the doctor uses determines whether it is a light peel—which affects light surface wrinkles—or a deep peel—which works on the deeper wrinkles. The deeper the peel, the more intricate the procedure.

Just remember that after these procedures, skin is ever so vulnerable to sunlight, and sunscreens are a necessity. Make sure that you choose an experienced dermatologist who performs chemical peels often.

Retin-A: Not for Everybody

Blushers and Scots, beware. Despite its proven ability to erase years from the face, the vitamin A–derivative cream called tretinoin (Retin-A) can wreak havoc on oversensitive skin. Research shows that the following people will probably have high sensitivity to topical tretinoin therapy.

- Fair-skinned, freckled, blue-eyed Celtic (such as Irish or Scottish) people who burn easily and tan poorly
- People with sensitive skin that stings strongly after use of perfumes, sunscreens or astringents
- Flush burners, whose faces turn red and feel hot when they are embarrassed or drinking alcohol
- Middle-aged people who generally have been heavy users of cosmetics, cleansers and toiletries and complain of dry skin
- People who have had previous skin disorders such as eczema, rosacea or seborrheic dermatitis

Some Light on Laser Surgery

Doctors wearing protective goggles, aiming the tip of a handheld laser beam at those vertical lines around your mouth. No, this isn't a scene from "Star Trek: The Dermatology Years." It's today's reality.

A growing number of doctors are using lasers—concentrated light that can cut tissue and destroy some tumors. Some doctors have been using the same technique to smooth away wrinkles. "It's really a much better way to deal with wrinkles than chemicals are," says Laurence David, M.D., president of the International Society of Cosmetic Laser Surgeons in Hermosa Beach, California. "We're able to very accurately, predictably and precisely remove wrinkles rather than rely on acid

and hope it goes where we want it to go," he says.

The laser emits a rapid series of beams that are half the size of a pencil eraser. The wrinkle is vaporized during a series of sharply directed, split-second exposures. Lasers work best on wrinkles of the lower and upper lips, the eyelids and the backs of the hands, says Dr. David.

For lip lines it takes about ten minutes, and the procedure can be done while you are awake. It feels like a series of little pinpricks. "You'll have brand-new baby skin—kind of pink at first—that fades to normal color," says Dr. David. "If you avoid the sun, the effects should last the rest of your life."

Skin Care Basics

When it comes to caring for your skin, take the sage advice of Henry David Thoreau: Simplify, simplify, simplify. Here are some ways to go about it.

Be selective. "Two or three products will do everything that you need," says Dr. Weiss. "Otherwise, you're drying the skin out just to put moisture back in." For one simple cleanser to use all over your body, Dr. Weiss suggests Dove, Basis, Neutrogena, Cetaphil, or Oil of Olay—none of which contains harsh, irritating ingredients.

Go easy. Women often make the mistake of scouring their skin with loofah-type scrubbers, according to Dr. Weiss. "I recommend just using your hands." He warns that scrubbers are too abrasive for facial skin.

Get yourself into warm water. Hot, steamy water might feel like it cleans your skin better, but warm is the way to go. "Hot water tends to dry out skin," says Dr. Weiss.

Don't rough yourself up. When drying your face after washing, rubbing roughly could eventually lead to saggy skin, says Leonard Engelman, makeup artist and president of Taut Cosmetics in Chatsworth, California. "Just dab yourself dry. The concept is that rubbing roughly around your eyes can break down the skin to a certain degree."

Avoid skin booze. Astringents are alcohol-based skin toners that strip skin of natural oils, says Engelman. "The original reason for astringents goes back decades to when women used heavy cleansing creams. Astringents were needed to remove excess oil from the skin's surface." Since today's cleansers are light, astringents aren't really necessary.

Keeping Up with Moisture

You've seen all the glossy ads hyping miracle eye creams and ultra-rich moisturizers that take years off your skin. These concoctions promise to do everything but scrub your kitchen floor.

Unfortunately, a wrinkle is a wrinkle, and short of cosmetic surgery, it's there to stay.

What a moisturizer can do is help hydrate the skin, which plumps it up a bit, says Dr. Bilkis. "If the skin is dehydrated, it shrinks down and looks more wrinkled."

If your skin is dry, moisturizers replace

Super Care for Your Skin

Whether it's dry, oily or combination, your skin deserves some tailor-made treatment. Here's how to find out what type of skin you have along with some special recommendations on its care from skin specialists.

Andrew Scheman, M.D., assistant professor of clinical dermatology at Northwestern University Medical Center in Chicago, suggests that you take this simple test to determine your skin type: Wash your face with soap and water and wait two hours. Then, take a piece of lens paper—that crinkly tissue used to clean glasses—and press it for ten seconds each to your forehead, nose, eyelids and cheeks. Check to see how oily the paper is. If your paper is dark with oil, you have oily skin. If there's just a bit of oil, you have normal skin. No oil means dry skin.

Nearly everyone has combination skin, which means the T-zone (the nose and forehead) is oilier than the rest of the face, says Dr. Scheman. Someone with more oil than normal in the T-zone as well as oily chin and cheeks has oily skin.

If the T-zone is dry, then the other areas of your face are even drier. Dry skin usually has small pores and is dry all over. It has a tendency to be finer and show fine lines, because it doesn't have the moisture

necessary to plump up the affected areas.

Here's what experts recommend when you have to care for different types of skin.

Cleansing. Combination skin should be washed morning and night with either a liquid or a cream cleanser. Use a very fine scrub every second or third day, but avoid a scrubber with very large particles, which can be too abrasive.

For oily skin, use a liquid cleanser that's meant for oily skin. Wash your face gently to remove facial oils without drying. Use a scrub every other day to keep pores clean. And remember, it's vital not to overdry oily skin, which causes it to produce more oil.

If you have dry skin, use a cream cleanser twice a day. Only use a mild scrub once a week to help exfoliate dead skin.

Moisturizing. For all skin types, eye cream should be used at night. Moisturizers could cause puffiness in the fine-pored eye area.

For combination skin, apply a water-based moisturizer after washing.

For oily skin, you should moisturize with an oil-free moisturizer wherever you see surface lines and wrinkles. Do it twice a day.

If you have dry skin, use a light-weight moisturizer in the morning and a heavier one at night.

lost oils, adds Dr. Coleman. The moisture soaks into your skin and adds volume to it. "It actually occupies space in the top layer of your skin."

Relative newcomers to the skin care world are alpha hydroxy acids (AHAs), which contain active exfoliators like glycolic and lactic acids. AHAs work by lightly peeling the top layer of skin, removing dead cells. Unlike the chemical peels given by some dermatologists, AHAs don't penetrate beyond the epidermis and thus are much gentler to the skin.

Antioxidant skin creams are another development in skin care technology. The makers of the creams claim that they neutralize free radicals—the molecules formed by sun exposure that destroy healthy skin cells. Containing vitamins C and E, these creams are touted as the answer to aging. The jury is still out, however, according to Lorraine Kligman, Ph.D., research associate professor of dermatology at the University of Pennsylvania School of Medicine in Philadelphia. "There is some evidence that they can prevent some of the acute damage done to the skin. Sunburn causes cells in the epidermis to die, and some of these preparations can reduce the number of sunburn cells. But what they do over the long term is under speculation."

Sometimes a Great Lotion

If you're using any kind of moisturizer, here are some ways to make it most effective.

Make a sandwich. When applying moisturizer, do it while your skin is still damp to help seal the moisture in. "You need to make a skin, water and moisturizer 'sandwich,' " says Dr. Resnik. "The moisturizer is like a roof that prevents evaporation of water."

Go for the grease. Did your mother recommend petroleum jelly as the moisturizer of choice? Well, guess what? She was right. It still can't be beat, says Dr. Kligman.

According to a study that Dr. Kligman did in 1992 using hairless mice, four weeks' application of the coal tar–based product actually thickened the epidermis. A mouse epidermal cell is usually condensed-looking, but treated with petroleum jelly, it gets larger and plumper, with an expanded cytoplasm (the juice of the cell).

"Not only are there more cells, but they're more juicy-looking," she says. "Enough of it gets into the intercellular layers—it does something to turn on the production of more cells."

Okay, so we're not hairless mice. But even so, Dr. Kligman recommends putting petroleum jelly on your face and around your eyes each night before going to bed. Keep it on for five minutes and gently wipe off any excess with a tissue.

Use one all over. Women don't need five different moisturizers for five different body parts, says Dr. Kligman. "There is no reason not to use the same one from head to toe." The only exception is, if you plan on being out in the sun, use a moisturizer that includes a sunscreen. It only takes 20 minutes of sun exposure for someone with fair skin to get burned.

Makeup for the Best Look

As your face ages—ever so gracefully, of course—you need to make adjustments in how everything is put together. Suddenly, thick, black eyeliner doesn't cut it. Frosted shades of eye shadow are a no-no.

"As we get older, the less we apply, the better we look," says Carole Walderman, president of Matrix Essentials in Solon, Ohio. "Heavy liners and bright colors draw attention to the very features that you're trying to soften."

Here are some ways to create your master-piece.

Tone down your eyes. Stick with subtle earth tones like brown, beige, gray and taupe. Metallic or pearlized colors reflect light, which emphasizes eye wrinkles, says Engelman.

Smooth on foundation. As you age, your pores appear larger, notes Walderman. When you apply foundation, it skips over the pores, leaving dark holes. "Use a water-based, liquid foundation on the skin first. Work it into your pores like a liquid putty. Over that, apply oil or water-based foundation for a smoother-looking surface."

Always keep the layers very thin, or you'll end up with foundation-caked wrinkles. For that same reason lighter shades are best as well. Use a sponge while applying to ensure light coverage.

Do some brows-ing. Your brows need to get lighter in color as you age, to soften the look of your face. Dark eyebrow pencil clashes with older skin tones. Use a light brown pencil rather than tweezing out white eyebrow hairs.

Just blush it on. If you have large pores or skin irregularities, cream blushes are best. With a powder blush, you hit the surface of your skin and rim the pores and wrinkles, so you end up accentuating the wrinkles. The cream blush, on the other hand, blends into the pores and around the irregularities, which makes them a lot harder to see.

Apply it just under your cheekbone and blend it up slightly. Also, use a touch of blush at your temple area as shown in the illustration. By darkening above your cheekbone at the temple and below your cheekbone by the jaw, you automatically make the cheekbone lighter, which accentuates it.

Don't overshadow. As you apply eye shadow, move across your eyelid from the outer corner by your temple to the inner cor-

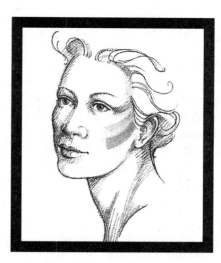

Apply the darkest blush to the area beneath the cheekbone, blending up to a lighter shade along the cheekbone. Another area of light blush goes near the temple as shown.

ner by your nose and keep the eye shadow high. If you bring the shadow too far down on the eyelid area, it will appear to drag your whole eye down.

Stay in lines. The same theory applies to eyeliner. Make small dots where you want the line and smudge them with a cotton swab or the spongy end of the eye pencil. To avoid accenting a droopy lid, stop short of the outer corner of your eye on the upper lid.

Pucker up with color. Use a lip liner pencil on your entire lip as a base and then apply lipstick over it. Corals are the safest colors as you age, because they go with many skin tones.

Skin-Deep Troubles

Oh, no. Not again.

And you thought that it was only teenagers who had what we call—so euphemistically—complexion problems.

Well, grown-ups have the same hormones—as well as the oil glands, sweat glands and all those other skin constituents—that can cause these problems.

But adult acne isn't the only skin problem on the books. As you get older, you may find other skin symptoms that leave you wondering, "Why me?" Psoriasis, eczema, dermatitis—even a fairly rare problem called rosacea—sometimes crop up when we least expect them.

You might not be able to reverse these problems, especially if you have a skin type or family history that predisposes you to certain skin conditions. But it helps to understand why these things happen and what you can do to reduce the discomfort.

Why Zits Happen

No one is immune to acne. Even if you sailed through your teens blemish-free, pimples could still be a big part of your mature years. "It's a myth that acne is just a teenage problem," says Mary Stone, M.D., associate professor of dermatology at the University of Iowa in Iowa City.

So what is to blame for your trip down acne lane?

A lot of the cause is hormonal, says Dr. Stone. Hormones trigger most acne flare-ups in the first place by causing the skin's oil glands to overproduce a substance called sebum, which comes up through the hair follicles to lubricate the skin. The passageway from the hair follicle to the skin's surface gets plugged up. The sebum combines either with keratin particles that are sloughed off in the hair follicles or with bacteria that reside there. The result: a shiny red pimple.

But acne isn't just zits; it's blackheads and whiteheads, too. Blackheads, which look like trapped flecks of dirt on the skin, are actually oxidized sebum or oil that has backed up and blocked the opening of the oil duct. Whiteheads are tiny, waxy looking white lumps made up of blocked sebum. They're like blackheads but are covered by a thin layer of epidermis, which prevents the sebum from oxidizing.

The hormones behind much of this acne are called androgens. They are produced by the ovaries and adrenal glands in females. (In men, androgens are produced by the testes.) These hormones first show up during adolescence. Hormonal imbalances can occur anytime in your life after puberty kicks in—hence, the replay of acne woes.

Heredity also can tip the scales for or against you. Check your parents' breakout quotient. If one of your parents had acne, you're far more likely to develop it yourself, says Dr. Stone. Other causes are stress, which triggers the adrenal gland to overproduce hormones, or simply having oil glands that are more active than average.

Although it is not always possible to discover what factor, or combination of factors, is behind your breakouts, Dr. Stone offers one guideline: "If you have irregular periods and excessive facial hair, there is a good chance that your acne is hormonal." Your physician should be able to determine if you have a treatable endocrine, ovary or adrenal gland problem.

Getting Free and Clear

In their teen years some girls were led to believe that they somehow brought acne on themselves. Too much junk food. Not washing their faces enough. Gorging on chocolate. All these "sins" have been blamed for outbreaks.

Well, enough blaming. Research shows that none of these factors is particularly important. Even though you can't control acne, however, there are several steps that you can take to make it a minimal part of your life.

Hands off. Resist squeezing pimples or blackheads, says Dr. Stone. "You're pushing material back down that can actually break the follicle wall. You can create new pimples and cause scarring."

If a pimple has a large yellow or white head and looks ready to pop, apply a warm, wet towel or washcloth for about ten minutes. When it's really white, you can take a sterile needle and pop the whitehead, then press with the compress. (Sterilize a needle over a match flame, but be sure to let it cool before using it.)

Be gentle. Don't think that roughing your skin up by scrubbing or using harsh soaps will prevent pimples. Scrubbing can cause the same trauma as squeezing can, says Dr. Stone. "Gently wash your face twice a day with a mild soap. Don't scrub your skin—that's abrasive."

Go easy on the moisturizer. Use an oil-free moisturizer only where your skin is dry. If your skin is oily enough for acne, you probably don't need much moisturizer. "I have found that all moisturizers aggravate acne if used on a daily basis," says Dr. Coleman.

Mellow out. Stress throws your body's system out of balance—which can lead to the overproduction of hormones, according to Dr. Bilkis. "This reaction can either directly cause a breakout or make your skin supersensitive and prone to rashes. You have hormone releases of all sorts linked to what's going on in your body. Your skin reflects everything."

For his patients Dr. Bilkis recommends healing from the inside out, by practicing methods of relaxation, such as meditation, journal keeping and bubble baths. His belief is that if you are healthy and at peace inside, your skin will be healthy as well.

Go for the benzoyl peroxide. Applying an over-the-counter drying agent like benzoyl peroxide or salicylic acid after you wash your face helps make a pimple go away faster, says Paul Zanowiak, Ph.D., professor of pharmacology at Temple University School of Pharmacy in Philadelphia. "It's a mild peeling agent that cuts back the inflammation."

Eczema: The Big Itch

Imagine a dash of mosquito bite along with a dab of poison ivy, topped off with a layer of itchy wool. Makes you want to scratch up a storm, doesn't it?

That kind of discomfort, to varying degrees, is a fact of life for people with eczema, the catchall term for a wide range of itchy discomforts in the dermatitis family.

The most common type of eczema is atopic dermatitis, which is an inherited tendency to get skin rashes as well as asthma and hay fever. While itchy skin doesn't guarantee that you'll be sneezing and wheezing a lot, your chances of getting those ailments goes up if you have atopic dermatitis.

Atopic dermatitis can be triggered by almost anything, including heat, wool fabrics and soaps or detergents, according to George Murphy, M.D., Herman Beerman professor of dermatology and professor of pathology at the University of Pennsylvania in Philadelphia. "People who get atopic dermatitis just have really sensitive skin. The immune system in the skin is a very potent thing. If it's overly stimulated, anything that is likely to cause eczema is more likely to cause it for them."

A close relative to atopic dermatitis is contact dermatitis, which is an allergic reaction to an external irritant. Hairdressers, for example, might gradually become sensitized to the shampoos that they use and get a rash on their hands. Or you could suddenly get itchy skin around the finger where you wear a nickel-plated ring.

If you can't link a rash to an obvious cause, you might have to do your own detective work, says Dr. Murphy. "The patient has to try and sort out what in her environment might be new or in some way related." A dermatologist can do a patch test: Up to 30 different allergy-causing proteins are put in small patches onto your back, and the doctor looks at your skin's reaction. The result could reveal what is causing the problem.

Steps to Stop Scratchiness

The most important steps in clearing up and preventing eczema are the simple, daily ones that become part of your routine. Here's what doctors recommend.

Load up on moisturizer. Because people with eczema have drier-than-average skin, keeping it well-moisturized is vital, says Nelson Novick, M.D., associate clinical professor of dermatology at the Mount Sinai School of Medicine in New York City and author of *You Can Look Younger at Any Age*.

After bathing, coat your skin with something scent-free and hypoallergenic, like Curel Moisturizing Cream. Make sure that you apply it when you are fresh from the shower or tub. Spread it on your still-damp skin so the moisture will lock in.

Choose shower power. Because it's easier to jump quickly in and out of a stall, showering doesn't dry out the skin like a bath can, says Dr. Novick. If you have eczema, he recommends that you shower in lukewarm water, set a timer for three minutes—and don't exceed that. He advises showering every other day, using this routine.

Don't be a washout. When you shower, "cleanse very gently," says Dr. Novick. "Let the water run over most of your skin. Your face, feet and underarms are the only naturally oily spots in your skin anyway."

Hydrate the air, too. A humidifier can help moisten dry air, which can alleviate eczema, says Dr. Novick. Keep the air at around 40 or 50 percent humidity, he advises. To check the humidity in your home or office, you can get a humidity gauge for less than $20 at a hardware store.

Go soft on the soap. Many people with eczema are allergic to the harsh chemicals found in standard soap, cautions Dr. Murphy. Hypoallergenic soaps or cleansers for sensitive skin, such as Oil of Olay sensitive skin bar, are your best bet.

Slip on your gloves. Since contact dermatitis is aggravated by soaps, detergents and household chemicals, always wear latex gloves while doing housework, says Dr. Novick. Better yet, wear cotton liners under the gloves. The rough lining inside the latex can trap accumulated dirt and sweat that can irritate skin.

Take a shine to cotton. Anything with a prickly surface, like wool or polyester, can irritate the skin, says Dr. Murphy. When it comes to clothes, cotton is best, because it lets the skin breathe.

Don't scratch that itch. Scratching your skin—even if it's not inflamed—can cause eczema, warns Dr. Murphy. "The more it itches, the more you scratch; it's a vicious cycle," he says. "Keep your hands off it. You're making it worse by creating more eczema."

One tip for easing the itch is to lay a damp strip of gauze, cotton or linen on the affected skin. Moisture evaporates from the dressing, which helps stop the itching. Repeat the cycle every few minutes for 15 to 30 minutes, several times a day.

Psoriasis

Commercials have referred to the "heartbreak of psoriasis." Whether it breaks your heart or hurts your psyche, psoriasis is definitely a pain to be reckoned with.

These patches of raised, red skin covered by silvery white scales can affect virtually any part of the body. Although psoriasis usually hits people in their twenties, it can strike at any age. It can be either mild or severe. And because no one knows its cause, there is no known cure—only treatment.

The best way to describe what causes psoriasis is to picture the skin's top layer, the epidermis, as being stuck in overdrive. Instead of the skin cells replacing themselves every month as they normally do, the cells of someone with psoriasis reproduce every four or five days. Once the turnover starts, blood flow to the area increases to support the process. The result is an abnormal layer of skin that takes the form of round or oval red patches—most commonly on the elbows, knees and scalp.

Although no one knows just why, sometimes a cut, burn or abrasion can bring about the onset of psoriasis. So, too, can stressful situations.

Whether or not you'll get psoriasis has to do mostly with luck. Because it is partly hereditary, your odds of getting it are increased if you have a parent or sibling who has it. If one parent has it, you have a 10 percent chance; if a parent and a sibling have it, you have a 16 percent chance; and if both parents have it, you have a 50 percent chance.

If you need to ease an outbreak, here are several treatments to try.

Cream it. The best way to manage psoriasis is to keep your skin well-moisturized, says Pamela Morgan, R.N., director of the Psoriasis Treatment Center in Seattle. If your skin starts to crack from dryness, that could set the stage for an outbreak. Moisturize two or three times a day with a light lotion that feels comfortable. If you've just finished bathing, leave water on your skin, shake off the excess and put on moisturizer to trap moisture in your skin.

Be a lukewarm bather. Warm showers or baths are better than piping hot, because of

the danger of overdrying skin with hot water, says Morgan.

Grease the skins. A warm bath moisturized with mineral oil is a perfect skin soother, says Glennis McNeal, public information director of the National Psoriasis Foundation, which can be reached at 1-800-723-9166. She recommends that you use extra-light mineral oil, available at any pharmacy. This mineral oil is the consistency of baby oil but has no coloring, preservatives or fragrances. McNeal suggests getting in the bath and letting your skin soak up water before dumping the oil in.

Bathe in breakfast. Oatmeal products are also very soothing, notes McNeal. You can buy oatmeal in powder form at a pharmacy, where it's sold under brand names like Aveeno. Just add the powder to your bathwater and soak for 15 to 20 minutes.

Love your loofah. Soaking in a tub gently exfoliates, or removes, the scales if you use a washcloth, sponge or loofah, says Morgan. "Be sure not to injure the skin by scrubbing too vigorously."

Don't dry with soap. Don't use soap on your affected skin unless you've fallen in a mud puddle, advises Morgan. It's far too drying—even the liquid cleansers. The only places where you need to soap up are the oil- or odor-producing spots like your face, crotch, armpits and feet.

Go over-the-counter. If you have a mild form of psoriasis, coal-tar products can help: Tegrin, Oxipor and MG217 are just a few topical medicines that slow down skin cell reproduction.

Skin Doctoring

If your psoriasis can't be controlled with moisturizers or coal-tar products, your doctor will probably prescribe either topical steroids or a calcipotriene ointment (such as Dovonex), which is made from a synthetic vitamin-D derivative.

Michael Holick, M.D., Ph.D., director of the Clinical Research Center at Boston University School of Medicine and chief of the section of endocrinology, diabetes and metabolism at Boston University Medical Center, calls Dovonex "the treatment of choice for the nineties." Its big advantage over steroids is that extended use of Dovonex doesn't thin the skin out like steroids do.

Yet another treatment—prescribed for about one-third of psoriasis patients—is ultraviolet light therapy, according to McNeal. One form of UV therapy involves going into a light booth and being exposed—sometimes as briefly as a minute—to UVB rays, which are 1,000 times stronger than the shorter tanning rays, UVAs. UVBs actually turn off the skin's ability to reproduce cells, notes Morgan.

Another form of light therapy, PUVA (psoralens and ultraviolet-A light) exposes you to UVA rays. Before the PUVA light treatment, you'll be given a booster drug called methoxypsoralen, which is either swallowed, dissolved in bathwater or painted onto the skin.

It can take months of UV treatments—administered two or three times a week—before the skin improves, but the benefits are often dramatic, says David Kalin, M.D., a physician in private practice in Largo, Florida. "I've had people with psoriasis for eight or ten years who have had no outbreaks since starting it. With some people, it goes away completely."

But it's a trade-off: Doctors caution that UV treatment increases the danger of getting skin cancer. And since UV rays are an aging factor in sunlight, the treatments can age your skin the same as sun exposure.

Rosacea: The Unwanted Bloom

We all know women whose skin looks like it's lit from within. Dewy skin graced with rosy cheeks that never requires foundation or concealer. You just have to hate them, don't you?

But having fine-pored, quick-to-color skin can also be a drawback. It's usually those peaches-and-cream complexions that are most vulnerable to rosacea, a skin condition marked by persistent flushing in the cheeks, nose and sometimes the chin and forehead.

The first sign of rosacea is usually intermittent flushing and blushing, which later develops into persistent redness in the cheeks, nose and chin and sometimes the eyes. In rosacea's inflammatory form, acne lesions in the form of little red bumps and pustules develop. The eyes can be affected as well—becoming red and itchy, with a feeling of grittiness.

Just who gets this blushing disease? Women—most often between the ages of 30 and 50—develop it three times more often than men, but men tend to get the more severe, inflammatory form. It often strikes fair-skinned people of Celtic background, usually those who have had a lifelong history of blushing easily or who have broken blood vessels around the nose or cheeks.

The appearance of rosacea is actually the result of what occurs in the underlying blood vessels, notes Diana Bihova, M.D., clinical assistant professor of dermatology at New York University Medical Center in New York City. People who get rosacea usually have unstable, superficial facial blood vessels that tend to dilate very easily and, eventually, remain permanently dilated. These are broken capillaries.

In most cases rosacea outbreaks are treated with topical and oral antibiotics. If the redness is persistent and severe, it can be zapped away with a dye laser, using a wavelength of light that is absorbed by one of the components of blood.

Since rosacea is triggered by a variety of aggravators, you may be able to avoid the condition with just a little diligence. Here are some hints from doctors.

Cool it. Hot foods and drinks dilate the facial blood vessels, which aggravates rosacea, says Dr. Bihova. Spicy foods have the same effect. So let your soup cool and stay away from the jalapeños. "You should always have a glass of cold water with your food to counter the hotness." Also, avoid activities that heat you up, such as doing heavy aerobics, taking a sauna or sitting for a prolonged period of time in a hot tub. On hot days, turn on the fan or air conditioner.

Split with those bananas. Some foods have chemical ingredients like histamines and tyramine, which aggravate rosacea, says Dr. Bihova. A few to watch out for are bananas, plums, raisins, citrus fruits, tomatoes, spinach, soy sauce and chocolate.

Don't abrade your derm. When you wash your face, the key word is *gentle*, says Joshua Wieder, M.D., a dermatologist in Santa Monica, California, and clinical instructor at the University of California, UCLA School of Medicine. Use gentle cleansers and handle the skin with kid gloves as well. "Abrasive cleansers cause trauma to the skin that aggravates redness."

See a doc. If you look in the mirror and see red, get a diagnosis, says Dr. Wieder. Sometimes rosacea can be confused with acne. A more serious diagnosis could be lupus, a disease of the immune system characterized by a red facial rash similar to rosacea. If your doctor isn't sure after an exam, blood tests or a skin biopsy can say for sure.

See also Moles, Nervous System

Skull

DID YOU EVER WONDER WHY, when you see a man dressed in drag, you can still tell he's a man?

Okay, so he's a little taller and a lot broader than most women you know. Then there's that hint of a five o'clock shadow. And let's face it, he's just not doing a very good job in those three-inch heels.

Those things aside, there's still a giveaway clue.

Take a look at the shape of his head.

There are small but significant differences between women's and men's skulls, says Susan Larson, Ph.D., assistant professor of anatomy at the State University of New York at Stony Brook. Those differences are significant enough that we can usually tell the difference between the faces of guys and gals. "Females have very vertical foreheads," she says. They "do not have a bony ridge above their eyes. Whereas males tend to have foreheads that slope back a bit and often have what are called brow ridges—sort of a bony protrusion right where their eyebrows are."

A Super Dome

Even though the skull seems like a single unit, it's actually an amalgamation of 22 different bones.

There's the cranium, or top part of the skull, that surrounds the brain like a helmet. It's made up of 8 immovable connected bones. The cranium encloses and protects the brain, eyes and ears and also provides a place for the muscles of the head to latch on.

Then there's the facial skeleton—made up of 14 bones, including the mandible, or jawbone, which is also considered part of the skull. The facial bones determine the shape of the face. The bones of the face are also the anchoring place for the facial muscles that are used to express feelings. Their structure also includes the pockets that hold the organs responsible for sight, smell and taste. Other cavities, the sinuses, are air pockets within the skull, lined with mucous membrane. Because of this air space, the skull is lightweight for its size.

The skull is less than a half-inch thick in most areas—and even thinner than that at the base of the skull and near the temples. It's tough bone, but even so, your skull is susceptible to lumps and bumps as well as more serious injuries such as concussion or fracture.

If you fall or bang your head so hard that you get a concussion, this is actually an injury to the brain rather than the skull. You've shaken up the brain enough to disrupt its function, says Kim Edward LeBlanc, M.D., clinical assistant professor of family medicine at Louisiana State University Medical School in New Orleans.

The most common cause of a concussion around the home is a fall, says Dr. LeBlanc—slipping on ice or snow in winter or losing your footing on a wet bathroom floor. You might lose consciousness for a few minutes. Depending on the severity of the concussion, the knockout blow may be followed by nausea, dizziness, headache, ringing in the ears or disorientation that can last as long as 24 hours. This type of injury can also cause bleeding. So just because nothing is broken doesn't mean that everything is all right inside your skull.

How do you know if you need medical attention? It's pretty simple: Any time that

No More Bike Bonk

If you are bicycling, wearing your helmet could reduce your risk of a head injury by as much as 85 percent, says Jeffrey Sacks, M.D., medical epidemiologist in the Division of Unintentional Injury at the National Center for Injury Prevention and Control, part of the Centers for Disease Control and Prevention in Atlanta. The illustration below shows the proper fit for a bike helmet.

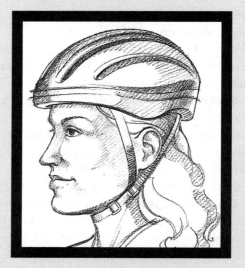

In the correct position, the helmet should be level, covering the forehead. Adjust the straps to the position shown.

you've been knocked unconscious, you should see a doctor, says Dr. LeBlanc. Even if you weren't out cold, call the doctor if you experience dizziness, nausea or headache or if you feel disoriented after a knock on the head.

More severe than concussions are skull fractures. When the bone actually breaks, the skull can mend, but the real danger is damage to the brain. Fortunately, these are the rarest of head injuries. The most vulnerable area is right around the temples where the bone is thinnest, according to Bruce Janiak, M.D., director of the Emergency Center at Toledo Hospital in Ohio.

The reason why this kind of fracture can be dangerous is that broken bone can break open a blood vessel that runs through that area, causing a brain hemorrhage. For both a concussion and a skull fracture, your doctor will check for evidence of brain damage, which is the most important consideration with these types of head injuries.

Tackling Safety Head-On

Statistics show that the number one cause of injuries to the head is automobile accidents. Nearly half these accidents involve the use of alcohol, according to Andrew Dannenberg, M.D., assistant professor at the Injury Prevention Center at Johns Hopkins University School of Hygiene and Public Health in Baltimore. So you're helping safeguard your noggin every time you buckle up, drive the speed limit and elect a designated driver. In addition:

Harness right. Don't ever put the shoulder harness behind you, says Dr. Dannenberg. When you're in an accident, the harness is what really holds you in place.

Buy bags. If you're in the market for a new car, get one with air bags on both the driver and passenger sides, says Dr. Dannenberg. Don't give up the seat belt, however. "Some people say, 'Oh I have an air bag; I don't need the seat belt.' You really need both." The air bag won't prevent side-to-side motion—and it won't stop you from banging your head on the side window or door.

See also Skeletal System

Spine

█ **CONSIDER THE CONTORTIONIST'S SPINE.** Pulled, bent, twisted, compressed, more snake's than woman's, more pretzel's than girl's.

What gives? How can contortionists—whether male or female—achieve those impossible shapes? "Very often the ligaments that support the bones in the spine are very loose and allow a lot more motion than normal at each joint. Many people are extremely flexible," says William Case, P.T., president of Case Physical Therapy in Houston.

Even if you're not as flexible as a contortionist, your spine is still a splendid thing. It handles heavy and light loads alike, trucking the bulky weight of your torso around and protecting the soft, delicate nerve tissue that makes up your spinal cord—the vital communication line from your body to your brain.

Your spinal column is made up of vertebrae, the bones that are stacked down its length like spools on a stick. "If you look at a person directly from the side, you can appreciate the engineering marvel of the human spine in the way it is curved," says Louis Sportelli, D.C., director of public affairs for the American Chiropractic Association and a chiropractor in Palmerton, Pennsylvania.

Those curves lend strength. "In physics, when you bend a rod, it becomes stronger and more resilient," he says. "And that's what happens with your spine, because of its curves. The curves act as shock absorbers and dissipate some of the forces that can compress the spine."

A Tilt for Better Curves

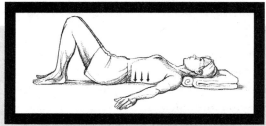

The
supine
pelvic
tilt.

You might have a great figure, but your greatest strength is in the curve of your back, not your front.

To help protect and support your spine and its natural small-of-the-back curve, you need to know how to tighten and strengthen your abdominal muscles. That curve is important, says Mary Pullig Schatz, M.D., yoga instructor and author of <u>Back Care Basics</u>. If the curve is either too flat or too pronounced—creating the flatback or swayback postures shown below—it weakens the spine and leads to pain and even degeneration.

To begin the fortifying process and learn what a tight, supportive abdomen feels like, practice Dr. Schatz's instructions for the supine pelvic tilt.

1. Lie on your back with your knees bent and your feet parallel on the floor. Let your arms lie comfortably at your sides, with your palms up. Place a flat pillow or folded towel under your head and a rolled-up towel under your neck for support.

2. Inhale fully into your chest and abdomen, letting your chest and belly expand. Then exhale. As you exhale, pull your navel toward the floor using your abdominal muscles. This action will move your lower back toward the floor as well.

3. Inhale again into your abdomen; on the exhalation, again press your navel and lower back toward the floor. At the same time, press your shoulders, elbows and the back of your head toward the floor, keeping your legs completely passive.

Repeat the tilt slowly at least ten times. Work toward being able to hold the position for 10 to 20 seconds. When you finish, roll to your side and then sit up.

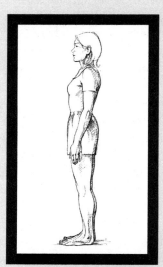

Check your profile. If you have a normal spine position, your posture looks like this.

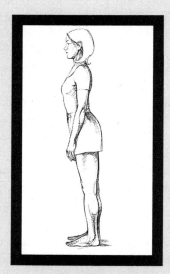

If your spinal position is "swayback," the curve in the back is pronounced—as shown above.

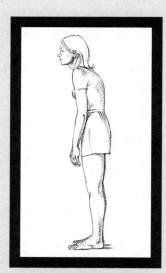

A "flatback" spine position thrusts your shoulders forward.

A spine can also curve too much. "If the angle of the lumbar curve in the small of the back is more than 30 degrees, it very likely will cause low back pain," Dr. Sportelli says. When that curve is even more pronounced, it's called lordosis or swayback.

The opposite is someone with no curve at all—resulting in the hunched appearance that's called kyphosis. Women with advanced osteoporosis—the bone weakening that usually comes with the onset of menopause—develop the condition that was commonly called dowager's hump.

Keeping Your Back Running

As for common back ailments, upper back pain is much less common than lower back pain. "Not much motion occurs in the midback," says Dr. Sportelli. "It is fixed in place by the spinal muscles and the stability of the rib cage."

Lower down in your back are the larger lumbar vertebrae that support most of the weight of your trunk. When your back aches, that's usually where it happens.

Between each of the bones, cushioning

Need a New Lineup?

Just mention back pain in a crowded room, and you're likely to hear—within seconds—someone say, "Oh, let me tell you about the most wonderful chiropractor!"

To believe or not to believe. For many people with back pain, that is the question.

Until recently, many M.D.s and Ph.D.s dismissed chiropractors as semiprofessionals with a status between quack and faith healer. Then a panel of medical experts convened by the federal Agency for Health Care Policy and Research pored through more than 10,000 studies of treatments for back pain. The panel looked at the reported results of spinal manipulation—the most common treatment offered by chiropractors—which includes touch, pressure and movement of the spine. Based on the research, the experts concluded that spinal manipulation was one of the very few treatments that relieved acute back pain—except for the pain associated with sciatica.

"The guidelines on back treatment issued by the panel raised the prestige of chiropractic considerably," says Scott Haldeman, M.D., D.C., Ph.D., associate clinical professor of neurology at the University of California, Irvine, and adjunct professor at Los Angeles Chiropractic College in Whittier. "Spinal manipulation looks very good compared with the other treatments for low back pain." Other treatments didn't hold up under scrutiny, including traction, acupuncture, steroid injections and the use of lumbar belts or corsets.

What are you getting when you visit a chiropractor? "Chiropractic is a profession that deals with conditions of the spine through nonsurgical and usually nonmedical means," explains Dr. Haldeman. This means that a doctor of chiropractic (D.C.) doesn't prescribe muscle relaxants or painkillers and doesn't do surgery.

"The more modern chiropractic approach is to include elements of physical therapy and exercise in addition to the hands-on approach," says Edward Hanley, M.D., chairman of the Orthopaedics Department at Carolinas Medical Center in Charlotte, North Carolina.

your every bend and sway, is a squishy spinal disk, sort of like a jelly doughnut. In fact, spinal disks, the dedicated shock absorbers, make up about one-quarter of your back-bone. They're good at what they do—protecting the bones and the spinal nerves—but they are not perfect. When we bend, twist and lift anything heavy—like a 30-pound toddler, for instance—that spinal maneuver can rupture a disk. This condition is called a herniated disk. The disk pops open, and some of the cushioning "jelly" squirts into the spinal canal.

It's the combination of twisting and bending that does the dirty work on the disks. "You have to be careful when you bend and twist to pull up even a weed," says John E. Dunn, M.D., clinical professor of orthopedic surgery at the University of Washington School of Medicine in Seattle.

Pressure from other movements and motions, stresses and strains—and poor posture—can also cause a disk to bulge and sometimes rupture. The popular term, slipped disk, refers to either case.

Bulging or ruptured, a disk can press against any of the spinal nerves that thread their way out of the main cord and between each vertebra. That's a pinched nerve—which spells pain. If the disk presses against any of the nerves feeding into the longest nerve in the body—the sciatic nerve—you have the particular form of punishment known as sciatica.

Dodging Disk Damage

Surprisingly, a sloppy disk doesn't necessarily cause pain. When researchers studied 98 people at a hospital in Newport Beach, California, none of them had any back pain, but only 36 percent of them had completely normal spinal disks. The rest all had at least one disk that bulged against the cartilage. Some people even had ruptured disks. So you may be harboring a disk or two that's looking for trouble—and not even know it.

Maybe you'll never be troubled by pain even if you have disk problems. That bulge can shrink back to normal, and often your body can reabsorb the pulp that escapes the disk's crust when it gets compressed.

Whether or not your disks are now in perfect order, there are ways to keep your disks and the rest of your backbone from slowing you down. Here's what experts recommend.

Above all, exercise. Your spinal disks are like hungry sponges feeding on the nutrients squeezed into their pulp by the movements your body makes. The more you move, the better that they're fed. It's that simple. Everyone should be in a regular, reasonable exercise program, says John D. Loeser, M.D., professor of neurologic surgery and director of the pain center at the University of Washington School of Medicine .

Crush out trouble. Smoking and not exercising are the two worst things a woman can do to her back, according to Stanley J. Bigos, M.D., professor of orthopedic surgery at the University of Washington School of Medicine. Smoking decreases blood flow to the back, and that—combined with lack of exercise—leaves your disks in a blood-starved state. In fact, research has shown that smoking speeds the aging of your disks that can lead to herniated disk. That's another reason to stub out the smokes before your health gets burned.

Do the bone stroll. The specific exercise to maintain a healthy back is walking, says James W. Simmons, M.D., orthopedic surgeon with the Alamo Bone and Joint Clinic in San Antonio. "You don't have to run a six-minute mile. Just the physical stress of walking alone will strengthen both your bones and disks."

As you walk you increase blood circulation: In effect, you're feeding energy to your spinal disks. And it's a risk-free exercise. As long as you're in generally good health, you can shape a walking program that will suit your schedule—a 20-minute daily walk, an hour every other day or an hour a day, according to Dr. Simmons. Other ideas for exercise? "Swimming is the number two thing to do. Biking is number three."

Work off some weight. Weight lifting builds strong bones. But if you're carrying excess body weight around, that payload can alter the mechanics of your spine, change your center of gravity and strain your spinal disks. That's why obesity, like smoking, also raises your chances of getting a slipped disk.

Luckily, you can lose weight doing the same thing that you do to ensure healthy disks: aerobic exercise. Working out helps you twice over, according to Mary Pullig Schatz, M.D., yoga instructor and author of *Back Care Basics*.

If you're overweight, however, you should always consult your doctor on how to get

(continued on page 386)

Normal Wear without the Tear

The spine's multitude of joints, called facet joints, are prey to the wear and tear of age, just like every other joint in your body. As you age you might begin to worry about the classic joint disease that many people get—called osteoarthritis, or degenerative joint disease. Many doctors don't use those alarm-bell words, however. "I'm more likely to call it simply an aging process—wear and tear," says Louis Sportelli, D.C., director of public affairs for the American Chiropractic Association and a chiropractor in Palmerton, Pennsylvania. "It's normal, natural. Anyone who is over 50 has a little bit of it."

Actually, wear and tear starts moving in at about the time you hit age 40. If your joints have been taxed hard during your sprightly youth, the aging process can wear your joints down even earlier. "It can show up in young people who play football or weight lift or do gymnastics," says Dr. Sportelli.

With so many facet joints, the spine is a true tattletale. "You can tell how old a person is by an x-ray of her spine. There are a wide variety of changes in the structure of the bones and joints and in the water content of the spinal disks, says John D. Loeser, M.D., professor of neurologic surgery and director of the pain center at the University of Washington School of Medicine in Seattle.

Those changes have to do solely with age—not with significant symptoms, notes Dr. Loeser. In other words, it's perfectly normal for the spine of a 45-year-old woman to show some worn-down areas in x-rays. Unfortunately, many radiologists think that the x-ray of a 20-year-old spine is the only normal one.

As aging spinal disks become drier and more brittle, the vertebrae themselves take on the weight that the disks used to bear. That added pressure of bone on bone can produce bone spurs on the vertebrae or on the edges of the degenerating disks. The bony outgrowths can press on spinal nerves and cause pain. Most cases, however, are so mild that you wouldn't even know they exist.

Bone: The Thick and Thin of It

If your spine could sing, one of its favorite tunes would be a blues number: "Oh, Oh, It's Hard to Be a Woman." That's because women develop osteoporosis at four times the rate that men do. In fact, 45 percent of all Asian and Caucasian women in America over the age of 50 are in some stage of the bone-thinning disease. And the bones in the spine can suffer the most.

What makes osteoporosis so sexist? No one knows, but the loss of estrogen at menopause plays a large role in bone depletion. Bone loss can start as early as age 30 in some women—and in all women, osteoporosis gathers speed during the first five years of menopause.

If you get an adequate supply of bone-building calcium in your food as you grow, you can establish an unwavering balance between the buildup and the breakdown of bone cells. With menopause, however, you hit the accelerator on the breaking-down process, so it's crucial to build up a calcium deposit big enough to see you through that change.

Women who do develop advanced osteoporosis have bones so porous that they can be fractured just from bending over. A brittle spine may develop a network of tiny fractures, essentially fragmenting under its own weight.

"These compression fractures are a very common source of back pain in older women," says John D. Loeser, M.D., professor of neurologic surgery and director of the pain center at the University of Washington School of Medicine in Seattle. In extreme cases the collapsing spine curves over into what's called a dowager's hump and pushes the inner organs around—interfering with normal breathing if the lungs are compressed. The abdominal organs can pouch out, too, into a prominent belly.

Your Chance of Encounter

Some women are at particular risk of osteoporosis. The leaders are Caucasian and Asian women. But any small-framed woman is more likely to get osteoporosis than someone who is large-boned or heavy-framed to begin with. No matter what your race, frame or body type, however, the risks shoot up for all women around the time of menopause.

Researchers have also found what may be an early warning signal of increased risk: premature gray hair. Based on studies at the Maine Center for Osteoporosis Research in Bangor, where scientists studied the bone scans and gray hair of 63 men and women, early gray hair might turn out to be a very significant indicator. The folks who went at least half gray before the age of 40 had four times the chance of showing low bone density as the people with normal graying.

A Bone-Tone Plan

Whatever risk group you're in, you need to know how to fatten up your bone account and build up your spine deposit. If you haven't reached menopause, the more you can do now, the better. Even if you're in menopause or past it, these bone-saving tactics may help you build toward a fracture-free future.

Walk a mile a day. In a study of 239 women at Tufts University in Boston, researcher Elizabeth Krall, Ph.D., and her colleagues learned that those who walked at least a mile a day had up to seven more years worth of bone on deposit than nonwalkers. They concluded that women who start a walking program during and after menopause can help stave off the bone loss that occurs then.

Walking is a weight-bearing exercise. "What happens when you do weight-bearing exercise is that your muscles pull on your bones and stimulate new bone formation," says Stephanie Beling, M.D., medical director of Canyon Ranch in the Berkshires, a health spa in Lenox, Massachusetts.

Capture that calcium. The National Institutes of Health in Bethesda, Maryland, recommends that you get 1,000 milligrams of calcium a day before you reach menopause and 1,500 milligrams per day after menopause.

The champion food sources are dairy products that have little or no fat (so that you won't put on weight), such as skim milk, nonfat or low-fat yogurt and low-fat cheese. Some leafy green vegetables, such as Chinese cabbage (bok choy) and mustard greens and broccoli, are other good sources.

You'll add some calcium whenever you have canned fish with bones, like sardines or sardines, or if you have cooked kidney beans, dried figs and prunes, toasted unblanched almonds, hazelnuts and Brazil nuts. Remember, though, that nuts are high in fat and dried fruits are loaded with calories.

Tag a Tum. If your diet doesn't take care of your daily calcium needs, "just take one or two Tums a day," says James W. Simmons, M.D., orthopedic surgeon with the Alamo Bone and Joint Clinic in San Antonio. "It's so simple. Tums carry as much free calcium as any calcium tablet. That will give you all the calcium you need."

Get a bone mineral density test. At the first signs of menopause ask your physician where to get a test that will measure your bone mineral density. If your bone is thin, you'll want to beef up your bone-building efforts by getting more calcium and more exercise. Consult your doctor to find out whether you should take medication to help prevent further bone loss, suggests Dr. Beling.

Start strength training. Another important way to build bone is through strength training, sometimes called toning or weight training. Strength training can be done with any kind of weights—dumbbells, plastic bottles weighted with sand or water or weight machines found at a gym. See the toning routines beginning on page 446 to learn how you can target specific body parts—the back, the hips, the legs and so on.

Consider hormone replacement therapy. If your bone mineral density has tested low, you may want to begin hormone replacement therapy (HRT). Women on an HRT program get a combination of estrogen and progestin, the synthetic form of the hormone progesterone. HRT has been found to be the most effective weapon against bone loss during the first five years of menopause, when bone loss is most rapid.

started with weight loss before you get into any heavy-duty exercising.

Save the tough stuff. When you sleep, your spinal disks soak up fluid from the tissues surrounding them. So much fluid is absorbed that your spine can increase in length overnight by as much as an inch, says Dr. Schatz.

You may have experienced this phenomenon. If you've ever worked out vigorously soon after getting up in the morning, you know that you are stiffer then. That's because your disks are still tight with overnight fluid. That also makes them more tense and prone to irritation, according to Augustus A. White III, M.D., professor of orthopedic surgery at Harvard Medical School and former orthopaedic surgeon in chief at Beth Israel Hospital in Boston. If you can, Dr. White suggests waiting until later in the day before any strenuous workout. By then, the tissues will have given up their bloat.

Sciatica—Pulp Friction

Take a look at your five closest friends. Chances are that two of them will have an episode of sciatica at some time in their lives. Sciatic pain follows a course all the way along the sciatic nerve, from your lower back down one thigh and into a foot. In its mildest form, sciatica can feel like nothing more than pins and needles running along that track. But when you have it bad, the pain can rival any toothache.

"Sometimes people are so frightened, and they hurt so much, that they'll do anything, even if it's surgery, to try and get out of the pain," says Annie Pivarski, orthopedic physician's assistant and supervisor of ergonomics and injury prevention at St. Francis Memorial Hospital in San Francisco. Sometimes people

with sciatica have loss of bowel or bladder control, or they're unable to lift their feet to walk. If you have these symptoms, call your doctor immediately. Once you've seen your doctor, however, try to wait before making the decision to have surgery—even if you're frightened by the severe symptoms, Pivarski advises.

Sciatica can be caused by a herniated disk pressing against any of the nerves that make up the large sciatic nerve. Indeed, a common back operation in America is a discectomy to remove the pulp pressing on a nerve. There are 142,000 discectomies performed on women each year, according to the National Center for Health Statistics National Hospital Discharge Survey.

"But lumbar (lower back) surgery is frequently unsuccessful," says Dr. Schatz. In fact, the federal Agency for Health Care Policy and Research found that only 1 person in 100 has back problems that can be helped by back surgery.

"People need to recognize that back pain is not usually a disease that requires a surgeon or specialist," says Dr. Loeser. "The vast majority of people with episodes of pain lose their symptoms within 30 days. Only 10 percent have pain after 90 days. And after that the figure eventually falls to 3 or 4 percent—the people with chronic pain."

Outwitting by Outwaiting

Sciatic pain usually responds to the same measures that you take for any back pain. That is, time and limited treatment. So there are lots of steps to consider before you start dreading the scalpel. Here's what doctors recommend.

Don't panic. Many people think that sciatica is an automatic reason for back surgery.

But that isn't so. Actually, medical experts say that only about 5 to 10 percent of people with sciatica will need surgical intervention.

So ease up on the panic button. Don't let sciatica, or any acute back pain, scare you into a hasty decision. Stop, wait and cogitate "even when pain has you frazzled," says Jeffrey Susman, M.D., member of the U.S. Public Health Service Agency for Health Care Policy and Research and vice-chairman of family medicine at the University of Nebraska College of Medicine in Omaha.

Stall four, six or even eight weeks. If your sciatic pain starts to subside within a day or two, you may not even need to call a doctor. The federal guidelines for back care say that you don't need x-rays or fancier tests, like MRIs (magnetic resonance imaging) or CAT (computerized axial tomography) scans, unless your back pain hasn't cleared up in four to eight weeks, and you're considering surgery.

"To keep your body well, stay away from the doctor," says Dr. Loeser. He's only half-joking.

Be normal. Resume regular activity as soon as you can, says Dr. Loeser. In fact, a study of 186 people in Finland with low back pain found that the 67 folks who continued as much ordinary activity as they could tolerate had shorter bouts of pain and less intense pain than the 52 people who were put on a back-mobilizing exercise program. The 67 people who spent two days getting straight bed rest took the longest to recover from pain.

"The best thing to do is get up and get active," says Dr. Susman. "Let nature heal you naturally."

Avoid reinjury. If you know what activity has triggered your sciatica, avoid it until you heal, suggests Dr. Susman. If you increased your workout schedule, for instance, or if you were doing heavy lifting when sciatica struck, make sure that you don't exercise as hard for a while.

You should also be aware that vibrations from a moving car can set off sciatica. Though it may be tough to avoid driving as much, try to reduce your time in the car, at least until your pain is gone, he says. "Time, plus avoiding the stressful activity, makes all the difference."

Know your red flags. Not all sciatica or back pain benefits from the wait-it-out method. There are a few symptoms that should prompt a phone call to your doctor.

Weakness or numbness in your legs is one. So is loss of bladder or bowel control. If you have a fever or abdominal pain or if the sciatica doesn't start to subside within 72 hours, you need a medical exam. You may have a fracture, tumor, infection or more serious nerve problem. "These are the symptoms that would call for more aggressive treatment," says Dr. Susman.

See also Nervous System, Skeletal System

Spleen

IMAGINE A RECYCLING STATION that does double duty as a defense barracks, and you have a picture of the mighty spleen.

A purplish, soft slab about five inches long, the spleen is tucked under the lower rib cage on your left side. "It's fairly well-behaved and unobtrusive most of the time," says DuPont Guerry, M.D., professor of medicine at the University of Pennsylvania School of Medicine in Philadelphia. Normally, the spleen keeps busy by retiring old red blood cells that wear out about every four months and have to be pulled from service.

"It culls the exhausted cells from the herd, and it's quite good at doing that," Dr. Guerry says. Once the spleen has snagged the exhausted red cells, it also salvages the iron out of them. It shuttles the extracted iron along to the bone marrow, where the mineral is reused in the making of the oxygen-bearing protein hemoglobin.

Defensive Action

The spleen is a fighter as well as a recycler. When someone coughs in a crowded room and bacteria and viruses make a beeline for our systems, the purple protector goes into action, making white blood cells and antibodies to attack warmonger germs. "The spleen helps defend our bodies against the sudden invasion of microorganisms," says Dr. Guerry. "It can recognize and filter out bugs in the blood."

Some infections and autoimmune disorders—like mononucleosis, malaria and lupus—enlarge the spleen. Mononucleosis can make it big and soft, so that it could easily burst.

Mostly, though, when you hear about spleens, it's because of an athletic injury or an automobile accident. "It's a fragile organ," says Janice Rothschild, M.D., general surgeon and assistant professor of surgery at Tufts University School of Medicine in Boston. "It's near the ribs, so rib fractures can be associated with spleen injuries."

When injured, the spleen can bleed profusely, according to Dr. Guerry. A bleeding spleen is a medical emergency. A surgeon will most likely remove it—an operation called a splenectomy.

Once the spleen is gone, the liver and bone marrow take up the slack. Despite its fine function as a filter, we barely miss the soft, spongy wedge. There is one serious risk that grows larger in its absence, however: the danger of getting certain bacterial infections. "It's more a problem with kids and their developing immune systems," says Dr. Guerry. "Anybody who has had her spleen removed should be vaccinated against certain infections, though."

Immunization is especially important to battle the bacteria that cause some kinds of pneumonia. So is immunization against the bacteria that cause meningitis, a potentially dangerous inflammation of the membranes surrounding the brain and spine. "You'll probably need booster shots periodically," adds Dr. Rothschild.

See also Lymphatic System

Stomach

YOUR STOMACH IS NOT SHY about letting you know that it's there. When you're hungry, it grumbles like the Grinch who stole Christmas. When you're nervous or anxious, it feels like an Olympic gymnast is in there practicing her latest round of back handsprings.

The stomach has a big job to do. Its main function is to break down the food we eat so our bodies can use it. Sometimes the stomach can do that without a hitch. Other times, it brews up trouble. Digestion can be impaired, or the stomach wall can get irritated—which is what happens when you have indigestion. Or, worse yet, if the lining of the stomach erodes, you can end up with a stomach ulcer.

The Belly Curve

Sitting between the esophagus and the small intestine, the stomach is a J-shaped, balloonlike sac that can expand and shrink as food enters and leaves. An empty stomach is about the size of a one-liter bottle, says Frank Hamilton, M.D., director of the Gastrointestinal Disease Program Branch at the National Institutes of Health in Bethesda, Maryland.

Quest for the Cause of Queasiness

The word <u>nausea</u> derives from the Greek word <u>nautes</u>, which means "sailor." Probably, in the old days a lot of seafaring mates were getting seasick. What a bummer for the captain, when in the place of "land ho!" all he kept hearing was "heave ho!"

Nausea lets us know that all is not well below deck. Sometimes a warning is all we get, and then the stomach settles down again. Other times, stomach contractions lead to mass evacuation, better known as vomiting. At that point, of course, we ask why.

In women of childbearing age who are sexually active, pregnancy is one of the first things that must be considered when nausea and vomiting arise, says David Peura, M.D., associate professor of medicine and acting chief of gastroenterology at the University of Virginia in Charlottesville. Take a pregnancy test or see your doctor. If you are not pregnant, your doctor can look for other causes.

Food poisoning? People usually experience nausea, vomiting and diarrhea about 6 to 12 hours after eating contaminated food, says Christina Surawicz, M.D., associate professor of medicine at the University of Washington School of Medicine in Seattle. To prevent food poisoning, don't leave perishable food unrefrigerated for more than four hours, be careful about eating picnic foods containing mayonnaise and make sure to cook meat thoroughly, suggests Dr. Surawicz.

As for seasickness, the problem is actually one of disturbed equilibrium in your middle ear, not a problem with your stomach. (See page 87 for some tips on preventing motion sickness.)

Expanded by Thanksgiving dinner, however, a full stomach can hold as much as two to three liters of food.

The stomach is a highly efficient Tupperware container and Cuisinart all in one. We need this storage container for food; without it we would have to eat about every 20 minutes.

As a food blender the stomach operates on pulse mode. Its rhythmic, food-churning contractions occur about every 20 seconds. The lining of the stomach also releases strong gastric juices that help break down food. "The stomach basically contains battery acid," says David Peura, M.D., associate professor of medicine and acting chief of gastroenterology at the University of Virginia in Charlottesville. Fortunately, the stomach lining also releases a mucus that usually protects the stomach wall against the bite of this high-power acid.

Burn Baby Burn

One of the biggest complaints among women over age 30 is a condition called dyspepsia, says Dr. Hamilton. This is a condition in which, for reasons not yet known, the stomach doesn't empty properly. Women complain of an uncomfortable fullness right after eating a normal-size meal. Other symptoms may include burping, bloating and nausea. Dyspepsia usually goes away if you take an antacid.

Another way that the stomach protests is with indigestion, or gastritis. That's when the lining of the stomach becomes inflamed, usually in response to fatty, spicy or acidic foods or medications or alcohol. Foods and alcohol can trigger increased acid secretion, while medications can interfere with the stomach's ability to produce protective mucus. The result is an uncomfortable burning sensation in the gut that can last for several hours. Avoiding these triggers can help prevent the problem, and taking an antacid can often provide relief, says Dr. Hamilton.

A Whole Other Matter

Another problem that women are at risk for is stomach ulcers, which occur when the lining of the stomach gets eroded and damaged. While ulcers used to be thought of as pretty much a man's problem, doctors are starting to see ulcers more often in women, especially in the 30- to 45-year-old age bracket, says Dr. Hamilton.

Ulcers are related to acid production, which can be triggered by nicotine, alcohol,

The New Culprit on the Block

It used to be that stress got the rap as an ulcer inducer. Now researchers are putting the spotlight on another culprit—a bacterium called Helicobacter pylori.

The bacteria itself doesn't cause the ulcer, says David Peura, M.D., associate professor of medicine and acting chief of gastroenterology at the University of Virginia in Charlottesville. Its presence can make the stomach more susceptible to stomach acid, however.

H. pylori is transmissible and tends to run in families, says Dr. Peura. If someone in your family has an ulcer caused by the bacteria, there's a good chance that you got the bacteria when you were a child.

Researchers find that when they treat infected people with a regimen aimed at eradicating the bacteria, ulcers are less likely to recur.

fatty foods and spicy foods—and a bacterium known as *Helicobacter pylori*. When too much acid is produced, the protective mucus is overpowered and can no longer defend the stomach lining. The acid eats away at it, and an ulcer forms.

One reason why women in the 30- to 45-year-old age group may be getting ulcers more is because more women are smoking, Dr. Hamilton observes. There is evidence that nicotine stimulates a nerve in the stomach called the vagus nerve, and that triggers increased acid production. In addition to contributing to ulcer development, smoking can interfere with ulcer healing. "We find that patients who smoke in excess of a pack of cigarettes a day have a harder time healing," he says.

Medications, particularly nonsteroidal anti-inflammatory drugs (NSAIDs), may be another contributing factor. Since many women take NSAIDs for menstrual cramps and premenstrual syndrome, they tend to use more of these medications than men, observes Christina Surawicz, M.D., associate professor of medicine at the University of Washington School of Medicine in Seattle. Women also take more steroid medications—another ulcer-inducing factor—since they suffer with immunologic diseases such as rheumatoid arthritis and lupus more than men do.

Usually, ulcers make themselves known. Signs that an ulcer may be present include a point-specific pain about the size of a silver dollar, pain that's located just below the breastbone, pain that doesn't move and pain that occurs at night. You don't get that kind of pain when you have an ulcer caused by NSAIDs, however, says Dr. Surawicz. In fact, women who are getting an ulcer from NSAIDs may not even be able to tell that they're getting one.

Up Your Ante against the Acid

Because specific foods and substances help produce more acid, you can discourage potential ulcers every time you bypass an acid generator. Here are some experts' tips on dodging the chief culprits.

Make your next puff your last. Since nicotine appears to contribute to ulcer development, do your best to quit, says Dr. Hamilton.

Read the label. NSAIDs can contribute to ulcer development when taken too frequently or improperly. "All over-the-counter medications have warnings on them," says Dr. Peura. There are dosage limits that you should not exceed, so read the label and follow the instructions.

Follow it with food. If you need to take NSAIDs frequently and regularly, do not take them on an empty stomach, says Dr. Hamilton. These medications should be taken with food or an antacid to buffer the stomach.

Censor your drinks. "Alcohol stimulates gastric secretions," says Dr. Hamilton. The higher the concentration of alcohol, the more damage that it can cause to the mucosal lining. So exercise moderation when drinking.

When Stomach Pain Strikes

If you experience stomach pain that you suspect may be an ulcer, the first step is to try an antacid, says Dr. Peura. Antacids come in several forms, including tablets, liquid and caplets. For stomach problems, Dr. Peura finds the liquid form to be most effective. If your symptoms do not get better, see a doctor.

See also Digestive System, Muscular System

Stress

FOR SOME PEOPLE, simply having to greet a stranger on the elevator is stressful. For others it's giving a speech in front of 100 people that gets the old sweat glands pumping.

Then there are those hardy hard-to-stress few who can handle it all at once—juggling deadlines at work, managing wayward children and dealing with the basement being submerged under two feet of water—without batting an eye.

Or so it seems. It's just that different people react differently to problematic, unexpected or even disastrous situations. Some of us—as many as one out of every five people tested—are hot reactors, which means that we experience dramatic and rapid increases in blood pressure when we run up against stress inducers. That hot reaction could be produced by something as mundane as missing a green light, standing in a grocery line or running out of dental floss.

What You're Facing

Women have their work cut out for them in today's world, notes Jerome Markovitz, M.D., assistant professor of medicine at the University of Alabama at Birmingham. "Working women are playing multiple roles and are therefore under more stress. They have to compromise certain roles in life in order to do it all. One role isn't fulfilled as well as the others in their lives. The result is a low-level neuroticism as to how to handle life, be a wife and mother, work at a job and be part of the community."

Whether or not these are your stress loads, you may be thinking, "Yeah, I have a little trouble unwinding, but it isn't going to kill me." Well, indirectly, it could. Stress has been linked to heart disease, high blood pressure, stroke, cancer and numerous other illnesses. Surveys show that 75 to 90 percent of all visits to primary care physicians—such as family doctors—are for stress-related complaints or disorders, according to Paul J. Rosch, M.D., president of the American Institute of Stress in Yonkers, New York.

Winding Down a Bit

There are a number of basic ways to keep from getting wound too tight. The first is to add balance to your life. Make a special attempt to seek out leisure activities that are different from your work.

"Our bodies require variety and change," says Keith Sedlacek, M.D., medical director of the Stress Regulation Institute in New York City. "We have to shift gears—readjust our speed—or our nervous systems will keep racing right into the next day."

The second method sounds contradictory: Work up a sweat once in a while. Research by Robert Thayer, Ph.D., professor of psychology at California State University, Long Beach, shows that 30 minutes of intense aerobic exercise immediately reduces body tension—and does it more effectively than moderate exercise like walking. But if moderate exercise is all you can handle, you can still expect to see an effect on your stress level—and it's the best for increasing your energy, which also helps reduce stress. New research at Hofstra University in Hempstead, New York, has also shown that weight lifting counters anxiety and depression and boosts self-esteem as well as or better than aerobic exercise.

Finally, you have to make little breaks into your schedule. "You need to put together a relaxation package, a set of techniques that will calm you down," says Allen Elkin, Ph.D., director of the Stress Management and Counseling Center in New York City.

Ways to Cool It

You don't need to get stressed out trying to put together a relaxation package. Here are some easy ways to do it.

Pad your schedule. "Realize that nearly everything will take longer than you anticipate," says Dr. Elkin. By allotting yourself enough time to accomplish a task, you cut back on anxiety. In general, if meeting deadlines is a problem, always give yourself 20 percent more time than you think you need to do the task.

Go to the bathroom. You can vent your emotions and get some of the tension out of your system while you are alone in the bathroom, says Roger Thies, Ph.D., associate professor of psychology at the University of Oklahoma Health Sciences Center in Oklahoma City. "By yelling and screaming while you're in the shower, you may head off that adrenaline squirt in your heart, and no one will hear you." Other times to let off steam in private: when you are driving in the car alone or when you are cooped up in the house.

Get all wet. Want to really relax your muscles? Soak in a tub of hot water. To get the most relaxation from a hot bath, Dr. Elkin suggests soaking for 15 minutes in water that is just a few degrees warmer than your body temperature, about 100° to 101°F. But be careful: If the water is too hot, it may stress your body even further.

Get a grip. If you're at a desk all day, keep a hand exerciser or a tennis ball in your drawer and give it a few squeezes during tense times. If you're at home most of the day, keep that de-stressor handy. "When stress shoots adrenaline into the bloodstream, that calls for muscle action," says Roger Cady, M.D., medical director of the Shealy Institute for Comprehensive Health Care in Springfield, Missouri. "Squeezing something provides a release that satisfies our bodies' 'fight or flight' response."

Serve soup, live longer. Be a volunteer, suggests Dr. Elkin. Isolation only magnifies your worries. Helping other people will give you a sense of accomplishment and self-respect—and remind you that, relatively speaking, your own troubles don't amount to a hill of beans in this world.

Learn to breathe. Most of us tend to be shallow breathers, which means that we breathe from our chests, says Dr. Elkin. This doesn't supply our bodies with enough oxygen to keep us relaxed. He suggests learning to breathe more slowly and more deeply from your abdomen. Just imagine that you have a small beach ball behind your belly button, which you slowly inflate and deflate.

Pop a bubble. One study found that students were able to reduce their feelings of tension by popping two sheets of those plastic air capsules used in packaging. "Now we know why people hoard those things," says Kathy M. Dillon, Ph.D., professor of psychology at Western New England College in Springfield, Massachusetts, and the author of the study.

Trade in the BMW for a Hyundai. Living beyond your means can actually make you sick. A researcher at the University of Alabama studied British census data on 8,000 households and found that families that tried to maintain a lifestyle they couldn't afford were likely to have health problems. So everything that you can do to cut down expenses is a step in the right direction.

Carry a humor first-aid kit. Laughter is a tremendous release, says Linda Welsh, Ed.D., director of the Agoraphobia and Anxiety Treatment Center in Bala Cynwyd, Pennsylvania. "You're changing your brain chemistry and putting yourself in an altered state," she says. "It works physically as well as emotionally, in that it lets go of the tension and improves your outlook."

How can you develop a funny bone? It's a matter of practice, notes Lee Berk, Ph.D., professor of preventive medicine and pathology at Loma Linda University School of Medicine in Loma Linda, California. "You can watch funny movies or TV shows, go to comedy clubs, listen to humor tapes in your car and really notice what makes you laugh." Learning to appreciate humor is much like developing an appreciation for music or reading: With repeated exposure, you develop your sense of humor even more.

Give yourself a time-out. Spend some quiet time at least once a day, says Scott Vrana, Ph.D., associate professor in the Department of Psychological Sciences at Purdue University in West Lafayette, Indiana. All you need to do is find a quiet room where you won't be disturbed, turn the lights down, close your eyes, focus on one thing and push all other thoughts out of your way.

Find a comforting word and say it over and over. As other thoughts come into your mind, let them passively go away. Do it once or twice a day for 15 to 20 minutes. "This is more preventive than anything. It helps reduce chronic anxiety," he notes.

Smell the apples. Keeping a green apple on your desk may calm your nerves, says Alan Hirsch, M.D., psychiatrist, neurologist and neurological director of the Smell and Taste Treatment and Research Foundation in Chicago. Though a green apple doesn't have a strong scent, you do smell it a little bit if it's right on your desk. Dr. Hirsch's current research shows that the scent of green apples significantly reduces stress and anxiety levels in women.

Jog your brain. At least 20 to 30 minutes of aerobic exercise three times a week is a great prescription for stress, notes Dr. Berk. "You can condition yourself cardiovascular-wise and change the hormone responses in your body that lead to stress as a result."

Students who ran twice a week for 20 minutes scored higher on creativity tests than did students who were required to sit through lectures, according to researchers at Baruch College of the City of New York. The researchers say that running induces a relaxed-brain state in which thoughts are thrown together randomly and new ideas often emerge.

Resign from that committee. Look at your life. Are you doing too much? If you're on the company softball team, volunteering on a church committee and chauffeuring kids to piano lessons and Girl Scout outings, and you don't have a weeknight free, you're choking on more than you can chew. "Prune your activity branches," says Dr. Elkin. Decide what gives you the most satisfaction and do only those things.

See also Emotions

Sweat Glands

■ **WE'RE KIND OF AMBIVALENT** when it comes to sweat. A glistening shine from a Nautilus workout is something to be proud of. Yet a similar sheen on your forehead during a meeting with the Big Cheese can be pure embarrassment. Some folks even use different words to talk about sweat: Men sweat, but women, well, they perspire.

Whether you flaunt sweat or pat on powder, it's all water under the bridge. In fact, sweat is 99 percent water with a dash of sodium chloride. It all comes from the three million–plus sweat glands scattered throughout your body.

When it comes to sweat production, men have the edge. Women usually produce less sweat than guys do, says Richard L. Dobson, M.D., professor of dermatology at the Medical University of South Carolina in Charleston. In women, the amount of sweat can vary at different phases in the menstrual cycle. Sweating tends to be more profuse after ovulation and premenstrually. At menopause, women often experience night sweats and hot flashes as their hormonal milieu shifts.

How Your Glands Act

You have sweat glands just about everywhere, but they are particularly abundant in your palms, underarms, forehead and soles of your feet. Each gland consists of a coiled tube, where the sweat is secreted, and a narrow passageway, or duct, that carries the sweat to the surface of the skin.

Not all sweat glands are the same, though.

One type, called eccrine glands, is found all over the body and serves as a hidden temperature control system. When the body heats up, these glands release the watery secretion we know as sweat. When the sweat evaporates, that helps cool the skin.

Eccrine glands located in the armpits also

No Sweat

Minutes before standing to speak in public, you may suddenly discover sweat glands that you never knew existed. Ask any new member of Toastmasters International—a club where people regularly practice public speaking—and they'll know what you're talking about.

One thing that can really help is confidence and experience, says Richard L. Dobson, M.D., professor of dermatology at the Medical University of South Carolina in Charleston who has been doing public speaking for 40 years. "When I first started speaking, I got sweaty palms, but now I can get up in front of three to four thousand people, and my palms are dry." Getting lots of practice and having well-rehearsed presentations are important for increasing confidence.

In addition, some form of relaxation technique can make a difference. Try yoga for 10 to 20 minutes a day to see if it makes a difference, suggests Lenise Banse, M.D., a dermatologist at Northeast Family Dermatology Center in Clinton Township, Michigan. Or you can practice progressive relaxation, where you release tension in every part of your body as you concentrate on relaxing stage-by-stage from the top of your head to the tips of your toes.

respond to emotional stimulation, says Dr. Dobson. That's why stressful situations such as public speaking can trigger sweating.

The second type of sweat gland, apocrine glands, is found in the armpits, genital area and around the nipples. These glands produce a milky white substance that, when mixed with bacteria, creates that smell known as body odor.

When the Heat Is On

A common sweat gland problem is prickly heat, a rash that forms when the ducts of the glands get plugged up. When sweat can't escape to the skin's surface, irritation develops. Here's what doctors recommend.

Chill out. Since hot, humid weather usually triggers prickly heat, get out of the sun and cool off, says Anita Highton, M.D., medical director of clinical research at Westwood-Squibb Pharmaceuticals in Buffalo. Take a lukewarm shower or bath or apply compresses that are 10 to 20 degrees below body temperature to soothe the itching.

Find an igloo. If you go back into the heat, you might have a flare-up. Stay in air-conditioned rooms as much as possible for at least a day after the rash subsides.

Loosen up. Tight clothing sets you up for prickly heat, because it traps sweat next to your skin and keeps it from evaporating, Dr. Highton says. To avoid that, wear loose-fitting cotton or polypropylene garments and avoid snug nylons or polyesters.

Take a vinegar plunge. To relieve itching, pour a cup of white vinegar into a lukewarm bath and soak in it until you feel comfortable, says Dr. Highton.

Slather up. Over-the-counter moisturizers such as Moisturel that contain dimethicone can help relieve the itching, says Dr. Highton.

Too Much of a Wet Thing

Another problem that some people experience is excessive sweating, referred to by doctors as hyperhidrosis. Only about 1 out of every 100 people has this condition, according to Dr. Dobson.

Excessive sweating can be treated with a prescription medication called Drysol, which contains aluminum chloride. Another effective treatment is iontophoresis, in which a mild electrical current is applied to the skin. Battery-operated devices are available without prescription that allow you to do iontophoresis at home, says Dr. Dobson. For excessive sweating, people generally use these devices to treat the underarms, hands or feet one or two times a day for about ten days. Since these machines may be difficult to find, contact a dermatologist for availability in your area.

See also Underarms

Tailbone

EVOLUTION IS A MESSY ARTIST. Left behind from her paint box are an appendix, wisdom teeth—and sometimes tiny tails. Rarely, but occasionally, a baby greets this brave new world with a tail peeping up from her tailbone.

"It's a pretty rudimentary tail—a funny little appendage of skin and fat and occasionally, some bone. It's just a disorganized hunk of tissue on the bottom of the butt," says John D. Loeser, M.D., professor of neurologic surgery and director of the pain center at the University of Washington School of Medicine in Seattle.

Dr. Loeser snips off about one tail a year—"a trivial operation." That's probably the only case in the state of Washington, he says. "They really are quite rare."

Even if you weren't born with a tail, you were born with a vestigial tailbone. It is the backbone's caboose. "It doesn't seem to do very much, except form an attachment for the pelvic ligaments," says Scott Haldeman, M.D., D.C., Ph.D., associate clinical professor of neurology at the University of California, Irvine, and adjunct professor at Los Angeles Chiropractic College in Whittier.

A Cuckoo Knock

The coccyx—the tailbone's proper name—is actually a little triangle of bone made up of four fused vertebrae. It sits below the sacrum, a much larger and more useful triangle of five fused spinal bones supporting the base of the spine.

The Greek word for "cuckoo" gave the coccyx its name. That's not because it's a crazy little bone, but because it reminded someone of a cuckoo's beak.

You'd have to take a hard fall to actually injure your tailbone. "The tailbone curls under," notes Dr. Haldeman. If you do fall down, you usually land on your buttocks—where the padding is—rather than hit the tailbone. Most women have a little more protection in this area than men. "The female pelvis has a little flare that protects the coccyx somewhat," he says. "Also, women have more fat on their buttocks, which protects the coccyx."

Tail Care

If you do land just so and happen to crack, displace or bruise your coccyx, the injury is called coccydynia. "But that just means pain in the tailbone," says Dr. Loeser. "A fracture hurts, but it heals relatively painlessly. Permanent pain in the tailbone, however, is hard to explain."

"For a while doctors used to cut out fractured tailbones if there was chronic pain, but that wasn't successful," says Dr. Haldeman. "If there is pain, a 'doughnut pillow' can be used for sitting. Luckily, coccydynia resolves itself for the majority of people."

If you do start to tumble, and if you have time to react, you can protect your tailbone. "Clearly, the way to fall is by using the martial arts technique," says Dr. Haldeman. "You want to curl and roll, rather than plop. You don't want to take all the force on any one part of your body. If you bend your legs and roll, that takes the force of the fall through multiple body parts and dissipates some of the shock."

See also Skeletal System

Tear Ducts

WHEN YOU STOP TO THINK ABOUT IT, crying is really a mixed signal. You win the lottery and cry tears of joy. You lose the whole pot playing the slot machines in Vegas, and you shed tears again—this time, tears of regret. As you hitchhike across the Nevada desert toward home, you get sand in your eye—fueling yet more tears.

Tears are salty, watery secretions that keep two parts of the eye constantly moist. They flow over the cornea—the transparent coating of the eye—and they lubricate the conjunctiva—the membrane covering the white of the eye and lining the inside of the eyelids. Doing their job on the cleanup crew, tears also wash away stray bits of dust and grit and help keep your eyes infection-free with a natural antiseptic called lysozyme.

Even though one tear is as good as another, they come from different sources. The tears that constantly keep your eyes moist, called the basic tear secretions, are produced on the conjunctiva and also in the eyelids. The tears that you cry over spilled milk, lost loves and squandered savings are reflex tears, generated from what's called a lacrimal gland in the upper, outer corner of your upper eyelid. These tears spring into action when you get something in your eyes as well.

Some of this overflow ends up in your tear ducts, the pinpoint-size holes located in the inside corners of your lower and upper eyelids. Rather than produce tears, tear ducts act as the drainage ducts through which the tears get washed into your nasal passages. That's right—when you blow your nose after a good cry, you're actually sending a spray of tears into your tissue.

Dry Times

You're not likely to pay much attention to everyday tear activity until the wells go dry. When your eyes are dry, however, they feel scratchy or irritated, or they burn. About 90 percent of dry eye cases are caused by a condition called keratoconjunctivitis sicca (KCS), which is just an elaborate name for what happens when you have a deficiency in tear production.

Although researchers don't know why, the change in the balance of hormones during pregnancy or menstruation can change women's tears. Menopausal or postmenopausal women are most often affected by KCS. "The tear film may be related to hormonal status," says Mary Gilbert Lawrence, M.D., ophthalmologist at Yale University School of Medicine and instructor of ophthalmology at the Manhattan Eye, Ear and Throat Hospital. "Many of my women patients find that during pregnancy they can't wear their contact lenses or that they need to use more lubricating drops in order to be more comfortable. In fact, many women say that their eyes feel dry at certain times of the month."

If you have dry eyes, and hormonal changes aren't the culprit, maybe you can blame medications. A few of the drugs that have this effect are the antihistamines, tricyclic antidepressants and other medications as well, so check with your doctor or pharmacist.

What, if anything, can you do about dry eyes? Here are some tear tips.

Steam up the air. Using a humidifier set at about 80 percent humidity helps moisturize the air, says Thomas Gossel, R.Ph., Ph.D., professor of pharmacology and toxicology and dean of the College of Pharmacy at Ohio Northern University in Ada. If your humidifier does not mark off percentages, set it at the maximum steaming level. Since the cornea is always exposed to the air, you're putting moisture on the cornea when you add moisture to the air, he notes.

Drop in. Over-the-counter artificial tears are the best remedy for dry eyes, says W. Steven Pray, R.Ph., Ph.D., professor of nonprescription drug products at Southwestern Oklahoma State University College of Pharmacy in Weatherford. Follow the manufacturer's directions when you're using the drops. Usually, that means two or three drops in each eye. It's not harmful to use more, but not helpful either, he notes. The excess will just run out of the eye.

Keep some drops out. Avoid any eye care products that constrict the eye's blood vessels, advises Dr. Pray. These drops only aggravate dry eyes.

Drip the drops correctly. The best way to apply eyedrops is to pull your lower eyelid down, says Dr. Pray. Then tilt back your head until you're looking up at the ceiling and drop in the artificial tears without touching your eye or eyelid with the applicator.

When you flood your eye with drops, the drops will run down your tear ducts and go down into your nose, so you end up swallowing them. To avoid that, after you put in the drops, place your thumb and forefinger in the corners of your eyes, tilt back your head and squeeze gently for about five minutes. Try to hold this position for the full five minutes, adds Dr. Pray. The drops will be less effective if you give them less time.

See also Eyes

Teeth

OVER THE CENTURIES, wars have been fought, kingdoms won and lives sacrificed for the sake of the Crown. But without any fanfare at all, most of us tote 32 crowns all our lives.

Every healthy tooth has a crown of gleaming enamel, the body's hardest substance. Underneath that enamel hard hat, and sheltered by it, is living pulp. Nerves and capillaries (tiny blood vessels) fill the pulp and descend into the parts of the teeth that we don't see—the roots and the root canals that tap into tooth sockets all around the upper and lower jaw.

Over the moats and canals of this multi-crowned kingdom, there falls a perpetual rain of that destructive marauder known as plaque. This is the fine, sticky film of bacteria, mucus and food particles that coats our teeth and makes them feel fuzzy to the touch of our tongues a few hours after brushing. It may be difficult to see the plaque that attacks both teeth and gums, but our entire crown kingdom sure feels the fallout.

The Plaque Attack

If we don't brush and floss the fuzz off, the plaque traps even more bacteria. And bacteria love the sugars in our food.

The marriage of bacteria and food breeds acid, which can eat through the enamel of our teeth and burrow through the layer of hard tooth that lies underneath, called dentin. And if that acid gets through the dentin, it will pummel the pulp. Then we get cavities. When the bacteria inflame the pulp, the result is a toothache. If bacteria eat away too much of the tooth, we can even lose it.

We can avoid all that, though, just by brushing and flossing our teeth and gums to clean out the food and bacteria. Dental disease may be our most widespread health problem, but it's probably the most preventable, too.

"Any dental disease is almost an optional disease. You can choose to have it, or not, by brushing and flossing or not brushing and flossing," says Richard H. Price, D.M.D., clinical instructor of dentistry at Boston University Henry Goldman School of Dentistry.

Your Basic Tooth Tool

Aristotle took a twig from a tree to use for a toothbrush. Not a bad approach for a fourth-century dental student—but better was yet to come. Around 1850, someone invented the first brush specifically intended for teeth, which had a wooden handle and boar bristles.

Toothbrushes have come a long way since the twig and the boar were pressed into service. Walk into any drugstore and scan the variety of toothbrushes. Not only do they come in every color but they also come in every shape. Here are some twentieth-century dentists' guidelines to help make sense of your choices.

Floss Right

Flossing and toothbrushing are inseparable buddies. Unless you floss daily, you're just asking for gum trouble—eventually. "There's no way around it—you have to do it," says Barry G. Dale, D.M.D., a cosmetic and general dentist in Englewood, New Jersey, and assistant clinical professor of dentistry at the Mount Sinai Medical Center Department of Dentistry in New York City. Here's how to give your pearlies a careful floss.

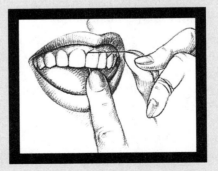

2. Using your thumbs and forefingers, slide about an inch of taut floss between your teeth. Curve the floss in a C shape around the tooth at the gum line.

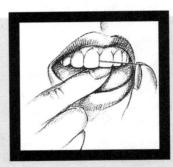

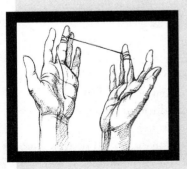

1. Break off about 18 inches of floss and wind most of it around one middle finger. Wind the rest around the middle finger of your other hand.

3. Gently slide the floss up and down between the tooth and gum, making sure that you go beneath the gum line. Repeat on the rest of your teeth with clean sections of floss.

Give 'Em the Brush-off

It's easy to get sloppy about toothbrushing. When we're doing it daily, we're on automatic pilot. But it's never too late to brush up on proper technique, says Jeffrey M. Shubach, D.M.D., a family dentist in private practice in Voorhees, New Jersey. Here's how to get the biggest payoff from your toothbrush time.

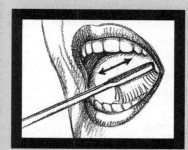

3. Brush the chewing surfaces of your teeth.

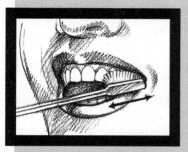

1. To clean the outside of your teeth, aim the brush at a 45-degree angle to the gum line. Use a back-and-forth motion and gently work the brush in short strokes.

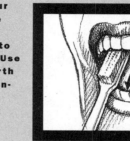

4. Clean the inside of your front teeth by holding the brush perpendicular to them. Brush from the gum to the biting edge—up on your lower teeth, down on your upper teeth.

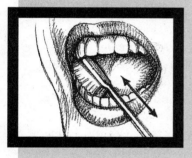

2. Then repeat on the inside of your teeth, using the same technique.

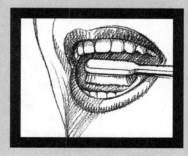

5. Many dentists believe that you should brush your tongue, because it can harbor bacteria and encourage bad breath.

Look for the seal. Narrow your search by looking for the American Dental Association (ADA) seal of acceptance on the toothbrush package. "The ADA seal means that studies have been done and submitted to the ADA panel. The manufacturer has to prove that the product does what it says it does—and that it's safe," says Barry G. Dale, D.M.D., a cosmetic and general dentist in Englewood, New Jersey, and assistant clinical professor of dentistry at the Mount Sinai Medical Center

Department of Dentistry in New York City.

Be a softy. After you have checked for the ADA seal, look for the words "soft bristles." Hard bristles can wear down your enamel and shove your gums away from your teeth—especially if you're the type who tends to brush too hard.

Get a grip. Check how it feels when you hold the brush. When you get it home and try it out, "make sure that the toothbrush feels comfortable in your hand," says Dr. Price. If it doesn't feel friendly, you won't be able to manipulate it easily around your mouth. Try out different brands, shapes and sizes until you find one that fits the bill.

Toss it out. A toothbrush only performs well for three to four months, at most. You can see when a toothbrush goes bad—the bristles around the edge start veering off to the side. "After that, throw it away," says Dr. Price.

Set an egg timer. Speed is fine for roller coasters, but whiz-brushing your teeth will eventually send you speeding to the dentist. "The average person spends only 51 seconds brushing," says Dr. Price. The time you should spend? About three minutes.

To slow down your brush rate, take a three-minute egg timer into the bathroom and leave it there. "Just brush your teeth until the sand runs out," he suggests.

Empower your brushing. Every time the dental hygienist cleans your teeth and looks at your gums, does she show you yet again the right way to brush and floss? Maybe you need some assistance from the power brushes in the tooth department.

"Electric toothbrushes give good results," says Dr. Price. In a study of 70 healthy adults at the University of Alabama School of Dentistry in Birmingham, researchers compared the effectiveness of electric toothbrushes with manual brushing. Using an electric toothbrush, they found, significantly reduced the incidence of swollen gums. (The less your gums swell, the better your brushing technique.)

"One advantage that electric toothbrushes have is that people cannot rush them. They require a little bit of time. The brush heads are smaller, so people spend more time brushing their teeth," says Dr. Price. Does that mean you should automatically switch to power? That's probably not necessary if you're a patient brusher. "You can do a fine job with a toothbrush if you do it right."

Using Fluoride to Cement 'Em

Fluoride isn't just a kid thing. "Adults with a high cavity index need fluoride, too," says Jeffrey M. Shubach, D.M.D., a family dentist in private practice in Voorhees, New Jersey. "It helps kids and adults whose home care and diets aren't up to par. In addition, it strengthens teeth to fight root cavities, which we get when we're older and our gums recede."

Receding gums expose the roots of our teeth, which are covered, not with hard enamel, but with a sensitive sheath called cementum.

Fluoride, a compound made from the chemical element fluorine, is so effective at preventing tooth decay that more than half of America's communities now add it to their water supply. Most toothpastes contain fluoride, as do some mouthwashes.

"Fluoride works by making cellular changes in the tooth," says David F. Halpern, D.M.D., a dentist in Columbia, Maryland, and a spokes-dentist for the Academy of General Dentistry and the state of Maryland. "This can happen, because the teeth can lose and gain valuable minerals. Fluoride can help replace what's lost. It restores minerals to the teeth, and it can heal tiny cavities."

Here's how to find out if your water supply has fluoride—and how to make this compound work for you.

Ring the water department. To find out if your community has fluoridated water, call your local water authority or public health department. Either department can tell you what levels are in your town supply. If you are getting it in your tap water, the fluoride level should be in the range of 0.7 to 1.2 parts per million parts of water.

If your community doesn't have fluoridated water, make extra sure that your toothpaste and mouthwash both list fluoride on their labels. Even if your water supply is fluoridated, getting an additional dose from other sources is a benefit for your teeth.

If your teeth are already showing the effects of fluoride deprivation, your dentist might prescribe a fluoride toothpaste such as PreviDent gel. The dental hygienist may treat your teeth with a fluoride gel or with varnish twice a year.

Rub it in. If you are age 35 or older, your dentist may have told you that your gums have started to recede, exposing the roots of your teeth. You can protect the exposed roots by rubbing in fluoridated toothpaste.

"The soft cementum covering tooth roots has a myriad of tiny tubules containing nerve fibers. That makes the roots very sensitive, too. But if you rub an ADA-approved toothpaste for sensitive teeth into the gum line, it will reach into those little tubules," says Dr. Price. Fluoride at the gum line works two ways: It helps prevent root cavities and decreases the natural sensitivity of the exposed root.

Dodging Cavities

For some people every tooth is a cavity just waiting to happen. But it doesn't have to be that way. Here are four wise ways to foil the black holes.

Grasp at straws. Sugar isn't the only enemy of enamel. The citric acid in juices and sodas can soften and erode the enamel of your pearly whites. Citrus-flavored soda, grapefruit juice and apple juice are serious offenders.

But juices are titans of nutrition, so you probably don't want to give them up. Instead, sip your citrus drink through a straw. "That way you don't bathe your teeth in acid or sugar. The juice goes directly to the back of your throat," says Dr. Halpern.

Swish some water. Let's get real: You can't always brush your teeth after you eat. If you're at a working lunch, chained to your desk or enjoying a picnic, toothbrushing is the last thing on your postlunch mind. At least do the next best thing: Swish some water around in your mouth.

"The water helps flush food and debris away from your teeth. It dilutes some of the bacterial activity," says Dr. Halpern. Later on, when you have access to a bathroom, pull out your toothbrush and toothpaste and complete the cleaning job.

Chew sugarless gum. A dentist recommending gum? That's like a doctor recommending smoking, isn't it? Well, not really—if the gum is sugarless.

Dr. Halpern recommends chewing sugarless gum after you eat, when you can't brush right away. "It mixes up the bacteria and dilutes them, making them less concentrated before they have a chance to organize. Once they get organized in one place, they can do a lot of damage."

Schedule your sweets. "The decay clock starts the moment that sugar enters your mouth, and it continues for about 20 minutes after your mouth is cleaned by saliva," says Dr. Dale. This means that it's not only important to watch what you eat or drink, but also how often you do it.

In terms of decay, it's far worse to eat one tiny Life Savers every 20 minutes all day long than a slab of chocolate cake once a day, Dr. Dale says. The Life Savers regimen would drape the teeth in a constant veil of

How Lipstick Tints Teeth

How are your teeth like chameleons, those little lizards that change colors to match their surroundings? "Lipstick color can affect how the color of your teeth looks," says Barry G. Dale, D.M.D., a cosmetic and general dentist in Englewood, New Jersey, and assistant clinical professor of dentistry at the Mount Sinai Medical Center Department of Dentistry in New York City.

"Any lipstick that has yellow or gold in it will make your teeth look more yellow," he says. "The violet range works much better. And, while you'd think that anything dark would make your teeth look whiter by contrast, that isn't so. Really dark red lipstick makes your teeth look darker."

If you're concerned about yellowing teeth, avoid the gold-tinged coral and mocha shades lined up at the pharmacy or department store. Instead, zero in on the pinks and light plums—the violet range. And forget savage-red Bette Davis lips.

sugar—bacterial food. In comparison, it's possible for sticky chocolate cake to be eaten and cleared from the mouth in less than an hour.

Saving Your Ivories

Sugars, starches and acids aren't the only bullies on the tooth block. Normal life is demanding and sometimes dangerous, too, says Dr. Price. "Every time we bite, we generate 40,000 to 50,000 pounds of pressure per square inch," he says.

Pressure like that, your munchers don't need. Here are two things that you can do to help guard your teeth.

Don't chomp ice. Chewing ice is one of the worst things we can do to innocent teeth, says Dr. Price. "People used to get blenders and ice crushers for shower gifts. Those machines are specially designed to crush ice—that's how hard ice is. We shouldn't be mashing ice with our molars. In fact, I had a patient who broke a tooth eating ice cubes."

If you tend to finish not only iced drinks but also the ice cubes in them, resist the temptation. Instead of crushing big chunks of ice with your teeth, go for the smaller slivers—and let them melt in your mouth like candy.

Guard your mouth. "Chew with your mouth closed," Mom used to say. But she didn't say to do that in your sleep—did she?

If your teeth gnash away when you sleep, it could be caused by stress. That's one of the major reasons for bruxism, the medical name for tooth grinding, says Dr. Shubach.

Short-term stress doesn't usually pose a problem. We adjust to new jobs, new houses or new babies, and we stop grinding our teeth before we hurt them.

But sometimes stress is prolonged—we nurse an aged parent, we start medical school, the baby is Dennis the Menace. "We take it out on our teeth," says Dr. Shubach. Long-term grinding can irritate the tooth nerve or wear the enamel away.

If your spouse says, "You've been grinding again, dear," it's time to talk to your dentist about it. She may prescribe a mouth guard, which is made out of hard acrylic plastic from a mold of your teeth. The mouth guard acts as a protective reminder to discourage grinding as you sleep.

"They can be cumbersome and awkward initially. But people generally get used to them," says Dr. Shubach.

The Kayoed Tooth

Maybe you've taken up in-line skating and spilled yourself onto a curb. Or the front doorknob got you in the kisser when you tripped on the top step. Suddenly, there's a throbbing in your jaw and something that looks like a kernel of corn in the palm of your hand. Amazingly enough, you may be able to save that lost front tooth and restore it if you stay calm and act fast.

"Do not let the tooth dry out," says Martin Trope, D.M.D., chairman of the Department of Endodontics at the University of North Carolina School of Dentistry at Chapel Hill. "You can put it back in the socket and hold it there until you get to a dentist, which should be as soon as possible. Or you can put it in a suitable storage liquid."

Milk is one suitable liquid, because it's relatively free of bacteria. The best liquid, however, is a nutrient-rich over-the-counter solution available in drugstores, called Save-A-Tooth. "It should be in every first-aid kit," says Dr. Trope. "Then, if you get to a dentist quickly, the tooth can be reimplanted."

Getting Back Your Tooth Youth

Yes, there is such a thing as age reversal. Making your teeth look younger can be done in just a few visits to the dentist. When you see the results, you might find yourself with a whole new image—especially when you smile in the mirror and a younger you smiles back.

The trick is all in the color. As we age, our teeth tend to darken. All the brushing in the world won't lighten them significantly, especially if you've been taking proper care of your teeth. But there is a procedure that can restore your pearlies almost to their state of original perfection. It's called whitening—and many who have had the procedure say that it does wonders for self-esteem.

If you're feeling older than your years because of yellowing, darkening or discolored teeth, you might want to check out a whiter

A Bracing Experience

Whoever thought that the old metal-mouth look of our childhoods would turn out to be fashionable when we grew up?

"Braces are 'in,' " says Barbara J. Steinberg, D.D.S., professor of dental medicine at the Medical College of Pennsylvania in Philadelphia. "The baby boomers are aging; they want nice smiles."

It's not just vanity, either. Crooked or crowded teeth can cause malocclusion—a bad bite that could stress the teeth and break down their supporting structure. Crowded teeth are also hard to keep clean enough to deter cavities and gum disease.

Metal braces are still the best kind, although they're smaller now. Invisible braces—with acrylic used on the front of the teeth and metal on the back—sometimes interfere with biting and chewing, and they're almost twice as expensive as metal braces. Tooth-colored ceramic braces look nice, but the ceramic material is more brittle and breakable than metal.

Braces work by gradually pushing your teeth into place. The bone beneath them adapts by breaking down on one side, allowing the teeth to move, and building up on the other side to hold them in place. The usual course of treatment time is about two years.

future. It's a two- to three-week process, and, though you need your dentist's supervision, you can do it at home.

The bleaching process begins with a visit to the dentist's office. She makes a mold of your teeth—usually just the upper teeth, since they're the most visible. Then the dental lab makes a clear, soft plastic tray from the mold. It fits over your teeth and looks like a little mouth guard.

At home you use a syringe to squirt a small bit of bleaching gel (carbamide peroxide, which breaks down into hydrogen peroxide) onto each tooth you want to lighten. Then you fit the tray over your teeth and wear it for the prescribed amount per day. "You can hardly see it. I wore mine while I was treating patients," says Dr. Price.

"It used to taste kind of bleachy. But it comes flavored now, although there's almost no taste," says Stephen Sylvan, D.M.D., associate professor of dentistry at State University of New York at Stony Brook.

Bleaching your teeth at home can cost from $150 to $600 or more. It's not permanent—you'll probably need a touch-up treatment two or three times a year. Some people may get side effects—gum irritation or tooth sensitivity—that clear up when they stop using the bleach. "But patients love it," says Dr. Sylvan. "Everybody wants whiter teeth."

Dentists warn to stay away from the tooth-whitening kits sold in drugstores or through TV ads. "They may dissolve away some of the tooth structure," says George Freedman, D.D.S., director of postgraduate programs in esthetic dentistry at Baylor College of Dentistry in Dallas and the State University of New York at Buffalo. "The kits can do major damage if they are used improperly or for too long."

See also Gums, Jaw, Tongue

Throat

YOU SWALLOW EVERY 15 SECONDS or so, whether you realize it or not. It's a reflex action: Unless you're doing something fun like eating, you aren't even aware that your throat is in action.

The throat is a muscular tube lined with mucous membrane that connects the back of the mouth and the nose to the esophagus, the tube that carries food from the throat to the stomach. Providing a passageway for both food and air, the throat is something that we can't live without.

One thing that we can live without, though, is a sore throat. That's when we become painfully aware of how often we swallow.

Colds and Strep

Some sore throats are caused by swallowing hostile substances, like a fish bone that scratches the throat's lining. But more often your throat gets red and inflamed because you have a virus—usually, the rhinovirus, which is responsible for the common cold, says Frederick Godley, M.D., otolaryngologist with the Harvard Community Health Plan of New England in Providence, Rhode Island.

Another culprit is the *beta-streptococcus* bacteria, better known as strep throat.

In children, strep can sometimes lead to rheumatic fever, a serious inflammatory disease that can affect the joints and heart, according to Michael S. Benninger, M.D., chairman of the Department of Otolaryngology at Henry Ford Hospital in Detroit and

Morning Soreness

Suppose you wake up every morning with a mild sore throat that usually goes away about the time you're having your glass of milk. The cause of this morning sore throat could be a little trickle of acid from your stomach, which backs up into your esophagus and into the larynx, says Michael Benninger, M.D., chairman of the Department of Otolaryngology at Henry Ford Hospital in Detroit and author of <u>Vocal Arts Medicine</u>. "It makes you wake up with a mild sore throat or a sense of a lump in your throat."

If this is your problem, Dr. Benninger advises that you don't eat just before bedtime. Also, avoid alcohol and caffeine and eat smaller meals during the day. For some people, taking an antacid like Rolaids, Mylanta or Tums can help ease the fire in their bellies before it can become painful burning in their throats.

Another possible cause of morning sore throat could be your in-house environment. Particularly in the winter, the air in your bedroom might rival the Sahara Desert, says Dr. Benninger. If that's the case, use a humidifier at night. Set the control at about 30 to 40 percent humidity.

author of *Vocal Arts Medicine*. But Dr. Benninger says that he has never seen rheumatic fever result from strep throat in an adult.

Unfortunately, you can't distinguish a sore throat from strep throat on your own. Both produce similar symptoms—redness, soreness and swelling and even bad breath. If you come down with a sore throat that lasts more than two days, visit your doctor for a throat culture to test for strep. If it is strep, you can take a course of antibiotics to get rid of it.

Smoother Soothers

If it's sore throat of the common variety, here's what you can do to soothe the soreness.

Go gargle. Mix a quart of warm or cold water with a tablespoon of salt and gargle, says George Simpson, M.D., professor and chairman of the Department of Otolaryngology at State University of New York at Buffalo. When you gargle, it's like cleaning out a dirty wound, so it could promote healing.

Squeeze a lemon. This sour citrus fruit helps stimulate saliva production, which is the natural moisturizer of the throat, says Dr. Benninger. "Have herbal tea with lemon. Both the tea and the lemon work to coat and soothe the throat. Or even a sugarless lemon drop would be good."

Try real tea. Dr. Simpson recommends regular tea as a throat helper. It is effective because it has a combination of caffeine, which is a mild stimulant, and tannic acid, which has a soothing effect.

Warm it up. "Applying a hot-water bottle or a towel soaked in hot water to the front of the neck would be effective," says Dr. Benninger.

Suck a lozenge. Medicated lozenges like Cepacol have a numbing effect, says Dr. Simpson. They also work by stimulating saliva flow, which eases throat pain.

See also Respiratory System, Tonsils

Thyroid

██ THE SKINNY KID GORDIE TELLS THE STORY about a fat kid who seeks revenge against his tormentors by provoking the "ultimate barf-a-rama" at his town's pie eating contest.

That's when the subject of the thyroid gland comes up.

"He was fat. Reeeeeal fat," says Gordie, trying to create a picture for his three fireside pals.

"Yeah," replies Vern with a sneer, "my cousin is like that. They say it's 'cause of his kyroid gland."

Vern got more than the word wrong. The notion that the thyroid gland is responsible for someone's being overweight is a common misconception, says Martin Surks, M.D., director of the Division of Endocrinology at the Montefiore Medical Center in New York City and author of *The Thyroid Book*. "Big-time obesity is rarely from the thyroid."

Your Regulator

The butterfly-shaped gland located at the base of your neck does play a role in your body's metabolism, says Dr. Surks. "It regulates how your body uses fuel."

Your body "burns" food much the way a car burns gas, and the thyroid basically regulates how your "motor" is set. The gland does this by releasing thyroid hormones: With the right amount of hormones, your body burns fuel at the proper rate. Those hormones help get other systems working properly, too—including heart rate, body temperature and menstrual cycles.

High Gear

When the gland produces too much hormone—a condition called hyperthyroidism—it's as if the gas peddle to your motor were pressed to the floor, says Dr. Surks. Your motor—including your metabolism—gets revved up, and you are basically thrown into overdrive.

A woman who has hyperthyroidism may have a rapid heartbeat, increased body heat and perspiration, nervousness, weight loss or

How to Slow That Baby Down

If you have a hyperthyroid condition—an overactive thyroid—there are a number of treatment options.

Pills. You'll need to take thyroid pills consistently and be monitored regularly by your doctor, says Martin Surks, M.D., director of the Division of Endocrinology at the Montefiore Medical Center in New York City and author of The Thyroid Book. Drug reactions to these pills are rare.

Radioactive iodine. Capsules containing radioactive iodine destroy part of the thyroid gland. The treatment always works, is safe and usually requires only a one-time treatment, says Dr. Surks. Radioactive iodine has been used for 50 years, and it's safety has been shown over and over again. Radioactive iodine is safe to use before pregnancies but never during pregnancy, he says.

Surgery. Surgery, though once a common treatment, is really inappropriate in this day and age, says Dr. Surks. So if it is the only option that your doctor offers, that should be a red flag. The one scenario where surgery may be the only option is if you are allergic to thyroid drugs.

a decrease in her menstrual flow and muscle weakness, among other things, says Kay McFarland, M.D., professor of medicine at the University of South Carolina School of Medicine in Columbia.

Just as revving the engine on your car isn't good for it, living with a hyperactive thyroid isn't good for your body. So it's important to see your doctor about treatment options.

Low Gear

When the thyroid gland is underactive and produces too little hormone—called hypothyroidism—everything is in low gear, says Dr. Surks. That's why people with hypothyroidism tend to experience fatigue, constipation, weight gain, chilliness and mental sluggishness. Other symptoms can include dry skin, coarse hair, hearing loss and puffiness.

A Gland Plan

Women get thyroid disease—leading to hyper- or hypothyroidism—ten times more often than men do. Though doctors say that there is not much that you can do to prevent thyroid disease, it's important to recognize it and get it treated. Here's what they recommend.

Know the symptoms. If you experience a rapid heart rate, increased nervousness or changes in your menstrual cycle or if you lose weight without really dieting, these may be signs of hyperthyroidism, so you should see your doctor, Dr. Surks says. By contrast, if you experience sluggishness, weight gain, fatigue and an increasing intolerance to cold, that could be hypothyroidism. You need to get that checked and treated, too.

Keep track of history. Thyroid disease can be inherited, experts say. So if you have a

Get a Boost from Hormone Pills

Doctors treat hypothyroidism—the condition in which your thyroid produces too little hormone—by replacing the lacking hormones with thyroid hormone pills that you take once a day for the rest of your life, says Martin Surks, M.D., director of the Division of Endocrinology at the Montefiore Medical Center in New York City and author of The Thyroid Book. While there are natural forms of thyroid hormone, most doctors advocate using a synthetic form. Often it takes a while to get the dose of thyroid hormone adjusted, so you'll need to be patient and not expect results overnight. Also, different drugs can affect your thyroid hormone medication, so notify your doctor about any other medications that you are taking.

family history of it, tell your doctor.

Take the test. Your doctor can detect thyroid disease by doing a blood test that measures your thyroid hormone levels, says Dr. McFarland.

Be sure to tell your doctor if you are currently taking oral contraceptives, though, because you would need a different kind of blood test, says Dr. Surks.

See an expert. When it comes to treating thyroid disease, the doctor's experience is really important, says Dr. Surks. For detection and treatment of thyroid disease, you want a doctor who is board certified in endocrinology, diabetes and metabolism from the American Board of Internal Medicine. Don't hesitate to get a second opinion, either.

See also Endocrine System

Toenails

THEY MAY LOOK PRETTY IN POLISH and sexy in sandals. But basically, toenails are vestigial claws left over from our simian ancestors, says Rodney S. W. Basler, M.D., assistant professor of internal medicine (dermatology) at the University of Nebraska Medical Center in Omaha. Although the big toenail may provide some strength, "toenails have practically no value," he observes.

Toenails grow more slowly than molasses pours. In fact, it takes the same time for a toenail to grow out as it does to have a baby: nine months. Unlike childbirth, however, toenails hardly ever hurt.

That is, unless you have an ingrown nail. This can happen when you jam your feet into

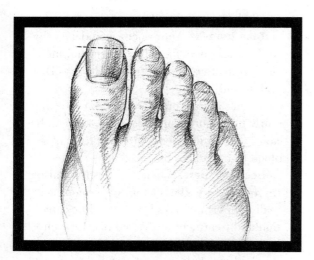

A good trim will help you prevent an ingrown toenail. Soak your foot in warm water for up to ten minutes, then clip your nail straight across, as shown. Leave at least one-sixteenth of an inch of white in the center of the nail. Finish by filing the edges of the nail to remove any rough ends.

tight shoes (or stockings) or give them bad clip jobs (which leave the edges of the nail ragged or curved). When the edges of the nail detour into the flesh, you can expect either a prickle or a blast of pain.

Women get ingrown toenails more often than men. Twice as many women as men over age 65 have ingrown toenails, because of years spent in high-heeled, pointed shoes, says S. W. Balkin, D.P.M., attending assistant professor of podiatry, podiatry section, in the Department of Orthopedics at Los Angeles County–University of Southern California Medical Center.

Another common toenail problem is fungus. Fungus spores abound in the world we live in, and the greedy little species called *Trichophyton mentagrophytes* feasts on the protein that makes up our toenails, called keratin. To a fungus spore, keratin is manna. Those microscopic plant forms eat it like junk food.

Toe fungus is painless, but it's also unsightly. The organism that turns nails yellowish and thick affects about 5 percent of the population, according Paul Kechijian, M.D., associate clinical professor of dermatology and chief of the nail section at New York University Medical Center in New York City. It's a glitch in the immune system, he says. "Some people just don't fight it off well."

"So far, there is really no way to kill the fungus organism," says Dr. Basler.

There are two things you can do that might help prevent fungus growth, however.

Dust your shoes. Antifungal powder, such as Tinactin, dries sweaty shoes and helps poison fungus spores. Get a container at the drugstore and shake a little into each pair of your shoes. When you get ready to wear a pair, tap out the powder, wear them, then sprinkle more powder in them before you put them away. (You can dust the inside of your

Give Your Nail a Lift

To coax an ingrown toenail into growing out properly, here's a method recommended by Rodney S. W. Basler, M.D., assistant professor of internal medicine (dermatology) at the University of Nebraska Medical Center in Omaha.

First, soak your foot for ten minutes in a basin of warm water to soften the nail. Then, with a rounded toothpick, carefully lift the softened edge of the ingrown nail as much as you can tolerate. Slip a small piece of gauze or cotton under the ingrown nail. That will encourage it to grow out and over the cotton instead of down into the flesh of your toe. Change the cotton daily until your toe heals. (If you see any pus or redness, call your doctor.)

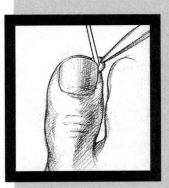

To give first-aid to an ingrown toenail, you'll need tweezers, a rounded toothpick and a small piece of gauze. Insert the gauze under the nail as shown.

socks with antifungal powder before you wear them, too.)

Dry your toes. Fungus thrives in dark, moist places, like the spaces between your toes, so keep your feet dry. One clever way to do this is to blow-dry your toes after each shower or bath with a hair dryer set on cool.

See also Feet

Tongue

DID YOU EVER SEE AUDREY, the lodge owner's daughter, on the TV series *Twin Peaks?* If so, you'll never forget the way she could tie a cherry stem with her tongue.

Equal talent: Someone who can touch her nose with the tip of her tongue.

The rest of us, though, just do run-of-the-mill things with our talented tongues: talk, taste, chew, swallow, give Bronx cheers.

"All our basic instinctual drives relate to the mouth," says Gerald Shklar, D.D.S., professor of oral pathology at Harvard School of Dental Medicine. A baby explores her little universe with her tongue, suckling milk at her mother's breast, then going on to suck her thumb. "In adults, the tongue plays an important role in erotic stimulation," he says.

Tongue Tasks

The secret of the tongue's talent lies in its muscle. In fact, the tongue is mostly a mass of muscles covered by mucous membrane. That musculature means that we can make it longer, thicker, shorter and thinner. And when the dentist tells you to relax your tongue, it can curl up on the floor of your mouth and rest like a dog.

All over the surface of the tongue are skinny, hairlike stubs of tissue called gustatory papillae. They're part of the mechanism commonly known as taste buds. At the tip of the tongue are the papillae cells that are shaped like cones. These cells give the front two-thirds of the tongue its whitish cast.

(continued on page 414)

A Matter of Taste

Two friends are having lunch in the Happy Hacienda. Allison orders a diet soda. Brenda says "Ick" to that and opts for a lightly flavored seltzer water.

When they order entrées, Allison chooses the Four-Alarm Devil's Tongue Chili. Brenda orders the No-Alarm Angel's Breath version. "What a food wimp!" laughs Allison.

"Well, hot things hurt my tongue," Brenda replies reasonably.

Two different women, two different food tastes. Brenda is a supertaster. That's a researcher's term for someone who has more than the average allotment of 10,000 taste buds. Armed with extra buds, a supertaster tastes foods almost twice as intensely as the average person.

Allison, is probably at the opposite end of the tasting spectrum. Scientists would call her a nontaster. She not only likes the jalapeño kick that pains her buddy but also needs it to feel as if she's having food that really tastes like something.

Of course, these are extremes—and many of us are somewhere in the midrange of the taste spectrum, where medium-hot chili seems completely satisfying.

Taste buds are the receptor cells on your tongue that get excited by food molecules. Your cheeks, soft palate and throat contain a few taste buds, too. But mostly, they're clustered in little heaps on your tongue around the tiny, hairlike, projecting papillae cells.

The receptors that are located on the tip and on the forepart of the tongue start jangling at the first tingle of sweet and salty flavors. Receptors along the sides of the tongue pucker up at signals of sourness. And if you've ever winced at the taste of bitter fruit, it's because the receptors on the back of your tongue pick up the sensations of bitterness.

Sweet, sour, salty and bitter are the four basic tastes that are familiar to many of us.

Taste experts also include a fifth, called unami, which is a different kind of bitter still considered a basic taste, according to Alan Hirsch, M.D., psychiatrist, neurologist and neurological director of the Smell and Taste Treatment and Research Foundation in Chicago. (Japanese horseradish has the taste of unami.) But it's not just your tongue that picks up these tastes; your nose gets in the picture, too.

All in Good Taste

True, Allison and Brenda have different numbers of taste buds. But research shows that all those tongue-tied buds behave the same, no matter whose mouth they're in.

Smart Tongue

"Taste is the true nutritionally wise sense," says Linda Bartoshuk, Ph.D., taste psychophysicist at Yale University School of Medicine.

In order to study the phenomenon of

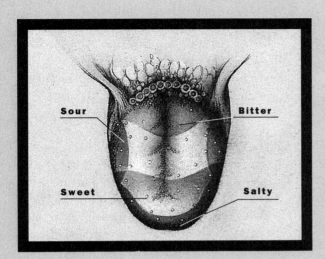

Different parts of your tongue are particularly sensitive to the basic tastes, as shown here.

how people register tastes, Dr. Bartoshuk has studied groups of supertasters, regular tasters and nontasters—including men, women and children in all three groups. Her findings show that women are better tasters than men: In fact, about three-quarters of those identified as super-tasters were women.

It's not such a blessing to be a super-taster, Dr. Bartoshuk says. "It narrows your food world considerably. You might not eat foods that are quite healthy, like vegetables, because they taste bitter to you." If you know someone who hates the taste of coffee, it could be that her super-taste sense responds overwhelmingly to its basic bitter taste—and the rich aroma isn't enough to counteract that basic aversion.

Getting More Yum on Your Tongue

Even if you can't improve your taste buds, you can enhance the taste of your food. Here are some pointers offered by experts.

• To get the most flavor out of your en-trée, take a bite and then chew it slowly and thoroughly, says Dr. Hirsch. Slow chewing heats up food molecules and re-leases the most flavor compounds. "The first bite of food always tastes best. After that, your taste buds adapt." If you alter-nate courses, chew thoroughly and clear your palate between dishes, however, you can avoid adaptation and get maximum pleasure out of your food.

• Chew your chocolate; don't suck on it until it melts on your tongue. With chewing you'll get the most flavor out of those warmed-up, chocolaty molecules.

• The best time of day to really taste is morning, according to Dr. Hirsch. Being hungry helps a lot in terms of tasting.

• Eat artichokes last. Artichokes have a sweet-tasting chemical that makes changes in your taste sensations, according to Dr. Hirsch. The aftermath of these changes—what Dr. Hirsch calls the artichoke effect—lasts about 15 minutes. After eating artichokes, everything you eat for the next 15 minutes is likely to taste sweet.

• Your breakfast orange juice will taste better if you brush your teeth after you drink it, according to Dr. Hirsch. The other way around will make your OJ decidedly bitter.

Underlying that, and accounting for the tongue's main coral-red shade, is a rich network of blood vessels.

Except when you get the occasional canker sore, the tongue is generally a contented—if muscle-bound—body part. Nothing much goes wrong with it, and we rarely give it a thought.

"A normal, healthy tongue is very resistant to infection," says Dr. Shklar. That's because it is bathed in saliva. "Saliva contains enzymes to fight bacteria. It also contains the immune substance IgA—immunoglobulin A," he says, which boosts our immunity to disease.

The tongue needs that battalion of fighters, since each surface cell on it is home to about 100 bacteria.

Does It Need a Brush-Off?

All those bacterial hordes have fueled a debate over tongue brushing among dental experts. Dr. Shklar and others think that saliva does a fine job of cleaning the tongue without any further assistance from your toothbrush. But other experts include tongue brushing as part of daily home dental care.

Some companies are even marketing tongue scrapers, devices to help you clean your tongue, says Richard H. Price, D.M.D., clinical instructor of dentistry at Boston University Henry Goldman School of Dentistry. In the physician-heal-thyself department, he adds, "I scrape my tongue right down to the last supper."

Whether or not you choose to brush and scrape your tongue, there are other things that you can do to help keep it wagging well.

How to Read Your Tongue

Usually, minding the tongue is no problem. It's just there, doing what it does. On occa-

sion, though, the tongue can turn white or black or green or red, depending on what bacteria or food it is responding to.

Also, there may be changes in the size of the papillae that sprinkle the surface of the tongue. They've been known to grow as much as twenty times their usual size—springing from 1 or 2 millimeters to a height of 20 millimeters, which is about three-quarters of an inch.

Generally, these changes are less alarming than they look. Even the ailment that sounds like it belongs to a werewolf—black hairy tongue—isn't a big deal, says Dr. Shklar. The tongue doesn't actually get hairy, but the papillae turn an interesting shade of charcoal. "It comes from a fungus or a particular pigment-producing bacteria that moves in after antibiotics kill off many of the mouth bacteria that repress it," he says. It goes away by itself, however.

Fungus isn't the only thing that can turn your tongue a darker hue. In rare cases certain foods with dark dyes such as licorice or other dark candy can also stain the tongue. Even chewing tobacco can cause staining. Here are some other tongue conditions that might not sound so familiar.

Geographic tongue. Your tongue literally looks like a map, with bald red patches mingled with healthy-looking regions. And the boundaries keep shifting; one patch returns to normal and another goes bald.

The bald, red areas are actually places where the papillae have disappeared. In these areas the tongue is noticeably more sensitive, according to Dr. Shklar. It's not serious. It just sits around for a while, and then it goes away."

Glossitis. When you have this condition, your whole tongue is inflamed, and it looks smooth and red all over.

"Streptococcal bacteria might be the problem in unusual cases," says Dr. Price, "or irritation from an injury or habit such as biting or rubbing the tongue." This tongue inflammation can also be caused by a vitamin B or iron deficiency. Once the cause is discovered, glossitis can be easily treated and cured.

Fissured tongue. If you're among the 10 percent of men and women who have extra deep grooves or pits in your tongue, you have a completely harmless condition called fissured tongue. There is only one potential complication: Food debris can build up in the grooves, which can then become stained with tea or coffee. So it can become unsightly.

It's a simple cleanup job, though. Here is Dr. Shklar's recipe: "Mix one part hydrogen peroxide (you can get it at the drugstore) with two parts water. Rinse out your mouth well with it. The rinse gets down into the grooves and fizzles and kills whatever bacteria is in them. It doesn't taste great—but it works."

Cancer-Conscious

More than 30,000 people get mouth cancer every year. The tongue is a common site, especially along the sides.

"Oral cancer used to be quite rare in women," says Dr. Shklar. "But then they started drinking alcohol and smoking as frequently as men do. Smoking and drinking alcoholic beverages are the main causes of oral cancer." Tongue cancer looks like a lump or a bump on the tongue. "It can be a raised tumorlike thing or an ulcer—an open sore—that doesn't heal."

A trip to the doctor's office can quickly tell the story. The rule of thumb is that if a sore on your tongue doesn't go away in two weeks, you should see your doctor.

See also Mouth, Teeth

Tonsils

■ **AS A KID, YOU PROBABLY ASSOCIATED** tonsils with a cool, creamy dessert that you could never get enough of.

After all, it seemed as though every child on the block had her tonsils taken out, and the war stories were always the same: "It was great! I got to eat all the ice cream I wanted for a whole week!" You practically envied them their diseased tonsils.

Now that you're an adult, however, any kind of surgery—even a minor one like a tonsillectomy—sounds about as appealing as ketchup on a rocky road sundae.

Like you, the medical profession has gradually changed its mind about tonsillectomies, says Frederick Godley, M.D., otolaryngologist with the Harvard Community Health Plan of New England in Providence, Rhode Island.

Over the past few decades doctors have come to the conclusion that removing tonsils surgically could result in bleeding and other complications and isn't always the answer for recurring sore throats. "In the 1950s and 1960s a lot of tonsillectomies were performed. It was almost a rite of passage for a child," says Dr. Godley. "Now we're much more selective."

New Tonsil Policies

These days, doctors remove tonsils for more specific reasons: tonsils that are chronically seriously inflamed or unusually enlarged, Dr. Godley notes. In addition, a doctor will consider removing the tonsils if they have an infection that might spread to other areas of the throat—or if enlarged tonsils are interfering with breathing.

So what good are the little troublemakers, anyway? The almond-size structures curve inward like slim half-moons on either side of the back of the throat. They're a small part of the lymphatic system, a complex network of specialized cells and supporting tissue that plays a major part in defending the body against infection. Though doctors and researchers still have not pinpointed the exact role of the tonsils within this lymphatic system, they do know that tonsils become expendable as we reach adulthood, according to Dr. Godley. "Because there are so many lymphatic tissues in the throat besides the tonsils,

we have come to learn that children and adults can safely live without them."

Shaped for Trouble

It's the tonsils' shape that causes trouble, notes Dr. Godley. "Their anatomy allows bacteria to hide in the folds of the surface of the tonsil, so that you either get infections easily or harbor bacteria there."

The result is tonsillitis, an ailment in which the tonsils swell and the throat gets red and sore. The symptoms of this condition are virtually the same as those for strep throat, which is caused by a bacteria called *Beta-streptococcus*, notes Dr. Godley.

Like strep throat, tonsillitis hits mainly

When to Bid Tonsils Good-Bye

Even among doctors, opinions are divided as to the effectiveness of removing tonsils.

The decision to perform surgery depends on what kind of sore throats the patient has been getting, according to Michael Benninger, M.D., chairman of the Department of Otolaryngology at Henry Ford Hospital in Detroit and author of <u>Vocal Arts Medicine</u>. "If the tonsils are the focus of bacterial infection, removing them will dramatically decrease the incidence of sore throats.

"But if you get a sore throat every time you get a cold or flu, it usually won't make any difference if you have your tonsils taken out," he notes. That's because the common cold and flu are viral and tend to affect other tissues in the throat, not just the tonsils.

"There's a small group of people who

benefit from a tonsillectomy," says Frederick Godley, M.D., otolaryngologist with the Harvard Community Health Plan of New England in Providence, Rhode Island.

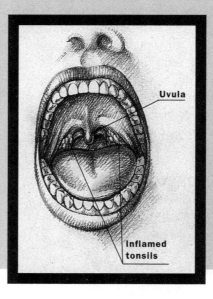

Uvula

Inflamed tonsils

In this tonsillitis sufferer, the inflamed tonsils are swollen to a point where the airway is partially obstructed.

young people. "Tonsillitis is 20 times more likely to occur in a child than in an adult," says Michael Benninger, M.D., chairman of the Department of Otolaryngology at Henry Ford Hospital in Detroit and author of *Vocal Arts Medicine*. "Tonsils start to shrink as the child ages, and at puberty they shrink substantially." Less than 10 percent of all tonsillectomies are performed on adults.

How do you know if your tonsils need the heave-ho? Here's a general guideline from Dr. Godley. If you've had six episodes of strep within one year, four episodes within each of two years or three a year for three years in a row, you're a candidate for tonsillectomy. It is always important to see your doctor, however, and have a throat culture taken to diagnose strep throat, which can be treated with antibiotics. Often chronic sore throats are caused by viruses, in which case removing your tonsils will not stop the infection.

See also Lymphatic System, Respiratory System, Throat

Underarms

THEY SWEAT. THEY SMELL. They're hard to shave. It's no wonder we call them The Pits.

We're talking underarms here. And let's face it: They're just downright high-maintenance, at least for American women. In our overly sanitized, hairless-is-sexy society, underarms require a lot of attention.

Day in and day out, you wash them, dry them, dust them and crust them with the deodorant or antiperspirant of your choice. And somewhere in there, you manage to flick your Bic razor, all in the name of staying dry, sweet-smelling and smooth.

Not that it has to be that way. In Europe women sport hairy underarms all the time, and it's no big deal. Washing is done with less frequency and body odor is less of a big deal. Here in the States, however, that fashion just hasn't quite caught on.

Quelling the Smell

Armpits have glands that produce sweat, but they also have other glands that produce a milky kind of secretion that mixes with bacteria to cause body odor. If you're enjoying the great outdoors, it doesn't matter how much you sweat—the bears and bees are quite happy with how you smell. Indoors, of course, it's a different matter. To keep your pits dry and sweet-smelling, here are some recommendations from Richard L. Dobson, M.D., professor of dermatology at the Medical University of South Carolina in Charleston.

Pick the right product. If your main objective is to discourage moisture, look for an antiperspirant. Antiperspirants contain aluminum chlorhydrate or aluminum zirconium complexes. These substances prevent sweating by clogging the superficial pores, says Dr. Dobson. They can help fight odor, too, since smell-producing bacteria can't thrive on dry skin. If you buy a deodorant, on the other hand, it will fight off odor by killing bacteria, but it won't prevent you from sweating.

Cool your pits. If you work out during the day, make sure that you take 10 to 15 minutes to cool down after your workout before putting on a deodorant, says Dr. Dobson.

Stay smooth. Underarm hair gives bacteria a place to hang out. So keeping your underarms shaved is one way to stay fresh, Dr. Dobson says.

Shaving for a Sweaty Day

If you're used to shaving under your arms, you're probably used to underarm rash. There are ways to avoid it, however. Here's what Dr. Dobson recommends.

Go for a night shave. Every time a woman shaves her underarms, she removes some of the outer protective layer of skin. If deodorants or antiperspirants are applied right away, that can be irritating. So allow a little bit of recovery time, says Dr. Dobson. If you're shaving under your arms, do so at night, and then wait until morning to apply your underarm product.

Make sure it's moist. When you shave, use water along with shaving cream or a mild soap. That gives the hair a chance to soften, says Dr. Dobson.

See also Skin

Urinary System

The urinary system arranges your body's garbage disposal, flushing out waste through the medium of urine, which it produces and excretes. To take care of processing, the kidneys filter foreign matter out of the blood, and ureters transport urine from the kidneys to the bladder. The bladder keeps the urine in temporary storage until you are ready to pass it along via the canal called the urethra.

■ The **bladder** is a muscle-walled balloon that collects and releases approximately two to three pints of urine a day. Unluckily, it is close to the bacteria-rich vagina and anus, so it is ripe for recurrent infections, called cystitis. (For ways to prevent these common infections, see "A Better Bladder" on page 27.)

■ The **urethra** is the pipe that carries urine from the bladder out of the body. A woman's urethra is shorter than a man's—only 1½ inches long—and because infection doesn't have as far to travel, women are more likely to get urinary tract infections (UTIs). (To sidestep those pesky UTIs, see "Bladder" on page 26.)

■ The two **kidneys** filter floating waste from the body's blood supply about 40 times a day. This is the site where you may develop kidney stones—crystals of salt and minerals that can become pea-size or larger. But there are ways you can reduce your risk of getting them. (For more information and some prevention tips, see "Pebble Passing" on page 190.)

■ The **urine** produced by the urinary system can reveal a lot about your health.

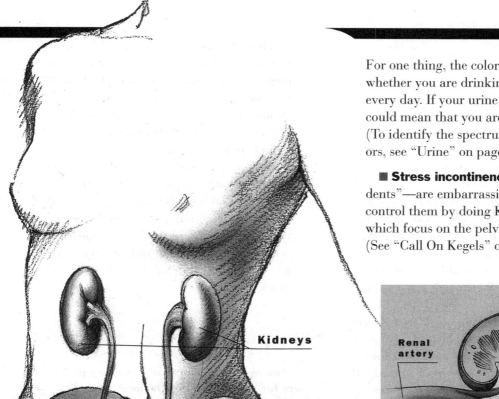

Kidneys

Pelvis

Ureters

Bladder

Urethra

For one thing, the color of urine shows whether you are drinking enough water every day. If your urine is dark yellow, it could mean that you are dehydrated. (To identify the spectrum of urinary colors, see "Urine" on page 420.)

■ **Stress incontinence**—little "accidents"—are embarrassing. But you can control them by doing Kegel exercises, which focus on the pelvic floor muscles. (See "Call On Kegels" on page 420.)

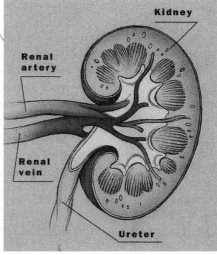

Kidney

Renal artery

Renal vein

Ureter

The renal artery brings blood from the heart to the kidneys. A rich bed of tiny arteries—capillaries—filters that blood. As blood runs through the capillaries, waste products get separated out, then flushed out in your urine. The cleaned-up blood flows out of the kidneys through the renal vein and back to the heart.

Where to Look

To find out how to keep your urinary system working well and how to avoid infections, see:

Bladder   page 26
Kidneys   page 190

Urine

PASSING WATER, it's sometimes called. That euphemism is about right, since urine is actually 96 percent water.

But that yellow fluid is also made up, in part, of substances that your blood and body don't need. It's filled with clues about how your body is working. So your urine can reveal a lot about your health, as well as whether you're getting enough water each day, says Alice Stollenwerk Petrulis, M.D., director of clinical nephrology at Metrohealth Medical Center and associate professor of medicine and reproductive biology at Case Western Reserve University in Cleveland. "If you're drinking enough fluids, your urine should be clear. If it looks yellow in the morning, that's just because you probably haven't urinated all night long, and it's more concentrated." Consistently dark yellow urine means that you're dehydrated and aren't getting enough liquids.

Here are what a few other colors could mean.

• Cloudy yellow: This could be normal, or it could indicate the presence of pus, blood or fat droplets. If you're on a strict vegetarian diet, your urine may often be this color.

• Smoky with a grayish cast: This indicates remnants of old red blood cells or yeasts.

• Red: This might be blood, which could indicate a kidney infection, bladder infection or bladder or kidney cancer. Eating beets, as well as taking Ex-Lax, can make your urine reddish as well.

• Dark brown: Cola-colored urine could indicate liver disease or hepatitis.

There are also a few smells to be aware of. If your urine has the odor of dead fish, that means that the ammonia level is high, and you could have a bladder infection. This strong odor can also signify vaginitis. In either case, you should check with your doctor to find out what is causing it.

If there is a peculiar smell that is not like ammonia, think about what you had at your last meal. If you recall having asparagus, that pungent odor is from leftover oxalates—a type of chemical that results from the breakdown of certain acids in your system. Don't give it a second thought: The odor will quickly disappear.

Call On Kegels

The most common kind of urinary problem for women in their thirties and forties is stress incontinence, which may result from pelvic muscles being weakened by childbirth or excess weight. You might be able to avoid stress incontinence, however, by strengthening the muscles involved in urination.

The best known method is Kegel exercises, in which you tighten and relax the muscles of the pelvic floor, says Mark Zilkoski, M.D., family practice physician at Trinity Hospital and Listerud Health Clinic in Wolf Point, Montana. While you're urinating, stop your urine midstream for five seconds; repeat five times. Try this a few times to get the feel of where these muscles are. Then do the Kegel exercises when you're not urinating until, with practice, you can do 20 to 30 repetitions three or four times a day.

See also Bladder, Kidneys, Urinary System

Uterus

IT EXPANDS. IT CONTRACTS. And part of it rebuilds itself every month.

No, it's not the economy.

We're talking about a body part that's located above the knees and below the breasts and—hint, hint—guys don't have one.

It's the part that yields the monthly menstrual blood and lower abdominal cramps that can send women (or their partners) to the round-the-clock-convenience store at midnight in search of tampons and Midol.

It's also the part that makes women groan in pain during childbirth and moan in ecstasy during lovemaking.

Unfortunately, this part of the body can develop benign growths, bleeding problems, infections and cancer.

Yes, all these things, and more, the uterus can do. The more you know about how it works and what the problems are, the better you will be able to make the decisions that affect the health of your uterus.

An Ever-Changing Organ

The uterus is an incredibly dynamic organ, says Alvin F. Goldfarb, M.D., professor of obstetrics and gynecology at Jefferson Medical College of Thomas Jefferson University in Philadelphia. It changes each month as a woman's body goes through the different phases of her menstrual cycle.

But there's more. The uterus is also capable of the amazing transformations that occur during pregnancy.

Before a woman has her first baby, the total size of the uterus is about the equivalent of a small clenched fist. Located above the vagina, behind the bladder and in front of the rectum, the organ consists of a whirl of overlapping muscular tissue. These are the muscles that contract during a woman's menstrual cycle and when she has an orgasm. When a woman is in labor, these muscles help deliver the baby.

Within this muscular wall is an internal clear area called the endometrial cavity. Before a woman ever has a child, this cavity is less than an inch wide and an inch in length. It is lined with specialized material called endometrial cells. These cells are replaced daily under the influence of the hormones that the ovaries produce.

Branching off from the top of the uterus are the fallopian tubes. The ovaries are also attached to the uterus with ligaments that help hold them in place. The lower portion of the uterus narrows to form the cervical canal and cervix, which extend down into the vagina.

Major Expansion

Stimulated by the sex hormones estrogen and progesterone, the uterine lining of a reproductive-age woman builds up and prepares itself for a potential pregnancy.

If the traveling egg doesn't get fertilized, there is a sharp plunge in the production of hormones. The uterine lining stops proliferating and sheds. It is the shedding process that creates menstrual blood.

If pregnancy does occur, the fertilized egg implants itself in the uterine lining and starts to grow. The muscular walls of the uterus stretch and enlarge, much the way a balloon expands when inflated with air. That one-inch cavity in the uterus expands until it can hold a six- to ten-pound baby.

Then, during childbirth, the muscular

walls of the uterus expand and contract. This motion is what propels the fetus out of the uterus, through the cervix and vagina and into the outside world.

Fibroids: The Common Problem

As early as their mid-thirties or forties, women may get fibroids, says J. Victor Reyniak, M.D., director of reproductive surgery at Mount Sinai Medical Center in New York City. Fibroids are the most common type of benign tumor.

While some fibroids, particularly the ones that grow into the uterine cavity, cause bleeding and discomfort, others produce no symp-

Fibroids may develop in many areas in and around the uterus—sometimes obstructing the fallopian tube, projecting into the uterine cavity or even protruding through the cervix.

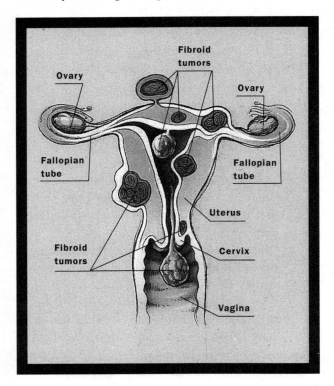

toms at all, according to Dr. Reyniak. The symptomless ones don't have to be removed. But if the fibroids produce bleeding, pain and pressure—and have grown to the size of a grapefruit—they should be taken out.

Researchers don't fully understand what causes fibroids. But "there is a genetic predisposition," says Dr. Reyniak. So if your mother has fibroids, there is a strong likelihood that you may develop them, too.

Reading the Bleeding

While fibroids are one possible cause of heavy bleeding, there could be some other uterus-related problem. If you are in your thirties or forties and have heavy bleeding, your doctor should check you for an ectopic pregnancy or miscarriage as well as fibroids, says Dr. Reyniak.

What about the other extreme—very light bleeding or none at all?

Lack of bleeding could be caused by anovulation, or the failure to ovulate, according to Dr. Goldfarb. Anovulation might result from some kind of imbalance in your endocrine system. Other causes could be a big change in weight or even heavy-duty stress. (Lack of bleeding might not be related to the uterus, however: Some women stop bleeding because of polycystic ovarian syndrome, a condition in which multiple cysts form inside the ovaries.) Whenever your bleeding is unusually heavy or light, consult your doctor.

The Chance of Cancer

The very word *cancer* is scary—there is no denying it—and many women worry about the chances of uterine or endometrial cancer. These are the cancers that occur either in some part of the uterus or in the endometrium, the uterine lining. There are several different types of cancer that can appear in this area, according to William Hoskins, M.D., chief of the gynecology service at the Memorial Sloan Kettering Cancer Center in New York City.

Doctors refer to one type as epithelial tumors. This kind of cancer starts to grow in a part of the uterine lining called the epithelial layer, which includes the endometrium. While this type of cancer makes up 95 percent of the cancers that develop in the uterus, says Dr. Hoskins, it is not frequently seen in women ages 30 to 45. Instead, it is more common in women over 50 years of age.

The second type of cancer that can develop in the uterus is uterine sarcoma. This cancer can arise from either the lining of the uterus or from the muscular wall, Dr. Hoskins says. It represents only about 5 percent of all uterine cancers, but it is more likely to show up again after it has been removed. Fifty percent of certain types of uterine sarcomas will recur, and that's higher than the recurrence rate for epithelial tumors. So the chance of surviving a sarcoma is lower than the chance of surviving an epithelial tumor.

The Estrogen Factor

Because the sex hormone estrogen has a great influence over cell production within the endometrium, the hormone can play a big role in cancer that affects the cells of the uterine lining. In the past, when estrogen replacement therapy was recommended for many postmenopausal women, they would receive unopposed estrogen. But researchers learned that when only estrogen is given, a woman's chance of endometrial cancer would increase seven- to eightfold over what her risk would be if she took no hormone replacement therapy or if she took estrogen with progesterone, says Dr. Hoskins.

Why does progesterone help balance the equation, reducing the risk of cancer?

Lining Out

Normally, the uterine lining begins building up each month prior to ovulation. Following ovulation, progesterone is released, helping prepare the lining to receive the egg. If an egg doesn't arrive, the progesterone will help shed the lining. Without progesterone the endometrial lining hangs around longer—and because it doesn't shed properly, the risk for cancer is greater.

Today, hormone replacement therapy (HRT) will normally include progesterone as well as estrogen, unless a woman has had her uterus removed during a hysterectomy. Yet there are other factors as well that can increase your risk of endometrial cancer. Women who have been diagnosed with a condition called polycystic ovarian syndrome are at greater risk, because their bodies release estrogen but do not produce progesterone. Obese women are also at greater risk, because when a woman has a lot of fat cells, she is more likely to produce excess estrogen.

Since abnormal vaginal bleeding is one symptom of uterine cancer, it is yet another reason to check with your doctor if your bleeding is unusual. Other symptoms include lower abdominal pain and lower back pain.

If you do have endometrial cancer, many doctors will recommend a hysterectomy. That's because the disease can spread to other areas of the body unless the uterus is removed. Not all hysterectomy procedures are the same, however. Doctors recommend that women be aware of and explore their different options before they decide what to do.

Hysterectomy— And Other Options

The exams are done, and the tests are in. You're sitting in your doctor's office listening to the verdict. Suddenly, there's one word that jumps out from all the rest.

Hysterectomy. It zaps you like an electric shock. Your doctor's words become a blur as she continues talking. Something about success rates. Then she's asking you what you want to do.

What do you do?

First off, try not to panic.

Hysterectomies are common, with an estimated 600,000 performed each year. In fact, they are the second most common type of surgery performed in the United States. (Cesarean section is first.)

The question is, why is the major surgery performed so often? Some women advocates and members of the health profession have claimed that hysterectomies are sometimes performed unnecessarily, and some doctors agree.

Is This the Way to Go?

It's important to keep in mind that just because your doctor has recommended a hysterectomy doesn't mean that you necessarily have to have one.

Before you make up your mind, you might want to consider the alternative methods for treating a host of gynecological problems, including fibroids, abnormal bleeding and chronic pelvic pain. "There are many medical and minor surgical alternatives to hysterectomy that should be considered prior to making your final decision," says Jack M. Lomano, M.D., director and president of the South Florida Woman's Center in Fort Myers, Florida.

Start by asking your doctor if there are any medications that can help alleviate your problem, says J. Victor Reyniak, M.D., director of reproductive surgery at Mount Sinai Medical Center in New York City. For example, certain drugs called GnRH agonists are used to treat a host of gynecological problems. GnRH stands for gonadotropin-releasing hormone. These medications can be used to treat large fibroids. They work by depriving fibroids of the estrogen that feeds them—and when estrogen is lacking, the fibroids shrink.

The GnRH medications can also be used to help stem abnormal bleeding and relieve the pain and discomfort of endometriosis and other chronic pelvic pain problems, says Dr. Reyniak. And if you're having painful periods or severe bleeding, be sure to ask your doctor about nonsteroidal anti-inflammatories such as Motrin and Advil, he suggests. Or you might be helped by oral contraceptives or hormone replacement therapy.

You can also ask your doctor if there is another surgical option that will help your condition. For instance, large fibroids that cause pain and pressure can be treated with myomectomy, a procedure in which the fibroid alone is removed and the uterus is left in place.

Protecting the Womb

With so much going on—and so many chances for problems—your uterus deserves first-class service. Here's how to make sure that you are doing all you can to keep it healthy and free of problems.

Get checked. To safeguard the health of

Before the Cut Is Made

Suppose you decide to have a hysterectomy, having concluded that it's really your best option. There is more than one kind of procedure—and some hysterectomies are more extensive than others. Here are three different types to consider before you make a final decision.

<u>Total hysterectomy with bilateral salpingo-oophorectomy.</u> This is the most extensive. The surgeon removes the uterus, the cervix, both ovaries and both fallopian tubes.

After this type of hysterectomy, you can no longer bear children. And because you won't ovulate, you won't produce ovarian hormones. For a woman of reproductive age, the result is early menopause—what doctors refer to as surgical menopause.

<u>Total, or complete, hysterectomy.</u> The doctor removes the uterus and cervix but leaves the fallopian tubes and ovaries in place. After this procedure you will not have menstrual periods or be able to bear children, since the uterus is removed. You will ovulate, however, if you are still in your reproductive years.

Your ovaries will still produce hormones that influence your health—estrogen, which affects the functions of your bones and heart, and androgen, which influences your sex drive.

<u>Supracervical hysterectomy.</u> The ovaries and fallopian tubes are left in place, but the uterus is removed. Most of the cervix, the lower portion of the uterus, stays in place.

Doctors have a reason for removing part of the cervix but leaving the rest in, according to Dr. Reyniak. The part of the cervix that is removed, called the transformation zone, is the area where cancerous cells can develop. By leaving the rest of the cervix in, the doctor ensures that a woman can still have sexual sensation in that area.

In addition to different kinds of hysterectomy, there are also a number of more moderate surgical approaches. They include:

<u>Abdominal hysterectomy.</u> The uterus is removed through an incision in the abdomen. This type of surgery is usually necessary when the uterus is too large to be removed through the vagina, says Dr. Reyniak.

<u>Vaginal hysterectomy.</u> The uterus is removed through an incision in the vagina. This leaves no scars, since all the stitches are made internally, says Dr. Reyniak.

<u>Laparoscopic-assisted vaginal hysterectomy (LAVH).</u> An instrument called a laparoscope is inserted through four to five small incisions in the abdomen. Through this instrument the physician cuts the ligaments that attach the uterus to the abdominal cavity. This releases the uterus, which is then removed through the vagina.

LAVH is a relatively new technique. "Some doctors may be more experienced with it than others," says Dr. Lomano. Before you have LAVH, ask your doctor how many of these surgeries that she has performed; twenty or more indicates a good level of experience.

her uterus, a woman should plan on having an annual exam, says Dr. Goldfarb. During a pelvic exam your doctor may be able to detect any unusual growths or masses in your uterus.

Watch for signals. "Above all, know your body," says Dr. Goldfarb. That way, if anything changes, you can consult your doctor. Any signs of unusual bleeding or pain are cause for concern, and you should let your doctor know about them.

Also, if you start missing periods and know you are not pregnant, talk to your doctor, says Dr. Goldfarb. Your ovaries may not be releasing eggs because of polycystic ovarian syndrome. Because this problem of not ovulating may increase your risk for the development of endometrial cancer, it's important to ask your doctor about the different medications that can induce ovulation. (If you're not ovulating because you are taking the Pill, you don't have to worry: In fact, the Pill actually protects against the development of the disease, he says.)

Of course, another possibility could be that you're starting menopause, which some women can experience as early as their mid-thirties.

Find the right doctor. Take the time to find a doctor you like, says Dr. Goldfarb. If you can't communicate with your physician, find one you can talk with openly. One way to begin the search is to ask your friends about gynecologists that they have been to and like.

Many hospitals also have physician referral services. By calling a special telephone number, you can find out what doctors are available at a particular hospital and hear comments from other patients who have seen them.

Consider the Pill. "The single most important thing that a woman can do to protect against ovarian and uterine cancer is to take birth control pills," says Dr. Hoskins. In addition to decreasing the risk of endometrial cancer, taking the Pill for five years or more will decrease the risk of ovarian cancer by 50 percent.

Watch your weight. By eating a low-fat diet and exercising, women can help prevent endometrial cancer, says Dr. Hoskins. That's because obesity is such a risk factor.

Be informed about HRT. If you've gone through menopause and you're currently getting HRT, you should find out what your HRT regimen includes or ask your doctor to explain it. If you've had a hysterectomy, then you're eligible to receive unopposed estrogen. For anyone else, however, the therapy should include progesterone as well as estrogen in order to avoid raising your risk of endometrial cancer.

Call on the experts. If you are diagnosed with cancer, see a gynecological oncologist, says Dr. Hoskins. Gynecological oncologists are the doctors who, through years of training, specialize in treating cancers of the reproductive tract. You can call the Society of Gynecological Oncologists at 1-800-444-4441 for a listing of gynecological oncologists in your area.

See also Pregnancy, Reproductive System

Vagina

WHEN IT COMES TO HUMAN REPRODUCTION, the vagina certainly has a great track record. It's where sperm first enter a woman's body to begin working their way through the cervical canal and into the uterus to hook up with an egg and produce life. It's also the route that most of us took into the Great Wide Open, pushing through a canal that during labor and childbirth had expanded to many times its size to accommodate a safe trip.

The vagina is a place for endings as well. In nonpregnant women, menstrual blood passes through the cervix and vagina, washing away all of the wasted cells that have built up in the lining of the uterus in false anticipation of conception.

For all of its importance, however, the vagina is a rather unassuming body part: a three-inch-long canal, lined with mucous membrane, that runs from the vulva up to the cervix, which is the neck of the uterus.

The adult vagina usually slopes upward and backward and has muscle and fibrous tissue forming its walls. When it's relaxed, the vagina is about one-half to three-quarters inch around, with the walls touching. Luckily for us, the size isn't steadfast. During pregnancy, changes take place that allow the vagina to do an impressive feat of expansion during labor and childbirth.

The Discomfort Zone

Television commercials euphemistically call it feminine itching. You've come to know it as the nagging, burning feeling that you sometimes get in one of your body's hardest-to-reach spots.

Its official name is vaginitis, and most women are intimately familiar with it. About half of the visits to gynecologists are prompted by this disorder, which is characterized by abnormal vaginal discharge, pain, itching and irritation. If you have vaginitis, intercourse may become painful and you may feel pain when you urinated.

The working definition of *normal secretions* is partly related to your menstrual cycle. Secretions turn thick and sticky just before and at the end of your period. As a woman's estrogen level drops after menopause, vaginal cells decrease in size, and the amount of normal vaginal secretion goes down.

In other words, the amount of secretion or discharge varies. "Everyone is different," notes Patti Jayne Ross, M.D., associate professor of obstetrics and gynecology at the University of Texas Medical School at Houston. "Go by whatever applies to you. Any amount of discharge is normal if it's what you're used to."

The Beast Infection

When it comes to pure set-your-teeth-on-edge itching, nothing quite compares with the intensity of a form of vaginitis known as a yeast infection. The vagina is a fertile breeding ground for yeast, says Eva Arkin, M.D., chief of gynecology at Scottish Rite Hospital in Atlanta. "The vagina is the perfect incubator. It's warm, dark, moist and rich in sugars," she notes.

Candida, a fungus in the yeast family, can be found in the mouth, rectum and vagina. In the vagina, candida starts growing out of control when the balance of normally occurring organisms—the vaginal flora—is somehow

How Dry I Am

It's the female equivalent of impotence. You're in bed with your partner, he's kissing and caressing you all over, and your vaginal area is as dry as year-old bread. He often feels like a failure. And you might, too.

But rather than indicating lack of arousal, vaginal dryness may be a physical disorder, says Patti Jayne Ross, M.D., associate professor of obstetrics and gynecology at the University of Texas Medical School at Houston. "It can happen before menopause, but it's usually associated with menopause and a decrease in estrogen," she notes. "The skin in the genital area gets thinner, red, irritated and tender."

Treatment is simple: See your doctor about starting hormone replacement therapy. Either estrogen or progestin, or a combination of both, is given orally, says Dr. Ross.

Short of hormone replacement therapy, there are still several things you can do if vaginal dryness puts a damper on your sex life. Here are some tips from top docs.

Pass the jelly. Using an over-the-counter lubricant is a quick and easy way to solve dryness, notes Dr. Ross. K-Y jelly is popular, but that brand can actually cause drying and irritation, she warns. Instead, she recommends a lubricant called Astroglide because it's more like an oil. "I've recommended baby oil to patients," she says. "But beware if you're using a condom." The problem is that baby oil is petroleum-based and can damage the latex in a condom, making it ineffective.

E's into it. Vitamin E is another good lubricant, says Eva Arkin, M.D., chief of gynecology at Scottish Rite Hospital in Atlanta. "I tell some people who have dryness on the labia to make a pinhole in a vitamin E capsule and apply it to the labial skin. That works well," she says.

Check out your pills. Birth control pills can create hormonal changes that affect vaginal secretions, notes Dr. Arkin. "Talk to your physician about possibly raising the estrogen level in your pills," she suggests.

Don't smoke. Smoking destroys estrogen, which in turn could make the vaginal area less healthy and moist, says Ellen Yankauskas, M.D., director of the Women's Center for Family Health in Atascadero, California. "You would find nicotine in a Pap test if you checked for it. That's how deeply it can penetrate," she says.

---

disturbed. "Yeast grows because of an upset in bacteria within the vagina and because of a change in vaginal pH," says Dr. Arkin. Often the use of antibiotics or birth control pills starts a mini-epidemic of candida. Yeast is transmitted mainly sexually and sometimes by sharing moist towels.

The distinct symptoms of candida vaginitis go beyond itching. There is a white, curdy discharge that resembles cottage cheese, along with a yeasty odor and redness in the vagina, the vulva and sometimes even the anus.

From Yeast to Rest

If you think you have a yeast infection, your doctor can diagnose you by examining a wet smear of your vaginal discharge for yeast-like organisms. A fast, simple treatment is the prescription drug fluconazole (Diflucan), given in pill form. In addition, here are strategies that some doctors recommend.

Scoop some plain yogurt. Eating a container of yogurt a day helps control vaginal yeast, notes Ellen Yankauskas, M.D., director of the Women's Center for Family Health in Atascadero, California. Yogurt has cultured bacteria that help control the yeast and keep it in line, she says. "It's a truce, or a balance. They keep the bad bacteria in control, so they don't flare up," she explains. Yogurt that contains the necessary *Lactobacillus acidophilus* bacteria will say "active cultures" on the label. But if yogurt isn't your cup of tea, you can also get acidophilus pills: Two a day will do the same thing as a cup of yogurt.

Cream that itch. An over-the-counter cream is a sure cure for most yeast infections, notes Dr. Yankauskas. Relief used to be available only by prescription. Now you can get over-the-counter brands such as FemCare and Gyne-Lotrimin, which contain clotrimazole, and Monistat 7, with miconazole.

"I usually tell people to use the cream until the symptoms stop, then use it one more day for good measure," says Dr. Yankauskas. "A yeast infection usually takes three to five days to get rid of."

Sack the sugar. Sugary foods help make your body a hospitable place for yeast, notes Dr. Arkin. "There are people with chronic yeast infections who break the cycle with very stringent no-sugar diets," she says. But if you don't want to do that, you can try to just cut down on carbohydrates, including pastas breads and high-sugar products.

Check out the spermicide. One common culprit behind yeast infections is the lubricant in condoms, notes Dr. Yankauskas. "Some lubricants contain nonoxynol 9, the spermicide that kills the AIDS virus, and some women are sensitive to these chemicals," she notes. If

your partner is using condoms with spermicide, Dr. Yankauskas recommends that you stick to whatever product your body tolerates.

Watch the Pill. Another candida-raiser could be the birth control pill, which works by raising your body hormone level and can alter vaginal secretions, says Dr. Yankauskas. "That just might trigger a yeast infection," she suggests.

C how good it is. Vitamin C helps make your vagina less appealing to yeast, notes Dr. Arkin, because it contains ascorbic acid, which acidifies the vaginal walls. She recommends taking 500 milligrams twice a day.

Don't douche. Overdouching is a major cause of yeast infections, notes Dr. Arkin. "It destroys the normal flora within the vagina, not to mention that all of the bacteria grow back 20 minutes afterward," she says.

Dr. Yankauskas says douching is never necessary. Women who douche have higher rates of pelvic infection, because douching pushes the germs deeper inside, she notes.

Stay dry. Don't make a habit of staying in a wet bathing suit or sweaty exercise clothing, notes Dr. Ross. "Change out of wet clothes," she says. "A moist environment promotes the growth of yeast."

Wear cotton panties. Wearing cotton panties provides much-needed absorption in the vaginal area, says Dr. Yankauskas. Cotton gives you a bit more air down there, helping to cut down on the accumulation of wetness that happens with nylon underwear.

Bathe it away. Another way to make your vagina more acidic and less friendly toward bacteria is by taking a boric acid bath, notes Dr. Arkin. Put two tablespoons of boric acid (which is available in powder form in most pharmacies) in a tub full of warm water and soak. If you have sensitive skin, a boric acid bath may be irritating, warns Dr. Arkin.

Is It Itis or Osis?

Pesky yeast infections can be the most maddening form of vaginitis. But another irritation that causes a bevy of discomforts is a bacterial infection called vaginosis. This is characterized by a thin, watery, grayish white discharge. With vaginosis, you may have intense burning, occasional redness of the vagina and vulva and a fishy odor. Oral antibiotics as well as prescription vaginal creams and gels are good treatments.

Just what causes vaginosis is debatable, says Dr. Arkin. "The bacteria may normally be found in small quantities in the vagina, and at opportune times, they grow," she says.

Another theory is that the bacteria are sexually transmitted, notes Dr. Arkin. The more partners you have, the greater your chances .

If you've had vaginosis and you want to protect yourself from getting it again, have your partner wear a condom to stop re-infection, suggests Dr. Arkin.

When Making Love Makes You Uptight

The lights are dim. Your favorite mood music is on the stereo. The satin sheets are glistening in the candelight. He's wearing nothing but a smile.

It sounds like an ideal setting for most women. But for those dealing with the daily trauma of vaginismus, a love nest can quickly turn into a hornet's nest of doubts and fears.

Vaginismus is the involuntary spasm of the muscles surrounding the vaginal opening, which causes the vagina to contract so tightly that intercourse is impossible.

"It's a psychological problem largely among women who are fearful of sexual activity," notes Barbara Levinson, R.N., Ph.D., a licensed marriage and family therapist and owner of the Center for Healthy Sexuality in Houston. "They have problems not with sexual arousal but with the actual act itself."

Often vaginismus may be the result of fear, especially if a stern moral upbringing or a sexual trauma early in life has made a woman afraid of the sex act. This reluc-

tance can affect her subconsciously, resulting in the tightening of the vagina, says Dr. Levinson.

The most important solution to vaginismus is to try to get to the root of any psychological problem with the help of counseling. Then you can start working on the mechanics of the problem.

Dr. Levinson recommends the following exercise: Start by inserting just two fingers into your vagina, calming yourself and taking deep breaths as you do so. Use lubrication if necessary. If you prefer, have your partner do it, inserting his fingers gently and slowly. Once you're comfortable with that, you can use dilators, which are tube-shaped devices sized from one-half inch in diameter to the size of a penis.

If this kind of manual stimulation doesn't make you nervous or afraid, you can advance to having your partner insert his penis and then move on to gentle intercourse, says Dr. Levinson. "Something like this can really be reversed with care and understanding," she notes.

Veins

IT'S BETTER THAN ROUTE 66. The circulatory system is your very own trans-body highway: 60,000 miles of arteries, veins and capillaries that handle five quarts of blood every minute of the day.

While your arteries take care of the outgoing traffic, your veins route it back to your heart. Way out at the edge of the system are the one-cell-wide capillaries. These are where the transfer of goods—oxygen and nutrients—from blood to tissues takes place.

The capillaries merge into venules, which converge on the veins, which wend their way through the body's town dumps, such as the kidneys and liver. There the waste is left behind, before the blood makes its way back through your veins to your heart.

The toughest part of this journey is up your legs. Given a chance to relax, your veins would stop fighting gravity and just let their load of blood pool at your feet. But the muscles in your legs help nudge the blood up the Matterhorn of your calves and thighs. And your arteries help, too. Running deeper than veins but parallel to them, the arteries pulse steadily, enhancing the work of your leg muscles.

Luckily, your veins are also equipped with one-way valves that act as roadblocks. As soon as the blood goes through, these valves momentarily slam shut to prevent any backsliding.

Pressure to Perform

Despite the long return trip that the blood has to make, the pressure in the veins still is much lower than that in the arteries. If you're unfortunate enough to slice open a vein, it won't spurt blood the way an artery would. In fact, most of what can go wrong with veins is more aggravating than dangerous.

Some women are alarmed by the sight of threadlike blue tracings on the sides of the nose, which are actually tiny capillaries showing through the skin. For others, the worst sight is spider veins on the thighs or knots of thick varicose veins on the back of the calves. But none of these appearances is life-threatening.

One great concern, however, is phlebitis. It's an inflammation that happens when a vein is bruised or becomes infected and a clot forms in the vein wall. If your doctor treats it with heat and anti-inflammatory medication, your accommodating body will eventually re-absorb the clot.

The veins can also host one killer worthy of a Quentin Tarantino movie. Deep-vein thrombosis can take a clot, or thrombus, and hurl it to the lungs, resulting in a condition called a pulmonary embolism. If the clot blocks circulation to the lung area, it can lead to death. Deep-vein thrombosis sometimes occurs when someone is hospitalized and flat on her back for a long time. That's why doctors are always eager to get patients up after surgery or any immobilizing illness.

Blaming Mom Again

Any veins that you see on your skin's surface and sigh about probably are just dilated or enlarged blood vessels. "Those tiny red veins that you see on your nose or cheeks aren't really broken blood vessels. They're tiny, dilated veins," says Brian McDonagh, M.D., founder and director of the Vein Clinics of America, based in Schaumburg, Illinois.

Something in a Different Vein

Think of all of the bathing suits that Victoria's Secret could sell if spider veins didn't exist. If you happen to be heir to this delicate red paisley of tiny, sprawling veins, almost always located somewhere on the luckless leg or thigh, then you think twice about flaunting the legs that bear them.

There is, however, a procedure that can put the reins on telltale veins. It's called sclerotherapy. With payment of several hundred dollars, one to a few office visits and a little bit of discomfort, you can have the family curse removed.

Sclerotherapy is usually performed by a dermatological surgeon, a vein specialist called a phlebologist or a vascular surgeon. A sterile, corrosive chemical solution is injected into the chosen veins. As the chemical enters the veins, the walls dissolve and the veins essentially disintegrate. These nonfunctional veins are then absorbed back into the body. The injection requires no anesthesia, but you'll need to wear support stockings until the site heals. Healing can take two to six weeks, according to David Green, M.D., a dermatologist at the Varicose Vein Center in Bethesda, Maryland, and a vein specialist on the staff of both Howard University Hospital in Washington, D.C., and the National Naval Medical Center, also in Bethesda.

You can also have larger varicose veins removed with sclerotherapy. But some surgeons still "strip" the largest, a procedure called phlebectomy.

If you do have a phlebectomy, it usually involves general anesthesia. A surgeon pulls a flexible wire through the unwanted vein. A hook is attached to the wire. When the surgeon draws the wire out of the body, it pulls the vein along with it. The cost for this procedure can run from $500 to several thousand dollars.

Tiny blood vessels in the face can be removed with a much more delicate treatment: a laser. The laser's light heats up the blood until it destroys the veins that hold it. Then the amazing body absorbs the remains.

Fear not: You won't be bedridden or wrapped in bandages after any of these treatments. "Side effects are minimal," says Dr. Green. "You may experience some temporary discoloration, but that will disappear in a few months."

Even better news: Once the veins are gone, they're gone. "The only chance you have of seeing them again is if they are not completely removed at the time of treatment," says Dr. Green.

Women who are nursing or pregnant should wait until they are through before having varicose veins removed, Dr. Green advises. "Although the chemical solution used for sclerotherapy is not of any danger to the woman, it may potentially be dangerous to a developing fetus," he says. "Many times the condition of varicose veins improves after a woman has finished the birthing process. Given time, they just might go away on their own."

Women who get these visible capillaries usually are fair-skinned and tend to blush easily, says David Green, M.D., a dermatologist at the Varicose Vein Center in Bethesda, Maryland, and a vein specialist on the staff of both Howard University Hospital in Washington, D.C., and the National Naval Medical Center, also in Bethesda. While too much sun or alcohol may provoke them, if you have them, it's probably because you inherited them from one of your parents.

The same goes for varicose veins. "I would say that at least 90 percent of varicose veins have some sort of genetic basis," says Dr. Green. But that doesn't mean that it's certain you'll have them or that they'll be as prominent as your mother's or father's may have been.

"You're not necessarily doomed," says Eugene Strandness, Jr., M.D., professor of surgery at the University of Washington School of Medicine in Seattle. "We see a lot of women with very mild varicose veins. But if they run in your family and you don't take care of them, they will get bigger."

But even if they do get bigger, that doesn't mean you're at greater risk of having severe circulatory problems. "It's important for women to understand that even if they have family histories of varicose veins and they do develop varicose veins, it doesn't mean that they'll go on to develop complications," says Dr. Strandness. "It's rare for anyone with primary varicose veins to develop skin color changes or leg ulcers."

Keeping Glorious Gams

Nutrition and exercise are just as important to your veins as to any other body part. Exercise keeps your circulation shipshape. Good nutrition helps keep your weight on target. "Being significantly overweight is thought to be a risk factor that can worsen an inherited predisposition to varicose veins," says Alan Kanter, M.D., medical director of the Vein Centers of Orange and Torrance Counties in California.

"If your legs are in good shape, there's less pressure on your bad veins, and your good

veins work better," says Dr. Kanter.

Here are some other suggestions that might help your veins stay in hiding.

Shake a leg. Standing or sitting for more than an hour can make anyone's legs uncomfortable. When your legs are quiet for too long, the valves in your veins get sluggish, and the blood grows stagnant. "When blood is out of circulation like that, the oxygen content of the blood is very low and more acidic. So it acts as an irritant, and your legs ache," says Dr. McDonagh.

"People with varicose veins have to move around at least once an hour," says Dr. Strandness. If you have a job that involves lots of sitting or standing in one place, get up and stretch.

Rock 'n' roll. Here's an exercise to stimulate circulation in your legs. Stand erect, keeping your weight well-balanced over your feet. With slow movements, lift your toes, return them to the floor, then rock forward and lift your heels. "This is especially helpful when you must stand in one spot for a long time," says Dr. Kanter.

Wear tight tights. If you jog or otherwise work out on your feet a lot, and if varicose veins run in your family, seek out tight tights in a sporting goods store or department store. Before you buy workout tights, try them on to make sure they'll put some pressure on your legs and thighs. The pressure keeps blood flowing up your legs and helps prevent them from feeling tired and cramped, according to Dr. Green. "Buy comfortable but snug exercise clothing. Any kind of compression will squeeze in the veins," he says.

Try some lightweights. Stockings can be leg-savers. There are a number of types to choose from, offering various grades of compression. Nonprescription stockings can be lightweight, providing low to moderate compression, or heavy, providing greater compression. (You can find both kinds of stockings in drugstores and medical supply stores.)

Lightweight therapeutic stockings can be just as attractive as regular stockings, and Dr. Strandness suggests that you wear them—especially when you're active—if you have a strong family history of varicose veins. "We don't know for sure, but it makes good sense that they would keep superficial veins compressed and not permit distension," says Dr. Strandness. "Distended veins don't go back to normal. They keep getting worse."

Look for gradients. Gradient, or graduated, versions of lightweight compression stockings are also available. "The compression is greatest at the ankles. Then the grading of the stockings milks the blood up the legs and thighs back to the heart," explains Dr. Green. "So the farther north you go, the less compression there is."

Or go for the heavies. If you feel that you're in need of even more support, try heavy support hose. They may not look as snazzy as the lighter ones, but there are times when you may need to wear them. Many women get their first varicose veins when they're pregnant and carrying all of that extra weight. "If you have a family history of varicose veins and you're pregnant, it's extremely important that you wear heavy gradient compression stockings during the third trimester," says Dr. Strandness.

Try what the doctor orders. Best of all, you can also get a prescription for support stockings from your doctor to make sure that they have the correct fit and strength, says Dr. Kanter. If they're too tight, he says, "they could act like a tourniquet."

Because precise fit is so important, some doctors do not recommend over-the-counter stockings to anyone. "Proper strength can be prescribed only after a knowledgeable examiner determines the medical need of a patient," says Dr. Kanter.

Put up your feet. For a woman with varicose veins, there's nothing comic about a stand-up routine. If you're standing anywhere—on cold linoleum, hard concrete or the carpet-lined floor at the bank—for too long, your legs will start to hurt and feel tired.

Take the weight off whenever you can. Lie on a couch and prop your hurting leg on pillows so that it's above chest level. Or lie on the floor and prop your leg against a wall for comfort. The blood in your leg will immediately start flowing to your heart, helped on its way by gravity. That will take the pressure off your overstrained veins, says Dr. Strandness.

Make a motion. Exercise is good, no doubt about it. "But a lot of vein specialists have the impression that certain high-impact exercises will aggravate varicose veins," says Dr. Kanter. While no studies have been done on this subject, Dr. Kanter recommends that women with varicose veins avoid jogging on hard surfaces (grass and cinders are okay). And he suggests doing low-impact aerobics instead of high-impact if you have varicose veins.

Lifting heavy weights can also aggravate varicose veins, says Dr. Kanter. If you have to strain so hard that you grunt, it's too much pressure. Use smaller weights and do more repetitions, he suggests.

What's safest of all? "You can walk on pretty much any surface," says Dr. Kanter. "Walking is excellent exercise. It's what we are built for."

See also Circulatory System

Vulva

CAN YOU IMAGINE IF WOMEN took their sex organs as seriously as men take theirs? What if the size of your labia was an indication of sexual prowess? Imagine teenage girls sitting around at sleep-overs, measuring the length of their vaginas. Can't you just hear it? "Wow, mine's a half-inch longer than yours! How about you, Jennifer?"

This scenario isn't just preposterous; it's unthinkable. For most women, the nether region of the female body is uncharted territory. We don't look at it, we don't explore it very much, and some of us don't even know exactly what's where.

In fact, some women might not even know that the vulva itself isn't an organ. *Vulva* is actually the name given to the entire outer area of a woman's genital-urethral organs. It's made up of the labia majora (or large lips), the labia minora (or small lips), the clitoris, the urethral opening and the vaginal opening.

Getting to Know Yours

Because of the way they're constructed, it's not as easy to get a gander at a female's genitalia as at a male's. You have to really make an effort.

"It's amazing how many women are afraid to look at their genitals," says Barbara Levinson, R.N., Ph.D., a licensed marriage and family therapist and owner and director of the Center for Healthy Sexuality in Houston. "How do you expect to guide your lover to give you pleasure if you don't know what you look or feel like?" When you have some free time, Dr. Levinson advises taking a handheld mirror and exploring until you have a complete picture.

The labia majora are the large lips on the outside of all of the genitalia. They contain deposits of fatty tissue and are covered with hair. Their purpose: completely covering the vagina so that no dirt or sweat can enter it.

The labia minora are the smaller, hairless lips inside the larger lips. They are a backup vaginal protection system for the labia majora. It's the labia minora that fill with blood during sexual arousal. With the swelling that accompanies that rush of blood, your labia get a tighter grip on the penis, enhancing sexual pleasure.

The most common problem that women have with their labia is vulval itching, which is usually caused by an allergic reaction to chemicals in deodorants, spermicides, creams and douches. It's also very common during menopause, when there is a reduced level of estrogen in the body. Antibiotics and hormones, both of which are taken orally or sometimes applied in cream form, are the best treatments.

Wrists

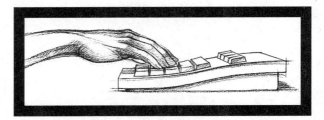

To avoid carpal tunnel syndrome, your hand should be in the position shown—with the wrist flat and even with the keyboard.

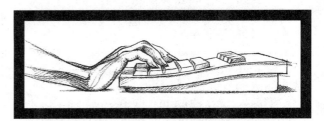

You're more likely to get carpal tunnel syndrome if your wrist is in this "cocked" position below the keyboard. If your fingernails are too long, your hand may be forced into this position.

WONDERING WHAT TIME IT IS?

Better check your armwatch.

Technically, that's what it is. The wrist area is actually lower than the spot where you sport your Timex or Seiko.

If you could use your x-ray vision for a quick wrist exam, you'd see that it looks like an eight-bone pileup occurred between the bones of your arm and those of your hand. The short, marble-size bones of your wrist, called carpal bones, sit in two uneven rows, each less than one-half inch wide, between where your arm ends and your hand begins.

That's not a whole lot of room for all of those bones. But somehow they find space to shift and glide against each other, allowing the wrist a lot of play.

If you rest your palm and forearm flat on a table, the carpal bones inside your wrist form an upside-down U. Underneath that U runs a ligament called the flexor retinaculum. In between the carpal bones and this ligament is a space, or tunnel (thus the name *carpal tunnel*), that houses nine tendons and a very sensitive median nerve.

The Biggest Offender

For women between 30 and 45 years of age, carpal tunnel syndrome is by far the biggest problem in the wrist area, says Anthony Foley, M.D., assistant professor of family medicine at Wright State University in Dayton, Ohio. The nerve and tendons inside the tunnel get irritated, inflamed and swollen, causing wrist pain, numbness and tingling.

Repetitive motion, particularly at work, is the major cause of carpal tunnel syndrome, says Dr. Foley. Experts estimate that approximately five times as many women as men develop this condition. Although that may be because of a combination of different things, there are probably more women engaged in activities such as keyboarding, according to Robert Sallis, M.D., assistant program director of the family medicine residency program at Kaiser-Permanente Medical Center in Fontana, California. Also, other health problems, such as thyroid disease, can trigger carpal tunnel syndrome, and more women than men have those problems.

But whatever the cause of carpal tunnel syndrome, here's what some experts recommend to help relieve it.

Find a new angle. If you work at a keyboard, make sure your wrists aren't cocked, says Pekka Mooar, M.D., assistant professor of orthopedic surgery and chief of sports medicine at the Medical College of Pennsylvania and Hahnemann University School of Medicine, both in Philadelphia. Your wrists should be even with the keyboard. If your desk isn't the right height, get a slide-out tray to hold the keyboard at the correct level.

Break the repetition. If you work at a keyboard all day, take frequent breaks, says Steven Stuchin, M.D., director of the Arthritis Center at the Hospital for Joint Diseases Orthopedic Institute in New York City. For some people, working at the keyboard for about 30 minutes and then taking a 5-minute break is a good preventive measure. "Find a system that works for you and never work to fatigue," recommends Dr. Stuchin.

Cut your fingernails. When you have long fingernails, you force your wrists into the cocked position that can aggravate carpal tunnel syndrome, says Dr. Sallis.

Protect your wrist at night. One of the first lines of treatment for carpal tunnel syndrome is wearing a wrist splint at night, says Dr. Mooar. The doctor who diagnoses the problem should be able to fit you for a comfortable splint.

Thumb Kind of Pain

DeQuervain's disease is another kind of problem that can develop from overusing the wrist. The pain is felt above the base of the thumb, in the area right next to the wrist, and radiates up the radial, or inner, side of the arm, says Dr. Stuchin.

The same swelling during pregnancy that can put pressure on the median nerve and contribute to carpal tunnel syndrome can also put pressure on tendons, says Dr. Stuchin. This can lead to the development of deQuervain's. "The biggest complaint is 'It hurts when I pick up the baby,'" says Dr. Stuchin.

An Exodus from Bible Cysts

Wrist pain can be caused by ganglia, little fluid-filled cysts that develop on the back or palm side of the wrist, according to Robert Sallis, M.D., assistant program director of the family medicine residency program at Kaiser-Permanente Medical Center in Fontana, California.

In the past, people called ganglia Bible cysts, says Pekka Mooar, M.D., assistant professor of orthopedic surgery and chief of sports medicine at the Medical College of Pennsylvania and Hahnemann University School of Medicine, both in Philadelphia. That's because ganglia used to be treated by whacking them with a Bible, he says.

Fortunately, the Bible-thumping days of wrist whacking are a thing of the past. Now ganglia are often treated by aspirating the fluid from them, a procedure performed in the doctor's office. While ganglia on the back side of the wrist are pretty safe to aspirate, those on the palm side need to be treated very carefully, since they may be near a main artery, says Dr. Sallis.

Sometimes the deQuervain's that develops during pregnancy subsides after childbirth. But other times, women continue to have trouble. As they constantly pick up their children, an activity that requires using their thumbs, they may feel the pain more acutely than they did during pregnancy.

If you feel pain at the base of your thumb and think you may have deQuervain's, don't ignore it, says Dr. Sallis. See your doctor for treatment. She might apply a splint or recommend periodic ice treatments to soothe the pain. Anti-inflammatory medication such as ibuprofen can also help, according to Dr. Sallis.

See also Skeletal System

Toning Your Body

Shaping Up

INSIDE EVERY WOMAN is a lean, sleek model of herself. A woman whose curvy muscles have thrown off their blanket of body fat. A shapely woman. A strong woman. Maybe even a superwoman who could paint a big capital *S* high on her toned chest.

This isn't wishful thinking. Every woman can uncover her inner model, given a little time and effort. The process is a program of exercise called toning—or body shaping, body sculpting or, most accurate of all, strength training. Whatever you call it, toning involves exercises such as tried-and-true push-ups, partial sit-ups called crunches, lunges and squats. It utilizes weights or dumbbells (usually five to ten pounds) and often elastic exercise bands. You also have the option of using weight machines for toning if you belong to a gym or a health club or you have them in your own home.

Toning routines work on specific muscles or muscle groups, such as the quadriceps and the hamstring muscles in the front and back of the thighs as well as the abdominal muscles, which support the front of the torso like a girdle.

"The nice thing is that you don't have to strength-train as frequently as you do aerobic exercise," says Michael Yessis, Ph.D., president of Sports Training in Escondido, California, and co-author of *Body Shaping*. Brisk aerobic exercise such as running, walking, swimming, working out on a treadmill or doing aerobics usually takes an hour or so three or four times a week if you want to see results. With strength training, however, "you can get by on 30 minutes twice a week," says Dr. Yessis, "although three days a week is preferred."

"You'll see a significant difference in your body after six weeks of body shaping," says Rebecca Gorrell, a certified fitness instructor and wellness education director at Canyon

Ranch in Tucson, Arizona. "It's one of the very few natural ways you can change the way you look," adds Larry A. Tucker, Ph.D., professor and director of health promotion at Brigham Young University in Provo, Utah.

In fact, change comes so predictably that it builds self-esteem in addition to better bodies. Researchers at Brigham Young, led by Dr. Tucker, conducted a 12-week study of 60 women with an average age of 42. Half of the women were assigned to exercise by walking; the rest of the women were assigned to a strength-training group. The scientists found that the body images of the walkers improved during the 12 weeks. But they also discovered that the body images of the women who strength-trained improved significantly more. "We saw substantial mental, emotional and physical changes," says Dr. Tucker.

The Miracle of the Muscle

Why is toning so much faster than aerobic exercise when it comes to showing results? Strength training increases the size of your muscles by increasing the number of myofibrils, the threadlike strands that form each muscle fiber. The long, slender muscle fibers are about the width of a hair, and they can grow as long as 12 inches. Bundles of about 150 fibers, combined with connective tissue, make up muscles such as the biceps on the front of your upper arms and the triceps on the back of them.

Until fairly recently, though, most women associated muscles with muscleheads. We were afraid if we lifted any weights at all, we'd start to look like Olive Oyls with Popeye arms. So weight training, another name for strength training, has sort of snuck into health clubs under the guise of toning and body-shaping classes.

As you gain muscle and lose fat, your body composition changes—even if your weight stays the same, Dr. Yessis has discovered. The percentage of body fat drops, and the amount of lean muscle rises. (You don't actually turn fat into muscle, though, because you can't turn a fat cell into a muscle cell.)

And since muscle burns more calories than fat does when your body is at rest, strength training to increase muscle size actually speeds up your metabolism (the rate at which you burn calories) by 2 to 3 percent, researchers say. Each pound of muscle you make burns about 30 to 50 more calories than a pound of fat. Even after a strength-training workout, calories continue to be burned at a high rate for many hours, according to Dr. Yessis. What all of this means is that you get a bonus almost as big as winning a body lottery: Either you can eat more good food without weight gain or you can lose weight more quickly if you need to.

That's not the only benefit of body shaping, either. Early research shows that strength training may have some effect on building strong bones to help thwart osteoporosis, or bone loss.

Working Out the Whole You

To help you get started, Gorrell has put together a time-conscious Total Body-Shaping Workout that Dr. Yessis agrees will be beneficial. You'll get the biggest benefits by doing the workout on two or three nonconsecutive days each week. In addition to the Total Body-Shaping Workout, this section has exercises to help tone certain muscles of your body, if you want to focus more on specific areas.

But before you jump into the workouts, here are two toning commandments.

Check your breath. You need to fight two tendencies: not thinking about how you breathe and holding your breath for too long when you lift, says Dr. Yessis.

When you lift light weights, such as the ones used in these workouts, Dr. Yessis says you should inhale and briefly hold your breath during the movement in the exercise with the most exertion—the actual lift, for instance. Then exhale as you lower the weights or perform the easier motion. "As long as you don't hold your breath too long, you breathe properly while you do the movements and you lift and lower the weights in a smooth, controlled manner, you should be fine," says Dr. Yessis.

One warning: People with heart, blood pressure or circulatory problems should never hold their breath when lifting weights, since blood pressure rises temporarily, warns Dr. Yessis.

Be progressive. "Muscles adapt so quickly that you have to frequently increase the amount of weight or resistance (if you're using an exercise band) that you use in order not to plateau," says Dr. Yessis. Increase the weight as soon as an exercise gets to be a little easy to perform. The last repetition of any exercise should be hard to do. To tone and firm continuously, your muscles need constant challenge.

Fitness experts say that after three to six weeks of any toning routine, you should change your program in some way in order to progress. "Besides increasing the weight or adding more repetitions of an exercise, switch to a different exercise that uses the same muscles in a slightly different way," says Gorrell. "Switch to weight machines if you belong to a gym, or switch from the machines to free weights (dumbbells). They each use your muscles a little differently."

The Total Body-Shaping Workout

GORRELL'S TIME-EFFICIENT Total Body-Shaping Workout takes 20 minutes two or three times a week. To do some of these exercises, you'll need a set of two-pound dumbbells and a set of five-pound dumbbells—or one set that allows you to gradually increase the amount of weight you're lifting. A set of single-piece dumbbells generally costs under $10. The kind that allows you to add more weight to increase resistance costs about $15 to $30 per set in most sporting goods stores. Or if you don't want to make any investment at all, you can fill plastic jugs or bottles with just enough sand or water to make your own two- and five-pound weights. (Remember: Sand will weigh more than water.)

For some of the exercises that are done on the floor, you'll probably want to use an exercise mat. A folded blanket works just as well. And a few of the exercises call for an exercise band, which is a strip of flexible rubber you can buy in most sporting goods stores. Exercises calling for a bench can be done on a padded exercise bench or a low bench with a cushion.

Do each exercise, except those in the warm-up and the cooldown, 8 to 12 times (you can start with 8 repetitions and work your way up to 12). This is called a set. If you cannot complete 8 repetitions, or reps, that means you're lifting too much weight. If you can do 12 reps without feeling muscle fatigue, you should be lifting more. If you have been doing the routine for several weeks and it feels comfortable, you can begin doing a sec-

ond set of all of the exercises. Progress from five to ten pounds gradually, as an exercise starts to feel easy.

Following the Total Body-Shaping Workout, you'll find exercises that help tone different parts of your body. (These begin on page 450 with the abdominal exercises.) Start with the total workout, then add or substitute some of the other exercises as you progress.

Beginning and Ending the Workout

Begin each session with the following series of warm-up exercises, which will loosen up the muscles you're going to use and help you avoid injury. Each of these warm-ups should be done ten times.

Once you've completed the warm-up, you're ready to begin the workout exercises. Reminder: Each exercise should be done 8 times to start, working up to 12 times as you advance.

At the end of the workout, after you've done enough repetitions of all of the exercises, you should cool down. Shake your arms and legs a little and walk around for five minutes. Then stretch.

Stretching elongates your muscles. It keeps them from tightening up and also keeps them flexible, which helps prevent soreness as well as pulling and tearing. Just make sure you do each of the two stretches shown slowly and deliberately, reaching and bending without bouncing.

No-Strain Warm-Up

To begin the warm-up, extend your arms out to the sides, slightly below the height of your shoulders as shown in **Figure 1.** Press your shoulders and arms forward and back, turning your arms over slightly as you move so that your palms face back when your arms are forward and forward when your arms are back (see **Figure 2**).

Warm up your lower back by bending at the waist and placing your hands on your thighs. Your knees should be slightly bent, so they're not locked straight. Arch your back upward, like a mad cat, as shown in **Figure 3**. Then, keeping your hands on your thighs, relax your back to a normal position.

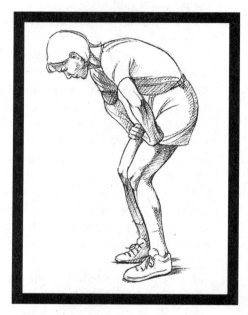

Figure 3

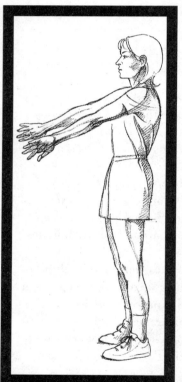

Figure 1

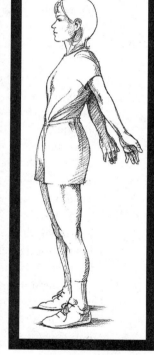

Figure 2

Stand up straight. With your right hand, reach toward the left, up over your head and in front of you on the diagonal as in **Figure 4**. Feel the stretch along the right side of your rib cage.

Pull your right arm down and back (a little to the back of your waist) while bending your arm and making a fist with your hand (**Figure 5**). Repeat with your left arm.

To finish the warm-up, put your hands on your hips and slowly bend from your waist toward your right side. Straighten, then bend toward your left side. Keep your knees slightly bent, and make sure your trunk is erect and you don't twist it.

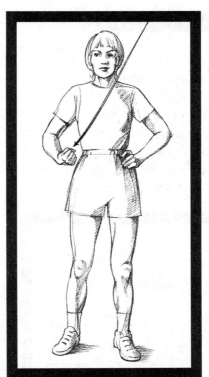

Figure 5

Place your hands on your hips and shift your pelvis from side to side.

Tighten your abdominal and buttocks muscles and tilt your pelvis backward. Then as you relax those muscles, tilt your pelvis forward. The movement is like a controlled swing.

Figure 4

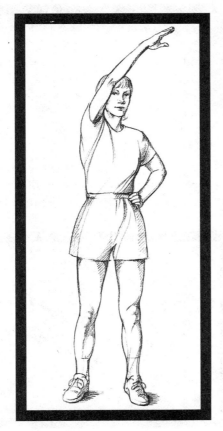

Single-Arm Row

This exercise tones your shoulder and back muscles.

With your left foot on the floor and your left knee slightly bent, position your right knee on a bench so that your knee is directly under your hip. Lean forward, placing your right hand on the bench, with your back flat

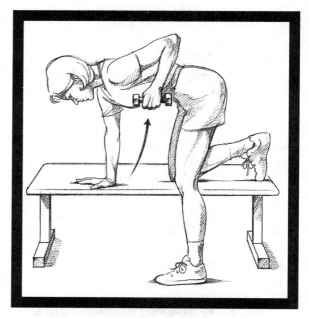

Figure 7

like pulling the cord on a lawn mower.) Return to the starting position and repeat. After you complete 8 to 12 repetitions, switch sides and repeat.

Push-Up

This helps tone your entire chest, even if you start with a half rather than a full push-up. Kneeling on an exercise mat, lean forward

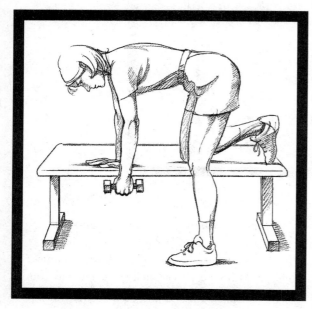

Figure 6

and parallel to the floor (**Figure 6**). Grasp a dumbbell in your left hand, with your arm fully extended downward and your palm facing in.

Squeezing your shoulder blades together, pull your left arm up, bending your elbow until the point of your elbow is a few inches above your back (**Figure 7**). (The motion is

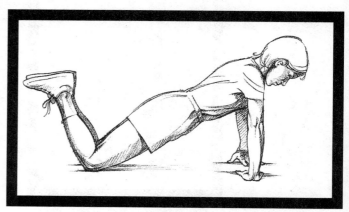

Figure 8

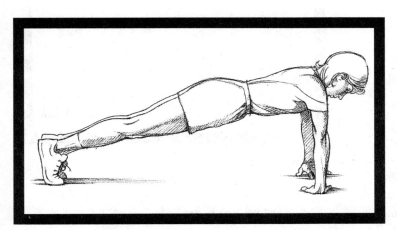

Figure 9

Lateral Shoulder Raise

This tones your shoulder muscles. Stand with your feet spread apart about as wide as your hips. Hold a two- or three-pound dumbbell in each hand, with your palms turned toward your thighs. Bend your knees slightly, so they're not locked. Now bend your elbows slightly. Keeping your trunk erect and your elbows bent, raise your arms out to the sides until your elbows are just slightly higher than your shoulders (**Figure 10**). Lower the dumbbells to your sides and repeat.

and place your hands shoulder-width apart on the mat. Your fingers should be pointing inward and your elbows outward (**Figure 8**). When you're in the upright position, your arms and back should be straight, and your knees should touch the floor. Lower your chest to the floor, keeping your upper body rigid. Then push up, straightening your arms.

When you've mastered the half push-up, you can progress to the full push-up. Begin in the raised position but with your knees off the floor, so you're balanced on your hands and toes and your back is straight (**Figure 9**). Remember to keep your fingers in and your elbows out. Lower your whole body until your chest lightly touches the floor. Then raise yourself until your arms are once again straight. Repeat in the same manner as the half push-up.

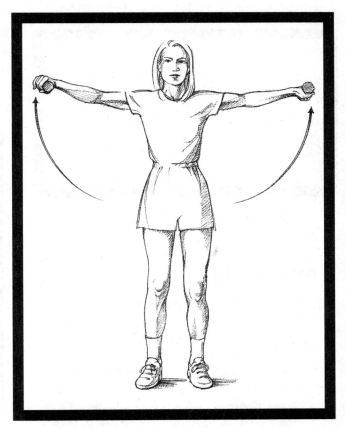

Figure 10

Abdominal Crunch

This exercise tones your upper abdominal muscles.

Lie on your back on a mat, with your knees bent and your feet flat on the floor. Place your fingertips behind your ears, with your elbows winged out as wide as they'll go. Tighten your stomach muscles to curl your trunk, lifting your shoulders until they clear the floor (**Figure 11**). Keep your elbows out, not in near your ears, so the lift comes from your abdominal muscles rather than by straining your neck, arms and back. Hold the crunch for a few seconds at the top of the lift. Then lower your upper body and repeat.

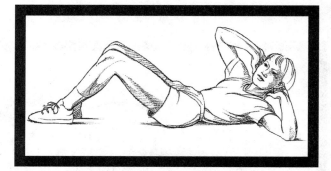

Figure 12

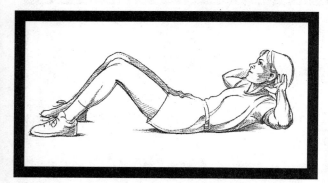

Figure 11

Rotating Crunch

This crunch tones the oblique muscles along the sides of your abdomen.

Start in the same position as for the abdominal crunch. Then leading with your right shoulder (not with your right elbow), lift your upper body on a diagonal toward your left knee (**Figure 12**). Keep your left shoulder on the floor. Hold the crunch for a few seconds, then lower. Complete the repetitions to your left side, then switch sides, leading with your

left shoulder to lift your body on a diagonal toward your right knee.

Squat

This exercise tones your thighs and buttocks.

Stand with your feet approximately shoulder-width apart and your toes pointed straight ahead or slightly out to the sides. With your feet flat on the floor, lower yourself

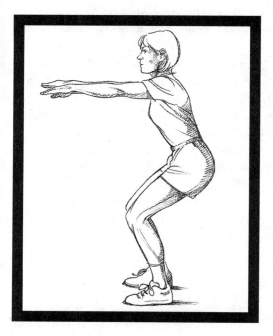

Figure 13

into the squat position, extending your arms straight ahead as you do so. You're in the right position when your trunk leans forward (up to 45 degrees), your butt moves back slightly and your thighs and arms are almost parallel to the floor (**Figure 13**).

While squatting, you want to look forward at all times and keep the natural curvature in your spine. Do not lower yourself so that your knees extend beyond your feet. Keep your heels glued to the floor to avoid stress on your knees. Then begin to raise yourself to a standing position.

Figure Four Stretch

Sit on the floor on a mat, with your right leg straight in front of you and your toes pointing up. Bend your left knee to place your left heel against the inside of your right thigh, close to your crotch. Meanwhile, try to keep your left knee as close to the floor as possible.

Bending from your hips, not from your waist, slowly reach out with your right hand as though trying to touch your right toes or ankle (**Figure 14**). Don't arch your back; just maintain the natural curve of your spine. Hold the position for 30 seconds, return to the start, then reverse leg positions and stretch your left hand toward your left toes for another 30 seconds. Finally, repeat this stretch, starting with your right leg bent and your left leg straight.

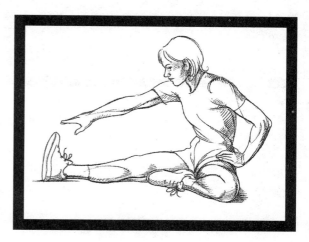

Figure 14

Lying Side Stretch

Lie on your back on a mat with your feet together and your arms straight out to the sides. Keeping your left leg fully extended on the floor, slowly lift your right leg in the air, keeping your right knee slightly bent. Then without bending your left knee, rotate your right hip and stretch your right leg straight across your body. Keep both hands on the floor (**Figure 15**). Hold this position for 30 seconds, continuing to stretch without bouncing. Return to the start and repeat the stretch a second time. Then do the same exercise again with your left leg, repeating it twice.

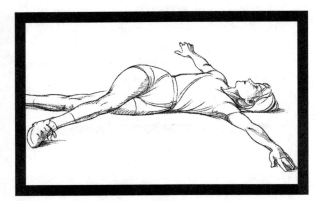

Figure 15

Abdominals

HERE ARE THE FIRST of the optional toning exercises that can be added to the Total Body-Shaping Workout or substituted for exercises in that workout.

Outside the belly, you have four abdominal muscles that demand attention. They include the long rectus abdominis, running from the lower border of the rib cage to the crotch, and the oblique muscles, located along the sides of the torso. In the Total Body-Shaping Workout, the abdominal crunch and the rotating crunch are good ways to start toning this area.

Remember, these exercises are a little more vigorous than those in the previous workout. Be sure to follow the directions closely and to stop if you feel strain or pain in any area. Also, be aware that while toning will firm the abdominal muscles, aerobic exercise will burn off the coat of fat that covers them.

Equipment: exercise mat (can substitute a rug or folded blanket).

Full Crunch

Lie on your back and lift your legs up and off the floor, with your knees bent, your ankles crossed and your calves parallel to the floor. Put your fingers behind your ears and aim your elbows toward your knees. Curl up your torso, bringing your knees and elbows toward each other until they touch at the top of the lift (**Figure 16**). (You may find it easier to raise your shoulders off the floor if you shoot your extended arms past your knees and toward your feet as you rise.) Lift your hips and shoulders off the floor as you tighten your abdominals. Hold the crunch for a few seconds,

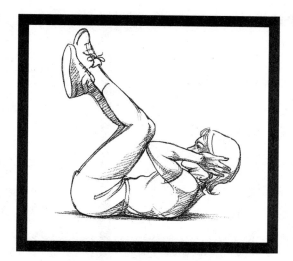

Figure 16

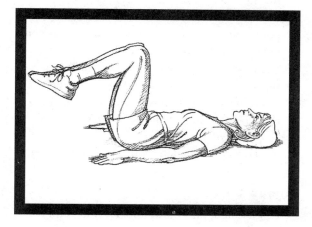

Figure 17

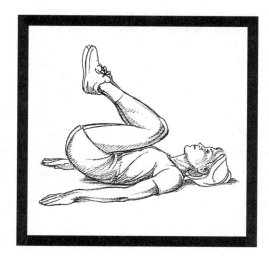

Figure 18

verse sit-ups with your arms down at your sides, do them with your arms stretched above your head on the floor to give your lower abdominals the maximum workout. Increase the number of repetitions until you get to 20, then gradually add a second set of 30 to 40 repetitions.

then slowly lower to the starting position. Start with two sets of eight repetitions each and work your way up to three sets of ten repetitions each. (*Note:* Be careful not to yank or pull yourself up by your neck or head.)

Reverse Sit-Up

Lie on your back, with your arms flat by your sides and your palms down. To start, bend your knees and raise your legs so that your thighs are vertical (**Figure 17**).

Then raise your buttocks off the floor, keeping your knees bent and bringing them toward your chest as your hips rotate upward (**Figure 18**). (When you first do this exercise, you may push down with your hands to help get your hips off the floor and your knees close to your chest.) Return to the starting position.

Be sure to rest for a second or two before you repeat the exercise. But don't lower your feet to the floor until you've finished four or five repetitions in your beginning set. (Remember: You are using your abdominal muscles, not momentum, to contract and pull your lower body toward your chest.)

Once you become proficient at doing re-

Biceps

LOCATED ON YOUR UPPER ARMS, the biceps are the muscles you use to lift boulders, babies and bowling balls. A sturdy set of biceps will also help you yank heavy bags of cat litter out of the trunk and hoist five-gallon bottles of water into the house. Just what you always needed, right?

Since none of the exercises in the Total Body-Shaping Workout is designed to help build biceps, the following are good to add to the basic routine whenever you can.

Equipment: five-pound dumbbells (to start), exercise bench (can substitute a chair).

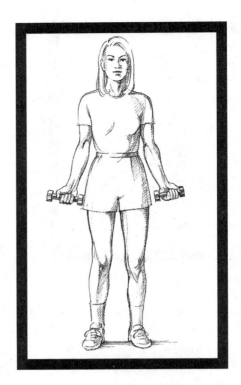

Figure 19

Biceps Curl

Figure 20

Pick up a pair of dumbbells and stand in a normal upright position, maintaining the normal curvature of your spine. Keep your elbows and upper arms along the sides of your body, and hold the dumbbells with your palms facing up (**Figure 19**). Raise the dumbbells toward your shoulders (**Figure 20**). Don't swing the dumbbells or arch your back. Slowly lower the dumbbells until they're in the starting position.

Do 8 repetitions, with beginners using 5- to 8-pound dumbbells and those at an intermediate level using 10- to 12-pound dumbbells. Do two sets, with a rest of about 30 seconds between sets. Gradually work your way up to 10 to 15 repetitions. Increase the weight when the curls start to feel easy.

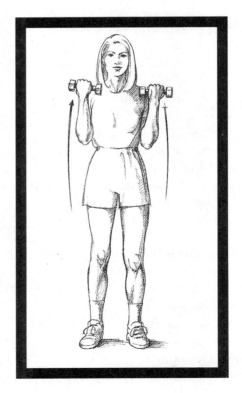

Concentration Curl

Sit on an exercise bench or a chair so that
your knees are at 90-degree angles. Place
your feet so that they're just a little more than
shoulder-width apart. Grasp a five-pound
dumbbell in your right hand, then rest your
right elbow against the inside of your right
thigh near your knee. Hold your arm so that
it's perpendicular to the floor, with your palm
facing your left calf (**Figure 21**).

Without moving your shoulders, bend your
right elbow and lift the dumbbell toward your
right chest-shoulder area (**Figure 22**). Slowly
return the dumbbell to the starting position.
Do eight repetitions with your right arm before switching to your left arm.

Do two sets of eight repetitions per arm.
Gradually increase the weight to ten pounds.
Progress to three sets, with ten repetitions per
arm in each set.

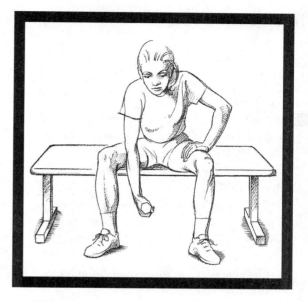

Figure 21

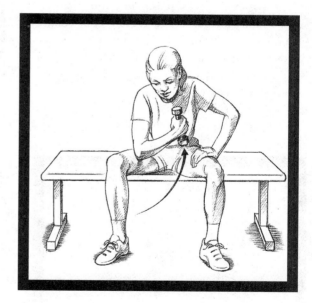

Figure 22

Buttocks

THE GLUTEUS MAXIMUS is the bulkiest—and, for some of us, the balkiest—muscle in the body. It's the muscle in each buttock; the more we shape the glutes, the less we leave to chance in this area.

The following exercise really works the hips, since this is where the outside strip of each glute is attached. But the net effect is to shape the whole hip and buttock area.

Equipment: exercise mat, exercise band.

Hip Extension

Loosely tie an exercise band into a half-bow (only one has a loop) around both ankles as shown in **Figure 23**. Kneeling on a mat, lower yourself until your elbows and forearms rest on the mat and your weight is balanced on your knees and forearms.

Slide part of the band down your left foot and "latch" it over the top of that foot. Ex-

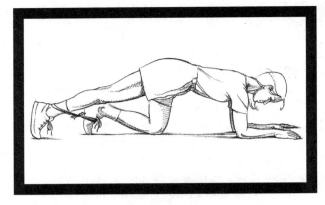

Figure 24

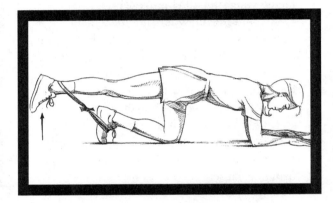

Figure 25

tend your right leg straight back so that your toes rest on the floor (**Figure 24**). Slowly lift your right leg no higher than your buttocks and hold it in the raised position for a few seconds, resisting the pressure of the exercise band (**Figure 25**). Slowly return your right toes to the floor.

Do one set of eight repetitions with your right leg, then switch to your left leg. Gradually increase the number of sets until you're doing three sets with each leg, switching from your right leg to your left leg for each set. And gradually decrease the length of the band so that it offers you more resistance. To protect and strengthen your back, hold your midsection in a tight contraction and keep your back straight while you do the exercise.

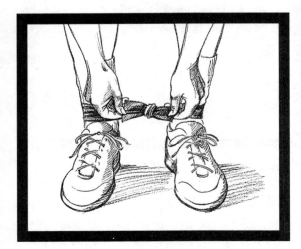

Figure 23

Calves

IT'S A GARGANTUAN WORD: *gastrocnemius.*
So fitness folks call the big muscles in the
back of the calves the gastrocs for short. If
you build and firm both of these babies,
they'll make your ankles look slim—even if
you have naturally thick anklebones and
Achilles tendons. The bottom line is a shape-
lier leg line.

Equipment: exercise step (can substitute
the bottom step of a staircase), exercise
band, exercise mat.

Heel Raise

You can do this exercise with an exercise
step or on the bottom step of a staircase. It
requires good balance, so keep your hand on
a wall or railing until you get used to bal-
ancing yourself.

With the balls of your feet on the edge of
the step and your heels hanging off the edge,
lower yourself as far as you can without tot-
tering backward. Sink until you feel a slight
stretch in both your calf muscles and your
Achilles tendons (**Figure 26**).

Then raise your heels as high as you can,
while keeping your back and legs straight
(**Figure 27**). Hold this position for a second
or two, then return to the starting position
and repeat.

Start with one set of 3 to 4 repetitions.
Gradually increase the number of reps to 15
to 20. Work your way up to three sets: 10 reps
in the first set; 15 reps in the second set, holding an eight- to ten-pound dumbbell in one
hand at your side; and 20 to 25 reps in the
third set, still holding the dumbbell.

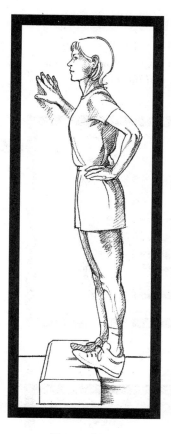
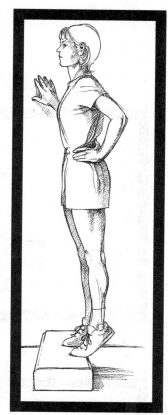

Figure 26   **Figure 27**

Toe Press

For this exercise, you'll need an elastic exercise band.

Sit on a mat with your legs straight out in
front of you, together but not touching, and
your toes pointing up. Holding each end of the
exercise band, loop it over the balls of your
feet. Point your toes back toward your shins as
far as you can without letting the band slip
free (**Figure 28**, next page). Then point your
toes away from you (**Figure 29**, next page).
Hold the position for a few seconds. Return to
the starting point, then repeat.

Do one set of eight repetitions. Gradually
increase the load until you're doing three sets

of eight repetitions. And gradually decrease
the length of the band that you hold between
your hands, so it offers you more resistance.

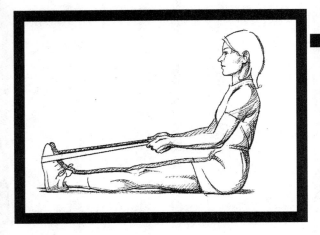

Figure 28

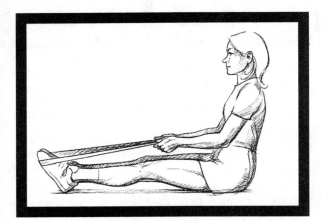

Figure 29

Chest

SORRY, YOU CAN'T INCREASE the actual size
of your breasts by body shaping. But you can
firm and tone the pectoral muscles that lie beneath them, and that will make your breasts
look fuller. Toning your chest muscles will
give you a natural breast lift.

Equipment: exercise band, exercise bench,
five-pound dumbbell (to start).

Horizontal Chest Press

While either standing or sitting, place an
exercise band across your back so that it
stretches horizontally across both shoulder
blades. Your hands should be positioned near
your armpits as they grip the ends of the
band, with your palms facing down. Take up
the slack until the band feels snug across your
back (**Figure 30**). Then slowly press your
hands and arms forward, keeping your palms
down (**Figure 31**). Return to the starting po-

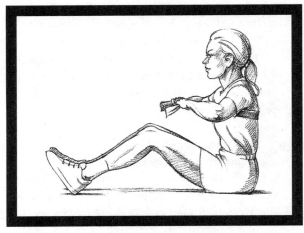

Figure 30

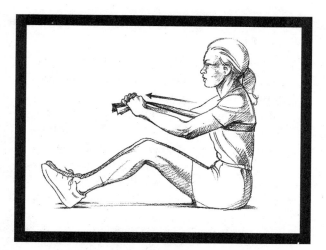

Figure 31

sition with a single, fluid motion.

Do one set of eight chest presses. Gradually increase to three sets of eight repetitions. And shorten the band to make it more snug, so it offers more resistance.

Pullover

Lie on your back on a padded exercise bench, with your head near one end of the bench and your feet flat on the floor, positioned shoulder-width apart. Grasp one end

of a five-pound dumbbell with both hands. Raise it directly overhead, with your arms fully extended as shown in **Figure 32**. This is your starting position.

Now lower your straight arms backward until the bottom end of the dumbbell reaches a point even with or slightly below the level of your back. Allow your arms to bend just enough to prevent uncomfortable stress on your elbows (**Figure 33**). Then return the dumbbell to the overhead position. Relax and repeat.

Start with 2 or 3 repetitions. Gradually increase to 15 reps using a ten-pound dumbbell. To progress beyond that, work up to three sets: 10 reps using a five-pound dumbbell for the first set; 8 to 10 reps using the heavier dumbbell for the second set; and 15 reps using the heavier dumbbell for the third set.

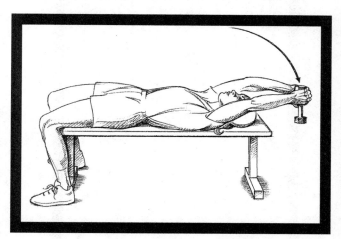

Figure 33

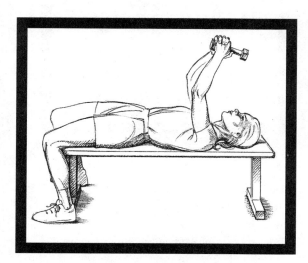

Figure 32

Forearms

STRONG FOREARM MUSCLES help you unscrew even the most stubborn lid from a marinara jar. And if you do office work that includes a lot of repetitive keyboard action, strengthening the forearm muscles is your best protection against carpal tunnel syndrome. Last but never least, working these muscles helps build up your wrists. For women who have osteoporosis, especially after menopause, this muscle building may be good insurance against wrist fractures.

Equipment: two- to five-pound dumbbells (to start).

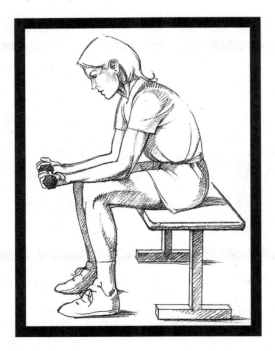

Figure 34

Wrist Curl

Use two- to five-pound dumbbells. Sit on an exercise bench or a chair, with your forearms resting on your thighs and your palms curled around the dumbbells and facing up. Your hands should extend beyond your knees, with your wrists straight to start (**Figure 34**). Lower the dumbbells by bending your wrists, allowing your hands to fall backward as far as they can go (**Figure 35**). Immediately lift the dumbbells back up, then repeat.

Start with one set of 4 or 5 repetitions and work your way up to 20 reps. You can add

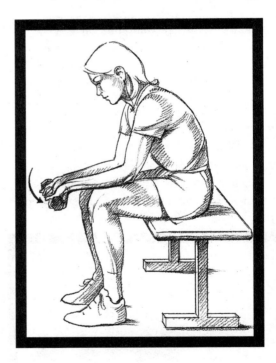

Figure 35

two more sets during subsequent workouts. When you begin doing three full sets in one workout, reduce the weight of the dumbbells by half. (If you've been using two-pound dumbbells, for example, use one-pounders instead.) Do 10 reps in the first set, 10 to 15 reps in the second set and, finally, 20 reps in the third set.

Reverse Wrist Curl

This is the same as the wrist curl, but it's done with your palms facing down rather than up.

Sit on an exercise bench or a chair, with your forearms resting on your thighs and your palms curled around the dumbbells and facing down. Lower the dumbbells as far as you can, keeping your forearms in contact with your thighs and bending at your wrists. Immediately lift the dumbbells as high as you can without raising your forearms (**Figure 36**). Do this at a moderate pace. For the number of reps and sets, follow the directions given for the regular wrist curl.

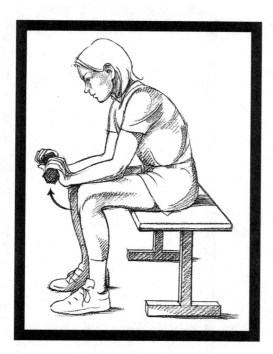

Figure 36

Neck

AT THE TOP OF YOUR NECK, not far behind your ear, the upper tip of the trapezius muscle is attached to the lower part of your skull. From there, the trapezius zigzags from neck to shoulder to back. As exercise tones this area, your neck becomes an elegant column for your head.

Neck Press

With your right hand, reach over your head and curve your hand above your left ear (**Figure 37**). Press your head to the left without tilting your head too far toward your shoulder, tensing against your hand's resistance for a count of six. Repeat with your left hand above your right ear.

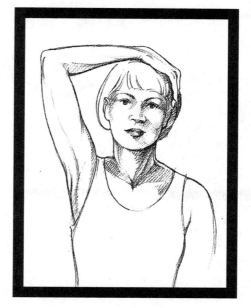

Figure 37

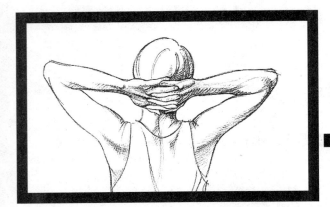

Figure 38

Then clasp your hands behind your head, with your fingers interlocked and your elbows flared. Steadily press your head back against your hands for a count of six (**Figure 38**).

Now place both hands, with your fingers still interlocked, against your forehead and press your head forward for a count of six (**Figure 39**).

Do one set of eight to ten repetitions of each of these movements.

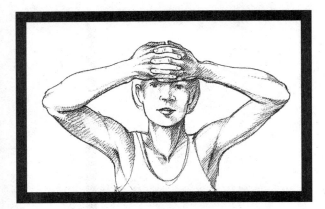

Figure 39

Shoulders

A GOOD SET OF SHOULDERS in a backless sundress is one of summertime's sassiest sights. With toned shoulders, you're virtually assured of a prouder bustline. You can banish round, stooped shoulders with the following workout.

Equipment: five-pound dumbbells (to start).

Overhead Press

Stand and grip a five-pound dumbbell in each hand, with your elbows bent so that your arms form Vs at your sides.

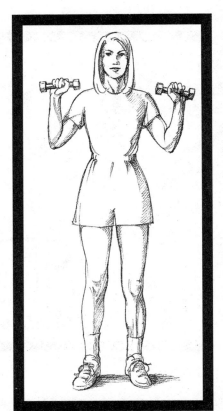

Figure 40

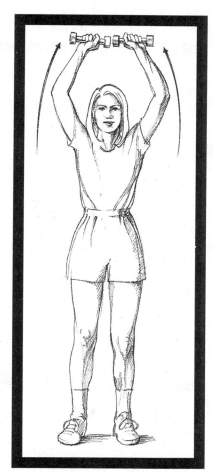

Figure 41

Thighs

THEY'RE SURELY THE FRONT-RUNNERS in the contest for least popular body parts. But thunder thighs were once assets—long ago, that is, lost in the mists of time.

Early in evolution, active women leading nomadic lives or working the fields needed Thor thighs that were powerful and agile, especially during pregnancy, when they had more weight to carry. Only the strongest-thighed survived.

Despite natural selection, you can still shape your thighs into limbs that are fit, firm and fine-looking.

What needs work are the quadriceps muscles, or quads, on the front of your upper legs. And here's how you can help your thighs shape up.

Equipment: two-pound ankle weights (to start).

Lunge

Stand in a well-balanced position, with your feet slightly more than hip-width apart. Step forward with your right leg, using as long a stride as possible (**Figure 42,** next page).

Keeping your trunk erect, lower yourself until your hip muscles begin to feel taut (**Figure 43**, next page).

When you've developed good flexibility in doing this exercise, you should be able to lightly touch the floor with the knee of your rear leg in a relaxed, slightly bent position. Shift your weight backward and take as many small steps as needed with your right leg to return to a standing position. Repeat with your left leg.

The dumbbells should be slightly more than shoulder-width apart, and your palms should face forward as shown in **Figure 40**.

Keeping your back straight, raise your arms and press the dumbbells up over your head so that the heads of the dumbbells touch at the top (**Figure 41**).

Be sure that you don't lean back while you're making this motion.

Slowly lower the dumbbells to the starting position, then repeat.

Do two sets of eight repetitions each. Then slowly increase to three sets of ten reps each, using ten-pound dumbbells.

Start with 3 repetitions per leg and work your way up to 20 reps per leg. To progress further, gradually work up to these three sets: 5 to 8 reps per leg for the first set; 10 reps per leg using five-pound dumbbells if you're a beginner or ten-pound dumbbells if you're at an intermediate level for the second set; and 15 to 20 reps per leg using five-pound dumbbells for the third set.

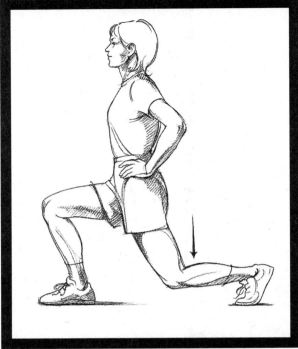

Figure 43

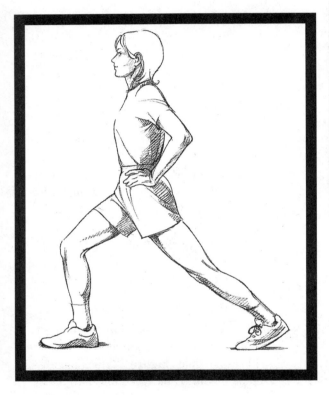

Figure 42

Leg Curl

Attach a two-pound ankle weight to each leg and stand facing a wall, with your feet about six inches apart (**Figure 44**). (To help keep your balance, touch the wall with your palms for support.) Bend your left knee and raise your left shin backward until it is approximately parallel to the floor or even slightly above the horizontal (**Figure 45**). Then slowly lower your leg to the floor.

Do one set of 4 repetitions, then repeat with your left leg. Gradually work your way up to 15 reps per leg, using five-pound ankle

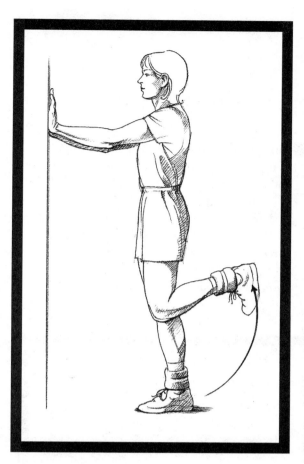

Figure 45

weights instead of the two-pounders. To progress further, build up to these three sets: 10 reps per leg with two-pound weights for the first set; 10 to 20 reps per leg with five-pound weights for the second set; and 20 to 25 reps per leg with the five-pounders for the third set.

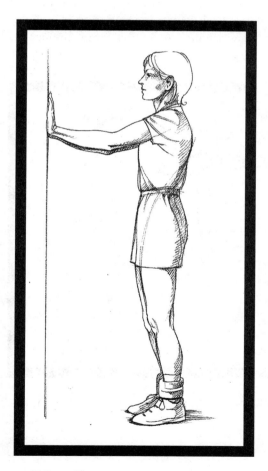

Figure 44

Triceps

THE MUSCLES along the back of your upper arms are called the triceps. If they become too flabby, though, some people might jokingly call them bat wings.

Good news, however: You can turn the back of your arms shapely fast, if you do the strength-building exercises described here.

Equipment: exercise bench, two-pound dumbbell (to start), five-pound dumbbell (to start).

Triceps Kickback

Stand with your right side next to a bench and hold a two-pound dumbbell in your left hand. Bending at your hips, lean forward and grasp the top edge of the bench with your right hand (**Figure 46**). Make sure your back is flat and parallel to the floor. Keeping your left foot flat on the floor, place your right knee along the edge of the bench as shown, making sure your knee is directly under your hip.

At the start, lift the dumbbell up to your side, squeezing your shoulder blades and bending your elbow up behind you as shown in **Figure 47**. Pause for a moment. Then move your forearm down, back and up in an arc, straightening your elbow as much as possible for maximum

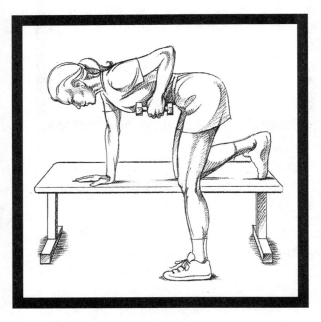

Figure 46

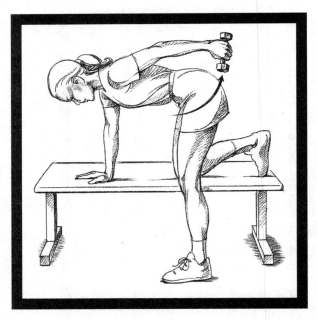

Figure 47

Triceps

results. The final position of the dumbbell should be well above the level of your back, but it should get there with lifting, not swinging. Slowly lower your arm to the starting point.

Do one set of 4 repetitions, then repeat with your right arm. Gradually increase the routine to 20 reps per arm using a five-pound dumbbell. To progress further, work up to three sets: 10 reps per arm with a five-pound dumbbell for the first set; 8 to 10 reps per arm with an eight-pound dumbbell for the second set; and 15 to 20 reps per arm with a five-pound dumbbell for the third set.

French Press

Standing with your feet shoulder-width apart, grasp one end of a five-pound dumbbell with both hands. Lift the dumbbell overhead, with both of your arms fully extended (**Figure 48**).

Slowly lower the dumbbell behind your head as far as possible, keeping your elbows pointed upward (**Figure 49**).

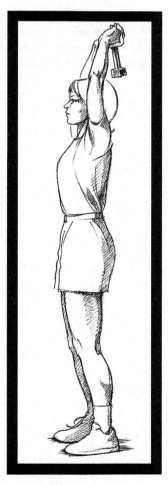

Figure 48

When you've lowered the dumbbell as far as you can, do not pause. Instead, begin to raise the dumbbell immediately, so your arms are once again extended. Pause for a second or so, then repeat.

Do one set of 4 repetitions to start. Gradually increase your weight to eight to ten pounds and your reps to 20. To progress, work up to three sets: 10 reps with an eight-pound dumbbell for the first set; 10 reps with a ten-pound dumbbell for the second set; and 15 to 20 reps with a five-pound dumbbell for the third set.

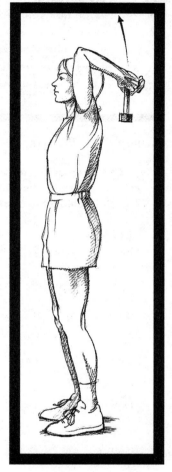

Figure 49

Aerobic Conditioning

AEROBIC EXERCISE IS AN ESSENTIAL ELEMENT of the total fitness picture. What fitness instructors call aerobic activity means 20 to 30 minutes of continuous exercise that significantly speeds up your heart rate and, because you're breathing and exercising steadily, sends an increased level of oxygen racing around the delivery route in your circulatory system. This kind of activity works your heart and your lungs, and it burns up fat. Most experts recommend doing it at least three times a week.

Where It Helps

This chart tells you which parts of your body are conditioned by various activities. Find the activity in the first column and the body parts that benefit from that activity in column 2. The third column lists other body parts that are conditioned, but to a lesser extent.

Activity	Conditions . . .	Also Conditions . . .
Ballroom dancing	Upper body (shoulders, arms, chest, back, waist, abdomen)	Lower body (hips, buttocks thighs, calves, ankles)
Biking	Hips, buttocks, thighs	
Boxing/boxercise	Upper and lower body	
Canoeing	Shoulders, back	Chest, abdomen, legs
Country line dancing	Lower body	
Cross-country skiing	Entire body	
Downhill skiing	Oblique muscles, buttocks, legs	Shoulders, arms, chest, back
Gardening	Shoulders, lower back, buttocks	Abdominals
Golfing	Lower body (if you don't use a golf cart)	Shoulders, arms, waist
Hiking	Midsection, lower body (hips, buttocks, thighs)	
Horseback riding	Back, lower abdominals, lower body	
Jumping rope	Wrists, lower body, calves, feet	Back, abdominals
Karate	Arms, hips, thighs, calves	
Race-walking	Lower body, oblique muscles	

Aerobic Conditioning

When it comes to building muscles, however, aerobics is the tortoise to toning's hare, says Canyon Ranch wellness education director Rebecca Gorrell. Aerobic activity doesn't target the muscles as directly as toning does. So if you rely solely on aerobic exercise to tone your muscles, it's a long haul. In their own slow fashion, though, various aerobic activities can help tone different parts of your body.

See also Muscular System

Activity	Conditions . . .	Also Conditions . . .
Rowing (on machine)	Entire body, especially arms, back, buttocks and legs	
Running	Midsection, lower body	
Scrubbing and polishing	Shoulders, chest, back	
Sculling	Entire body	
Skating	Lower body, especially the hips	
Slide (a plastic or rubber runner mat fitted with a hard plastic bumper at each end)	Hips, inner and outer thighs	
Stair climbing/ bench stepping	Lower body, especially the thighs	
Swimming	Entire body	
Tennis, squash	Playing arm, lower body	
Vacuuming	Shoulders, arms, lower body	
Volleyball	Entire body, especially the legs and oblique muscles	
Walking	Lower body	Lower abdominals

Five Super Videos

Good body alignment—proper form—is crucial if you want to prevent injury when you're doing strength training. While it may be best to learn from a skilled, certified class instructor, you don't have to, if you have guidance from a well-qualified instructor with a clear video program. Now there are a number of very good video training programs that demonstrate the proper technique for each exercise and help you avoid injury. You'll also discover ways to vary your routine and learn brand-new routines when you want to progress.

Here's a list of toning videos that are highly recommended by Carole Gorman-Swift, fitness director and owner of the fitness and dance studio Dancebeat in Haddonfield, New Jersey. Gorman-Swift is a certified aerobics instructor with a graduate degree in dance; she has been teaching dance aerobics since 1980.

Except for *Connie Love: Ultra Toner Workout*, these programs are usually available from video stores by special order or from Collage Video Specialties (1-800-433-6769).

Connie Love: Ultra Toner Workout, Beginner to Advanced

A top-notch fitness instructor, Love leads 30 exercises using an elastic exercise band. Although this is an instructional tape designed for fitness instructors, it is appropriate for beginners as well. Love demonstrates how to use the exercise band properly, and the exercises are simple and nonstrenuous. She understands the body's muscles and proper technique. Her cueing (words or motions the instructor uses to alert you to an upcoming change in movement) is perfect for both first-time exercisers and seasoned veterans. To order, call 1-800-222-7774.

Nike's Total Body Conditioning, Start-Up to Intermediate

Includes three step sequences and three slide sequences, mixed with elastic band exercises. (A slide is a plastic or rubber runner mat that is fitted with a plastic bumper at each end.) You can substitute dumbbells for the elastic band. For a great low-impact workout, follow along with the step and slide sections, which are adapted for people without equipment. The soundtrack is upbeat, and the three fitness experts—Donna Richardson, Andre Houle and Alison Lowe—are fun. The tape finishes with abdominal and stretch workouts.

Kathy Smith's Secrets—Upper or Lower Body, Intermediate

Two separate and terrific videos, beautifully filmed. They combine floor and standing free-weight routines. Every exercise is well-explained and well-filmed, so it's easy to follow. Smith adapts all exercises for all levels of ability. In each of the videos, she demonstrates using two different sets of weights—for example, three- and five-pound dumbbells.

Kari Anderson: Tone It Up,
Intermediate

Anderson, like Love, gives excellent cues, which makes it easier for you to follow along and learn a brand-new routine. This is a well-choreographed total body workout. When you order the tape, you get an elastic exercise band (Dyna-Band is the brand name), and Anderson shows how to use it in many exercises. Most of the upper-body toning exercises are choreographed with lower-body movements, so you combine aerobic work with toning. There's a lot of variety in the routines, too.

Molly Fox Shape Up! Total Body
Workout, Beginner to Intermediate

A friendly, top-notch teacher leads you through an inclusive upper- and lower-body workout using dumbbells and ankle weights. Recommended use: twice weekly. Fox, always upbeat, is excellent at explaining what to do and what to feel.

Index

Note: <u>Underscored</u> page references indicate boxed text. **Boldface** references indicate illustrations. *Italic* references indicate tables. Prescription drug names are denoted with the symbol Rx.

Abdominal aorta, **419**

Abdominal crunches

for muscle toning, 448, **448**, 450–51, **451**

for pelvic conditioning, 337

Abdominal fat, health risks from, 39, 64, 120–21

Abdominal muscles

back support from, 15

toning, <u>380</u>, 448, **448**, 450–51, **451**

Abdominal pain, from pancreatitis, 308

Acetaminophen

kidney damage from, 191

for pain relief, 11, <u>296</u>, <u>297</u>

Achilles tendon, 1–2, **1**

ACL tears, 197

Acne, 372–73

Acticipe R (Rx), for gum disease, 155

Acupressure, for pain relief, 293–94, **294**

Acupressure armband, for motion sickness, 87–88

Addison's disease, 3

Adhesions, pelvic, fallopian tube blockage from, 118

Adhesive capsulitis, 350–51

Adrenal cortex, <u>100</u>

Adrenal glands, 3, <u>100</u>, **101**, 182

Adrenaline, 3, <u>105</u>, 182

Advil. *See* Ibuprofen

Aerobics. *See* Exercise(s), aerobic

AFP screening, for birth defects, <u>311</u>

Age spots, 361

Aging, effect on

brain, 51–52

fertility, 142

spine, <u>383</u>

AHAs. *See* Alpha hydroxy acids

AIDS, 340, <u>344</u>, 345, 346

Airplane ear pain, <u>86</u>, <u>299</u>

Alcoholic beverages

breast cancer risk from, 64

breast lumps and, 55–56

as cause of

auto accidents, 379

decreased sexual desire, <u>338</u>

headaches, 299, 302, 303

increased stomach acid, 391

memory loss, <u>45</u>

folate absorption affected by, 32

heart disease prevention and, 175

pain and, 299, 302

Aleve, for pain relief, 181

Allergies, 356–57

asthma and, 208, 209

menstruation and, <u>239</u>

nasal polyps from, 263

Alpha-fetoprotein (AFP) screening, <u>311</u>

Alpha hydroxy acids (AHAs)

in lipstick, 203

for skin care, 370

Alveolar sac, **324**

Alveoli, **324**

Alzheimer's disease, 53

Amenorrhea, 246. *See also* Menstruation, cessation of

American Society for Reproductive Medicine, 146

Amniocentesis, for prenatal screening, <u>311</u>

Amoxicillin (Rx), for sinusitis, 355

Amoxil (Rx), for sinusitis, 355

Anemia, 30, <u>30</u>, 312

Anesthesia

for dental treatment, <u>301</u>

epidural, for childbirth, 74–75

Aneurysm, stroke from, 53

Anger, 94–95, <u>95</u>, 98, <u>176</u>, <u>340</u>

Ankle bones, **359**

Ankles, 3–5

slimming, <u>4</u>

sprains of, 4–5

strengthening, 3–4

Anovulation. *See* Ovulation, failure of

Antacids
   for heartburn, 107
   intestinal problems from, 184
   for ulcer pain, 391
Anterior cruciate ligament (ACL) tears, 197
Antibiotics, for sinusitis, 355
Antidepressants, tricyclic, for pain relief, <u>296</u>
Antihistamines, for allergies, 357
Anti-inflammatory medications. *See* Aspirin; Ibuprofen;
     Nonsteroidal anti-inflammatory drugs (NSAIDs)
Antioxidants
   benefits of, 271–73
   for preventing
      arterial disease, 8
      cataracts, 116–17
Antioxidant skin creams, 370
Antiperspirants, 417–18
Aorta, <u>80</u>, **81**
   abdominal, **419**
Apocrine glands, 396
Appendicitis, 5–6
Appendix, 5–6
Armpits, 417–18
   shaving, 37
Arms, toning exercises for, 452–53, **452–53**, 458–59,
     458–59, 464–65, **464–65**
Arteriosclerosis, 8
Artery(ies), 6–9
   blood clots in, 7, 53
   carotid, 7, <u>80</u>, **81**
   endometrial, **80**
   femoral, 7, **81**
   hardening of, 8
   narrowing of (*see* Atherosclerosis)
   preventing disease of, 8–9
   renal, **419**
   umbilical, **80**
Arthritis, 188–89
   osteoarthritis, 188, **188**
   rheumatoid, 180–81, 188–89, <u>358</u>
Artificial tears, for dry eyes, 399
Aspirin
   nasal polyps from, 263
   for pain relief, 11, <u>296</u>
   for preventing heart disease, 32, 176
   tinnitus from, 87
Astemizole (Rx), for allergies, 357

Asthma, 208–10, <u>209</u>, <u>210</u>, 211, <u>239</u>, <u>324</u>
Asthma inhalers, <u>209</u>, 210
Astringents, for skin care, 368
Astroglide, for vaginal dryness, <u>428</u>
Atherosclerosis, 7, 8
   from diabetes, 305
   heart disease from, 169
Atopic dermatitis, 373
Automobile safety, 379

Back. *See also* Spine
   anatomy of, <u>358</u>
   massage for, 292
Back pain, 9–18, <u>358</u>
   causes of, 10
   doctors who treat, <u>11</u>
   lifting and, 18, **18**
   low, 381
   posture and, <u>14</u>, **14**
   during pregnancy, <u>319</u>
   preventing, 15–17
   sexual positions and, 13
   sitting and, 17–18
   standing and, <u>14–15</u>
   treating with
      aspirin, 11
      bed rest, 13
      exercise, 13, 15
      spinal manipulation, <u>10</u>, 11, <u>11</u>, 13, <u>381</u>
      yoga, 12, **12**
Bactroban (Rx), for nasal lubrication, 261
Bad breath, <u>249</u>
Bangs, trimming, <u>163</u>
Barrier methods, of birth control, 20, 25, 343
Basal body temperature (BBT), as sign of ovulation,
     144, <u>286</u>
Basal cell cancer, 365
BBT, as sign of ovulation, 144, <u>286</u>
Beans
   fiber in, <u>278</u>, <u>279</u>
   iron in, 106
Bed boards, for back support, <u>17</u>
Bed rest, for back pain, 13
Belly button, 19
Bentyl (Rx), for diarrhea, 184
Benzoyl peroxide, for acne, 373

Beta-carotene
  as antioxidant, 271, 272
  for preventing
    arterial disease, 8
    breast cancer, 64
    lung cancer, 213
  sources of, 272
Biceps curls, for muscle toning, 452–53, **452–53**
Biceps muscle, **251**
Bicycle helmet, proper fit of, **378**
Bikini line, removing hair from, 35–37
Bilirubin levels, in blood tests, 32
Biofeedback, for pain relief, 298–99
Bioflavonoids, for breast tenderness, 63
Birth. *See* Childbirth
Birth centers, 69–70, 71
Birth control
  barrier methods, 20, 25, 345
  breastfeeding and, 78
  choosing method of, 20
  Depo-Provera, 20, 21, 23, 107, 245
  emergency methods of, 24
  intrauterine device, 19, 20, 21, 24–25, 24,
      143
  myths about, 19–25
  Norplant, 20, 21, 23
  in older women, 19–20
  during perimenopause, 227, 312
  Pill, the (*see* Birth control pills)
  sterilization, 19, 20–21, 21
  unplanned pregnancy and, 312–13
Birth control pills
  antibiotics and, 158
  breastfeeding and, 78
  conception after stopping, 24, 143
  for controlling heavy periods, 245
  effects of
    gum changes, 156
    heartburn, 106–7
    spotting, 244
    vaginal dryness, 428
    yeast infections, 429
  low-dose, as emergency contraception, 24
  during perimenopause, 227
  for protection against
    endometrial cancer, 323, 426
    ovarian cancer, 289, 323, 426

  for relieving menstrual symptoms, 242–43
  safety of, 19, 22–24
Birth defects
  folic acid for preventing, 271, 310–11
  prenatal screening for, 311
  from vitamin A excess, 272
Birthing rooms, 69–70
Birthmarks, 26
Black hairy tongue, 414
Blackheads, 372
Bladder, 26–28, 418, **419**
Bladder infections. *See* Urinary tract infections
      (UTIs)
Bleaching
  of body hair, 35
  of teeth, 405–6
Bleeding
  aspirin and, 296
  from fibroids, 422
  from hemorrhoids, 320, 321
  ibuprofen and, 296
  menstrual (*see* Menstruation)
  between periods, 243–44
Blisters, on feet, 133
Blood
  diseases of, 30–31
  functions of, 28–29
  maintaining health of, 29–32
Blood capillaries, **216**
Blood cholesterol test, 219
Blood clots, 7, 53, 431
Blood glucose levels, in blood tests, 32
Blood pressure. *See* High blood pressure
Blood pressure test, 218–19
Blood sugar levels, in blood tests, 32, 306
Blood tests, 32, 105, 218–19, 225–26
Blood transfusions, 29
Blood types, 29
Blood urea nitrogen (BUN) levels, in blood tests, 32
Blushes, 371, **371**
Body hair
  excess, from hormone imbalance, 37–38, 287
  removing with
    bleaching, 35
    depilatories, 37
    electrolysis, 35, 36
    shaving, 33, 37, 418

waxing, 33–34, <u>34</u>
underarm, 418
Body mass index, for measuring body fat, 123, *123*
Body shaping. *See* Body toning
Body toning, 43. *See also* Exercise(s); Weight training
  activities contributing to, *466–67*
  of individual muscles
    abdominals, <u>380</u>, 448, **448**, 450–51, **451**
    biceps, 452–53, **452–53**
    buttocks, 448–49, **448**, 454, **454**
    calves, 4, 455–56, **455–56**
    chest, 446–47, **446–47**, 456–57, **456–57**
    forearms, 458–59, **458–59**
    neck, 459–60, **459–60**
    shoulders, 446, **446**, 447, **447**, 461–62, **461–62**
    thighs, 448–49, **448**, 461–63, **462–63**
    triceps, 464–65, **464–65**
  Total Body-Shaping Workout for, 443–50
  videos for, <u>468–69</u>
Body type, 38–39, 42–43
  dressing for, <u>40–41</u>
Bone loss. *See* Osteoporosis
Bone marrow, <u>216</u>, **217**
Bone mineral density test, for assessing osteoporosis
    risk, 179, 229–30, <u>385</u>
Bones, broken. *See* Fractures
Bone scans, for detecting osteoporosis, 222–23, 224–25
Bonine, for Ménière's disease, <u>89</u>
Boric acid baths, for preventing yeast infections, 429
Boron, for memory, 49
Bowels, <u>83</u>
Bowel scintiscan, for detecting irritable bowel syn-
    drome, 225
Braces, orthodontic, <u>405</u>
Bradykinin, pain and, 291
Brain
  aging and, 51–53
  anatomy of, 45–46
  creativity and, <u>46–47</u>
  disorders of, 52–53
  factors causing memory loss, <u>45</u>
  female vs. male, 48–49, <u>258</u>
  functions of, 44–46
  hormones and, 47–48
  increasing power of, 49–51, <u>50–51</u>
  loss of cells in, 46–47
  regions of, **259**

Brain cells, 46–48, <u>258</u>
Brain stem, **259**
Bras
  to prevent breast sagging, 58
  proper fitting of, <u>55</u>
Braxton Hicks contractions, 73
Breakfast, 103
  food choices for, 103, 281
  skipping, <u>282–83</u>
Breast cancer, 60–61
  breastfeeding as protection against, 77
  detecting with
    mammography, 61, 62–63, 221–22
    RODEO, 224
  preventing with, 63–65
    fiber, <u>278</u>
    fruits and vegetables, 65, 280, <u>280</u>
    low-fat diet, 275
    soy products, 65, <u>281</u>
  risk factors for, 61–62
    birth control pills, 22
    hormone replacement therapy, 61, 65, 173–74,
      232, <u>233</u>
  survival rate for, 212
  treating, <u>57</u>, 61
Breastfeeding, 77–79
Breast implants, <u>60–61</u>
Breast lift surgery, 58
Breast reduction surgery, <u>56</u>
Breasts
  anatomy of, 54
  cysts in, 55
  examination of
    by health professional, 160, 221
    by self, <u>57</u>, <u>58–59</u>, 61, 62, 221
  fibroadenomas in, 55
  lumps in, 54–57
    discovery of, <u>57</u>
  pregnancy and, 315
  premenstrual tenderness in, <u>62–63</u>
  sagging, 57–58, 60, <u>250</u>
  toning muscles beneath, 456
Breathing
  asthma and, 208–10, 211
  for controlling hot flashes, 234
  diaphragmatic, 206, <u>324</u>
  for energy, 105

Breathing (continued)
   pursed-lip, 214–15
   for relaxation, 143, 206–7
   for vocal control, 201
   for weight lifting, 442
Breath test, for detecting ulcers, 225
Broken bones. See Fractures
Bronchi, 324, **325**
Bronchial tubes, 324, **325**
Bronchioles, **324**
Bronchitis, 210–11, 211, 324
   chronic, 214
Bruxism, 185, 186, 404
Bunions, 132, 133, 358
BUN levels, in blood tests, 32
Bursitis
   elbow, 92
   hip, 181
   knee, 195
Bustline, measuring, for bra fitting, 55
Butter
   saturated fat in, 171
   substitutes for, 279
Buttocks, toning exercises for, 448–49, **448**, 454,
      454

Caffeine
   breastfeeding and, 79
   breast lumps from, 57
   calcium absorption blocked by, 189, 231
   memory loss from, 45
Calcipotriene ointment (Rx), for psoriasis, 376
Calcium
   absorption of, 189, 231, 270–71
   food sources of, 269, 385
   high blood pressure and, 174
   for joints, 189
   menopausal requirement for, 236, 385
   parathyroid hormone and, 182
   pregnancy requirement for, 317
   for premenstrual syndrome, 241
   for preventing osteoporosis, 179, 269–71, 385
   in vitamin-mineral supplements, 272
Calcium supplements, 106, 179, 270, 270, 317
Calluses, on feet, 132
Calories, daily requirement for, 276

Calves
   pain in, from claudication, 9
   toning exercises for, 4, 455–56, **455–56**
Cancer. See also specific types; Tumors
   malignant moles, 246–47, 247
   preventing with
      beta-carotene, 64, 213
      exercise, 64
      fiber, 64, 278
      fish oil, 65
      folate, 345
      fruits and vegetables, 65, 280, 280
      low-fat diet, 308
      olive oil, 64–65
      soy products, 65, 281
Candida, yeast infections from, 427–28
Canker sores, 248–49, 248
Capillaries
   blood, **216**
   lymphatic, **216**
   renal, 419
   respiratory, **324**
Carbohydrates
   cravings for, 98
   for morning sickness, 315
   for premenstrual syndrome, 241
   as snacks, 103
Carbon dioxide levels, in blood tests, 32
Carotid arteries, 7, 80, **81**
Carpal bones, **359**
Carpal tunnel syndrome, 436–37, **436**
Car safety, 379
Cataracts, 116–17, 116
Cavities, dental, 403–4
CBC, 32
Cellulite, 126
Cerebellum, **259**
Cerebral cortex, 258, **259**
Cerebrum, **259**
Cervical cancer, 67
Cervical cap, for birth control, 25
Cervical dysplasia, 66
Cervical mucus, at ovulation, 286
Cervical nerves, 258, **259**
Cervicitis, 66
Cervix, 66–67, **322**, 323, **323**
Cesarean sections, 68, 77

Chemical peels, for wrinkles, 367

Chest, toning exercises for, 446–47, **446–47**, 456–57, **456–57**

Chest pain, from heart problems, <u>107</u>

Childbirth. *See also* Pregnancy

  cesarean section for, <u>68</u>, 77

  choosing health professional for, 68–69, <u>68</u>

  choosing setting for, 69–71, <u>71</u>

  episiotomy for, <u>68</u>, 75–77

  pain relief for, 74–75

  resuming sex after, <u>76</u>

  support persons for, <u>69</u>

Childbirth preparation classes, 71–73

Chin, 79

Chiropractors, back treatments by, <u>10</u>, 11, <u>11</u>, <u>381</u>

Chlamydia, 343, <u>344</u>

Chloride levels, in blood tests, <u>32</u>

Cholesterol, dietary, sources of, 171

Cholesterol, serum

  HDL, 9, 169–70, 231

  LDL, 169–70, 231

  lowering, 171–74, <u>278</u>

  risk ratio of, <u>169</u>, 170

  testing, 219

Chorionic villi sampling (CVS), for prenatal screening, <u>311</u>

Chronic obstructive pulmonary disease (COPD), 214–15

Chronic pain, 292, 295

Cigarettes. *See* Smoking

Cingulate gyrus, **259**

Circulatory system, <u>80–81</u>

Cirrhosis, 204–5

Claritin (Rx), for allergies, 357

Claudication, exercise therapy for, 9

Clavicle, **359**

Clitoris, 82

  orgasm and, 333, 334, 336

Clomiphene citrate (Rx), for inducing ovulation, 144

Clotrimazole, for yeast infections, 429

Clots, blood, 7, 53, 431

Cluster headaches, 303

Coal-tar products, for psoriasis, 375

Coccydynia, 397

Coccyx, **359**, 397

Codeine (Rx), for pain relief, <u>296</u>

Coffee, iron absorption and, 106

Colds, 355–56, <u>356</u>

Cold sores, 203–4, <u>239</u>

Collagen injections, for wrinkles, 366–67, <u>366</u>

Collarbone, 82

Colon cancer

  fiber for preventing, <u>278</u>

  tests for, 223–24

Complete blood count (CBC), <u>32</u>

Compression stockings, for varicose veins, 433–34

Computed tomography (CT) scans, for heart disease screening, 226

Computer use

  carpal tunnel syndrome and, 436–37, **436**

  eyestrain from, 112–13

  sitting posture for, 351, **351**, 352

Conception, timing of, 141

Concussion, 378

Conditioners, hair, 164–65

Condoms

  for birth control, 20, 25

  damage to, <u>428</u>

  female, <u>345</u>

  how to use, <u>342</u>

  for preventing sexually transmitted diseases, 25, 341, 343, 345

  yeast infections from, 429

Congestion, nasal, 352–57

Conjunctivitis, 113–14

Conscious sedation, for dental treatment, <u>301</u>

Contact dermatitis, 373–74

Contact lenses

  eye infection from, 114

  types of, <u>109</u>, 112

Contraception. *See* Birth control

Contractions, labor vs. Braxton Hicks, 73

Contraction stress test, for fetal monitoring, <u>311</u>

Cooldown stretches, in Total Body-Shaping Workout, 443, 449–50, **449–50**

COPD, 214–15

Corns, 132, **132**

Cortisol, 3, 182

Cortisone (Rx), for hip bursitis, 181

Cosmetics, 370–71

Cosmetic surgery. *See* Plastic surgery

Cough, smoker's, 214

Cough medicines, for bronchitis, 211

Cracking knuckles, <u>166</u>

Cramps, menstrual, 242–43
 ibuprofen for, 297
Cranberry juice, for preventing bladder infections, 27
Cranium, 359, **359**, 377
Cravings, food
 depression and, 98
 during pregnancy, 317
Creatinine levels, in blood tests, 32
Creativity, enhancing, 46–47
Cross-training, for preventing arthritis, 196–97
Cruciferous vegetables, cancer protection from, 280
Crunches, abdominal
 for muscle toning, 448, **448**, 450–51, **451**
 for pelvic conditioning, 337
CT scans, for heart disease screening, 226
Cushing's syndrome, 3, 100
Cuticles, 148
CVS, for prenatal screening, 311
Cystitis. *See also* Urinary tract infections (UTIs)
 interstitial, 28
Cysts
 breast, 55
 ovarian, 287
 in polycystic kidney disease, 191, 191
 wrist, 437

Dalkon Shield, pelvic infection from, 25
Dandruff, 328, 330
Decongestants
 for airplane ear pain, 299
 for sinusitis, 354
Deep-vein thrombosis, 431
Deltoid muscle, **251**
Dental floss, 155
Dentistry, pain-free, 300–301
Deodorant, 418
Depilatories, for hair removal, 37
Depo-Provera
 for birth control, 20, 21, 23
 for controlling heavy periods, 245
 heartburn from, 107
 spotting from, 244
Depression, 96–97, 98
 during pregnancy, 316
DeQuervain's disease, 437

Dermatitis
 atopic, 373
 contact, 373–74
 seborrheic, 328, 330
Dermis, sun damage to, 361
Dermoid tumors, 287
Deviated septum, 266
DEXA, for detecting bone loss, 224–25, 231
Diabetes, 100
 bladder infections with, 27
 exercise and, 307–8, 307
 gestational, 305, 310
 glucose monitoring for, 225–26
 preventing, 307–8
 risk factors for, 306–7
 types of, 304–5, 305
Diaphragm, **325**
 breathing from, 206, 324
 strengthening, for sexual pleasure, 336–37
Diaphragm, contraceptive, 20, 25
 for preventing sexually transmitted diseases, 67, 343
Diarrhea, 183, 184
Dicyclomine hydrochloride (Rx), for diarrhea, 184
Diet
 low-fat (*see* Low-fat diet)
 for menopause, 233, **235**, 236
 for premenstrual syndrome, 240–41
Dieting. *See* Weight loss
Diflucan (Rx), for yeast infections, 428–29
Digestive system, 83
Digital rectal exam, for detecting colon cancer, 161, 223
Dimenhydrinate, for Ménière's disease, 89
Disks, spinal, 258, **359**, 381–82, 386
Dizziness, causes of, 52
Doctors, choosing male vs. female, 222
DONA, 69
Douching
 before Pap smear, 161, 162
 pelvic inflammatory disease from, 118–19
 yeast infections from, 429
Doulas, for childbirth support, 69
Doulas of North America (DONA), 69
Dovonex (Rx), for psoriasis, 376
Dowager's hump, 381, 384
Down's syndrome
 maternal age and risk of, 310
 screening for, 311

Dramamine, for Ménière's disease, <u>89</u>

Dramamine II, for motion sickness, 88

Dressing, according to body type, <u>40–41</u>

Drugs. *See* Medications

Dry eyes, 398–99

Dry mouth, 327

Drysol (Rx), for excessive sweating, 396

Dual energy x-ray absorptiometry (DEXA), for detecting bone loss, 224–25, 231

Dyes, hair, 165

Dyspepsia, <u>83</u>, 390

Dysplasia, cervical, 66

Ear infections, 84–86

Ear pain, from flying, <u>86</u>, <u>299</u>

Ear piercing, risks of, <u>90–91</u>

Ears, 84–91

    cosmetic surgery for, <u>88</u>

    motion sickness and, 87–88

    ringing in, 86–87

Ear wax removal, <u>84–85</u>

Eccrine glands, 395–96

Ectomorphs, 39

Ectopic pregnancy, <u>119</u>

    birth control pills and, 22

    from chlamydia, 343

Eczema, <u>239</u>, 373–74

Elbow joint, **359**

Elbows, 92–93

Electrolysis, for hair removal, 35, <u>36</u>

Emergency contraception, <u>24</u>

Emotions, 93–99

    anger, 94–95, <u>95</u>, 98

    depression, <u>96–97</u>, 98

    jealousy, 99

    during pregnancy, 315–17

    sense of smell and, <u>262</u>

    sex and, 337, <u>338</u>

Emphysema, 214

E-Mycin (Rx), for sinusitis, 355

Endocrine system, <u>100–101</u>

Endometrial artery, **80**

Endometrial cancer, 22, 145, <u>323</u>, 422–23, 426

Endometrial tissue sample, 220–21

Endometrial vein, **80**

Endometriosis, 118, 145, 287–88, <u>322–23</u>

Endometritis, 145

Endometrium, **322**, <u>322–23</u>, **323**

Endomorphs, 39

Endorphin, as painkiller, 292, 293

Energy, 102–6

    eating for, 102–4, <u>103</u>

    exercise for, 104–5

    iron intake and, 105–6

Enkephalin, as painkiller, 292

Epidermis, sun damage to, 361

Epidural anesthesia, for childbirth, 74–75

Epiglottis, **198**

Episiotomy, <u>68</u>, 75–77

Epithelial tumor, 423

Erythromycin (Rx), for sinusitis, 355

Esophagus, **83**, 106–7, **198**, **325**

Estrogen, <u>100</u>. *See also* Hormone replacement therapy (HRT)

    in birth control pills, 22

    body fat and, 120

    bone loss and, 178

    brain cells and, 48

    breast cancer and, 61–62, 64, 65, 173–74, 232, <u>233</u>

    breast lumps from, 56

    endometrial cancer and, 423

    foods to replace, 233

    in menstrual cycle, <u>238</u>

    ovulation and, 286

    production of, 182

    side effects of, <u>234</u>

    topical, for vaginal dryness, 235

Estrogen replacement therapy. *See* Hormone replacement therapy (HRT)

Evening primrose oil, for breast tenderness, <u>63</u>

Exams. *See* Eye exams, frequency of; Gynecological exam; Medical tests

Exercise-induced asthma, <u>209</u>

Exercise(s)

    aerobic, 441, 466–67

        fat burning from, 127, 129

        for preventing breast cancer, 64

        for reducing stress, 392–93, 394

        step, avoiding Achilles tendon injury in, **2**

    ankle-strengthening, 3–4

    asthma and, <u>209</u>, 210

    for back health, 382–83

    brain activity and, 49–50

Exercise(s) *(continued)*
  breastfeeding and, 79
  calf-strenghthening, 4
  calories burned from, *128*
  cooldown, 443, 449–50, **449–50**
  diabetes and, 307–8, <u>307</u>
  eye, 112
  facial, 364
  for fatigue, 105–6
  for heart conditioning, 170–71, <u>170</u>
  hip pain and, 181
  jaw, 187
  Kegel, 236, 336, <u>419</u>, <u>420</u>
  kneecap pain from, 194
  knee-strengthening, <u>193</u>, 194
  lung disease and, 214
  during menopause, 233, **235**, 236
  neck, 79, <u>253</u>
  pelvic, 337
  during pregnancy, 317–18, 320
  for preventing
    arterial disease, 9
    breast cancer, 64
    osteoporosis, 179, 229
  pubococcygeal, for sexual pleasure, 335–36
  for reducing blood pressure, 176
  for relieving
    back pain, 12, **12**, 13, 15
    claudication, 9
    joint pain, 189
    menstrual cramps, 243
    premenstrual syndrome, <u>242</u>
    sinusitis, 355
  scents and, <u>264–65</u>
  shinsplints from, 347
  shoulder, <u>349</u>, **349**, 350–51
  spinal disks and, 386
  stretching (*see* Stretching)
  toning (*see* Body toning; Weight training)
  varicose veins and, 434
  walking (*see* Walking)
  warm-up, 2, 347, 443, 444–45, **444–45**
  for weight control, 285
  for weight loss, 126–27, *128*, 129–30, <u>282</u>
  yoga (*see* Yoga)
Exercise stress test, for detecting heart disease, 219–20
External oblique muscle, **251**

Eyebrow plucking, <u>117</u>
Eye debris, removing, 114–15
Eyedrops, for dry eyes, 399
Eye exams, frequency of, 115–16
Eyeglasses
  choosing, <u>111</u>, 112
  nasal congestion and, 355
Eye infections, 113–14
Eye makeup, 371
Eyes, 108–17
  dry, 398–99
Eyestrain, from computer work, 112–13

Facet joints, aging and, <u>383</u>
Facial bones, 378
Facial hair, removal of, 33–35
Fainting, causes of, 52
Fallopian tubes, 118–19, 145, **322**, **323**
Farsightedness, 108–10
Fat, body. *See also* Obesity; Overweight
  abdominal, health risks from, 39, 64, 120–21
  cellulite, <u>126</u>
  genetic influence on, 121–22
  health risks from, 120–21
  hormones and, 120
  liposuction for removing, <u>124</u>
  measuring, 122–24
Fat, dietary
  breast lumps and, 56
  calories from, 267, 275
  cancer risk from, 63–64, 275
  daily allowance of, <u>277</u>
  guidelines for cutting, 275–77, 279
  heart disease and, 274
  top five sources of, <u>275</u>
  types of, 171
Fat cells, 121
Fat-free foods, overeating, <u>282</u>
Fatigue
  eating to overcome, 102–4, <u>103</u>
  exercise to overcome, 105–6
  from iron deficiency, 105–6
Fecal occult blood test, 223
Feet, 131–40. *See also* Toenails
FemCare, for yeast infections, 429
Femoral artery, 7, **81**

Femoral neck bone, <u>358</u>, **359**
  fracture of, <u>178</u>, <u>358</u>
Femur, **359**
Ferritin test, serum, for measuring iron level, 105
Fertility, 141–46. *See also* Infertility
  threats to, 142–43
Fetal monitoring, <u>311</u>
Fever, medication for, <u>297</u>
Fever blisters, 203–4
Fiber
  health benefits of, <u>278–79</u>
  for lowering cholesterol, 171–72, <u>172</u>, <u>278</u>
  for preventing
    cancer, 64, <u>278</u>
    hemorrhoids, 321
  sources of, <u>278–79</u>
Fibroadenomas, breast, 55
Fibroids, uterine, 145, 245, 422, **422**
  treating, 245, <u>424</u>
Fibula, **359**
Figure four stretch, as cooldown exercise, 449,
  449
Fimbria, **322**
Finger bones, **359**
Fingernails, 146–50
Finger swelling, <u>167</u>
Fish, for preventing
  breast cancer, 65
  heart disease, 171
Fissured tongue, 415
Flat shoes, for Achilles tendon flexibility, 1, 2
Flatulence, 183, 184
Floss, dental, <u>155</u>
Flu, bronchitis vs., <u>211</u>
Fluconazole (Rx), for yeast infections, 428–29
Fluoride, for preventing tooth decay, 402–3
Folate. *See also* Folic acid
  absorption of, affected by alcohol, 32
  for healthy blood, 31
  for preventing
    arterial disease, 8–9
    cervical cancer, 345
  sources of, 271, 345
Folic acid, 67, 271, 310–11, 345. *See also* Folate
Follicles, ovulation and, 286
Follicle-stimulating hormone test, for detecting
  menopause, 229

Food cravings
  depression and, 98
  during pregnancy, 317
Food labels, fat content on, 276–77
Food poisoning, <u>389</u>
Foot, Achilles tendon and, 1–2
Foot bones, **359**
Foot massage, <u>138–39</u>
Foot odor, <u>140</u>
Foot pain
  causes of, 131–33, 136–37, 139
  preventing, 139–40
Footwear. *See* Shoes
Forearms, toning exercises for, 458–59, **458–59**
Fornix, **259**
Foundation makeup, 371
Fractures
  hip, 177, 178, <u>178</u>, 222, <u>358</u>
  pelvic, 309
  rib, 326
  skull, 378–79
  spinal, <u>384</u>
  tailbone, 397
Freckles, as birthmarks, 26
Free radicals, antioxidants and, 271–72
French press, for toning triceps, 465, **465**
Fructose, intestinal problems from, 183
Fruits
  fiber in, <u>279</u>
  increasing intake of, 281, 284
  intestinal problems from, 183
  for preventing
    arterial disease, 8
    cancer, 65, 280, <u>280</u>
    cataracts, 116–17
  protective compounds in, 280, 281
Fungus
  nail, <u>147</u>
  toenail, 410–11
  tongue, 414

Gallbladder, <u>83</u>, **83**, 151–53
Gallstones, <u>83</u>, 151–53
Gamete intrafallopian transfer (GIFT), for infertility,
  144
Ganglia, <u>437</u>

Gas, intestinal, 183, 184
Gastritis, 390
Gastrocnemius, toning exercises for, 455–56,
    455–56
Genital warts, 66, 67, 344–45
Geographic tongue, 414
Gestational diabetes, 305, 310
GIFT, for infertility, 144
Ginger
    for morning sickness, 315
    for nausea, 88
Gingivitis, 154, 239
Glasses. *See* Eyeglasses
Glaucoma, 115
Glossitis, 414–15
Glucose monitoring, for diabetes, 225–26
Gluteus maximus, toning exercises for, 448–49, **448**,
    454, **454**
Gluteus muscle, **251**
Gonadotropin-releasing hormone (GnRH)
    for gynecologic problems, 424
    ovulation and, 286
Gonorrhea culture, 344
G-spot, orgasm and, 333, 334
Gum, sugarless
    cavity prevention from, 403
    intestinal problems from, 183–84
Gum disease, 154–58, 239
Gum pockets, 156–57
Gums, 154–59. *See also* Teeth
Gynecological exam, 159–62, 220–21, 289,
    426
Gynecologic oncologists, how to find, 290, 426
Gyne-Lotrimin, for yeast infections, 429

Hair, 162–65
    body (*see* Body hair)
    trimming, 163
Hair coloring, 165
Halitosis, 249
Hammertoes, 132
Hand bones, **359**
Hands, 165–67. *See also* Fingernails
Hardening of the arteries, 8
HDL cholesterol. *See* High-density lipoprotein (HDL)
    cholesterol

Headaches
    acupressure for, 293–94
    causes of
        alcohol, 299, 302, 303
        specific foods, 299, 302, 303
        stress, 302–3
    cluster, 303
    medication for, 297
    migraine, 299, 302–3
    tension, 250, 302
Head injury, 378–79
Hearing, 84
Hearing loss, 90–91
Heart, 80, **81**, 168–76
    exercise for conditioning, 170–71, 170
    functions of, 168
Heart attacks, 168, 169
    from blood clots, 7
    hostile personality and, 176
Heartburn, 83, 106–7. *See also* Reflux
    sore throat from, 407
Heart disease
    causes of, 169
    chest pain from, 107
    diabetes and, 305
    hormone replacement therapy and, 232, 233
    incidence of, 168
    menopause and, 228, 229, 231
    preventing, 170–76, 278
    risk factors for, 175
    screening for, 226
Heel pain, 136–37, 139
    acupressure for, 294, **294**
Heel raise, for calf toning, 455, **455**
Helicobacter pylori, ulcers from, 225, 390, 391
Helmet, bicycle, proper fit of, **378**
Hemophilia, 31
Hemorrhoids, 320–21
Hepatitis, 204, 205, 205
Hepatitis B, pregnancy and, 314
Hernia, umbilical, 19
Herniated disks, 382, 386
Herpes simplex Type I virus, cold sores from, 203–4
High blood pressure
    diet therapy for, 174
    effects of
        cardiovascular disease, 80

kidney damage, 191
  memory loss, <u>45</u>, 52
  nosebleeds, 261
exercise for lowering, 9, 176
during pregnancy, <u>310</u>
from stress, 175–76
testing of, 218–19
High-density lipoprotein (HDL) cholesterol, 9, 169–70, 231
High heels
  Achilles tendon affected by, 1–2, **2**
  back pain from, <u>15</u>
  hip problems from, 180–81
Hip
  arthritis of, 180–81
  bursitis of, 181
Hip extension, for toning buttocks, 454, **454**
Hip fractures, 177, 178, <u>178</u>, 222, <u>358</u>
Hip joint, **359**
Hip replacement surgery, <u>180</u>
Hips, 177–81
Hirsutism, 37–38, 287
Hismanal (Rx), for allergies, 357
HIV. *See* Human immunodeficiency virus
Hoarseness, 198–201, <u>200</u>, <u>239</u>
Homocysteine, arterial disease and, 8
Horizontal chest press, for muscle toning, 456–57, **456–57**
Hormone replacement therapy (HRT)
  breast cancer risk from, 61, 65, 173–74, 232, <u>233</u>
  gallstones from, 152
  after hysterectomy, <u>338</u>, 426
  investigating, 426
  for lowering cholesterol, 173–74, <u>233</u>
  during menopause, <u>100</u>, <u>230</u>, 231–32
  for preventing
    heart disease, 232, <u>233</u>
    osteoporosis, 179–80, <u>385</u>
  progesterone in, 423, 426
  side effects of, <u>234</u>
  uterine cancer from, 231–32, <u>234</u>
  for vaginal dryness, <u>428</u>
Hormones. *See also specific hormones*
  adrenal, 3
  body fat and, 120
  brain cells and, 47–48
  as cause of
    acne, 372, 373

  excess body hair, 37–38
  gum changes, 155–56
  formation of, 182
  role of, in ovulation, 144–45
Hose, support, for varicose veins, 433–34
Hostility, heart attacks and, <u>176</u>
Hot flashes, 227–28
  controlling, 234
HPV. *See* Human papillomavirus
HRT. *See* Hormone replacement therapy
Human immunodeficiency virus (HIV), 340, <u>344</u>, 345–46
Human papillomavirus (HPV), 66, 67, 344–45
Humerus, **359**
Hyperhidrosis, 396
Hypertension. *See* High blood pressure
Hyperthyroidism, 408–9, <u>408</u>
Hypothalamus, **259**
Hypothyroidism, 409, <u>409</u>
Hysterectomy, 423, <u>424–25</u>
  sexual desire and, <u>338</u>
Hysterosalpingography, 145

Ibuprofen
  kidney damage from, 191
  for treating
    back pain, 11
    bronchitis, 211
    dental pain, <u>301</u>
    menstrual pain, 242, <u>424</u>
    pain, <u>296</u>, <u>297</u>
    shoulder pain, 350
ICSI, for infertility, <u>144</u>
Immunization, after spleen removal, 388
Imodium A-D, for diarrhea, 184
Impingement syndrome, 348, 350
  exercises for preventing, <u>349</u>, **349**
Incontinence, stress
  Kegel exercises for, <u>419</u>, <u>420</u>
  in menopause, 235–36
Indigestion, 390
Infections. *See specific infections*
Infertility
  assisted reproduction methods for, <u>144</u>
  causes of, <u>142–43</u>, 144–45, 287, 343
  help for, 145–46

Ingrown toenails, 410, **410**, 411, **411**
Inhalers, asthma, 209, 210
Inhibited sexual desire, 340
Insomnia
    menstruation and, 239
    pain and, 298
Insulin, 100, 182, 304, 305, 306
Interstitial cystitis, 28
Intestines, **83**, 183–84
Intrauterine device (IUD)
    for birth control, 19, 20, 21, 24–25, 24
    safety of, 24–25
    sexually transmitted diseases and, 143
Introcytoplasmic sperm injection (ICSI), for infertility, 144
In vitro fertilization (IVF), for infertility, 144
Iontophoresis, for excessive sweating, 396
Iron, sources of, 30, 105–6, 273
Iron-deficiency anemia, 30, 30, 312
Iron supplements, 106, 273
Irritable bowel syndrome, 225
Itching
    from eczema, 373–74
    from hemorrhoids, 321
    from prickly heat, 396
    from vaginitis, 322, 427, 429
    vulval, 435
IUD. *See* Intrauterine device
IVF, for infertility, 144

Jaw, 185–87
Jealousy, 99
Joints, 187–89
    care of, 189
    painful conditions of, 188–89
    types of, 187–88 *(see also specific joints)*
Jugular veins, **81**

Kegel exercises, 236, 336, 419, 420
Keratoconjunctivitis sicca, dry eye from, 398
Kidney failure, 191
Kidney infections, 27, 190
Kidneys, 190–91, 418, **419**
Kidney stones, 190, 418
Kneecap, 192, 194, **359**

Knee joint, 358, **359**
Knees, 192–97
    anatomy of, 192
    anterior cruciate ligament tears in, 197
    bursitis of, 195
    pain in, 192, 194–95, 250
        acupressure for, 294, **294**
    preventing arthritis of, 195–97
    strengthening exercises for, 193, 194
    stretching exercises for, 196
    tendinitis of, 195
Knuckles, cracking, 166
Kyphosis, 381

Labels, food, fat content on, 276–77
Labia majora, 435
Labia minora, 435
Labor. *See also* Childbirth
    preparation for, 71–74
    stages of, 73, **74–75**
Labyrinthitis, 88–89
La Leche League International, 77
Laparoscopy
    for gallbladder removal, 153
    for hysterectomy, 425
Laryngeal cancer, 199, 200
Laryngitis, 198–201, 200, 239, 324
Larynx, 197–201, **198**, 324, **325**
Laser surgery, for removing
    facial blood vessels, 432
    port-wine stains, 26
    wrinkles, 368
Lateral shoulder raise, for muscle toning, 447, **447**
Latissimus dorsi, 250, **251**
Laughing gas, for dental treatment, 301
LDL cholesterol, 169–70, 231
Leg curl, for toning thighs, 463, **463**
Leg lifts, reverse, for pelvic conditioning, 337
Legumes, fiber in, 278, 279
LES, heartburn and, 106, 107
Leukemia, 30–31, 216
Lifting techniques, for preventing back strain, 18, **18**
Limbic system, 258, **259**, 262
Lip balm, 202
Lip cancer, 204
Lipids. *See* Fat, dietary

Lip liner, 371

Liposuction, for removing fat, 124

Lips, 201–4

Lipstick, 203, 371, 404

Liquor. *See* Alcoholic beverages

Liver, **83**, 204–5

Liver spots, on hands, 166

Loperamide hydrochloride, for diarrhea, 184

Loratadine (Rx), for allergies, 357

Lordosis, 381

Low back pain, 381

Low-density lipoprotein (LDL) cholesterol, 169–70, 231

Lower esophageal sphincter (LES), heartburn and, 106, 107

Low-fat diet
   guidelines for, 275–77, 279
   for preventing
      cancer, 308
      heart disease, 229, 273–75
   switching to, 283

Lubricants, vaginal, 235

Lucy Peters, International, 36

Lumbar nerves, **259**

Lumpectomy, for breast cancer, 57, 61

Lunch, skipping, 282–83

Lung cancer, 212–14

Lunge, for toning thighs, 461–62, **462**

Lungs, 206–15
   asthma and, 208–10, 209, 210, 211
   breathing and, 206–7
   bronchitis and, 210–11, 211
   obstructive diseases of, 214–15
   pneumonia and, 215
   tuberculosis and, 215

Lupus, 188, 239

Luteinizing hormone, ovulation and, 286

Lying side stretch, as cooldown exercise, 450, **450**

Lymph, 216

Lymphatic capillaries, **216**

Lymphatic system, **216**, **217**

Lymph nodes, **217**

Lymphocytes, 216, **216**

Magnesium
   high blood pressure and, 174
   for premenstrual syndrome, 241

Makeup, 370–71

Malaria, 31

Mammography, for detecting breast cancer, 61, 62–63, 221–22, 222

Mammoplasty, reduction, 56

Mandible, **359**

Manicures, 149, **149**

Margarine, trans fats in, 171

Massage
   back, 292
   foot, 138–39
   neck, 292–93, **293**
   for pain relief, 292–93, **293**
   scalp, 328–29, **328**, **329**
   for sexual pleasure, 339
   shoulder, 293, **293**

Mastectomy, for breast cancer, 57, 61

Mastopexy, for sagging breasts, 58, 60

Mattresses, replacing, 17

Meat
   iron in, 105–6
   for morning meal, 103

Meclizine hydrochloride
   for Ménière's disease, 89
   for motion sickness, 88

Medical tests
   blood tests, 32, 105, 218–19, 225–26
   bone tests, 222–23, 224–25
   breast examinations, 221–222, 224
   colon cancer tests, 223–24
   for detecting
      heart disease, 226
      irritable bowel syndrome, 225
      ulcers, 225
   exercise stress tests, 219–20
   gynecological tests, 159–62, 220–21
   prenatal screening, 311

Medications. *See also specific medications*
   effects of
      bone thinning, 179
      dry eyes, 398
      heartburn, 106, 107
      ulcers, 391
   during pregnancy, 311–12
   sexual desire and, 338

Melanoma, 247, **247**, 365–66

Memory, improving, 49, 50–51

Memory loss
   from Alzheimer's disease, 53
   causes of, 45
Ménière's disease, 89, 89
Menopause, 227–36
   bladder infections after, 27
   diet for, 233, **235**, 236
   estrogen depletion during, 227, 228
   exercise during, 233, **235**, 236
   heart disease risk and, 228, 229, 231
   hormone replacement therapy during (see Hormone
      replacement therapy)
   hot flashes during, 227–28
   osteoporosis risk and, 178, 222, 223, 228, 229,
      230–31, 231, 384
   premature, 142, 143, 228–29
   symptoms of, 227–28, **228**
   timing of, 228–29
Menstrual cycle, 237–46. See also Menstruation
   changes in, 243–44, 244
   events of, 238
   fertile days of, 141
   pelvic exam and, 162
   tracking individual differences in, 238–40
   vocal cords affected by, 197–98
Menstrual period, 237. See also Menstrual cycle;
      Menstruation
Menstruation. See also Menstrual cycle
   birth control pills and, 22
   cessation of, 228, 246, 287, 426 (see also
      Menopause)
   cramps during, 242–43
   diarrhea during, 184
   health effects of, 239
   heavy, 244–46, 422
   light, 422
   premenstrual syndrome and (see Premenstrual
      syndrome)
Mesomorphs, 39
Metacarpals, **359**
Metatarsals, **359**
Miconazole, for yeast infections, 429
Micronutrients
   shortage of, 269
   sources of, 273
Midlife. See Menopause
Midwives. See Nurse midwives

Migraines, 299, 302–3
Mineral oil, for psoriasis, 375
Minerals, 268–73, 274. See also specific minerals and
      vitamins
Mittelschmerz, as sign of ovulation, 286
Moisturizers
   for eczema, 374
   for preventing wrinkles, 369–70
   for psoriasis, 375
Moles, 26, 246–47, 247
Monistat 7, for yeast infections, 429
Morning sickness, 314–15, 389
Morphine (Rx), for pain relief, 296
Motion sickness, 87–88, 389
Motor areas of brain, 258, **259**
Motrin. See Ibuprofen
Mountain pose, for back pain, 12, **12**
Mouth, 248–49
Mouth cancer, 248, 415
Mouth sores, 248–49, 248
Mouthwashes, antibacterial, 156, 158
Mucus
   cervical, at ovulation, 286
   for diagnosing nasal problems, 357
Multi supplements, 272, 274
Mupirocin (Rx), for nasal lubrication, 261
Muscle, calorie burning by, 442
Muscle pain, relieving, 295, 297
Muscle toning. See also Body toning
   for sexual pleasure, 335–37
Muscular system, 250, **251**
Mustache removal, 33–35
Myomectomy, for fibroids, 245, 424

Nail biting, 148
Nail care, 137, 147–50
Nail fungus, 147
Nails. See Fingernails; Toenails
Naproxen, for pain relief, 181
Narcotics, for pain relief, 296–97
Nasal congestion, 352–57
Nasal sprays, rebound problems from, 354–55
National Psoriasis Foundation, 375
Nausea, 389
   during pregnancy, 314–15
Navel, 19

Nearsightedness, 108–10, _110_
Neck, _250_, **251**, 252–57
    desk work and, 254–55
    exercises for, 79, _253_
    massage for, 292–93, **293**
    overtwisting of, _254_
    painful, 252–54, 351
    sleep and, 255
    stiff, 255–56
    toning exercises for, 459–60, **459–60**
    whiplash injury to, _250_, 256–57
    wrinkling of, 257
Neck press, for muscle toning, 459–60, **459–60**
Nerves, _258_, **259**
Nervous system, _258_, **259**
Neural tube defects
    folic acid for preventing, 310–11
    screening for, _311_
Neurologists, back treatments by, _11_
Neuromas, 131, 132
Neurosurgeons, back treatments by, _11_
Nicotine patch, for smoking cessation, _213_
Night splint
    for bunions, 133
    for carpal tunnel syndrome, 437
Night sweats, in menopause, 227–28
Nitrous oxide, for dental treatment, _301_
Nodules, on vocal cords, _200_
Nonoxynol-9
    for preventing sexually transmitted diseases, 343
    yeast infections from, 429
Nonsteroidal anti-inflammatory drugs (NSAIDs). _See also_ Aspirin; Ibuprofen
    for bursitis, 181
    for painful periods, _424_
    ulcers from, 391
Nonstress test, for fetal monitoring, _311_
Norplant
    for birth control, 20, 21, _23_
    breastfeeding and, 78
    heartburn from, 107
    spotting and, 244
Nose, 260–66
    cosmetic surgery for, _260_, 261
    deviated septum in, 266
    irritation of, 261, 263
    polyps in, 263

Nosebleeds, 261, 263
NSAIDs. _See_ Nonsteroidal anti-inflammatory drugs
Nuprin. _See_ Ibuprofen
Nurse midwives, 68, _68_, 69, 70
Nutrition, 266–85
    balanced diet for, 266–67
    food sources of, 280–81, 284
    low-fat diet and, 273–77, 279–80
    3-2-1 eating plan for, 267–68, _268_
    from vitamins and minerals, 268–73, _274_
        antioxidants, 271–73
        calcium, 269–71, _269_
        fiber, _278–79_
        folate, 271
        micronutrients, 273

Oatmeal powder, for psoriasis, 375
Obesity. _See also_ Overweight; Weight gain
    gallstones from, 152
    hormones and, 182
Ob/gyns, _68_, 69
Oblique muscles, _251_
    toning, 448, **448**, 450
Obstetricians, _68_, 69
Oil
    monounsaturated, 64–65, 171
    sautéing with, 279
    substitutes for, 279
Olive oil, 64–65, 171
omega-3 fats, for preventing
    breast cancer, 65
    heart disease, 171
Oncologists, gynecologic, how to find, 290
Oophoritis, 288
Orabase, for canker sores, 249
Oral cancer, _248_, 415
Oral contraceptives. _See_ Birth control pills
Orgasm, 332–34, 336
Orthopedic surgeons, back treatments by, _11_
Orthotics, for foot problems, _135_, 139
Osteoarthritis, 188, **188**
    of hip, 180–81
Osteopaths, back treatments by, _11_
Osteoporosis
    as cause of
        dowager's hump, 381

Osteoporosis *(continued)*
  as cause of *(continued)*
    hip fractures, 177, 178, <u>358</u>
    pelvic fractures, 309
    spinal fractures, <u>384</u>
  early detection of, 222–23, 224–25
  menopause and, 178, 222, 223, 228, 229, <u>230–31</u>,
    231, <u>384</u>
  preventing with
    calcium, 179, 189, 269–71, <u>385</u>
    hormone replacement therapy, 179–80, <u>230</u>,
      231–32, <u>385</u>
    strength training, <u>385</u>, 442
    weight-bearing exercise, 179, <u>384–85</u>
  risk factors for, <u>384</u>
Ovarian cancer
  protecting against, 22, 289–90, <u>323</u>
  risk factors for, 288–89, <u>288</u>
Ovarian cysts, 287
Ovaries, <u>100</u>, **101**, 285–90, **322**, <u>323</u>, **323**
  benign tumors of, 287
  functions of, 285–87
  sex hormones produced by, 182
Overeating
  from depression, 98
  of fat-free foods, <u>282</u>
Overhead press, for toning shoulders, 460–61, **460–61**
Overweight. *See also* Obesity; Weight gain
  diabetes risk from, 307
  heartburn from, 105, 106
  pregnancy and, 310
Ovulation, <u>322</u>
  failure of, 144–45, 287, 422
  fertility and, 141
  heavy periods and, 246
  menstrual cycle and, <u>238</u>
  signs of, <u>286</u>
  spotting with, 243
  steps in, 285–86

Pain. *See also specific pain sites*
  chemistry of, 291–92
  chronic, 292, 295
  foods triggering, 299, 302, 303
  mittelschmerz, as sign of ovulation, <u>286</u>
  referred, **291**

Pain relief, 290–303
  in dental treatment, <u>300–301</u>
  medications for, <u>296–97</u> *(see also specific pain relievers)*
  techniques for
    acupressure, 293–94, **294**
    biofeedback, 298–99
    folding and holding, 295
    massage, 292–93, **293**
    relaxation, 295, 298
  with Thera Cane, 298, **298**
  tryptophan and, 299
Pain relievers, <u>296–97</u>. *See also specific pain relievers*
  natural, 291–92
  tolerance to, <u>297</u>
Palms, sweaty, 166–67
Pancreas, <u>83</u>, **83**, <u>100</u>, **101**, 304–8
Pancreatic cancer, 308
Pancreatitis, 308
Pap test, 67, 160, 220, <u>222</u>
  for detecting human papillomavirus, 67, 344, 345
  increasing reliability of, <u>161</u>
  menstrual cycle and, 162
Paraffin dips, for moisturizing hands, 166
ParaGard, as intrauterine device, 25
Parathyroid glands, <u>100</u>, **101**
Parathyroid hormone (PTH), calcium balance con-
  trolled by, 182
Patella, 192, 194, **359**
PC muscles, strengthening, for sexual pleasure, 335–36
Peak flow meter, for asthma sufferers, <u>210</u>
Peas, iron in, 106
Pectoral muscles, <u>250</u>, **251**
  toning (*see* Chest, toning exercises for)
Pedicures, <u>137</u>
Pelvic adhesions, fallopian tube blockage from, 118
Pelvic exam, 160–61, 220, 289, 426
Pelvic fractures, 309
Pelvic infection, from Dalkon Shield, 25
Pelvic inflammatory disease (PID)
  causes of, 118–19, 343
  ovarian inflammation from, 288
  pelvic adhesions from, 118
Pelvic rolls, for increasing sexual pleasure, 337
Pelvis, 309, **359**
  exercises for, 337
  male vs. female, **358**
Perimenopause, 227, <u>227</u>, 312, <u>323</u>

Period, menstrual, 237. *See also* Menstrual cycle;
    Menstruation
Periodontitis, 154
Perspiration, 395–96
    palm, 166–67
    underarm, 417–18
Pesticides, breast cancer risk from, 65
Petroleum jelly
    for hemorrhoids, 321
    for lips, 202–3
    for nasal lubrication, 261
    for skin care, 370
Phalanges, **359**
Pharynx, <u>325</u>, **325**
Pheromones, sexual attraction and, <u>263</u>, <u>265</u>
Phlebectomy, for varicose veins, <u>432</u>
Phlebitis, <u>80</u>, 431
Physiatrists, back treatments by, <u>11</u>
Physical therapists, back treatments by, <u>11</u>
Phytochemicals, for preventing breast cancer, 65
Phytoestrogens, for menopause relief, 233
PID. *See* Pelvic inflammatory disease
Piercing, ear, <u>90–91</u>
Piles, 320–21
Pill, the. *See* Birth control pills
Pilocarpine, for dry mouth, 327
Pinched nerve, <u>258</u>
Pinkeye, 113–14
Pituitary gland, **100**
Placenta, <u>80</u>
Plaque, arterial, 7, **7**
Plaque, dental, 154, 156, 157, 159, 399–400
Plastic surgery
    for breasts, <u>56</u>, 58, <u>60–61</u>
    for ears, <u>88</u>
    liposuction, <u>124</u>
    for nose, <u>260</u>, 261
Plica pain, 194–95
PMS. *See* Premenstrual syndrome
Pneumonia, 215
Pockets, gum, <u>156–57</u>
Polycystic kidney disease, 191, <u>191</u>
Polycystic ovarian syndrome, 287, 422, 423, 426
Polycythemia, <u>31</u>
Polyps
    nasal, 263
    vocal cord, 199, <u>200</u>

Port-wine stain, as birthmark, 26
Posture, back pain and, <u>14</u>, **14**
Potassium
    high blood pressure and, <u>174</u>
    levels of, in blood tests, <u>32</u>
    for lowering cholesterol, <u>173</u>
    for preventing kidney stones, 191
Pregnancy, 309–20. *See also* Childbirth
    back pain during, <u>319</u>
    bladder infections during, <u>27</u>
    breast changes during, 315
    depression during, <u>316</u>
    diabetes during, <u>305</u>, <u>310</u>
    eating during, 317
    ectopic, <u>119</u>
        birth control pills and, 22
        from chlamydia, 343
    emotions during, 315–17
    exercise during, 317–18, 320
    folic acid and, 271
    gum care during, 158–59
    heartburn during, 106
    hepatitis B and, <u>314</u>
    morning sickness during, 314–15, <u>389</u>
    in older women, <u>310</u>
    prenatal tests during, <u>311</u>
    preparation for, 309–12
    sex during, 320
    shoe size after, 136
    after stopping birth control pills, 24, 143
    stretching exercise during, <u>189</u>
    stretch marks from, 315
    unplanned, 20, 312–13
    weight gain during, 313–14
    womb development during, **313**
Premenstrual syndrome (PMS)
    diet for relieving, <u>240–41</u>
    symptoms of, 240, 242
Prenatal tests, <u>311</u>
Presbyopia, 110, 112
Prickly heat, 396
Pro-Flow, for dry mouth, 327
Progestasert, as intrauterine device, 25
Progesterone
    in hormone replacement therapy, 423, 426
    ovulation and, 286
    polycystic ovarian syndrome and, 287

Progestin, side effects of, 234
Prophylactics. *See* Condoms
Pseudoephedrine
    for airplane ear pain, 299
    for sinusitis, 354
Psoriasis, 328, 330, 374–76
PTH, calcium balance controlled by, 182
Pubic hair, removing, 35–37
Public speaking, sweating and, 395
Pubococcygeal (PC) muscles, strengthening, for sexual
        pleasure, 335–36
Pullover, for toning chest, 457, **457**
Pulmonary artery, **81**
Pulmonary embolism, 431
Pump bumps, from high heels, **2**
Push-ups, for toning chest, 446–47, **446–47**

Quadriceps, 250, **251**

Radial keratotomy, for correcting nearsightedness,
        110
Radioactive iodine, for hyperthyroidism, 408
Radius, **359**
Radon, lung cancer from, 213–14
Rash, from contact dermatitis, 373–74
Rectal exam, digital, for detecting colon cancer, 161,
        223
Rectum, 320–21
Rectus abdominis, toning, 450
Referred pain, **291**
Reflux. *See also* Heartburn
    hoarseness from, 200
    sore throat from, 407
Relaxation
    breathing for, 143, 206–7
    for pain relief, 295, 298
    scents promoting, 264
    techniques for, 393–94
Relaxation response, for tension release, 298
Renal arteries, **419**
Renal capillaries, 419
Renal vein, **419**
Reproductive system, 322–23, **322**, **323**
Resistance exercise. *See* Body toning; Weight training
RESOLVE, 146

Respiratory system, 324–25, **324**, **325**
Retin-A (Rx), for wrinkles, 257, 367, 367
Reverse leg lifts, for pelvic conditioning, 337
Rhagades, on lips, 202
Rhesus (Rh) factor, 29
Rheumatic fever, from strep throat, 406–7
Rheumatoid arthritis, 180–81, 188–89, 358
Rh factor, 29
Rhinoplasty, for reshaping nose, 260, 261
Ribs, 326, **359**
RICE, for ankle sprains, 4–5
Ring removal, from injured finger, 167
RODEO, for detecting breast cancer, 224
Root canal, 301
Rosacea, 376–77
Rotator cuff tendinitis, 348, 349, **349**, 350

Salicylic acid, for acne, 373
Saline breast implants, 61
Saliva, 327
Salivary glands, 327
Salt. *See* Sodium
Saphenous vein, **81**
Scalp, 328–30
Scapula, **359**
Scents, effects of, 264–65
Sciatica, 258, 386–87
Sciatic nerve, 258, **259**
Sclerotherapy, for spider vein removal, 432
Seasickness. *See* Motion sickness
Seborrheic dermatitis, 328, 330
Sedation, conscious, for dental treatment, 301
Seldane (Rx), for allergies, 357
Self-esteem, body image and, 39, 42, 441
Septum, deviated, 266
Serophene (Rx), for inducing ovulation, 144
Serotonin, as painkiller, 292
Serum ferritin test, for measuring iron level,
        105
Sex, 330–40
    attitudes about, 331
    bladder infections from, 27
    after childbirth, 76
    emotions and, 337, 338
    maximizing pleasure from, 337–40
    orgasm from, 332–34, 336

pleasure-enhancing exercises for, 335–37
positions for, 13, 334–35, 339
during pregnancy, 320
renewing excitement in, 333
statistics on, 331
Sexual attraction, sense of smell and, 263, 265
Sexual desire
factors affecting, 338
inhibited, 340
Sexually transmitted diseases (STDs), 341–46
chlamydia, 343, 344
effects on
cervix, 66, 67
fertility, 142–43
human immunodeficiency virus, 344, 345–46
human papillomavirus, 66, 67, 344–45
preventing, 25, 341, 343
testing for, 162, 341, 344
Shampoo
choosing, 164
dandruff, 330
Shaving, of body hair, 33, 37, 418
Shinbone, 346, **359**
Shins, 346–47
Shinsplints, 346–47
Shoes
athletic, 133, 135, 140
fit of, 135–36, **136**
flat, for Achilles tendon flexibility, 1, 2
foot pain from, 131–32
high-heeled
Achilles tendon affected by, 1–2
back pain from, 15
hip problems from, 180–81
for preventing
arthritis, 195–96
back pain, 14–15
shinsplints, 347
Shoe sizer, 133, 134, 135
Shoe stretcher, 139
Shortening, substitutes for, 279
Shoulder joint, **359**
Shoulder pinches, for maintaining good posture, 14, **15**
Shoulders, 348–52
dislocated, 350
frozen, 350–51
massage for, 293, **293**

rotator cuff tendinitis in, 348, 350
preventing, 349, **349**
subluxation of, 350
thoracic outlet syndrome and, 258, 326, 351–52
toning exercises for, 446, **446**, 447, **447**, 461–62, **461–62**
Sickle cell disease, 31
Sigmoidoscopy, for detecting colon cancer, 223–24
Silicone breast implants, 60–61
Single-arm row, for toning shoulders and back, 446, **446**
Sinuses, 325, **325**, 352–57
blocked by
allergies, 356–57
common cold, 355–56
sinusitis, 352–55
function of, 352
location of, **352**, 353
Sinusitis, 325, 353–55
Sitting, back pain prevention and, 17–18
Sit-ups
reverse, for abdominal toning, 451, **451**
yoga, for back pain, 12, **12**
Sitz bath, for hemorrhoids, 321
Sjögren's syndrome, 327
Skeletal system, 358–59, **358**, **359**
Skin, 360–77
care of, 368–70
makeup for, 370–71
moisturizing, 369–70
pregnancy and, 315
sun exposure and, 58, 360–64
types of, 369
Skin cancer, 246–47, 247
risk factors for, 362
self-examination for, 365, **365**
from sun exposure, 360
types of, 365–66
Skin prick tests, for allergies, 210
Skin problems
acne, 372–73
dermatitis, 328, 330, 373–74
eczema, 239, 373–74
psoriasis, 328, 330, 374–76
rosacea, 376–77
Skull, 377–79
fracture of, 378–79

Sleep
  back pain prevention and, <u>16–17</u>
  facial creases from, 364
  lack of, memory loss from, <u>45</u>
  neck pillow for, 255
  scents promoting, <u>265</u>
Sleep positions
  jaw pain from, 187
  during pregnancy, <u>319</u>, **319**
Sleep problems
  menstruation and, 239
  pain and, 298
Slimming. *See* Body toning; Weight loss
Smell(s)
  effects of, <u>264–65</u>
  sense of, <u>262–63</u>
Smoker's cough, 214
Smoking
  asthma and, 210
  bronchitis and, 211
  calcium absorption blocked by, 189
  as cause of
    cardiovascular disease, 7, 9, 175
    cataracts, 116
    gallstones, 152–53
    lung cancer, 212, 213
    ulcers, 391
    vaginal dryness, <u>428</u>
    wrinkles, 364
  cervical dysplasia and, 67
  effect on
    blood, 32
    fertility, 143
    skin elasticity, 58
    vocal cords, 199
  osteoporosis and, 179
  ovarian cancer and, 289
  pancreatic cancer and, 308
  pelvic inflammatory disease and, 119
  quitting, <u>212–13</u>, 312
  sinusitis and, 355
  spinal disks and, 382
Snacking, insulin levels and, <u>306</u>
Snacks
  energy-producing, <u>103</u>
  fruit and vegetable, 281, 284
Sneakers. *See* Shoes, athletic

Society of Gynecologic Oncologists, 290, 426
Sodium
  high blood pressure and, <u>174</u>
  levels of, in blood tests, <u>32</u>
Somatotypes, 38–43
Sorbitol, intestinal problems from, 183–84
Sores, mouth, 248–49, <u>248</u>
Sore throat, 406–7, <u>407</u>
  from tonsillitis, 416–17, <u>416</u>
Soy
  for lowering cholesterol, 172
  for menopause, 233
  for preventing breast cancer, 65, <u>281</u>
Sperm, infertility and, 145
Spermicides
  for preventing sexually transmitted diseases, 67
  yeast infections from, 429
Spider veins, <u>432</u>
Spina bifida, folic acid for preventing, 310–11
Spinal disks, <u>258</u>, **359**, 381–82, 386
Spinal manipulation, for back pain, <u>10</u>, 11, <u>11</u>, 13, <u>381</u>
Spine, 379–87. *See also* Back
  aging and, <u>383</u>
  curves in, 379, <u>380</u>, 381
  fractures of, from osteoporosis, <u>384</u>
  strengthening, <u>380</u>
Spirometer, for testing lung function, <u>210</u>
Spleen, **217**, 388
Splint, night
  for bunions, 133
  for carpal tunnel syndrome, 437
Spotting, between periods, 243–44
Sprains
  ankle, 4–5
  pain medication for, <u>297</u>
Squamous cell cancer, 365
Squats, for toning thighs and buttocks, 448–49, **448**
Standing, back pain prevention and, <u>14–15</u>
STDs. *See* Sexually transmitted diseases
Step aerobics, avoiding Achilles tendon injury in, **2**
Sterilization, for birth control, 19, 20–21, <u>21</u>
Sternum, **359**
Sties, 114
Stim-U-Dent, for gum care, 157
Stockings, compression, for varicose veins, 433–34
Stomach, **83**, 389–91

Stomach muscles. *See* Abdominal muscles
Stomach upset, <u>389</u>
   during pregnancy, 314–15
Stones. *See* Gallstones; Kidney stones
Stool, occult blood in, 223
Stool softeners, for hemorrhoids, 321
Strawberry mark, as birthmark, 26
Strength training. *See* Body toning; Weight training
Strep throat, 406–7, 416, 417
Stress, 392–94
   as cause of
      acne, 373
      energy loss, <u>105</u>
      headaches, <u>302–3</u>
      high blood pressure, 175–76
      infertility, <u>142–43</u>
      memory loss, <u>45</u>
      tooth grinding, 404
Stress incontinence
   Kegel exercises for, <u>419</u>, <u>420</u>
   in menopause, 235–36
Stress test
   exercise, 219–20
   for fetal monitoring, <u>311</u>
Stretching
   for Achilles tendon, 2
   of calf muscles, 4
   for good posture, 14, **15**
   for joint pain, 189
   during pregnancy, <u>189</u>
   for preventing knee pain, <u>196</u>
   for preventing shinsplints, 347
   before rising from bed, <u>16–17</u>
   in Total Body-Shaping Workout, 443, 449–50, **449–50**
Stretch marks, during pregnancy, 315
Stroke
   beauty parlor, <u>252</u>
   from blood clots, 7
   types of, 53
   warning signs of, <u>53</u>
Subzonal sperm injection, for infertility, <u>144</u>
Sudafed. *See* Pseudoephedrine
Sugar, energy loss from, 104
Sun exposure, skin damage from, 58, 360–64
Sunglasses
   for preventing cataracts, 116, <u>116</u>
   for protecting eye skin, 363

Sunscreen
   for lips, 202
   for neck, 257
   for protecting skin, 362–63
   vitamin D blocked by, 270
Supplements. *See specific supplements*
Support groups, infertility, 146
Support hose, for varicose veins, 433–34
Swayback, **380**, 381
Sweat glands, 395–96
Sweating, 395–96, 417–18
Sweaty palms, 166–67
Sweeteners, intestinal problems from, 183–84
Syphilis test, <u>344</u>

T 380A, as intrauterine device, 25
Tailbone, **359**, 397
Talcum powder, ovarian cancer and, 289
Tampons, toxic shock syndrome from, <u>245</u>
Tannin, iron absorption and, 106
Tanning salons, 364
Tarsals, **359**
Tartar, dental, 154, 158
Taste, sense of, <u>412–13</u>
Taste buds, 411, <u>412</u>, **413**
Tay-sachs disease, 312
TB, 215
Tea, iron absorption and, 106
Tear ducts, 398–99
Teeth, 399–406. *See also* Gums
   bleaching, 405–6
   braces for, <u>405</u>
   brushing, 158, <u>401</u>, 402
   cavities in, 403–4
   color of, <u>404</u>, 405
   flossing, <u>400</u>, **400**
   fluoride for, 402–3
   grinding, 185, 186, 404
   knocked-out, 405
   pain-free dentistry for, <u>300–301</u>
   plaque on, 399–400
Temperature, basal body, as sign of ovulation, 144, 286
Temporal lobes, <u>258</u>, **259**
Temporomandibular joint disorder (TMD), 185–87, 186

Tendinitis
   Achilles, 1
   knee, 195
   pain medication for, <u>297</u>
   rotator cuff, 348, 350
      exercises for preventing, <u>349</u>, **349**
Tendon, Achilles, **1**, 1–2
Tennis elbow, 92–93
Tension headaches, <u>250</u>, 302
Terfenadine (Rx), for allergies, 357
Testosterone, effect of, on brain cells, 47–48
Tests, medical. *See* Medical tests
Thera Cane, for pain relief, 298, **298**
Thighbone, **359**
Thighs, toning exercises for, 448–49, **448**, 461–63,
   462–63
Thoracic nerve, **259**
Thoracic outlet syndrome, <u>258</u>, 326, 351–52
3-2-1 eating plan, 267–68, <u>268</u>
Throat, 406–7
Thrombosis, deep-vein, 431
Thymus, **101**
Thyroid gland, <u>100</u>, **101**, 408–9
Thyroxine, <u>100</u>, 182
Tibia, 346–47, **359**
Tinnitus, 86–87
Tiredness. *See* Fatigue
TMD, 185–87, <u>186</u>
Toe bones, **359**
Toenails, 410–11
   pedicure for, <u>137</u>
Toe press, for calf toning, 455–56, **455–56**
Tofu, as soy source, 172, 233, <u>281</u>
Tongue, 411–15
Tongue cancer, 415
Tongue scrapers, 414
Toning, body. *See* Body toning; Weight training
Tonsillectomy, 415–16, <u>416</u>, 417
Tonsillitis, 416–17, **416**
Tonsils, <u>216</u>, **217**, 415–17
Toothaches
   acupressure for, 294, **295**
   ibuprofen for, <u>297</u>
Toothbrush
   choosing, 399–401
   for tongue brushing, 414
Tooth brushing, 158, <u>401</u>, 402

Tooth grinding, 185, 186, 404
Toothpaste
   fluoridated, 403
   for healthy gums, 158
Total Body-Shaping Workout, 443–50
   body-shaping exercises in, 443, 446–48, **446–48**
   cooldown stretches in, 443, 449–50, **449–50**
   warm-up for, 443, 444–45, **444–45**
Toxic shock syndrome, <u>245</u>
Trachea, **198**
Trans fats, <u>171</u>, 277, 279
Transvaginal ultrasound, for uterine examination, 220
Trapezius muscle, **251**
Tretinoin (Rx), for wrinkles, 257, 367, <u>367</u>
Triceps, **251**
   toning exercises for, 464–65, **464–65**
Tricyclic antidepressants, for pain relief, <u>296</u>
Triple testing, for prenatal screening, <u>311</u>
Tryptophan, for pain relief, 299
Tubal ligation. *See* Sterilization, for birth control
Tuberculosis, 215
Tumors. *See also specific cancers*
   benign ovarian, 287
   dermoid, 287
   epithelial, 423
   fibroid (*see* Fibroids, uterine)
Tums, calcium in, <u>385</u>
Tylenol. *See* Acetaminophen

Ulcers
   mouth, 248–49, <u>248</u>
   stomach, <u>83</u>, 390–91
   tests for detecting, 225
Ulna, **359**
Ultrafast computed tomography, for heart disease
      screening, 226
Ultrasound
   for detecting
      appendicitis, 6
      ovarian cysts, 287
   prenatal, <u>311</u>
   transvaginal, for uterine examination, 220
Ultraviolet light
   cataracts from, 116, <u>116</u>
   skin damage from, 360–61
   in tanning salons, 364

Ultraviolet light therapy, for psoriasis, 376
Umbilical arteries, **80**
Umbilical hernia, 19
Umbilical vein, **80**
Underarms, 37, 417–18
Ureters, **419**
Urethra, 418, **419**
Urethritis, 27
Urinary system, 418–19, **419**
Urinary tract infections (UTIs), 26–28, 27, 418
  kidney infections and, 190
  in menopause, 235
Urination
  frequent, in menopause, 235–36
  painful (*see* Urinary tract infections)
Urine, 418–19, 420
Uterine cancer, 422–23
  from hormone replacement therapy, 231–32, 234
Uterine lining, **322**, 322–23, **323**
Uterine muscle, strengthening, for sexual pleasure, 336
Uterine sarcoma, 423
Uterus, 322, **322**, **323**, 421–26
  anatomy of, 421
  development of, in pregnancy, **313**
  fibroids in, 422
  pregnancy and, 421–22
  protecting health of, 426
  removal of (*see* Hysterectomy)
UTIs. *See* Urinary tract infections

Vaccinations, after spleen removal, 388
Vagina, **322**, **323**, 427–30
Vaginal dryness, 428
  in menopause, 234–35
Vaginal infections. *See also* Vaginitis
  in menopause, 235
Vaginal orgasms, 333, 334, 335, 336
Vaginismus, 430
Vaginitis, 322, 427–29
Vaginosis, 430
Varicose veins, 80, 432, 433, 434
Vasectomy, vs. female sterilization, 21, 21
Vastus medialis, 250, **251**
Vegetables
  fiber in, 279
  increasing intake of, 281, 284

for preventing
  arterial disease, 8
  cancer, 65, 280, 280
  cataracts, 116–17
protective compounds in, 280, 281
Vein(s), 80, 431–34
  endometrial, **80**
  jugular, **81**
  renal, **419**
  saphenous, **81**
  spider, 432
  umbilical, **80**
  varicose, 80, 432, 433, 434
Vertebrae, **359**
Vertigo, 88–90, 89
Videos, body toning, 468–69
Vision, 108–10, 112–13, 115–17
Vitamin A
  as antioxidant, 271, 272
  for preventing breast cancer, 64
  toxicity of, 272
Vitamin B$_6$
  for brainpower, 51
  for morning sickness, 315
  sources of, 273
Vitamin B$_{12}$, for healthy blood, 30–31
Vitamin C
  as antioxidant, 271, 272, 273
  for healthy blood, 31–32
  for iron absorption, 106
  for preventing
    arterial disease, 8
    bladder infections, 28
    colds, 356
  sources of, 272–73
  for treating
    glaucoma, 115
    lung disease, 214
Vitamin D, for calcium absorption, 231, 270–71
Vitamin E
  as antioxidant, 271, 272, 273
  for healthy blood, 31
  for lowering cholesterol, 173
  for preventing
    arterial disease, 8
    breast lumps, 57

Vitamin E *(continued)*
  sources of, 273
  for treating
    canker sores, 249
    lung disease, 214
    vaginal dryness, 428
Vitamin-mineral supplements, 272, 274
Vitamins, 268–73, 274. *See also specific vitamins and*
    minerals
Vocal cords, 197–201, **198**
Voice
  improving, 198, 199
  preventing hoarseness of, 198–201
Voice box. *See* Larynx
Vulva, 435

Waist-to-hip ratio
  diabetes risk and, 306–7
  for estimating body fat, 124
Walking
  for back health, 13, 15, 382–83
  for conditioning heart, 170
  for diabetes control, 307
  for energy, 104–5
  for preventing osteoporosis, 384–85
  varicose veins and, 434
Warm-up exercises
  for Achilles tendon, 2
  for preventing shinsplints, 347
  in Total Body-Shaping Workout, 443, 444–45, **444–45**
Warts, genital, 66, 67, 344–45
Waxing
  of body hair, 33–34, 34
  of hands, 166
Weight, ideal
  finding, **125**, 284–85
  before pregnancy, 310
Weight control
  for avoiding health risks, 284–85
  for hormone balance, 182
  for preventing
    arthritis, 195
    diabetes, 307
Weight gain. *See also* Obesity; Overweight
  during menopause, 236
  during pregnancy, 313–14

Weight loss
  for back health, 383, 386
  breastfeeding and, 78–79
  eating plan for, 130
  exercise for, 126–27, *128*, 129–30
  guidelines for, 125, 282–83, 284–85
  for lowering cholesterol, 174
  before pregnancy, 310
  for preventing diabetes, 307
  rapid, gallstones from, 152
  scents promoting, 264
  skin elasticity and, 364
Weight training. *See also* Body toning
  fat burning from, 127, 129
  for preventing osteoporosis, 229, 385
  starting, 43
Wheat bran, for preventing breast cancer, 64
Wheezing, from asthma, 208, 209
Whiplash, 250, 256–57, **257**
Whiteheads, 372
Whole-wheat foods, fiber in, 278–79
Workouts. *See* Body toning; Exercise(s); Weight training
Wrinkles
  heredity and, 362
  around lips, 202
  neck, 257
  treating, 366–67, 366, 367, 368
Wrist bone, **359**
Wrist curls, for toning forearms, 458–59, **458–59**
Wrists, 436–37

Xerostomia, 327

Yeast infections, vaginal, 322, 427–29
Yoga
  for back pain, 12, **12**
  for relieving menstrual symptoms, 243, **243**
Yoga sit-up, for back pain, 12, **12**

Zinc
  for memory improvement, 49
  for premenstrual syndrome, 241
  sources of, 273
Zinc supplements, iron absorption and, 106
Zygote intrafallopian transfer (ZIFT), for infertility, 144